Handbook of Tourette's Syndrome and Related Tic and Behavioral Disorders

Second Edition

NEUROLOGICAL DISEASE AND THERAPY

1. Handbook of Parkinson's Disease, *edited by William C. Koller*
2. Medical Therapy of Acute Stroke, *edited by Mark Fisher*
3. Familial Alzheimer's Disease: Molecular Genetics and Clinical Perspectives, *edited by Gary D. Miner, Ralph W. Richter, John P. Blass, Jimmie L. Valentine, and Linda A. Winters-Miner*
4. Alzheimer's Disease: Treatment and Long-Term Management, *edited by Jeffrey L. Cummings and Bruce L. Miller*
5. Therapy of Parkinson's Disease, *edited by William C. Koller and George Paulson*
6. Handbook of Sleep Disorders, *edited by Michael J. Thorpy*
7. Epilepsy and Sudden Death, *edited by Claire M. Lathers and Paul L. Schraeder*
8. Handbook of Multiple Sclerosis, *edited by Stuart D. Cook*
9. Memory Disorders: Research and Clinical Practice, *edited by Takehiko Yanagihara and Ronald C. Petersen*
10. The Medical Treatment of Epilepsy, *edited by Stanley R. Resor, Jr., and Henn Kutt*
11. Cognitive Disorders: Pathophysiology and Treatment, *edited by Leon J. Thal, Walter H. Moos, and Elkan R. Gamzu*
12. Handbook of Amyotrophic Lateral Sclerosis, *edited by Richard Alan Smith*
13. Handbook of Parkinson's Disease: Second Edition, Revised and Expanded, *edited by William C. Koller*
14. Handbook of Pediatric Epilepsy, *edited by Jerome V. Murphy and Fereydoun Dehkharghani*
15. Handbook of Tourette's Syndrome and Related Tic and Behavioral Disorders, *edited by Roger Kurlan*
16. Handbook of Cerebellar Diseases, *edited by Richard Lechtenberg*
17. Handbook of Cerebrovascular Diseases, *edited by Harold P. Adams, Jr.*
18. Parkinsonian Syndromes, *edited by Matthew B. Stern and William C. Koller*
19. Handbook of Head and Spine Trauma, *edited by Jonathan Greenberg*
20. Brain Tumors: A Comprehensive Text, *edited by Robert A. Morantz and John W. Walsh*
21. Monoamine Oxidase Inhibitors in Neurological Diseases, *edited by Abraham Lieberman, C. Warren Olanow, Moussa B. H. Youdim, and Keith Tipton*

22. Handbook of Dementing Illnesses, *edited by John C. Morris*
23. Handbook of Myasthenia Gravis and Myasthenic Syndromes, *edited by Robert P. Lisak*
24. Handbook of Neurorehabilitation, *edited by David C. Good and James R. Couch, Jr.*
25. Therapy with Botulinum Toxin, *edited by Joseph Jankovic and Mark Hallett*
26. Principles of Neurotoxicology, *edited by Louis W. Chang*
27. Handbook of Neurovirology, *edited by Robert R. McKendall and William G. Stroop*
28. Handbook of Neuro-Urology, *edited by David N. Rushton*
29. Handbook of Neuroepidemiology, *edited by Philip B. Gorelick and Milton Alter*
30. Handbook of Tremor Disorders, *edited by Leslie J. Findley and William C. Koller*
31. Neuro-Ophthalmological Disorders: Diagnostic Work-Up and Management, *edited by Ronald J. Tusa and Steven A. Newman*
32. Handbook of Olfaction and Gustation, *edited by Richard L. Doty*
33. Handbook of Neurological Speech and Language Disorders, *edited by Howard S. Kirshner*
34. Therapy of Parkinson's Disease: Second Edition, Revised and Expanded, *edited by William C. Koller and George Paulson*
35. Evaluation and Management of Gait Disorders, *edited by Barney S. Spivack*
36. Handbook of Neurotoxicology, *edited by Louis W. Chang and Robert S. Dyer*
37. Neurological Complications of Cancer, *edited by Ronald G. Wiley*
38. Handbook of Autonomic Nervous System Dysfunction, *edited by Amos D. Korczyn*
39. Handbook of Dystonia, *edited by Joseph King Ching Tsui and Donald B. Calne*
40. Etiology of Parkinson's Disease, *edited by Jonas H. Ellenberg, William C. Koller, and J. William Langston*
41. Practical Neurology of the Elderly, *edited by Jacob I. Sage and Margery H. Mark*
42. Handbook of Muscle Disease, *edited by Russell J. M. Lane*
43. Handbook of Multiple Sclerosis: Second Edition, Revised and Expanded, *edited by Stuart D. Cook*

44. Central Nervous System Infectious Diseases and Therapy, *edited by Karen L. Roos*
45. Subarachnoid Hemorrhage: Clinical Management, *edited by Takehiko Yanagihara, David G. Piepgras, and John L. D. Atkinson*
46. Neurology Practice Guidelines, *edited by Richard Lechtenberg and Henry S. Schutta*
47. Spinal Cord Diseases: Diagnosis and Treatment, *edited by Gordon L. Engler, Jonathan Cole, and W. Louis Merton*
48. Management of Acute Stroke, *edited by Ashfaq Shuaib and Larry B. Goldstein*
49. Sleep Disorders and Neurological Disease, *edited by Antonio Culebras*
50. Handbook of Ataxia Disorders, *edited by Thomas Klockgether*
51. The Autonomic Nervous System in Health and Disease, *David S. Goldstein*
52. Axonal Regeneration in the Central Nervous System, *edited by Nicholas A. Ingoglia and Marion Murray*
53. Handbook of Multiple Sclerosis: Third Edition, *edited by Stuart D. Cook*
54. Long-Term Effects of Stroke, *edited by Julien Bogousslavsky*
55. Handbook of the Autonomic Nervous System in Health and Disease, *edited by C. Liana Bolis, Julio Licinio, and Stefano Govoni*
56. Dopamine Receptors and Transporters: Function, Imaging, and Clinical Implication, Second Edition, *edited by Anita Sidhu, Marc Laruelle, and Philippe Vernier*
57. Handbook of Olfaction and Gustation: Second Edition, Revised and Expanded, *edited by Richard L. Doty*
58. Handbook of Stereotactic and Functional Neurosurgery, *edited by Michael Schulder*
59. Handbook of Parkinson's Disease: Third Edition, *edited by Rajesh Pahwa, Kelly E. Lyons, and William C. Koller*
60. Clinical Neurovirology, *edited by Avindra Nath and Joseph R. Berger*
61. Neuromuscular Junction Disorders: Diagnosis and Treatment, *Matthew N. Meriggioli, James F. Howard, Jr., and C. Michel Harper*
62. Drug-Induced Movement Disorders, *edited by Kapil D. Sethi*

63. Therapy of Parkinson's Disease: Third Edition, Revised and Expanded, *edited by Rajesh Pahwa, Kelly E. Lyons, and William C. Koller*
64. Epilepsy: Scientific Foundations of Clinical Practice, *edited by Jong M. Rho, Raman Sankar, and José E. Cavazos*
65. Handbook of Tourette's Syndrome and Related Tic and Behavioral Disorders: Second Edition, *edited by Roger Kurlan*
66. Handbook of Cerebrovascular Diseases: Second Edition, Revised and Expanded, *edited by Harold P. Adams, Jr.*

Additional Volumes in Preparation

Handbook of Tourette's Syndrome and Related Tic and Behavioral Disorders

Second Edition

edited by

Roger Kurlan

CRC Press
Taylor & Francis Group
Boca Raton London New York

CRC Press is an imprint of the
Taylor & Francis Group, an **informa** business

CRC Press
Taylor & Francis Group
6000 Broken Sound Parkway NW, Suite 300
Boca Raton, FL 33487-2742

First issued in paperback 2019

ISBN-13: 978-0-8247-5316-0 (hbk)
ISBN-13: 978-0-367-39371-7 (pbk)

A CIP record for this book is available from the British Library.

Library of Congress Cataloging-in-Publication Data available on application

Visit the Taylor & Francis Web site at
http://www.taylorandfrancis.com

and the CRC Press Web site at
http://www.crcpress.com

Preface

When the first edition of this book was published in 1993, I commented how notions regarding Tourette's syndrome (TS) had undergone recent dramatic changes. Major shifts in views of the disorder included identification of its complex spectrum of clinical features (including tics and specific behavioral disorders, particularly obsessive-compulsive disorder and attention deficit hyperactivity disorder), establishment of heredity as a major etiological factor, and recognition that, rather than a rare disorder, it occurs quite commonly in the population.

Views of TS continue to evolve rapidly, resulting in the need to convey this important information in a second edition. New data suggest that the TS behavioral spectrum extends to include anxiety disorders and rage attacks. More and more complexities in the hereditary transmission pattern of TS are becoming apparent, posing new challenges in the longstanding research attempts to identify involved genes. Recent epidemiological studies indicate that perhaps 1% of all schoolchildren have TS, with up to 25% of children with school problems demonstrating tics. A novel potential cause of at least some cases of TS has been proposed, namely, a poststreptococcal autoimmune process, which remains highly controversial. There have also been major advances in the treatment of TS with the availability of atypical antipsychotic drugs, guanfacine, new long-acting stimulants, and more anti-obsessional drugs. In short, important developments have occurred in virtually all the topics covered in the first edition, making the publication of this second edition important and timely.

Appreciation and thanks are extended to the authors, who have provided clear, concise, and up-to-date information. I hope this book will help you appreciate TS as a fascinating condition that will help us learn about the most basic aspects of human behavior.

Roger Kurlan

Contents

V. GENETICS AND EPIDEMIOLOGY

VI. CLINICAL CARE

VII. SPECIAL TOPICS

Contributors

Karen E. Anderson University of Maryland School of Medicine, Baltimore, Maryland, U.S.A.

Cathy L. Barr University of Toronto, The Toronto Western Hospital Research Institute and The Hospital for Sick Children, Toronto, Ontario, Canada

Laurie Brown The University of Alabama at Birmingham, Birmingham, Alabama, U.S.A.

Richard Bruggeman University Hospital Groningen, Groningen, The Netherlands

Ruth Dowling Bruun New York University School of Medicine, Westhampton Beach, New York, U.S.A.

Cathy L. Budman New York University School of Medicine, New York and North Shore University Hospital, Manhasset, New York, U.S.A.

Barbara J. Coffey New York University Child Study Center, New York, New York, U.S.A.

Donald J. Cohen[†] Yale University School of Medicine, New Haven, Connecticut, U.S.A.

[†]Deceased.

Henry Colle St. Lucas Hospital Ghent, Ghent, Belgium

Peter G. Como University of Rochester School of Medicine and Dentistry, Rochester, New York, U.S.A.

P. Michael Conneally Indiana University School of Medicine, Indianapolis, Indiana, U.S.A.

Leon S. Dure The University of Alabama at Birmingham, Birmingham, Alabama, U.S.A.

Valsamma Eapen UAE University, United Arab Emirates and University College London Medical School, London, England

David Eidelberg North Shore-Long Island Jewish Research Institute, North Shore University Hospital, Manhasset and New York University School of Medicine, New York, New York, U.S.A.

Gerald Erenberg Cleveland Clinic Foundation, Cleveland, Ohio, U.S.A.

Stanley Fahn Columbia University College of Physicians & Surgeons and The Neurological Institute of New York, Presbyterian Hospital, New York, New York, U.S.A.

Andrew Feigin North Shore-Long Island Jewish Research Institute, North Shore University Hospital, Manhasset and New York University School of Medicine, New York, New York, U.S.A.

Diane Findley Yale University School of Medicine, New Haven, Connecticut, U.S.A.

Elisabeth M. J. Foncke Amsterdam Medical Center, Amsterdam, The Netherlands

Deborah Frisone McLean Hospital, Belmont, Massachusetts, U.S.A.

Loren Gianini Massachusetts General Hospital, Cambridge, Massachusetts, U.S.A.

Christopher G. Goetz Rush University, Chicago, Illinois, U.S.A.

Stacy Horn Rush University, Chicago, Illinois, U.S.A.

Joseph Jankovic Baylor College of Medicine, Houston, Texas, U.S.A.

Michael Johnson University of Utah, Salt Lake City, Utah, U.S.A.

Robert A. King Yale University School of Medicine, New Haven, Connecticut, U.S.A.

Roger Kurlan University of Rochester Medical Center, Rochester, New York, U.S.A.

Carolyn Kwak Baylor College of Medicine, Houston, Texas, U.S.A.

Anthony E. Lang Toronto Western Hospital, Toronto, Ontario, Canada

James F. Leckman Yale University School of Medicine, New Haven, Connecticut, U.S.A.

Sue Levi-Pearl Tourette Syndrome Association, Inc., Bayside, New York, U.S.A.

Michael P. McDermott University of Rochester Medical Center, Rochester, New York, U.S.A.

William M. McMahon University of Utah, Salt Lake City, Utah, U.S.A.

Jonathan W. Mink University of Rochester School of Medicine and Dentistry, Rochester, New York, U.S.A.

Karen Minzer Johns Hopkins University School of Medicine, Baltimore, Maryland, U.S.A.

Donna R. Palumbo University of Rochester School of Medicine and Dentistry, Rochester, New York, U.S.A.

David L. Pauls Massachusetts General Hospital and Harvard University School of Medicine, Boston, Massachusetts, U.S.A.

Tamara M. Pringsheim Toronto Western Hospital, Toronto, Ontario, Canada

Mary May Robertson The National Hospital for Neurology and Neurosurgery and University College London Medical School, London, England

Lori Rockmore Mount Sinai School of Medicine, New York, New York, U.S.A.

Maria C. Rosario-Campos Yale University School of Medicine, New Haven, Connecticut, U.S.A.

Oliver Sacks Albert Einstein College of Medicine, Bronx, New York, U.S.A.

Lawrence Scahill Yale University School of Medicine, New Haven, Connecticut, U.S.A.

Harvey S. Singer Johns Hopkins University School of Medicine, Baltimore, Maryland, U.S.A.

Caroline M. Tanner Parkinson's Institute, Sunnyvale, California, U.S.A.

Chris van der Linden St. Lucas Hospital Ghent, Ghent, Belgium

Lawrence A. Vitulano Yale University School of Medicine, New Haven, Connecticut, U.S.A.

William J. Weiner University of Maryland School of Medicine, Baltimore, Maryland, U.S.A.

Jessica W. Yakeley Maudsley Hospital, London, England

1

Motor and Vocal Tics

Stanley Fahn
Columbia University College of Physicians & Surgeons
and The Neurological Institute of New York
Presbyterian Hospital
New York, New York, U.S.A.

INTRODUCTION

Historically, the French used the term *tic*, or *tique*, for centuries to denote an "unpleasant gesture" (1). The term was first used to describe certain trick movements in horses in 1665 (2). Then it was used to refer to distasteful motor acts in humans, but in 1756, the term *tic douloureux* was coined (cited in Ref. 2) (trigeminal neuralgia in today's lexicon), thereby setting up the different, confusing meanings for the word *tic*. It seems preferable to remain with the original usage, namely, that *tic* refers to certain unwanted motor acts. The term *convulsive tic* (*tic convulsif*), as used by Charcot in Goetz (3) and Gilles de la Tourette (4), connotes the "abruptness and momentariness" of the abnormal movement (5).

Fahn (6) defined motor tics as consisting of patterned sequences of coordinated involuntary movements. Interestingly, the classic treatise on tics by Meige and Feindel (7) in 1907 and the earlier publication by Guinon (8) had a similar definition of tics—systematized, involuntary, coordinated movements. These definitions apply best for complex tics; for simple tics, a single myoclonic-like contraction is the common feature, and these are not coordinated movements, although they can be repetitive.

Because complex tics resemble stereotypies, the question arises as to whether tics should be listed as a subcategory of stereotypies rather than an independent category of hyperkinetic disorders. Meige and Feindel (9) distinguished between tics and stereotypies by describing the former as acts that are impelling but not impossible to resist, whereas the latter, although illogical, are without an irresistible urge. Shapiro et al. (10) prefer to reserve *stereotypy* for those movements seen in schizophrenia, autism, and mental deficiency. I also prefer to list tics in its own hyperkinetic dyskinesia category.

Although a complex tic often recurs, and thereby has features of a stereotypy, simple tics more closely resemble myoclonic jerks. Therefore, analogously, if complex motor tics are to be classified as a stereotypy, then simple motor tics should be classified as part of the myoclonias. It is this diversity of motor tics that sets their phenomenology apart from all others. Furthermore, as will be pointed out below, tics have many other features that aid in their diagnosis, such as their suppressibility, their accompaniment by an underlying urge or compulsion to make the movement, their variability, their migration from one body part to another, their abruptness, their brevity, and the repetitiveness, rather than randomness, of the particular body part affected by the movements.

As will be discussed below, tics as occurring in Gilles de la Tourette syndrome [usually referred to as Tourette's syndrome (TS)] can be somatic motor phenomena (motor tics) or phonic phenomena (equivalently referred to as phonic or vocal tics). These are sounds produced by moving air through the nose, mouth, or throat. In contrast to many other movement disorders, the movements and sounds are not constantly present (except when extremely severe), but occur out of a background of normal motor activity; hence, there is a paroxysmal pattern to them. Motor and vocal tics can be simple or complex. Meige and Feindel (11) emphasized motor tics as being either clonic or tonic. The more common clonic tics are rapid and brief in duration; the less common tonic (or dystonic) tics are contractions that are longer in duration.

PHENOMENOLOGY OF TICS

Motor Tics

Simple Motor Tics

Motor tics can be simple or complex (Table 1). Simple motor tics are abrupt, sudden, and usually brief movements. The most simple and brief would be an isolated jerk resembling a myoclonic jerk in speed (i.e., lightning-like). More often appearing as a single, isolated jerk, there would be a repetitive run of these fast movements, making their distinction from myoclonus easier. In addition, rather than the tic repeating in the same site, a different body part

Table 1 Phenomenological Characteristics of Tics

Motor tics

(1) Simple motor tics
- (a) Clonic tics
  - (i) Isolated, single movement
    Examples: eyeblinking, shrug, eye movement, nose flare
    Differential diagnosis: myoclonus, chorea
  - (ii) Run of simple movements
    Examples: repetitive eyeblinking, arm-jerking
    Differential diagnosis: blepharospasm
- (b) Dystonic tics
  - (i) Isolated, single movements
    Examples: prolonged oculogyric deviation, head deviation, mouth-opening
    Differential diagnosis: focal and segmental torsion dystonia, oculogyric crisis

(2) Complex motor tics
- (a) Clonic tics
  - (i) Nonpurposeful, appearing purposeful, acts
    Examples: tossing head, touching body, rubbing, spitting
    Differential diagnosis: stereotypies, mannerisms, akathitic movements, hyperekplexia
  - (ii) Acts not appearing purposeful
    Examples: head-shaking, trunk-bending, series of different facial twitchings
    Differential diagnosis: stereotypies, mannerisms, akathitic movements, hyperekplexia, and other exaggerated startle syndromes
- (b) Dystonic tics
  Examples: bruxism with sustained head tilt
  Differential diagnosis: segmental or generalized torsion dystonia

Vocal tics

(1) Simple vocal tics
Examples: throat-clearing, sniffing, grunting, barking, yelping, squeaking, clicking
Differential diagnosis: moaning with akathisia, parkinsonism; squeaking and grunting with oromandibular dystonia and Huntington's disease; humming with blepharospasm and Meige syndrome

(2) Complex vocal tics
Examples: whistling, belching, coprolalia, echolalia, palilalia
Differential diagnosis: palilalia with stuttering; echolalia with exaggerated startle syndromes; coprolalia with encephalitis; spitting with Huntington's disease and neuroacanthocytosis

may be involved with the next tic. This variation in location also helps distinguish simple tics from myoclonic jerks.

Examples of a simple motor tic that appears as an isolated movement are an eyeblink, shrug, head jerk, dart of the eyes, twitch of the nose or flare of the nostril, mouth-opening, and tongue protrusion. A run of any of these would result in, for example, several eyeblinks in a row, a series of arm jerks, or a run of facial twitches.

The single, isolated simple motor tic could also be difficult to distinguish from choreic jerks, which are slightly slower than myoclonus. Choreic movements do not tend to repeat immediately in the same site, but appear randomly in different muscles. Tics may repeat in the same site before appearing elsewhere. A run of the tic movements would be particularly helpful to distinguish simple motor tics from chorea.

Another hyperkinetic disorder that needs to be differentiated from tics is dystonia, particularly from dystonic tics and from eye-blinking tics. Repetitive blinking is seen in mild idiopathic blepharospasm, which is considered a form of focal dystonia (12). Fortunately, the blinking from tics and blepharospasm can usually be differentiated from each other by the presence of either other tics or dystonic movements at other sites. In addition, tics almost always begin in childhood, whereas blepharospasm is predominantly a disorder of the older adult population (13).

Dystonic tics are more difficult to distinguish from torsion dystonia. As emphasized by Meige and Feindel (11), tics not only may be rapid jerks (clonic tics) but may also present as sustained contractions. Sustained contraction is a characteristic feature of dystonic movements. Meige and Feindel called tics with sustained contractions *tonic tics*. The concept of dystonia had not yet been defined in those days, but today, these tics of sustained contractions are more commonly called *dystonic tics*. Examples of dystonic tics are sustained tilt of the head, sustained elevation of the shoulder, sustained abduction of the shoulder, sustained flexion of the trunk, and sustained opening of the mouth. A major differential feature is that torsion dystonia is a continual hyperkinesia, usually twisting in pattern, that can result in sustained, continuous abnormal postures. Dystonic tics, in contrast, are abrupt bursts of movement that are sustained in a posture, but usually for a relatively short duration. They do not tend to be continuous. The presence of the more typical clonic tics in other body regions indicates that the sustained contractions are probably dystonic tics rather than torsion dystonia.

Although dystonic tics are less common than clonic tics, Jankovic and Stone (14) reported that they occurred in 57% of 156 patients with TS, 100% of whom had clonic tics. The most common dystonic tics in this population were oculogyric deviations (43 patients), sustained closure of eyelids (23 patients), and neck-posturing (11 patients).

Perhaps the most helpful feature to differentiate simple tics from myoclonus, chorea, and dystonia is the fact that complex motor and vocal tics may also be present in the patient with simple tics, thereby allowing one to establish the diagnosis by "the company it keeps." However, occasional patients with dystonia may also have tics (15,16), and this association can make it especially difficult to discern simple dystonic tics from dystonia in some patients presenting with known tics and in others presenting with known dystonia.

Another important motor feature that helps differentiate tics from other dyskinesias is ocular deviation, if present. Ocular movements such as a jerk of the eyes (clonic motor tic) or a more sustained eye deviation (dystonic motor tic) may occur in patients with tics (18). When these ocular movements are present, they often suggest that the correct diagnosis is tics because few other dyskinesias involve ocular movements. The exceptions are: (1) opsoclonus ("dancing eyes"), which is a form of myoclonus; (2) ocular myoclonus (rhythmic vertical oscillations at a rate of approximately 2 Hz), which often accompanies palatal myoclonus and is considered a rhythmical segmental myoclonus; and (3) oculogyric spasms (a sustained deviation of the eyes), most often associated with neuroleptics or as a consequence of encephalitis lethargica.

Complex Motor Tics

Complex tics are abrupt, distinct, coordinated patterns of sequential movements. They may appear purposeful, as if performing a voluntary motor act, but they serve no purpose (save the relief of an urge or unpleasant sensation; see below). Examples of complex tics that appear purposeful include such acts as tossing the head as if to move hair off the face, touching the nose, touching other people, smelling objects, spitting, neck-cracking, rubbing, jumping, and copropraxia (obscene gestures). Examples of complex tics that appear nonpurposeful include head-shaking associated with shrugging, repetitive kicking, sequential display of a variety of facial movements, trunk-bending, and echopraxia (mimicking movements performed by others). A run of simple motor tics could be considered at the borderline between simple and complex motor acts.

Other movement disorders that present with clonic-like complex movements but are commonly considered distinct from tics are: (1) the repetitive complex movements, known as stereotypies, of patients with hyperactivity, mental retardation, or psychosis; (2) hyperekplexia, which is an excessive startle syndrome; (3) akathitic movements (initiated to overcome a feeling of inner restlessness); (4) the rituals of the obsessive–compulsive; and (5) the "hand-caressing" movements in Rett's syndrome (a syndrome in young girls with autism, dementia, and motor difficulties). All these other complex movements can sometimes be difficult to distinguish from complex motor tics, and the correct diagnosis of tics is usually made by exclusion of these or by finding an association with simple motor tics or with vocal tics.

Dystonic tics can also manifest themselves as complex acts. Examples would include a combination of bruxism (sustained jaw-clenching with teeth-gnashing) and sustained head-tilting, sustained trunk-bending with arm or leg deviation, and sustained facial distortion plus sustained trunk-twisting. Complex dystonic tics are rather uncommon, but an example can be seen on the videotape publication of Jankovic and Fahn (17). Dystonic complex tics could be mistaken for segmental or generalized torsion dystonia, or possibly paroxysmal dystonic choreoathetosis.

Vocal Tics

Simple Vocal Tics

Vocal tics, also referred to as phonic tics, are sounds produced by moving air through the nose, mouth, or throat. These sounds range from simple throat-clearing sounds and sniffing to grunts to verbalizations of syllables and words. Like somatic motor tics, vocal tics can also be divided into simple and complex tics. Single sounds, such as throat-clearing, barking, grunting, yelping, squeaking, snorting, clicking, and sniffing, represent simple vocal tics.

Complex Vocal Tics

When vocal tics are more complicated, such as whistling, panting, belching, or hiccupping, or include words, they can be considered complex vocal tics. Verbalizations (the expression of words) can be complete words, but more commonly are partial words or unintelligible words. Utterances of inappropriate, undesired statements or obscenities (more often than profanities) are known as coprolalia. Echolalia (repeating the words of others) and palilalia (repeating one's own words) are fairly common complex vocal tics.

Involuntary and voluntary phonations occur in only a few other neurological disorders. These include moaning in akathisia, severe parkinsonism, and progressive supranuclear palsy, and from levodopa toxicity; brief sounds in oromandibular dystonia, Huntington's disease, neuroacanthocytosis, and tardive dyskinesia; and the sniffing and spitting occasionally encountered in Huntington's disease and neuroacanthocytosis. The humming and coughing encountered in some patients with blepharospasm or Meige syndrome should be considered voluntary because they are used as tricks to suppress the dystonic movements.

Tics Status or Status Tics

Rarely, motor and vocal tics can be quite prolonged, usually as a series of clonic tics or dystonic tics that are continual, lasting tens of minutes. These episodes appear to have received little comment in the literature on tics. They are not continuous tics because there may be short periods of normal behavior between the episodes of ticking, rather than minutes of uninterrupted tics. The tics can be simple or complex, but the patient is unable to suppress them during these attacks. It is reasonable to consider them severe attacks of tics, with prolongation of continual tics. In analogy with status epilepticus, I refer to them as tics status or status tics.

Blocking Tics

Another type of tic phenomenology that is rarely, if ever, discussed in the literature is the feature described here as blocking tics. This is a motor phenomenon seen in some patients with tics in which there is a brief interference of social discourse and contact. There is no loss of consciousness and, although the patient does not speak during these episodes, the patient is fully aware of what has been spoken. These occurrences have the abruptness and duration of dystonic tics or a series of clonic tics, but they do not always occur during an episode of an obvious motor tic. I present them here as appearing in two situations: as an accompanying feature of some prolonged tics, including tics status, and as a specific tic phenomenon in the absence of accompanying obvious motor or vocal tics.

For the former, an example would be a burst of tics that is severe enough to interrupt ongoing motor acts, including speech (Refs. 19 and 20; published videotape with Ref. 17), so that the patient is not able to perform other activities. We may wish to consider these episodes "intrusions" because the interruption of activities is due to a positive motor phenomenon (i.e., severe, somewhat prolonged, motor tics).

As for the latter (i.e., inhibition of other ongoing motor activities without obvious "active" tics), we can consider these "blocking" tics. These events should be differentiated from seizures or other paroxysmal episodes of loss of awareness. There is never loss of awareness with blocking tics. Individuals with intrusions and blocking recognize that they have these interruptions of normal activity, and are fully aware of the environment around them, even if they are unable to speak at that time.

OTHER FEATURES OF TICS

Paroxysmal Nature

As mentioned in the introduction, the word *convulsif* applied to tics represents the abruptness and momentariness of the motor or vocal tic, out of a background of normal motor behavior. This paroxysmal nature of tics is characteristic, and only in severe states of tics, such as prolonged tics or tics status, are the tics continual. This paroxysmal feature is a most helpful clinical feature to distinguish tics from most other hyperkinetic movement disorders (Table 2).

Other paroxysmal dyskinesias usually present no difficulty in diagnosis. Paroxysmal kinesigenic choreoathetosis (or dystonia) is triggered by sudden movement or startle, lasts seconds to a few minutes, and is suppressed with anticonvulsant therapy. Paroxysmal dystonic choreoathetosis is induced by stress, prolonged exercise, alcohol, or caffeine, and lasts minutes to hours, too long to be confused with brief bursts of tics. Paroxysmal ataxia and paroxysmal tremor have the typical features of ataxia and tremor, respectively, which are easily distinguished from tics. Stereotypies, which can occur as bursts or can be more continual, could give the most difficulty in being discriminated from tics. As mentioned in the introduction, we are listing stereotypies as nonimpelling acts that would not be irresistible from being suppressed, and stating that these repetitive complex behaviors are associated with schizophrenia, autism, and mental retardation.

Table 2 Differential Diagnosis of Paroxysmal and Nonparoxysmal Hyperkinesias

Paroxysmal hyperkinesias	Continual hyperkinesias
Tics	Athetosis
PKC[a]	Ballism
PDC[b]	Chorea
Paroxysmal ataxia	Dystonia
Paroxysmal tremor	Myoclonus
Stereotypies	Tardive dyskinesia
	Tremors

[a] Paroxysmal kinesigenic choreoathetosis.
[b] Paroxysmal dystonic choreoathetosis.

Variability

A characteristic feature of tics is their variability in time, place, severity, and frequency of appearance. Patients with tics usually have remissions (and also exacerbations). This variability in time distinguishes tics from most other hyperkinetic movement disorders except for other paroxysmal dyskinesias (Table 2). Tics can move from one part of the body to another, which also distinguishes tics from other hyperkinetic movement disorders. Tics can wax and wane in severity, and have remissions and exacerbations. Severity can be best judged by the impact that tics have on the patient's daily functioning and how much effort is needed to try to overcome the tics. Tics may occur from very few per day to many times a minute, and this variability in frequency is another feature limited to paroxysmal disorders (Table 2).

On the other hand, for a period of time, a patient's tics will usually recur in the same parts of the body, and multiple regions of the body can be involved in this fashion. This pattern of repetition, until they change sites or remit again, can last from weeks to months or years, and has been referred to as "systematic" by Charcot [in Goetz (3), p. 57] and "systematized" by Meige and Feindel (7) and Guinon (8). The pattern of tics reappearing again and again in the same manner resembles the characteristic feature of stereotypies.

One feature of variability over the day is that it is quite common for individuals with tics to manifest more of them in the safety of their homes, especially at night, when relaxed while watching television. This may be because tics can be voluntarily suppressed for short periods of time (vide infra), and the patient makes this effort when in public.

Distribution

Tics occur predominantly in the upper part of the body. Data from Shapiro et al. (21) reveal that tics in the upper face (around the eyes and eyelids) occurred at least once in 80% of patients with TS. Reported frequencies of involvement of other body regions included the neck (69%), upper limbs (55%), lower limbs (26%), and torso (24%).

Premonitory Sensation and Urge

An inner feeling of a need to make a movement or a sound is experienced by the majority of patients with tics; executing the movement or sound relieves this urge. This psychic feature has long been recognized as part of the tic phenomenology (9,22,23). Wilson (22) has said that no feature of tics "is more prominent than its irresistibility. The strain in holding back is as great as the relief in letting go." The need to make the movement is as great as the need to scratch an itch.

More recently, the term *sensory tic* was composed by Shapiro et al. (24) to refer to "somatic sensations in joints, bones, muscles, or other parts of the body," which are relieved by the performance of a motor tic in that particular body part. These recurrent somatic sensations are those of pressure, tickle, warmth, cold, pain, or other dysphoric sensations in localized regions (24). How different and specific these focal sensations are compared to the generalized discomfort or urge often preceding a tic is not certain.

The use of the term *sensory tics* was accepted by Kurlan et al. (25). But Lang (26) argues against the use of this term, and I agree with him. As stated above, tics should apply to a motor phenomenon, not withstanding the inappropriate term *tic douloureux*. Although the term *sensory tics* was meant to describe motor tics that occur in response to a localized premonitory sensation, the terminology lends itself to ambiguity, and it could be mistaken to represent a pure sensory phenomenon without a motor component. Moreover, Shapiro et al. (24) initially thought these focal sensations were an uncommon circumstance, leading them to coin the term. However, Kurlan et al. (25) subsequently reported that 41% of their patients experienced a localizable sensation, and that 76% described any sensation or feeling preceding the tics.

Lang (26) specifically queried 170 patients with tics and other types of hyperkinesias. He found that 41 of 60 patients with tic disorders stated that all their motor and vocal tics were intentionally produced to relieve some sensation, whereas only 8 of 110 patients with other hyperkinetic disorders thought that (these eight patients had akathisia, an inner feeling of restlessness; it is characteristic of akathisia that moving about eliminates this unpleasant sensation).

Very few other movement disorders are preceded by sensory complaints. Akathitic movements are a response to akathisia, which most commonly occurs as a complication of neuroleptic medication. The restless legs syndrome is a disorder in which a crawling sensation occurs in the legs when the patient is sitting or lying down at night, to be relieved by the person walking about. Rarely, some myoclonic jerks in patients with essential myoclonus have an electrical-like sensation in the same body part that contains the myoclonus.

Suppressibility

Unless the disorder is very severe, most individuals with tics can voluntarily suppress them for varying periods of time (27). This is in contrast to other hyperkinetic movement disorders, which can be suppressed for only very short durations, if at all (27). But when tics are purposefully suppressed, an inner tension of discomfort builds up, which is relieved only by an increased burst of tics. This tension is the increase of the inner urge described above. It is a generalized or focal uncomfortable feeling that otherwise would be relieved by executing the movement or sound. Suppressibility is one aspect to be considered in rating the severity of tics (Table 3).

Voluntary, Involuntary, and "Unvoluntary"

Lang (26) discussed the terminology of tic movements and sounds as to whether they should be labeled "voluntary" or "involuntary." He pointed out that tics are typically listed as an involuntary movement disorder. Such a classification was probably originally based on the need to differentiate this neurological disorder from psychiatric disorders. However, one could argue today that psychogenic movement disorders, particularly those due to conversion reaction (28), are not truly voluntary. Therefore, labeling tics involuntary should be reevaluated, as Lang (26) has proposed.

With the knowledge that premonitory sensations and urges precede tics, that executing the tic relieves these unpleasant sensations, and that the majority of patients with tics state that the movements and sounds are voluntary, we should redefine the traditional concept that tics are equivalent to the classic abnormal "involuntary" movements, such as tremor, myoclonus, chorea, ballism, athetosis, and dystonia.

One concept is that the motor or vocal action in response to a premonitory sensation is "voluntary," and that the motor or vocal action

Table 3 Spectrum of Severity of Tics

Feature	Mild ◄		► Severe
Duration	Acute, brief	Intermediate length	Tics status
Motor tics	Simple	Complex	Copropraxia, echopraxia, self-mutilation
Vocal tics	None	Poorly audible noises	Loud noises, coprolalia
Variety of tics	Few	Multiple	Many
Suppressible	Easily	With concentrated volition	No
Interference with life's activities	No disruption	Mildly disruptible	Highly disruptible

Source: Ref. 6.

relieving the generalized discomfort or an urge is "involuntary" (24,25). But perhaps the term *unvoluntary* may be better used to describe most motor and vocal tics, meaning that the movement or sound is a response to relieve either an unpleasant sensation or uncomfortable urge. By definition, we should consider *unvoluntary* to mean automatic without conscious effort, as implied from studies of the *Bereitschaftpotential* in patients with TS (31). This premovement EEG potential does not preface the movements of simple tics. Furthermore, because patients have no ability to "will" away the tics, which are "irresistible" in the words of Wilson (22), neither *voluntary* nor *involuntary* seems entirely appropriate. Hence, an intermediate word such as unvoluntary, or its equivalent, can be used to better describe tics.

ASSOCIATED CLINICAL FEATURES IN PATIENTS WITH TICS

It has long been recognized that patients with tics, especially patients with TS, tend to be obsessive or compulsive (Refs. 22 and 29; Ref. 3, p. 58). Discussions of obsessive–compulsive disorder and attention deficit disorder are found elsewhere in this volume. For now, we need to note the association of compulsive personality in patients with tics for the purpose of aiding the differential diagnosis of tics from other movement disorders. As mentioned above, Meige and Feindel (9) used this feature to differentiate tics from stereotypies. We should also ask whether the need to respond to inner or somatic sensory feelings could be a feature of compulsive behavior. This question is beyond the scope of this chapter.

Table 4 Etiological Classification of Tics

- (I) Idiopathic
  - (A) Hereditary (TS)
  - (B) Sporadic
- (II) Symptomatic
  - (A) Neuroacanthocytosis
  - (B) Postencephalitic
  - (C) Head injury
  - (D) Carbon monoxide intoxication
  - (E) Vascular
  - (F) Drug-induced
    - (1) Stimulants (amphetamine, methylphenidate, pemoline, levodopa)
    - (2) Tardive tics (neuroleptics)

ETIOLOGICAL CLASSIFICATION OF TICS

Tics are usually considered pathological, whereas mannerisms and habit spasms are physiological (6). In this chapter, stereotypies have been considered a separate entity.

Etiologically, tic disorders can be classified as: (1) idiopathic, including hereditary (and including TS, which is considered hereditary) and (2) symptomatic (Table 4). Whether transient tic disorder and chronic motor or phonic tics should be considered entities distinct from TS can eventually be answered once the gene for TS is discovered. For now, I will not label these separate etiological entities, distinct from TS, although for research purposes, they should be so considered (30,31) until a final status can be assigned to these conditions. Tics due to brain insults are listed in Table 4 as symptomatic tics.

By far, the most common condition causing tics is TS, the focus of this monograph.

REFERENCES

1. Wilson SAK. Neurology 1940; Vol. II:. Baltimore: Williams and Wilkins, 1940:1629.
2. Meige H, Feindel E. Tics and Their Treatment (translated from French by SAK Wilson). London: Appleton, 1907:26.
3. Goetz CG. Charcot, the Clinician: The Tuesday Lessons. Excerpts from Nine Case Presentations on General Neurology Delivered at the Salpetriere Hospital in 1887–88 by Jean-Martin Charcot, Translated with Commentary. New York: Raven Press, 1987:56–70.
4. Gilles de la Tourette G. La maladie de tics convulsifs. Sem Med 1899; 19:153–156.
5. Meige H, Feindel E. Tics and Their Treatment (translated from French by SAK Wilson). London: Appleton, 1907:31.
6. Fahn S. The clinical spectrum of motor tics. Adv Neurol 1982; 35:341–344.
7. Meige H, Feindel E. Tics and Their Treatment (translated from French by SAK Wilson). London: Appleton, 1907:45.
8. Guinon G. Sur la maladie des tics convulsifs. Rev Med 1886; 6:50–80.
9. Meige H, Feindel E. Tics and Their Treatment (translated from French by SAK Wilson). London: Appleton, 1907:57–58.
10. Shapiro AK, Shapiro ES, Young JG, Feinberg TE. Gilles de la Tourette Syndrome. 2nd ed. New York: Raven Press, 1988:345.
11. Meige H, Feindel E. Tics and Their Treatment (translated from French by SAK Wilson). London: Appleton, 1907:118–124.
12. Fahn S. Blepharospasm: a form of focal dystonia. Adv Neurol 1988; 49:125–133.

13. Jankovic J, Orman J. Blepharospasm: demographic and clinical survey of 250 patients. Ann Ophthalmol 1984; 16:371–376.
14. Jankovic J, Stone L. Dystonic tics in patients with Tourette's syndrome. Mov Disord 1991; 6:248–252.
15. Shale HM, Truong DD, Fahn S. Tics in patients with other movement disorders. Neurology 1986; 36(suppl 1):118.
16. Stone LA, Jankovic J. The coexistence of tics and dystonia. Arch Neurol 1991; 48:862–865.
17. Jankovic J, Fahn S. The phenomenology of tics. Mov Disord 1986; 1:17–26. Video supplement.
18. Frankel M, Cummings JL. Neuro-ophthalmic abnormalities in Tourette's syndrome: functional and anatomic implications. Neurology 1984; 34:359–361.
19. Feinberg TE, Shapiro AK, Shapiro E. Paroxysmal myoclonic dystonia with vocalisations: new entity or variant of preexisting syndromes? J Neurol Neurosurg Psychiatry 1986; 49:52–57.
20. Fahn S. Paroxysmal myolonic dystonia with vocalizations [letter]. J Neurol Neurosurg Psychiatry 1987; 50:117–118.
21. Shapiro AK, Shapiro ES, Young JG, Feinberg TE. Gilles de la Tourette Syndrome. 2nd ed. New York: Raven Press, 1988:140.
22. Wilson SAK. Neurology. Vol. II. Baltimore: Williams and Wilkins, 1940:1631.
23. Leckman JF, Cohen DJ. Descriptive and diagnostic classification of tic disorders. In: Cohen DJ, Bruun RD, Leckman JF, eds. Tourette's Syndrome and Tic Disorders: Clinical Understanding and Treatment. New York: Wiley, 1988:4.
24. Shapiro AK, Shapiro ES, Young JG, Feinberg TE. Gilles de la Tourette Syndrome. 2nd ed. New York: Raven Press, 1988:356–360.
25. Kurlan R, Lichter D, Hewitt D. Sensory tics in Tourette's syndrome. Neurology 1989; 39:731–734.
26. Lang A. Patient perception of tics and other movement disorders. Neurology 1991; 41:223–228.
27. Koller WC, Biary NM. Volitional control of involuntary movements. Mov Disord 1989; 4:153–156.
28. Fahn S, Williams DT. Psychogenic dystonia. Adv Neurol 1988; 50:431–455.
29. Leckman JF, Cohen DJ. Descriptive and diagnostic classification of tic disorders. In: Cohen DJ, Bruun RD, Leckman JF, eds. Tourette's Syndrome and Tic Disorders: Clinical Understanding and Treatment. New York: Wiley, 1988:9–10.
30. Kurlan R. Tourette's syndrome: current concepts. Neurology 1989; 39:1625–1630.
31. Obeso JA, Rothwell JC, Marsden CD. Neurophysiology of Tourette syndrome. Adv Neurol 1982; 35:105–114.

2

Premonitory ("Sensory") Experiences

Tamara M. Pringsheim and Anthony E. Lang
Toronto Western Hospital
Toronto, Ontario, Canada

In 1980, Bliss (1) provided one of the first reports emphasizing the significance of sensory phenomena in Tourette's syndrome (TS) through an introspective analysis of his own personal experience with the disorder. After years of careful observation, he became aware of sensory signals preceding movements. "Each movement is preceded by certain preliminary sensory signals and is in turn followed by sensory impressions at the end of the action. Each movement is a voluntary capitulation to a demanding and restless urge accompanied by an extraordinarily subtle sensation that provokes and fuels the urge." "The intention is to relieve the sensation, as surely as the movement to scratch an itch is to relieve the itch." Based on this experience, Bliss emphasized that "the movement is not the whole message." "The movement, even if grotesque and miserable, is not the most important part of TS activity. Clinical evaluations have centered on the overt symptoms, but curiously they have stopped short of probing for the sensory events, the covert modes, that show before and at the end of the evident act. The sensory symptoms are there, and they tell more than the visible and audible actions."

This fascinating and detailed report led to increased interest in sensory phenomena in Tourette's syndrome, and to several larger studies that shall be discussed in this chapter. Indeed, the concept of premonitory or sensory experiences preceding tics has provoked much discussion on the phenomenology of tics, and the characterization of tics as a response to an irresistible urge, rather than a completely involuntary act.

In 1988, Shapiro et al. (2) introduced the term "sensory tics". By this they meant the occurrence of "recurrent involuntary somatic sensations in joints, bones, muscles, or other parts of the body," which evoke a dysphoric feeling causing the patient to intentionally respond with a movement or vocalization to relieve the abnormal sensation. Sensory complaints included heaviness, lightness, emptiness, tickle, temperature changes, or poorly described abnormal superficial or deep sensations. Shapiro et al. believed that the movements of sensory tics differed from the more typical varieties in that they were more prolonged (often lasting 1 sec or more) and usually consisted of tonic squeezing, stretching, or tightening of muscles. Vocalizations also differed from the usual simple phonic tics in being more prolonged, lower pitched humming, gurgling, or "mm" sounds. At that time, the authors felt that sensory tics were relatively uncommon. Through retrospective review of medical records, they found that only 8.5% (105 of 1237) of patients had antecedent sensory phenomena. The authors concluded that, although these symptoms were distinctly different from the more common tics seen in TS, these patients indeed represent a "sensory subtype of Tourette's disorder."

Subsequent studies carried out by direct interview of patients with TS have yielded much different results. The results of a survey of 34 randomly selected TS patients by Kurlan et al. (3) provided the first support that sensory phenomena are a common and integral component of the disorder. Seventy-six percent of their patients described a distinct sensation or feeling preceding their tics. Twelve percent described a variety of focal sensations including an itch, tightness, or a poorly characterized feeling. Thirty-five percent experienced generalized nonlocalizable sensations that were both *somatic*, including tightness, tension, and tingling, and *psychic* such as an urge, pleasure appreciated after the movement, surprise, tension, or apprehension. Twenty-nine percent experienced both focal and generalized sensations. One of the interesting differences between those with and without sensory antecedents was the observation that 96% of the former group reported the ability to suppress tics voluntarily compared to 63% of subjects who had no sensory experiences. Importantly, these authors found that the movements and vocalizations accompanying sensory tics were indistinguishable from those that lacked the subjective sensory antecedents.

Several studies on premonitory urges and sensory phenomena in TS have come from Cohen and Leckman (4). In their 1992 study of 28 patients by direct interview, 22 (79%) of the subjects reported that they experienced premonitory urges before their motor and phonic tics. In 13 cases (57%), the premonitory urges were experienced as being more bothersome that the tics themselves. Twelve (55%) also expressed the belief that the premonitory urges enhanced their ability to suppress tic symptoms. Seventy-one percent of the subjects felt that their tics were a voluntary response to the premonitory urges that they experienced.

In 1993, a second, larger study of premonitory urges by the same group was performed by questionnaire and follow-up telephone interview (if necessary) of 132 patients with TS (5). Ninety-three percent of respondents identified having a sensation (mental or physical awareness), such as "an urge," "a feeling," "an impulse," or "a need" to experience a tic during the past week, and 95% reported ever having had them. When asked to mark on a body diagram all of the locations where the patients had ever experienced these sensations, the shoulder girdle, palms, midline abdominal region, ventral thighs, feet, and eyes were regions of high sensory awareness.

The mean age at which respondents first became aware of the premonitory urges was 10.0 years, which averaged 3.1 years after the onset of tics. Eighty-nine percent of patients felt the sensation or urge was either partly or wholly a physical experience. Head, neck, and shoulder tics were most frequently preceded by premonitory urges, and most urges were judged to be felt in muscle. Ninety-two percent of subjects reported that they experienced their tics to be partly or wholly voluntary. Sensations and urges were altered by medication in 63 of 101 respondents, being reduced in frequency and intensity by neuroleptics. Stress and anxiety increased pre-tic urges and sensations, while relaxation and concentration decreased the urge, in 92 of 120 respondents. The authors concluded that premonitory urges are common among adolescents and adults with tic disorders, and that subjects with tic disorders often experience their movements as being a voluntary response to these unwanted urges.

A recent study at the Baylor College of Medicine Parkinson's Disease Center and Movement Disorders clinic sought to define the various sensory phenomena associated with motor tics. Using a questionnaire, 92% of patients with TS reported premonitory sensations, of which the majority identified as an "urge to move" or "impulse to tic." Premonitory sensations were most commonly experienced in the face (73%), followed by the neck (66%) and shoulders (56%), and were usually localized within the muscle, rather than joints or skin. Patients perceived that the motor tic would be eliminated without the premonitory sensation, and had a tendency to describe the motor tic as a voluntary movement (6).

Sensory phenomena in patients with obsessive–compulsive disorder (OCD) and/or TS have been studied to determine if sensory or premonitory symptoms help to differentiate tic-related OCD from non-tic-related OCD. Miguel et al. (7) interviewed 20 adult outpatients with OCD, 20 with OCD plus TS, and 21 with TS. They found that patients with OCD plus TS and patients with TS alone had significantly more sensory phenomena preceding their repetitive behaviors, including bodily sensations (e.g., an itch, tickle, or burning sensation) and mental sensations (urge, inner tension, or energy buildup). Sensory phenomena were found in 40% of patients with OCD, 100% of patients with OCD plus TS, and 95% of patients with TS. For each type of bodily sensation, the OCD group reported significantly fewer tactile (15%) and no muscular–skeletal/visceral sensations when compared with the TS (43%) and OCD plus TS (85%) groups. Differences between the OCD group and the TS and OCD plus TS groups were also more striking for the less-complex mental sensations such as urge only and energy release.

As previously mentioned, the identification of premonitory urges as a common experience among patients with TS called into question the very nature of tics themselves. In the late 1980s, most literature described tics as "involuntary," with little distinction between this and the involuntary nature of other hyperkinetic movement disorders. Some categorized tics with epilepsy and reflexes, because of their "involuntary" and "unintended" nature. In an effort to clarify the issue, patients at the Movement Disorders Clinic of the Toronto Western Hospital were interviewed with questions directed at the "voluntary" or intentional vs. "involuntary" aspects of their symptoms (8). One hundred two of the 110 patients with non-tic disorders (patients with dystonia, tremor, tardive dyskinesia, hemifacial spasm, chorea, myoclonus) responded that all their abnormal movements were completely involuntary. Four of sixty patients with tic disorders thought that all their movements and vocalizations were completely involuntary, while the vast majority (41/60) responded that all their movements and vocalizations were performed voluntarily, with the remaining 15 responding that their tics had both voluntary and involuntary components. The results of this study helped to confirm Bliss's personal experiences that a large proportion of the motor and phonic symptoms experienced by patients with tics are irresistibly but purposefully executed, unlike other hyperkinetic movement disorders with which tics are commonly grouped.

Kane (9), a graduate student with TS, published a report of his experiences with the disorder. He expressed the belief that the etiopathogenesis of TS is less "sensory" than "attentional," and that pre-tic sensations are manifestations of somatosensory hyperattention. According to his experience, he argued that the TS patient suffers from an oppressive hyperawareness of what his or her skin, muscles, and joints feel like, because of deficient attentional inhibition. "When sitting in a chair, I do not lose awareness of the tactile sensation of the seat against my body, nor can I ignore the deeper somatic sensations of what my back and legs feel like." "If all tics are suppressed, virtually all my joints and muscles begin to demand my attention. The TS state heightens to a stiffening feeling, such that my skin feels like a hardened casing and my joints feel as though they are becoming rigid. The intensity rises until it becomes so unpleasant and distracting that tics must be executed (with a compulsion that rivals the scratching of a severe itch)." Cohen and Leckman (4) also described a similar concept of "site sensitization" in 13 of 20 (65%) of patients with TS questioned about whether or not they felt that they had heightened sensitivity to sensory stimuli. Examples from patients included having to cut the tags out of every shirt they had because the tags rubbed their neck and constantly bothered them, being unable to wear blue jeans because of the way they feel at the waist or the back of the knee, and never being able to get their socks to feel comfortable because of the way the seams rub their toes.

The cause of Tourette's syndrome and the premonitory urges preceding tics remains unknown, although understanding of the pathophysiology of the disorder has considerably progressed in recent years. It is clear, given the prominence of premonitory urges and other sensory experiences, that this rather unique aspect of tics must be accounted for in any theories developed to explain the pathogenesis of TS. The 1993 study of Leckman et al. (5), indicating a latency of 3 years between the onset of tics and the awareness of sensory phenomena, might suggest that the latter are a secondary problem. However, this was retrospective historical data related to symptoms experienced many years earlier. It is our experience that although many children have considerable difficulty expressing their personal experience with tics, some are certainly able to provide a convincing account of preceding sensory experiences and the performance of the tic to relieve them from the onset of TS symptoms.

In their original paper on premonitory urges, Cohen and Leckman (4) hypothesized that TS is associated with a failure to inhibit subsets of corticostriatothalamocortical (CSTC) minicircuits. They state that the processing of somatotopically organized sensory information in parallel with adjacent circuits that process information associated with both the planning and performance of motor behaviors may provide the neuroanatomical basis for the premonitory urges of TS.

Fried et al. (10) have studied the supplementary motor area (SMA) using electrical stimulation mapping. They were able to elicit movement in specific anatomical locations by stimulating corresponding areas of the SMA. Subthreshold stimulation of certain areas of the SMA produced an urge to make a movement. This finding is of significance as the SMA is thought to have a key role in the planning and initiation of voluntary movements. This suggests that facilitation of SMA activity may be involved in the premonitory urges preceding tics. Indeed, studies using transcranial magnetic stimulation (TMS) have found decreased motor inhibition in patients with TS, which may relate to these findings (11,12). Whether the SMA is the origin of such symptoms or simply one component in the circuit responding to subcortical drives is unclear. The finding that tics may not be preceded by a normal Bereitschaftpotential, or readiness potential (13), which is believed to originate in the SMA, might argue against this hypothesis; however, the presence of premonitory sensory symptoms or urges have not been assessed in such studies.

Ziemann et al. (11) studied 20 patients with TS and 21 healthy controls with the application of focal TMS to the left motor cortex, and surface EMG from the right abductor digiti minimi muscle. These studies demonstrated that compared to healthy controls, patients with TS had normal motor thresholds, but a shortened cortical silent period and deficient intracortical inhibition. The authors felt that the normal motor threshold in patients with TS suggests that the deficient motor impulse control in TS is not because of hyperexcitability at the membrane level, while it is compatible with disordered inhibitory control through the CSTC circuit. The shortened cortical silent period may indicate a reduced inhibitory interneuronal control of the output cells in the motor cortex. This could be because of pathology within the motor cortex, deficient inhibition of subcortical afferents to the motor cortex, or enhanced motor drive or facilitated accessibility of the motor cortex by motor commands in TS.

The role of peripheral feedback mechanisms in maintaining the premonitory sensory symptoms was first suggested by the experience of a patient whose long-standing frontalis muscle tics and the preceding premonitory urge resolved in response to intramuscular botulinum toxin treatment. The urge (and tics) did not return over several months of follow-up, long after the focal weakening effect of the toxin had subsided (14). Subsequently, Jankovic et al. (15,16) carried out larger-scale, open-label studies confirming that botulinum toxin completely abolished or markedly relieved the premonitory symptoms in 45 patients with TS. Finally, in a randomized, double-blind, controlled clinical trial, Marras et al. (17) found that botulinum toxin significantly reduced both treated tic frequency and the urge associated with the treated tic, compared to placebo. The success of botulinum toxin injection in abolishing premonitory urges suggests that it may interrupt a normal peripheral feedback mechanism such as local muscular tension, which may be necessary for the generation of tics, and the accompanying sensory symptoms.

In conclusion, premonitory urges are a common and integral part of the experience of patients with TS. The recognition of this phenomenon has led to the classification of tics as a voluntary response to an irresistible urge. Although the pathophysiological basis of these symptoms is not fully understood, it appears that both peripheral and central mechanisms may play a role.

REFERENCES

1. Bliss J. Sensory experiences of Gilles de la Tourette syndrome. Arch Gen Psychiatry 1980; 37:1343–1347.
2. Shapiro AK, Shapiro ES, Young JG, Feinberg TE. Gilles de la Tourette Syndrome. New York: Raven Press, 1988.
3. Kurlan R, Lichter D, Hewitt D. Sensory tics in Tourette's syndrome. Neurology 1989; 39:731–734.
4. Cohen AJ, Leckman JF. Sensory phenomena associated with Gilles de la Tourette's Syndrome. J Clin Psychiatry 1992; 53:319–323.
5. Leckman JF, Walker DE, Cohen DJ. Premonitory urges in Tourette's Syndrome. Am J Psychiatry 1993; 150:98–102.
6. Kwak C, Jankovic J. Sensory phenomena in motor tics. Mov Disord 2002; 17(Suppl 5):339.
7. Miguel EC, do Rosario-Campos MC, da Silva Prado H, do Valle R, Rauch SL, Coffey BJ, Baer L, Savage CR, O'Sullivan RL, Jenike MA, Leckman JF. Sensory phenomena in obsessive–compulsive disorder and Tourette's disorder. J Clin Psychiatry 2000; 61:150–156.
8. Lang AE. Patient perception of tics and other movement disorders. Neurology 1991; 41:223–228.
9. Kane MJ. Premonitory urges as attentional tics in Tourette's syndrome. J Am Acad Child Adolesc Psych 1994; 33(6):805–808.
10. Fried I, Katz A, McCarthy G, Sass KJ, Williamson P, Spenser SS, Spenser DD. Functional organization of human supplementary motor cortex studied by electrical stimulation. J Neurosci 1991; 11:3656–3666.
11. Ziemann U, Paulus W, Rothenberger A. Decreased motor inhibition in Tourette's disorder: Evidence from transcranial magnetic stimulation. Am J Psychiatry 1997; 154:1277–1284.
12. Moll GH, Wischer S, Heinrich H, Tergau F, Paulus W, Rothenberger A. Deficient motor control in children with tic disorder: evidence from transcranial magnetic stimulation. Neurosci Lett 1999; 272:37–40.
13. Obeso JA, Rothwell JC, Marsden CD. The neurophysiology of Tourette syndrome. In: Friedhoff AJ, Chase TN, eds. Advances in Neurology. Vol. 35. Gilles de la Tourette Syndrome. New York: Raven Press, 1982:105–114.
14. Lang AE. Clinical phenomenology of tic disorders, selected aspects. In: Chase TN, Friedhoff AJ, Cohen DJ, eds. Advances in Neurology. Vol 58. Tourettes Syndrome: Genetics, Neurobiology, and Treatment. New York: Raven Press, 1992:25–32.
15. Jankovic J. Botulinum toxin in the treatment of dystonic tics. Mov Disord 1994; 9(3):347–349.
16. Kwak CH, Hanna PA, Jankovic J. Botulinum toxin in the treatment of tics. Arch Neurol 2000; 57:1190–1193.
17. Marras C, Andrews D, Sime E, Lang A. Botulinum toxin for simple motor tics. A randomized, double-blind, controlled clinical trial. Neurology 2001; 56:605–610.

3

The Natural History of Gilles de la Tourette Syndrome

Ruth Dowling Bruun
New York University School of Medicine
Westhampton Beach, New York, U.S.A.

Cathy L. Budman
New York University School of Medicine
New York
and North Shore University Hospital
Manhasset, New York, U.S.A.

INTRODUCTION

As Tourette's syndrome (TS) has been more widely and thoroughly studied, it has generally been acknowledged that cases consisting of tics alone are less common than those with comorbid emotional and behavioral disorders (1–4). More often than not, clinicians treating TS are realizing that tics are not the most severe problem that many of their patients must face. To be complete, therefore, an account of the natural history of TS must include TS-associated disorders along with the appearance, progression, and regression of tics.

Tics and associated symptoms naturally fluctuate over time in severity and in the extent of their interference with normal functioning. The symptomatic ebb and flow may be due to endogenous causes that are as yet poorly understood, or to external factors such as medications, stress, adaptability, and special assistance received (e.g., modified school programs). Sometimes causes for the fluctuations in severity of various symptoms can be identified. Often, they cannot. Nevertheless, there is general agreement among investigators on the nature of the average course of this complex neuropsychiatric disorder.

ONSET OF TS: CHILDHOOD

Tics of all kinds are quite common during childhood, occurring in 4–24% of school children and, in most cases, are transitory (5). By *Diagnostic and Statistical Manual of Mental Disorders* (DSM) convention, tics are classified by their nature as either motor or vocal and by their natural history as either transient (lasting less than 12 months) or chronic (persisting beyond 12 months). The presence of chronic, multiple motor, and vocal tics, varying in severity and character over time, is the essential feature of TS. However, considerable evidence exists to suggest that transient tic disorder (TTD), chronic tic disorder (CTD), and TS represent varying manifestations of the same genetic abnormality, falling on a spectrum with mild, transient tics at one end and TS at the other (4,6).

It should also be noted that the validity of the distinction between motor and vocal tics is often meaningless because vocal tics, with the exception of linguistically meaningful words and phrases, are simply produced by motor movements of facial, laryngeal, pharyngeal, or respiratory muscles (4,6,7).

Despite differing views on the precise definition of TS, there is general agreement that the mean age of onset of tics falls between 6 and 7 years of age (8,9). An international database of 3500 people diagnosed with TS at 64 sites recently established the mean age of tic onset to be 6.4 years. Forty-one percent of cases began below the age of 6 years and 93% were symptomatic before the age of 10 years. Only 1% of cases was said to have begun between the ages of 16 and 20 years (3).

The upper age limit for onset of symptoms has been controversial. By DSM-IV and DSM-IV-TR definition, the onset of the tics of TS must occur before the age of 18 years. However, it has varied from 14 years in DSM-III to 21 years in DSM-III-R.

Motor tics are most commonly the first symptom to appear. Reviews of a number of large studies composed of approximately 2400 patients indicate that 50–70% of TS patients experienced facial tics as their first symptom. The next most common presenting symptoms were simple tics of the neck and shoulders, followed by those of the upper extremities. Motor tics of the lower extremities and trunk were the least common presenting symptoms. Thus, in general, motor tics progress in a rostral–caudal fashion, involving the head and shoulders before the trunk or extremities. In the individual patient, however, the progression is rarely this orderly (10–12).

Simple vocalizations, most frequently reported as repetitive throat-clearings, occur as presenting symptoms in only 12–37% of subjects

(10,11). As a rule, these tics appear about 2 years later than motor tics (9). It is even less common (only 7–11% of patients) that presenting symptoms consist of complex, stereotyped movements or vocalizations. Coprolalia occurs as a presenting symptom in 2–6% of cases, commonly manifesting itself several years after the onset of other symptoms (10,11,13). In a series of patients evaluated by Shapiro et al. (5), the average age for onset of coprolalia was 13.5 years. In fact, this perplexing and difficult symptom occurs in only a third or less of patients (3,13).

Simple motor or minor vocal tics are often overlooked. Typically, children may blink excessively, grimace, sniff, cough, or clear their throats with unusual frequency but will probably never see a physician because of these symptoms. In some cases, a referral to an ophthalmologist or an allergist may be sought and, in other cases, the symptoms may be misperceived as attention-seeking behavior, prompting intervention by a psychologist or other therapist. A study done by Golden and Hood in 1982 demonstrated that more than 60% of TS patients were originally diagnosed with "nervousness," causing the diagnosis of TS to be delayed for many years (10,11). More recently, due to greater medical and public awareness of the disorder, such lengthy delays in diagnosis have been reduced. However, many cases are still missed by physicians and not diagnosed until a parent or the patient learns about TS from an acquaintance or through the media. Of the 3500 individuals collected by the international database in the years 1998–2000, 16% were not diagnosed until adulthood (3).

A study done by the authors and their colleagues sought to determine the course of children who initially presented to a psychiatrist or neurologist with the complaint of transient tics. Our group was able to obtain follow-up information on 58 children who had originally met the criteria (DSM-III and ICD 9) for a diagnosis of TTD. Sixty-two percent were reevaluated at follow-up by a structured telephone interview and 38% were reevaluated by personal interview. The time since the initial diagnosis of TTD ranged from 2 to 14 years. On follow-up, it was found that only 17% of the patients could still be diagnosed as having had TTD. Forty percent met the diagnostic criteria for chronic motor or vocal tic disorder (CTD) and the remaining 53% continued to experience tics that were chronic and episodic (either TS or tic disorder NOS by DSM-IV criteria). Although there were only four patients who had initially presented with vocal tics alone, it is interesting to note that all went on to have either CTD or TS. Of the patients who initially presented with motor and vocal tics, 47% were subsequently diagnosed with TS, whereas of those who presented with motor tics alone, only 5% subsequently met criteria for TS (8).

Although these were children who presented to specialists for a diagnosis, causing the study to be weighted toward the severe end of the spectrum of transient tics, it strongly suggests that an early presentation of vocal tics may bode a more persistent and complex course than motor tics alone (8).

Tics characteristically vary in intensity and frequency over time. Patients may experience periods of time when they are almost asymptomatic only to be disappointed by the return of relatively severe tics. Others will experience consistently severe tics for a period of years. Sometimes a certain tic will always be present whereas a variety of others will come and go, never to return (1,5,8,10,11).

Symptoms that may cause confusion between tics and compulsions include: touching, hitting (self or others), jumping, smelling one's hands, smelling other objects, retracing steps, twirling, and doing deep knee bends (13). Jankovic (6) calls these types of tics "compulsive" and stipulates that they are preceded by, or associated with, feelings of anxiety, or the fear that something "bad" will happen if a tic is not performed.

There is significant comorbidity of TS with attention deficit hyperactivity disorder (ADHD). School-based and clinic-based studies have identified the frequency of ADHD in TS patients to be between 24% and 75% (14–19). Symptoms of hyperactivity, impulsivity, distractibility, inattentiveness, and low frustration tolerance are most commonly first identified between the ages of 3 and 5 years, roughly 2–3 years before the appearance of tics (10,11). Hence, a significant number of children who have not yet developed tics but do have symptoms of ADHD will receive psychostimulant medication. Psychostimulants have been documented in some cases to exacerbate existing tics, or to provoke tics in susceptible individuals. Consequently, the use of stimulant medication for the treatment of ADHD in children with TS, or a family history of TS, has been a focus of concern and controversy (8,20–23). However, recent research has demonstrated that this is less common than previously believed and, at the present time, because symptoms of ADHD will often cause greater morbidity and social impairment than tics alone, there is considerable evidence that stimulants may be the drugs of choice for ADHD symptoms in the majority of TS children (22,25).

In addition to ADHD, specific learning disabilities are a frequent comorbid occurrence in children with TS. Neuropsychological testing may reveal discrepancies in verbal IQ and performance IQ, abnormalities in graphomotor and nonmotor visual perceptual abilities, or deficits in verbal receptive skills (26–28). Comings et al. (14) have reported a need for special education services that is five times greater than that of the general population. Moreover, a study of 200 TS children and adolescents conducted by Erenberg et al. (29) revealed that 22% had an identified learning disability and 20% received some special education classes.

A learning disability may be diagnosed at any age and may be successfully treated by helping the child (or the adult) to accommodate for the specific deficit. Because learning disabilities, along with ADHD, may contribute considerable morbidity in terms of low self-esteem, educational frustration, and failure, it is important that a child who is having school difficulties be given neuropsychological testing.

Although somewhat controversial in the past, there is now general agreement among investigators that obsessive–compulsive symptomatology (OCS) and obsessive–compulsive disorder (OCD) are commonly associated with TS and may even be an intrinsic part of the disorder (30). Probably due to varied interpretations of the definition of OCD, estimates of the incidence of OCD in TS patients have varied considerably, but a preponderance of recent studies finds an incidence between 30% and 60% (2,3,6,31).

Most typically, obsessive–compulsive symptoms develop at age 9 or 10 years, 2–3 years after the onset of tics (8,9). Many TS patients exhibit symptoms associated with classical OCD such as contamination and aggressive fears. However, many others describe a type of OCD that is particularly associated with TS—that of "evening up" rituals, the need to perform actions until they feel "just right," or the need to do things a certain number of times (2). Significant overlap is observed among compulsive behaviors, obsessive thoughts, and complex tics, thus complicating assessment of OCD in patients with TS. A diagnostic dilemma is apt to occur when, for example, a tic must be repeated a certain number of times, or a number of tics must be performed in a certain sequence before the patient is able to feel relief. Ultimately, the correct diagnosis of such a symptom may be important in the choice of a specific treatment (8).

Because OCS/OCD symptomatology may present considerably later than ADHD and tics, the possibility of its development in the future must be kept in mind when treating young patients. After OC symptoms have been established, they tend to wax and wane in a manner not dissimilar to the tics of TS.

Aggressive behaviors, rage outbursts, self-harming behaviors, immaturity, withdrawal, social problems, autism spectrum disorders, conduct disorders, affective disorders, anxiety disorders, stuttering, sleep disorders, increased incidence of migraine headache, restless legs, and inappropriate sexual behaviors have all been reported to occur with increased incidence in association with TS (1,3,9,19,31–37). These comorbid problems may have a profound effect on the severity of tics (36). In addition, new problems may be introduced by pharmacotherapy. Neuroleptics, for example, can cause sedation, dysphoria, weight gain, poor school performance, school phobia, and additional movement disorders such as tardive dyskinesia, akathisia, or acute dystonic reactions (38).

Children with TS are challenged by a myriad of symptoms that present during a developmental period when peer relationships and approval become increasingly important. Tics may lead to severe disturbances of self-esteem and isolation from social relationships with classmates. Tics and symptoms of ADHD may also result in severe disruption of classroom activities and underachievement. Failure to identify and diagnose TS can result in unnecessary threatening, punishing, bribing, and humiliation of children by their family, teachers, and peers. However, once the correct diagnosis of TS is made and it is understood that the child's tics are involuntary, barriers to obtaining appropriate treatment ad rehabilitation programs can be overcome.

In many cases, extensive educational meetings with teachers and school officials may be required to obtain necessary resources and support. In other instances, the child may require individual psychotherapy to work on improving self-esteem and coping skills for living with a chronic disorder. Family therapy may be indicated for working on maladaptive interactions, medication compliance, and feelings of guilt engendered, particularly in affected parents. Peer self-help and support groups may be helpful as children enter adolescence. However, because cases vary greatly in their characteristics, severity, comorbidity, and circumstances, treatment must be individualized based on the child's abilities and deficits, and within the context of the family and social milieu.

Peterson points out that, until the age of 10 or 11 years, most children with TS will report that they are unaware of any premonitory urges. Because they cannot predict when tics will happen, they feel unable to control them (9). This gradually changes as the preteen years progress and varying degrees of control over the expression of tics are developed. The power to hold back tics will depend particularly on characteristics such as on the child's social awareness and the degree of associated impulsivity or mood stability.

Preadolescence is also a time when OCS begins to be a problem for many children and may cause considerable internal distress.

ADOLESCENCE

By the time the average child with TS reaches adolescence, the child has had symptoms for 6–7 years. Adolescence is a time of both emotional and physical unpredictability. It is a difficult time in the lives of most people, with or without medical problems. Growth spurts, hormonal changes, development of secondary sexual characteristics, and increasing social demands all contribute to frequent emotional ups and downs. Not surprisingly, tics and associated TS symptoms may seem to become worse at this time and clinicians who treat TS often find that they are spending a disproportionate amount of their time with adolescents and their parents. In fact, tic symptoms may not actually be worse at this time; they may only be more problematic. It is not unusual for coprolalia to first present during early adolescence, and although scientifically this may not be considered to be a worse symptom than another kind of tic, it certainly seems worse for the patient and the family. Other tic symptoms that may not have been so problematic for a younger child now may also become acutely embarassing and it is not uncommon for adolescents to refuse to go to school when tics are severe.

Although a recent study seems to indicate that changes in estrogen and progesterone levels do not correlate with changes on the severity of tics and OCD symptoms, girls often experience a subjective worsening of tics during the onset of menstruation and prior to each menses (39).

Adolescence is also a time when associated behavioral problems become greater. Although irritability tends to wax and wane along with tic severity in younger children, more clear-cut behavioral problems emerge during adolescence. As temper tantrums become less age-appropriate, they are more likely to come to the attention of the physician and, as children grow to adult size, outbursts of rage become more threatening and less tolerable to families and schools. Whatever the cause, behavioral problems tend to increase in severity over time, even in the face of apparent improvement of tics. For example, when the incidence of behavioral and social problems in a group of TS patients aged 6–11 years was compared with a group aged 12–16 years, abnormal scores on the Child Behavioral Checklist were more common in the older group (19). Because obsessive–compulsive symptoms often reach a peak in severity at about the same age (mid to late teenage years) at which tics begin to wane, it is particularly important to look for OCD when behavioral problems develop later in the course of TS (2,10,13).

Although the natural history of various behavioral problems has not been well documented, there is some evidence that temper tantrums, aggressiveness, and explosiveness appear in the preadolescent period, become severe in the teenage years, and gradually recede thereafter. Trimble (40) has found a significant association between aggression and symptoms of compulsive touching and copropraxia. Comings and Comings (41) and Comings (42) feel that the incidence of aggressivity increases at about the same age that tics are receding in severity.

LATE ADOLESCENCE AND ADULTHOOD

Although many studies have been done to determine when and how TS symptoms begin and how they progress during childhood and adolescence, much less information has been gathered about the natural history of the disorder from late adolescence onward. More information is needed about the course of TS symptoms during pregnancy as well as menopause. Such data have been difficult to collect because many of the older patients have been lost to follow-up. Although this is likely to be because symptoms have grown milder and less disruptive as patients reach adulthood, there are few longitudinal studies to provide the proof.

Although genetic studies make an effort to identify all members of a family who are symptomatic, or even partially symptomatic, a longitudinal view is again lacking. Efforts to obtain a broader overview of the lives of TS patients have been made by sending questionnaires to all members of the Ohio chapter of the TSA (43,44). However, these studies almost certainly suffer from an ascertainment bias. Thus, until the diagnosis of TS is reliably made by the average family practitioner or internist, we may continue to have only a skewed sample of patients with which to define the later natural history of the disorder.

Twenty-five years ago, TS was considered a lifelong disorder (5). Although remissions were documented, these were only known to last for a few years at the most and were considered rare. As the diagnosis was made more frequently and many milder cases were identified, this view changed. At the present time, there is a general consensus that if one considers TS to be primarily a tic disorder (by DSM-IV criteria alone), the prognosis is quite favorable.

A follow-up study by Erenberg et al. (45) reported on anonymous replies to a questionnaire obtained from 58 patients, aged 15–25 years. Of this group, 26% reported that their tics had almost disappeared, 47% felt that tics had lessened considerably, 14% remained unchanged, and another 14% had become worse. The average age of the respondents was 18 years. There was no correlation in this group between the degree of improvement and maximum severity of tics or responses to therapy. Fifty-five of the 58 patients had originally been treated with medication. Eighty-one percent still under the age of 18 years continued to take medication, whereas only 41% of those over 18 years were still being medicated. It is interesting to note that only 14% of this group felt that their TS had been characterized by motor and vocal tics alone.

A study done on the patients of Bruun (10) focused on tic severity. Of 136 patients who had been followed from 5–15 years, 130 had been on medication. There was a marked improvement overall for these patients. Although 59% were rated as mild to moderate when first evaluated, 91% were so rated after 5–15 years and seven patients had no tics at all. Twenty-eight percent of those who had originally been medicated were off medication. Those who remained on medication were mostly on lower doses than they had originally required.

At the same time, 121 patients were questioned retrospectively about the course of their tics. Fifty-two percent stated that they had spontaneously improved. Thirty-six percent of these first experienced an improvement in their late teenage years. Nine percent did not experience a lessening of tics until their early 20s, and another 5% not until their late 20s or early 30s. Three patients noted relative remissions in their 50s.

Shapiro and Shapiro reported in 1989 that 5–8% of their patients recovered "completely and permanently" during puberty or adolescence. They also reported that tics became less or much less severe in about 35% of patients during adolescence and in most patients when they become adults. The exceptions were a few patients whose early symptoms were mild but became severe in early adulthood (20s or early 30s) (46).

Nee et al., in a retrospective study, found that 40% of 30 adult patients considered their symptoms to be worst during the first decade after onset. Sixty-seven percent of these patients experienced symptomatic relief during the second decade, and improvement continued gradually throughout life except for a period of slight worsening during the fourth decade (47).

Musisi et al. (48) contacted 33 of their patients after a period of 1–15 years (mean of 7 years). The patients ranged in age from 13 to 59 years at the time of follow-up. Ratings were done by the TS global scale, which includes tics and social functioning together (49). It was found that a poor prognosis was associated with birth trauma, mental retardation, obsessive–compulsive features, and attention deficit disorder. A better response to drug therapy (haloperidol or pimozide) was associated with a family history of tics (48).

A demographic study done in North Dakota by Burd et al. (50) also sheds light on the natural history of TS. Questionnaires were sent to all North Dakota pediatricians, psychiatrists, neurologists, family practitioners, mental health centers, psychiatric hospitals, state institutions for the mentally retarded, and the state comprehensive evaluation center. The investigators were able to get information (either by questionnaire or phone contact) from all but two physicians. It was found that the prevalence of TS among North Dakota children (19 years and younger) was 9.3–1.0 per 10,000 (boys and girls, respectively). The prevalence rate among adults, however, was considerably lower: only 0.77 for men and 0.22 for women per 10,000. Projecting from these figures, the investigators estimated that there were approximately 33,000 children and only 8000 adults with TS in the United States.

On the basis of these findings, it can be stated with assurance that the tic symptomatology of TS is ameliorated with age. After a review of the multitude of studies that have been done, a very general conclusion may be drawn that approximately one third of cases will remit completely during late adolescence or early adulthood, another third will show a significant improvement (in both amount and severity) of tics, whereas the remaining third will continue to be symptomatic throughout early adulthood and middle age (12).

Nevertheless, although tics may decline, associated problems may be less predictable. Comings (42) finds that panic attacks, depression, agoraphobia, and alcoholism reach the highest levels at ages 19–20 years, whereas a tendency toward obesity increases steadily with increasing age, particularly in women. Self-injurious behavior has been reported in TS, with an incidence varying from 7% to 40% (10,47). Most commonly, a self-injurious tic will be performed until a certain feeling of satisfaction is obtained. Most documented cases have occurred in the later teenage or adult years.

Antisocial behavior has been documented in TS by many investigators and is one of the behavioral problems often associated with adulthood. The incidence, however, is unclear, and the definitions vary from one study to another. Aggressive behaviors have been reported to be as high as 31% by Robertson et al. (51), 30% by Trimble (40), 21% by Van der Wetering et al. (52), 41% (patient reports) by Erenberg (45), and 42% by Comings and Comings (16). However, exact delineation of these aggressive behaviors is often lacking, and Robertson (13) suggests that there may be an ascertainment bias.

On the other hand, the patients studied by Erenberg et al. (45), although reporting a number of associated difficulties, appeared to have a better prognosis. Of the 58 patients who filled out their follow-up questionnaire, 62% reported learning disabilities and 76% admitted to behavioral problems. These consisted of: problems with concentration (57%), severe mood swings (52%), extreme anxiety (45%), severe temper outbursts (41%), and obessive–compulsive behavior (32%). At the time of follow-up, 19% indicated that learning or behavior problems were no longer interfering with their lives, 50% said that they were interfering to some degree, and 31% felt that these problems were interfering a great deal with their current adjustment. The 49 patients who had both tics and associated symptoms were asked to compare the impact of each on their lives. Forty-five percent felt that their behaviors and/or learning disabilities were more detrimental than their tics (45).

Also on the more optimistic side was a study done by Burd et al who, followed 39 of 54 TS patients from their prevalence study for an average of 13 years. They found that tic severity declined by 59%, global assessment of functioning improved by 50%, and the average number of comorbidities decreased by 42% (53).

GERIATRIC PERIOD

Although the most notable of Dr. Gilles de la Tourette's original nine cases, the Marquise de Dampierre lived to the age of 86 years (or more); there have been few other reports of TS patients in the geriatric age range. The Marquise is said to have been sequestered in her castle until her death due to the socially embarrassing nature of her symptoms. Unfortunately, we do not know if her symptoms had abated to any degree in her later years.

Very few other cases have been reported in people aged 70 years and over. There is a general impression, based mainly on anecdotal reports obtained by one of the authors, that tics and obsessive–compulsive symptoms tend to diminish in old age. In Bruun's TS case records of over 3000 patients, only 15 are 70 years or older and only one of these has symptoms that continue to interfere significantly with life. This is an area that deserves further investigation.

Finally, another way to learn about the natural history of TS is to examine the social and occupational status of adults with TS. Three surveys have been performed to determine various characteristics that may indicate how TS patients, in general, adjust to life (10,43,48). One, the Ohio study, involved a group of 114 adult patients who were members of the Ohio TSA chapter. The other two—by Bruun (10), involving 179 adult patients, and by Musisi et al. (48), involving 33 patients (both adolescents and adults)—were patients under the care of physicians. Musisi et al. found an overall downward shift in social class compared to that of the patients' parents. Thirty-three percent had discontinued school, 30% of the adults required ongoing social support, and 27% were unemployed. In averaging the statistics found in Bruun's group and the Ohio study, we find that: 39% of the adults were never married, 50% were married, and 9% were divorced or separated. Forty-eight percent were employed full time, 9% were employed part time, 29% were unemployed, 2% were retired, and 5% were homemakers. Of the patients who were employed, 32% were in professional, technical, managerial, or executive positions; 31% were in clerical or sales-level positions; 20% were laborers, operatives, service providers, or domestics; 12% were craftsmen or artists; and 6% were students. The Ohio study also surveyed educational status and found that, of the adults: 4% had 0–8 years of schooling, 18% had 9–11 years, 32% were high school graduates, 32% had had some college experience, 2% had graduated from college, 4% had some graduate school experience, and 10% had graduate or professional degrees.

CONCLUSION

In summary, the natural history of TS reveals the complexities of this disorder. At the present time, much of our understanding of this illness stems from the study of more severely symptomatic individuals. This is especially true for adult TS patients. As more studies evaluate milder cases, a more realistic understanding of the evolution and resolution of its diverse symptoms can be gained.

Future research into the interrelationship and biological significance of comorbid conditions will help clarify why some TS patients develop more protracted symptoms and impairment whereas others experience relatively complete remission of symptoms and go on to lead essentially normal lives.

REFERENCES

1. Shapiro AK, Shapiro E, Young JG, Feinberg TE. Gilles de la Tourette Syndrome. 2d ed. New York: Raven Press, 1988:356–360.
2. Frankel M, Cummings JL, Robertson MM, Trimble MR, Hill MA, Benson DF. Obsessions and compulsions in Gilles de la Tourette's syndrome. Neurology 1986; 36:378–382.
3. Freeman RD, Fast DK, Kerbeshian J, Robertson MM, Sandor P. An international perspective on Tourette syndrome: selected findings from 3500 individuals in 22 countries. Dev Med Child Neurol 2000; 42:436–447.
4. Marcus D, Kurlan R. Tics and its disorders. Neurol Clin 2001; 19(3):735–757.
5. Shapiro AK, Shapiro ES, Bruun RD, Sweet RD. Gilles de la Tourette Syndrome: Signs, Symptoms and Clinical Course. New York: Raven Press, 1978:261.
6. Jankovic J. Phenomenology and classification of tics. In: Jankovic J, ed. Neurologic Clinics. Vol. 15. Philadelphia: WB Saunders Company, 1997:267–275. No. 2.
7. Kurlan R. Diagnostic criteria for genetic studies of Tourette's syndrome. Arch Neurol 1997; 54:517–518.
8. Bruun RD, Budman CL. The course and prognosis of Tourette syndrome. In: Jankovic J, ed. Neurologic Clinics. Vol. 15. Philadelphia: WB Saunders Company, 1997:291–298. No. 2.
9. Peterson BS. Considerations of natural history and pathophysiology in the psychopharmacology of Tourette's syndrome. J Clin Psychiatry 1996; 57(suppl 9):24–34.
10. Bruun RD. The natural history of Tourette's syndrome. In: Cohen DJ, Bruun RD, Leckman JF, eds. Tourette's Syndrome and Tic Disorders: Clinical Understanding and Treatment. New York: Wiley, 1998:21–39.
11. Bruun RD, Budman CL. The natural history of Tourette's syndrome. In: Chase TN, Friedhoff AJ, Cohen DJ, eds. Gilles de la Tourette's Syndrome. Advances in Neurology. Vol. 58. New York: Raven Press, 1992:1–6.
12. Singer HS, Walkup JT. Tourette Syndrome and other tic disorders. Medicine 1991; 70(1):15–32.
13. Robertson MM. The Gilles de la Tourette syndrome: the current status. Br J Psychiatry 1989; 154:147–169.
14. Comings DE, Himes JA, Comings BG. An epidemiological study of Tourette's syndrome in a single school district. J Clin Psychiatry 1990; 51:463–469.
15. Kurlan R, Whitmore D, Irvine C, McDermott MP, Como PG. Tourette's syndrome in a special education population: a pilot study involving a single school district. Neurology 1994; 44:699–702.

16. Comings DE, Comings BG. Tourette syndrome: clinical and psychological aspects of 250 cases. Am J Hum Genet 1985; 35:435–450.
17. Park S, Como PG, Cui I, Kurlan R. The early course of the Tourette's syndrome clinical spectrum. Neurology 1993; 43:1712–1715.
18. Kurlan R, Daragjati C, Como PG, McDermott MP, Trinidad KS, Roddy S, Brower CA, Robertson MM. Non-obscene, complex socially inappropriate behavior in Tourette's syndrome. J Neuropsychiatry Clin Neurosci 1996; 8:311–317.
19. Singer HS, Rosenberg LA. Development of behavioral and emotional problems in Tourette syndrome. Pediatr Neurol 1989; 5:41–44.
20. Singer HS, Schuerholz LJ, Denkla MB. Learning difficulties in children with Tourette syndrome. J Child Neurol 1995; 10:858–861.
21. Erenberg G, Cruse RP, Rothner AD. Gilles de la Tourette's syndrome: effects of stimulant drugs. Neurology 1985; 35:1346–1348.
22. Gadow KD, Sverd J, Sprafkin J, Nolan EE, Ezor SN. Efficacy of methylphenidate for attention-deficit hyperactivity disorder in children with tic disorder. Arch Gen Psychiatry 1995; 52:444–445.
23. Peterson BS, Leckman JF, Lombroso P, Zhang H, Lynch K, Carter A, Pauls D, Cohen DJ. Environmental risk and protective factors. Tourette's Syndrome—Tics, Obsessions, Compulsions: Developmental Psychopathology and Clinical Care. New York: John Wiley and Sons, Inc., 1999:213–229.
24. Freeman RD. Attention deficit hyperactivity disorder in the presence of Tourette syndrome. In: Jankovic J, ed. Neurologic Clinics. Vol. 15. Philadelphia: WB Saunders Company, 1997:411–420. No. 2.
25. Kurlan R. Treatment of ADHD in children with tics: a randomized controlled trial. Neurology 2002; 4:527–536.
26. Incagnoli T, Kane R. Neuropsychological functioning in Tourette Syndrome. In: Friedhoff AJ, Chase TN, eds. Gilles de la Tourette Syndrome. New York: Raven Press, 1982:305–309.
27. Hagin RA, Beecher R, Pagano G, Kreeger H. Effects of Tourette Syndrome on learning. In: Friedhoff AJ, Chase TN, eds. Gilles de la Tourette Syndrome. New York: Raven Press, 1982:323–328.
28. Hagin RA, Kugler J. School problems associated with Tourette's syndrome. In: Cohen DJ, Bruun RD, Leckman JF, eds. Tourette's Syndrome and Tic Disorders. New York: Wiley, 1988:223–236.
29. Erenberg G, Cruse RP, Rothner AD. Tourette syndrome: an analysis of 200 pediatric and adolescent cases. Clevel Clin Q 1986; 53:127–131.
30. Alsobrook JP, Pauls DL. A factor analysis of tic symptoms in Gilles de la Tourette's syndrome. Am J Psychiatry 2002; 159:196–291.
31. Grad LR, Pelcovitz D, Olson M. Obsessive–compulsive symptomatology in children with Tourette's syndrome. Am Acad Child Adolesc Psychiatry 1987; 26:69–72.
32. Singer HS, Allan R, Brown J, Salam M, Hahn IH. Sleep disorders in Tourette Syndrome: a primary of unrelated problems? [Abstract]. Ann Neurol 1990; 28:424.

33. Barabas G, Mathew WS, Ferrari M. Somnambulism in children with treatments in children with Tourette's Disorder. Dev Med Child Neurol 1984; 26:457–460.
34. Kadesjo B, Gillberg C. Tourette's disorder: epidemiology and comorbidity in primary school children. J Am Child Adolesc Psychiatry 2000; 5:548–555.
35. Singer HS. Current issues in Tourette syndrome. Mov Disord 2000; 15:1051–1063.
36. Coffey BJ, Biederman J, Smoller J, Geller DA, Sarin P, Schwartz S, Kim GS. Anxiety disorders and tic severity in juveniles with Tourette's disorder. J Am Child Adolesc Psychiatry 2000; 39:562–568.
37. Budman CL, Bruun RD, Park KS, Lesser M, Olson M. Explosive outbursts in children with Tourette's disorder. J Am Acad Child Adolesc Psychiatry 2000; 39:1270–1276.
38. Bruun RD. Subtle and underrecognized side effects of neuroleptic treatments in children with Tourette's Disorder. Am J Psychiatry 1988; 145:621–624.
39. Kompoliti K, Goetz CG, Leurgans S, Raman R, Comella CL. Estrogen, progesterone, and tic severity in women with Gilles de la Tourette syndrome. Neurology 2001; 57:1519.
40. Trimble M. Psychopathology and movement disorders: a new perspective on the Gilles de la Tourette syndrome. J Neurol Neurosurg Psychiatry 1989; Suppl: 90–95.
41. Comings DE, Comings BG. A controlled study of Tourette syndrome, I–VII. Am J Genet 1987; 41:701–866.
42. Comings DE. Conduct. Tourette Syndrome and Human Behavior. Duarte, CA: Hope Press, 1990:131–149.
43. Stefl ME. The Ohio Study: Initial Report of Data Prepared for the Tourette Syndrome Association.
44. Bornstein RA, Stefl ME, Hammond L. A Survey of Tourette Syndrome Patients and Their Families: The 1987 Ohio Tourette Survey, A Report Written for the Tourette Syndrome Association.
45. Erenberg G, Cruse RP, Rothner AD. The natural history of Tourette Syndrome: a follow-up study. Ann Neurol 1987; 22(3):383–385.
46. Shapiro ES, Shapiro AK. Gilles de la Tourette Syndrome and tic disorders. Harv Med Sch Mental Health Lett 1989; 5(11).
47. Nee LE, Caine ED, Plursky RJ, Eldridge R, Ebert MH. Gilles de la Tourette's syndrome. Clinical and family study of 50 cases. Ann Neurol 1980; 7: 41–49.
48. Musisi S, Sandor P, Lang A, Moldofsky H. Gilles de la Tourette's Syndrome: a follow-up study. J Clin Psychopharmacol 1990; 3:197–199.
49. Harcherik DF, Leckman JF, Detlor J, Cohen DJ. A new instrument for clinical studies of Tourette's Syndrome. J Am Acad Child Psychiatry 1984; 23:153–160.
50. Burd L, Kerbeshian J, Wilkenheiser M, Fisher W. Prevalence of Gilles de la Tourette Syndrome in North Dakota adults. Am J Psychiatry 1986; 143:787–788.
51. Robertson M, Trimble MR, Lees AJ. The psychopathology of the Gilles de la

Tourette Syndrome: a phenomenological analysis. Br J Psychiatry 1988; 152:383–390.
52. Van der Wetering BJ, Cohen AP, Minderaa RB, et al. Het Syndroom van Gilles de la Tourette: Klinische Bevindingen. Nederlands Tijdschrijte voor Geneeskunde 1988; 132:21–25.
53. Burd L, Kerbeshian J, Klug MG, Barth A, Avery PK, Benz B. Long-term follow-up of an epidemiologically defined cohort of patients with Tourette syndrome. J Child Neurol 2001; 16:431–437.

4

Obsessive-Compulsive Disorder and Self-Injurious Behavior

Valsamma Eapen
UAE University
United Arab Emirates
and University College London Medical School
London, England

Jessica W. Yakeley
Maudsley Hospital
London, England

Mary May Robertson
The National Hospital for Neurology and Neurosurgery
and University College London Medical School
London, England

INTRODUCTION

In this chapter, we discuss obsessive-compulsive disorder (OCD), self-injurious behavior (SIB), and their relationships to Gilles de la Tourette's syndrome (TS). We begin with a historical perspective and then consider each of the behaviors separately.

The first clear description of TS in the scientific literature was in 1825, when Itard (1) reported the case of the Marquise de Dampierre, who developed symptoms of TS at the age of 7 and who, because of the socially unacceptable nature of her vocalizations, was compelled to live as a recluse until she died at the age of 85.

A convincing case has been made that the 18th-century literary figure, the worthy Dr. Samuel Johnson, suffered from TS (2,3). Miss Lucy Porter told Boswell (4) that when Dr. Johnson was introduced to her mother, "his appearance was very forbidding... he often had, seemingly, convulsive starts and odd gesticulations, which tended at once surprise and ridicule." He apparently had a wide repertoire of such motor tics as mouth opening, lip pursing, squinting, and perpetual convulsive movements of the hands and feet. He had several vocalizations, including "ejaculations of the Lord's prayer," whistling sounds, and sounds like the clucking of a hen and a whale exhaling (2–4). Dr. Johnson also exhibited echolalia and mild SIB in that he used to hit and rub his legs and cut his fingernails too deeply. It has also been suggested that he suffered from severe OCD: he felt impelled to measure his footsteps, perform complex gestures when he crossed a threshold, and involuntarily touch specific objects (3).

OBSESSIVE-COMPULSIVE DISORDER

Obsessive-compulsive disorder is characterized by recurrent obsessions or compulsions that are sufficiently severe to 1) cause marked distress, 2) be time-consuming (more than an hour a day), or 3) significantly interfere with the person's normal routine, functioning, social activities, or relationships (5). Obsessions are recurrent ideas, thoughts, images, or impulses that enter the mind and are persistent, intrusive, and unwelcome. Attempts are made to ignore or suppress these thoughts or to neutralize them with some other thoughts or actions. The person recognizes them to be a product of his/her own mind. Compulsions are repetitive, purposeful behaviors performed in response to an obsession and are designed to neutralize or prevent discomfort or some dreaded event or situation. However, the activity is excessive or not connected realistically to what it is designed to prevent, and the person recognizes that his/her behavior is unreasonable. Evidence that OCD and TS are related can be argued from several perspectives.

Historical Evidence

As said above, the first description of TS was in 1825 by Itard (1). Many years later, Charcot saw this same patient, and his observations were published in 1885 by his student, Gilles de la Tourette (6), in a paper describing a total of nine cases of the syndrome later to be named after him. In his account of the case of the Marquise, Gilles de la Tourette described obsessive thoughts that tormented her (7), as well as her tics and vocalizations. Charcot, however, was the first neurologist to identify involuntary "impulsive" ideas, such as doubting mania, double checking, touching, and arithmomania (counting rituals or an obsession with numbers), as part of the disorder and to link these to the impulsive movements or tics (8). Some of these "impulsions" would now be classified as compulsions (modern definitions specify that execution of an impulsive deed gives the patient some form of pleasure, satisfaction, or excitement, whereas the patient derives only relief from tension by carrying out the compulsive activity; that is, impulsive acts are ego-syntonic, whereas compulsive acts are ego-dystonic) (9).

Following Charcot and Gilles de la Tourette, many other 19th-century neurologists became interested in the relationship between these psychological aspects of the disease and its motor manifestations. In 1899, Gilles de la Tourette (10) noted the anxieties and phobias of his patients and acknowledged the ideas of Guinon (11), who suggested that *tiqueurs* nearly always had associated psychiatric disorders characterized by multiple phobias and agoraphobia. Grasset (12) also referred to the obsessions and phobias of patients, which were to him an accompaniment of the tic disorder, representing psychical tics. Robertson and Reinstein (13) translated, for the first time, these writings of Gilles de la Tourette, Guinon, and Grasset, illustrating how these early clinicians documented the psychopathology of people with "convulsive tic disorder" with particular reference to OCD, including checking rituals, arithmomania, *folie du doute*, *delire de toucher* (forced touching), *folie du pourquoi* (see below), and a "mania" for order.

Meige and Feindel (14), in "Tics and Their Treatment," described a patient "O," who was 54 years old and whom they consider to be the prototype of a tic patient. In retrospect, it is clear that this patient had TS. He had motor tics which began at the age of 11 years, echophenomena (copying behaviors), a "tic of phonation dating back to his 15th year," and "an impulse to use slang." In addition, he was impulsive and had suicidal tendencies and obsessive-compulsive behaviors (OCB). Meige and Feindel (14, pp. 82–83) later state: "The frequency with which obsessions, or at least a proclivity for them, and tics are associated cannot be a simple coincidence. Without defining the word obsession, let us be content to recall the excellent classification given by Regis, according to whom they mark a flaw in voluntary power, either of inhibition or of action. On the one hand we have *impulsive obsessions*, subdivided into obsessions of indecisions, such as ordinary *folie du doute*; of fear such as agoraphobia, of propensity such as those of suicide or homicide... In all these varieties of obsession, increase or diminution of volitional activity is undesirable... the physical stigmata of obsessional patients, if compared to the mental Equipment of the sufferer from tic, we cannot but notice intimate Analogies between the two, analogies corroborated by a glance at their symptomatology." They describe case histories of patients with typical features of OCD, including the relief of anxiety that accompanied the carrying out of a particular motor act. However, in addition to the close link between the motor movement and a compulsion, they noted that often, there was no direct connection between a patient's obsessions and the tics, the former occurring in the form of extraordinary scrupulousness, phobias, and excessive punctiliousness in their actions. They specifically mentioned arithmomania, onomatomania (the dread of uttering a forbidden word or the impulse to intercollate another), and *folie du pourquoi*, which is the irresistible habit of seeking explanations for the most commonplace, insignificant facts by perpetually asking questions.

In 1927, Wilson (15) also acknowledged a relationship between tics and OCD: "No feature is more prominent in tics than its irresistibility... The element of compulsion links the condition intimately to the vast group of obsessions and fixed ideas." Ascher (16) noted that all five of the TS patients he reported had obsessive personalities, while Bockner (17) commented that the majority of TS cases described in the literature had obsessive-compulsive (OC) neurosis. In summary, the relationship between TS and OCB/OCD has been documented since the 1800s and the first patient described (the Marquise de Dampierre) had significant OCB. Throughout the rest of the 19th and early 20th century, the relationship between OCB and TS continued to be documented with excellent clinical descriptions of individual cases.

Epidemiological Evidence

These historical speculations were based mainly on anecdotal descriptions of single case studies, and it was not until much later that larger groups of patients were extensively studied to reveal a more definite association between OC symptomatology and TS. Shapiro et al. (8) divide the history of TS into seven periods, starting in 1825. The increasing interest in psychological theories after 1900 resulted in the diverse and often confusing psychoanalytic explanations that dominated the second quarter of this century, the third period. The fourth period, called "Epidemiology and Reviews," began in 1954 with the retrospective studies of Zausmer (18), but it was not until 1962 that an observed frequency of obsessional symptoms, traits, or illness in a population of TS patients was recorded (19). Torup (19), in a study of 237 children treated for tics between 1946 and 1947 in Denmark, judged 12% to have a compulsive behavior pattern. Since then, many epidemiological studies have revealed significant percentages of such patient populations experiencing some form of OC phenomena, and these reported rates have, in general, tended to increase in recent years. Thus Kelman (20) in 1965, Fernando (21) in 1967, and Corbett et al. (22) in 1969 reported figures of 11%, 31%, and 12.5% in their studies, respectively. By the 1970s and 1980s, however, some researchers recorded rates reaching far higher figures: 32% (23), 33% (24), 38% (25), and as high as 60% (26), 66% (27), 68% (28), 71% (29), 74% (30), and as high as 80% (31). The earlier lower figures may have resulted from the use of less specific measures to assess OCD, differences in the definition of OCD, or an unusually high frequency of OCD in the control studies (8).

It should be borne in mind that Shapiro et al. (32–34), on the other hand, have consistently failed to observe an association between TS and any specific psychiatric syndrome or psychodynamic factors. In a controlled study using the Minnesota Multiphasic Personality Inventory (MMPI), a group of TS patients did not differ significantly from general psychiatric outpatients on factors such as overt and underlying psychosis, OC traits, inhibition of hostility, hysteria, and general maladjustment (8). They found OC traits in 12.8% of TS patients and in 14.6% of controls (8). They did, however, acknowledge that only one patient of 34 was free from psychiatric illness, the majority being diagnosed as having various types of "personality disorders." They also pointed out that there may be a subgroup of TS patients who has a great deal of difficulty with OC rituals (8).

Problems with case definitions of OCD and its differentiation from other psychiatric diagnoses, especially anxiety disorders and depression, which share similar features, have hampered attempts to accurately determine the prevalence of OCD in the general population, which is necessary for interpretation of the rates of OCD observed in TS patients. Like these figures, the reported prevalence rates of OCD in the general population have risen over the years. The early community surveys were unreliable, and in 1942, Roth and Luton (35) found a prevalence of OCD of only 0.3% in a Tennessee community. More recent community surveys are much more sophisticated. They comprise two types of interview schedules: the Present State Examination (PSE) studies and the stringent Diagnostic Interview Survey (DIS) Epidemiologic Catchment Area (ECA) studies (36). It has been suggested that the PSE is not the ideal instrument for the identification of OCD in the community (36), and indeed, only one PSE study has identified a case of OCD (37). The consensus from DIS ECA studies is that the lifetime prevalence of OCD ranges from 1.9% to 3.2% (38–48). Only one study from Taiwan yielded lower figures, possibly owing to different methods of analysis (49).

It therefore seems clear that the prevalence of OCD in patients with TS is much greater than would be expected by chance alone. It is of added interest that since 1987, the diagnoses of OCD and TS are no longer mutually exclusive according to accepted diagnostic conventions. In its definition of OCD, DSM-III stated that the obsessions or compulsions must not be due to another mental disorder, such as TS, schizophrenia, major depression, or organic mental disorder (50), whereas the current DSM-IV states that in some people with TS, an associated diagnosis is OCD (5).

In the late 1980s, investigators started to use specially designed inventories to assess the incidence of OCD among TS patients and normal controls

(51). Frankel et al. (52) used a questionnaire derived from the Leyton Obsessional Inventory (LOI) in their controlled study of British and American patients with TS, American patients with OCD, and normal control American subjects and found that 47% of males and 86% of females in the TS group of 16 patients met diagnostic criteria for OCD. Caine et al. (53) used a questionnaire developed by Carey and reported that 49% of the 41 patients in their epidemiological study of Monroe County schoolchildren had obsessional ideas or associated ritualistic motor behavior, although only 3 were significantly impaired to warrant a diagnosis of OCD. However, this study was limited in that it included only children. Van de Wetering et al. (54), in a controlled study, used a Dutch version of the LOI on their cohort of 66 Dutch TS patients and found that 47% admitted to obsessive rituals, 18% to obsessive thoughts, and 4% to obsessive imaging. Robertson et al. (55) used both the LOI and the Crown Crisp Experiential Index/Middlesex Hospital Questionnaire (CCEI) Obsessional Scale and found that 37% of their group of 90 TS patients in the United Kingdom reported OCB. In this study, coprolalia and echophenomena were significantly associated with OC phenomena. Robertson and Gourdie (56) interviewed 85 members of a multiply affected TS family. Fifty were diagnosed as TS cases, with four members having only OCB. Distinction between cases and noncases could be made on the basis of OC features and the trait score of the Leyton Obsessional Inventory (LOI). Furthermore, four Arab TS cases were described by Robertson and Trimble (57), where all four had OCB. In a New Zealand cohort of 40 TS cases, 20 of whom were evaluated in detail, half of the cases were found to have OCB (58). Pauls et al. (59) also reported that OCB occurs in approximately 40% of TS cases.

In this context, only a few studies have included control groups. Fifty-two percent of TS patients in one study were found to have OCB as compared to 12.2% of the controls (52) and, in another study, 45% of TS patients compared to 8.5% of controls (60). In yet another controlled study, TS patients were found to be disproportionately obsessional, which was not accounted for by depression (61). Similarly, Robertson et al. (62) found that TS patients have significantly more obsessionality than controls. Given that the population prevalence of OCD is between 1% and 3%, the prevalence of OCD in TS patients seems to be much greater than that is expected by chance. Zohar et al. (63) in an epidemiologic sample of 861 Israeli adolescents found 40 individuals with OC spectrum disorders. However, the use of different questionnaires/scales in these studies, as well as the varying sample sizes and cultural differences, may account for the diversity of figures obtained. In this regard, it is interesting to note that in a recently established multisite international database of 3500 individuals with TS from 22 countries, 27% and 32% were found to have comorbid OCD and OCB, respectively (64).

Other studies have examined the occurrence of tics and other associated features of TS such as coprolalia, echophenomena, and attention-deficit disorder (ADD) in primary OCD patients. Rasmussen and Tsuang (65) reported a prevalence of 5% of TS in OCD patients. Pitman et al. (66), in their study of 16 TS outpatients, 16 OCD outpatients, and 16 normal controls, reported that 6 patients (37%) of the OCD group met criteria for any tic disorder (only one patient met criteria specifically for TS) compared to only 1 subject in their control group, whereas 10 patients (63%) in the TS group met criteria for OCD. These figures would suggest that while OCD might now be considered an integral part of TS, the majority of OCD subjects do not suffer from a tic disorder and may represent a separate etiological group. In a review article, Rapoport (67) suggests that some 20% of OCD patients have tics.

In summary, the population prevalence of OCD is between 1% and 3%, whereas the prevalence of OCB/OCD in TS patients is much higher with rates of OCD in studies of TS patients ranging from around 11% to 80%. In addition, in several controlled investigations, cohorts of patients with TS have been shown to be significantly more obsessional than normal controls.

Phenomenological Evidence

The area of phenomenological evidence has not been as extensively explored to date, although several recent studies have attempted to define the precise phenomenology of the OC thoughts and behaviors that occur in TS patients, to relate these to other variables, and to compare them to the symptomatology that occurs in OCD patients without a tic disorder. A comprehensive study by Pitman et al. (66) reported that certain kinds of compulsive behaviors, such as touching and symmetry behaviors ("evening-up" rituals to ensure that the body was symmetrical or balanced), occurred more often in the TS patients than in the OCD group, although some TS patients exhibited the more common compulsions such as checking, washing, and counting. Similarly, the types of tics occurring in OCD patients suffering from a tic disorder were not unlike those commonly experienced by TS patients, including blinking and making noises such as humming, sniffing, and throat clearing. The authors noted other psychopathological phenomena that occurred at much higher rates in both the TS and OCD groups than in the control sample, such as pathological doubt, slowness, and depersonalization. Both groups also shared high rates of unipolar depressive illness and generalized anxiety disorder compared to the controls. These results led the authors to propose "the notion of a symptomatic continuum from simple tic to complex tic to compulsion." However, despite this large symptomatic overlap, the two conditions were by no means phenomenologically identical. Echo phenomena, history of ADD, and SIB occurred frequently in TS but not OCD patients, whereas phobic and panic disorders were much more common in the OCD patients (66).

Frankel et al. (52) also revealed considerable overlap in the type of OC symptoms experienced by TS and non-TS OCD patients, including checking and fear of contamination. They also noted that such symptomatology changed with age in the TS patients, with the younger patients exhibiting compulsive behavior related to impulse control and the older patients manifesting behaviors more classically associated with OCD, such as checking, arranging, and fear of contamination (52).

Montgomery et al. (27) suggested that the frequency of OC symptoms increases with the duration of TS. However, Robertson et al. (55) could not demonstrate a significant relationship of such symptoms to either age or duration of TS.

Coprolalia, which is one of the most distressing symptoms that can occur in TS, has rarely been described in OCD patients. However, Pitman and Jenike (68) presented a single case history of a man fulfilling DSM-III-R criteria for an OCD diagnosis who had manifested coprolalia since the age of 6, but did not otherwise satisfy criteria for a diagnosis of TS. The authors emphasized that this case further blurred the phenomenological distinction between the two disorders and remind us that Janet (69) and Meige and Feindel (14) also observed an association between coprolalia and obsessions almost a century ago. Meige and Feindel stated (14, p. 220): "And though the ejaculation be not audible, the first degree of coprolalia consists in the mental presentation of the objectionable phrase. Among those who suffer from obsessions, mental coprolalia is far from uncommon. A patient with Folie du doute, mentioned by Seglas, was afraid to pronounce indelicate words because he felt himself articulating them mentally, and sometimes he used to ask whether they had not really escaped him. One step more and these verbal hallucinations assume the characteristics of a genuine tic."

Others, including Nee et al. (28) and Cummings and Frankel (70), have also observed that TS and OCD share clinical features such as waxing and waning of symptoms, early age of onset, lifelong course, ego-dystonic behavior, worsening with depression and anxiety, and, in particular, their occurrence in the same families. However, despite some overlap in clinical features, available evidence suggests that the two conditions are not phenomenologically identical and that OCD may well be a heterogeneous entity, with one subtype related to TS (71).

Muller et al. (72) found that nearly 80% of the patients could be correctly classified as having TS or primary OCD diagnosis based on two items of the Hamburg obsessive-compulsive inventory, namely, "fearful obsessive thoughts" found in 90% of OCD patients and echophenomenon present in

56% of TS patients. Differences between OCD and TS patients were evident on the Maudsley Obsessive Compulsive Inventory (MOCI) subscales "checking" and "slowness/repetition" as well as on the total scores. While TS patients scored higher than controls, they reported fewer symptoms when compared to OCD patients.

Santangelo et al. (73) studied the role of gender and comorbid OCD on the phenomenology of TS. They reported that probands with OCD were more likely than those without OCD to onset with complex tics, and that females onset with compulsive tics more often than males. In a study of TS children and adolescents with TS, de Groot et al. (74) observed that presence of comorbid obsessions contributed to the prediction of learning problems, perfectionism, and antisocial behavior, while compulsions contributed to the prediction of hyperactivity, psychosomatic symptoms, and muscular tension.

However, nonobscene complex socially inappropriate behaviors (NOSI) occurring in TS were not found to be associated with obsessions or compulsions (75). George et al. (76) compared 10 OCD patients to 15 TS patients with comorbid OCD. It was found that more violent, sexual, and symmetrical obsessions as well as forced touching, counting, and self-damaging compulsions were more common in comorbid OCD/TS subjects. On the other hand, obsessions concerning dirt or germs and cleaning compulsions were more commonly encountered in OCD subjects. Furthermore, the TS group reported that the compulsions occurred spontaneously or de novo, while in the OCD group, this was preceded by guilt or worry. Iida et al. (77) compared TS patients with and without OCB and found that in contrast to OCB-free TS patients, TS + OCB patients had a higher incidence of volatile temper, compulsive tics, perinatal disorders, and brain-wave changes, as well as a higher prevalence of developmental disorders and a higher severity of TS. They suggested that TS + OCB may be more strongly associated with organic cerebral disorders.

Holzer et al. (78) reported that patients with a history of tic disorder had significantly more touching, repeating, self-damaging, counting, and ordering compulsions. Similarly, in an epidemiological study of OCD, Zohar et al. (63) reported that OCD subjects with tics had significantly more touching, ordering, repeating, counting, violent, sexual, and aggressive behaviors. Eapen et al. (71) compared the distribution of OC symptoms in 16 patients with OCD and 16 patients with TS and associated OCB. Among the obsessional symptoms, sexual and violent themes were more common in the TS group, while concern about contamination and fear of something going wrong or bad happening was more common among OCD group. With regard to compulsions, symmetry/evening-up behaviors, saying or doing things "just right," and forced touching were more prevalent in the TS group, while washing and cleaning were more common in the OCD group. Sex of the proband did not account for any of these differences. Cath et al. (79) in a recent study compared the symptomatology in TS + OCD, TS−OCD, OCD-tic, and control subjects. They found that specific nonanxiety-related impulsions discriminate between TS and OCD-tic individuals. Petter et al. (80) found that TS patients with comorbid OCD were significantly more likely to report obsessions involving nonviolent images, need for symmetry and excessive concern with appearance, and compulsions such as touching, blinking or staring, and counting. The authors suggested that the differences in symptomatology between TS and primary OCD may be linked to putative differences in pathophysiology.

Rasmussen and Eisen (81) reported two subtypes of OCD: one associated with abnormal risk assessment, high levels of anxiety, and pathologic doubt involving worry that something terrible might happen which may be relieved by checking and washing compulsions, and the other type associated with incompleteness and sense of imperfection that is relieved when a compulsion is performed "just right." The latter was often associated with tics, TS, onychophagia, and trichotillomania. McElroy et al. (82) proposed that all these conditions belong to a family of OCD spectrum disorders with the TS subtype having predominantly impulsive features.

However, a problem inherent in this approach of comparing OCD patients with or without tic disorder is the disagreement as to whether certain symptoms should be classified as compulsions or complex motor tics (83). Furthermore, Leckman et al. (84) found considerable overlap between TS and OCD symptoms in that 93% of their 135 subjects with a tic disorder reported experiencing premonitory urges before performing tics. Thus it seems that the common distinction based on the involuntary nature of tics as compared to OC symptoms is not entirely valid. Miguel et al. (85) reported that intentional repetitive behaviors in OCD differ from those in TS in that the former is preceded by cognitive phenomena and autonomic anxiety and the latter by sensory phenomena. In another study by the same investigators, it was found that like the TS group, the OCD + TS group reported more sensory phenomena and fewer cognitions than the OCD group (86).

In a factor analysis of symptom subtypes, Baer (87) found three factors—"symmetry/hoarding," "contamination/cleaning," and "pure obsessions"—of which only the first was associated with a lifetime history of tics or TS. In a cluster analysis of OC symptoms, Eapen et al. (71) found that the "TS cluster" was characterized by fear of harming self/others, obsessions with violent/aggressive themes, symmetry/evening-up, saying/doing things "just right," forced touching, and arranging, while the "OCD cluster" was characterized by obsessions about dirt, germs, and contamination as well as the need to tell/ask/know, fear of something bad happening, need to be neat and clean, and excessive washing and cleaning. In addition to such differences in the symptom profile, both research and clinical experience suggest that the OCB occurring in the context of TS is rather ego-syntonic causing less distress to the patients and is often associated with lesser levels of anxiety.

In summary, it does appear that there are significant differences between the OCB encountered in TS and OCD patients. However, some degree of overlap makes the absolute distinction and separation difficult. In general, the OCB in TS is ego-syntonic, while the symptoms in OCD are ego-dystonic.

Evidence from Family and Genetic Studies

If it has not yet been possible to demonstrate the biochemistry of an abnormal gene product in a disease of uncertain etiology, four other main types of study may be carried out to obtain evidence to suggest that genetic factors are involved. These are twin studies, family studies, adoption studies, and genetic linkage studies.

In 1964, Ellison (88) reported a 64-year-old twin with TS whose supposedly identical co-twin was discordant. However, the methods for determining zygosity in this case were questioned (8). In the TS twin study of Jenkins and Ashby (89), both twins were described as obsessional. Another triplet study in which the triplets were reared apart showed 100% concordance for TS but not OCD (90). In a comprehensive twin study by Price et al. (91), involving 43 pairs of same-sex twins in which at least one co-twin had TS, the authors found concordance rates of 53% for monozygotic pairs and 8% for dizygotic pairs. These rates rose to 77% and 23%, respectively, when the diagnostic criteria were widened to include any tics. Although the higher concordance rates for the monozygotic twins would suggest that genetic factors are involved in the etiology of TS, it was concluded that environmental factors must also be responsible for the expression of the disease, given that the concordance rates for the identical twins did not approach unity. Reexamination of the data revealed that each unaffected co-twin of all the discordant pairs had a higher birth weight than the affected twin. This led the authors to suggest that some prenatal nongenetic factors may be important in the development of TS. Furthermore, Wolf et al. (92) in a twin study reported considerable phenotypic variability even within monozygotic twin pairs.

Having established that TS was an inherited disorder (93), researchers went on to look for a genetic relationship between TS and OCD in several family studies. As part of a much larger family study of TS, Pauls et al. (94) interviewed 90% of all first-degree relatives (FDRs) of 32 TS probands, as well as compiling family history reports about each family member from all available data obtained. While the authors acknowledge the difficulties in making an accurate diagnosis of OCD, they found the frequency of OCD diagnoses among these first-degree relatives to be significantly higher (9–13 times) than the frequency of OCD estimated in the general population from the ECA study in which similar methodology was employed (39). Furthermore, the rates of TS and OCD in families of TS probands with OCD were virtually the same as in the families of TS probands without OCD. In addition, the frequency of OCD without TS among FDRs was significantly elevated, particularly among the female relatives, in both groups of families. Subsequent segregation analysis performed on these results gave further support to the autosomal dominant model for TS, but also indicated that, in at least a proportion of cases, TS and OCD constitute alternate expressions of the same gene, and that this expression may be sex-specific (95).

This evidence indicating that TS and OCD share a genetic etiology prompted the researchers to continue examining the evidence for a genetic basis for OCD alone (96). Family studies have also shown that OCD is significantly greater among first-degree relatives of patients with OCD than in the general population.

Two studies (97,98) that directly interviewed all first-degree relatives found the rates of OCD in the parents to be 15–20% and 17%, respectively, which were significantly greater than those obtained in the ECA study (39). Lenane et al. (98) personally interviewed, in a structured interview, 145 first-degree relatives of 46 children and adolescents with severe primary OCD who were consecutively referred to an NIMH study. They found that 30% of probands had at least one first-degree relative with OCD, a rate higher than that expected from a general population and than that found in parents with conduct-disordered patients. This rate is consistent with a genetic factor in OCD. Presenting OC symptoms of probands and their parents were usually dissimilar, arguing against any simple social or cultural transmission. Although all families in the study were asked about the presence of TS symptoms in the 147 FDRs, there were only 3 acknowledged suspicious cases. None of those was formally evaluated to make a definite diagnosis. Of the 18 families who were specifically questioned about the presence of tics at any time in their lives, 44% had a positive family history of tics in at least one first-, second-, or third-degree relative (98). Furthermore, the early-onset OCD is suggested to be more etiologically homogenous, with higher rates of OCD in the relatives (99).

When compared to population prevalence estimates, several family studies have reported significantly higher rates of OCD in parents and siblings of OCD probands, with rates among parents being 5–10 times higher (100). Two family studies have found remarkably similar risk rates in FDRs of young OCD probands. Lenane et al. (101), in a study of 145 FDRs of 46 children and adolescents with OCD, reported an age-corrected morbid risk of 35% in FDRs, when subclinical OCD was included. Similarly, Riddle et al.

(102) examined families of 21 children and adolescents with OCD and found that 35.7% of parents received a diagnosis of clinical or subclinical OCD. Bellodi et al. (103), on the other hand, studied 92 adult OCD probands and found that the rate of OCD among FDRs was only 3.4%. However, when probands were separated into two groups based on whether the age of onset was before or after 14 years, it was noted that the morbid risk for OCD among relatives of the early onset probands was 8.8% compared to 3.4% among the relatives of probands with a later age of onset.

Although Pauls et al. (104) and Black et al. (105) did not find an increased incidence of tic disorders among adult OCD patients, several other investigators have suggested that childhood onset OCD may be different from adult onset OCD and that the childhood onset subtype may be more closely related to TS (102,106,107).

Cavallini et al. (108), in a segregation analysis study of OCD families, suggested a dominant model of transmission. When the phenotype was widened to include TS and chronic motor tics, an unrestricted model of transmission became the best fit, and they proposed that the OCD phenotype probably presents a higher level of heterogeneity than the TS phenotype. Furthermore, the clinical and phenotypic heterogeneity may be linked to genetic heterogeneity, with some individuals having inherited the "TS + OCD genotype" and the others the "classic OCD genotype." Eapen et al. (71) in a family study of OCD probands and TS + OCD probands found that all the OCD probands who shared a similar symptom profile to that of TS probands had at least one first-degree relative with OCD, while none of the OCD probands with classic OCD symptoms had a positive family history. These authors concluded that the latter could be regarded as sporadic or nonfamilial cases. These observations may be consistent with genetic heterogeneity within both OCD and TS. In this regard, it is interesting to note that Lichter et al. (109) reported that OCB is less prominent in sporadic than in familial TS, perhaps reflecting a more restricted pathophysiology in this subgroup. These investigators also found that although bilineal transmission of tics is relatively infrequent in consecutive TS pedigrees, co-transmission of OCB from an otherwise unaffected parent is common and significantly influences the development of OCB and self-injurious behaviors, but not tics, in the offspring.

In summary, both twin and family studies strongly suggest that a genetic relationship exists between TS and OCB (110) and that, in some cases, OCB may be an alternative expression of the putative TS gene(s) (111–113). However, not all cases of OCD are associated with TS (59). The findings from both the genetic studies and the phenomenological data described before suggest that OCD can be divided into at least three categories: 1) sporadic (no family history), 2) familial (positive family history), and 3) OCD associated with a family history of tics or TS (59). This challenges traditional assumptions of etiological homogeneity in OCD.

Neurochemical and Neuroanatomical Evidence

The evidence presented so far would suggest that TS and OCD share a common neurochemical and neuroanatomical basis. In TS patients, no gross neuropathological lesions have been recognized, but there is some evidence to suggest that the condition is due to dysfunction of dopaminergic transmission in the basal ganglia or limbic system (114,115). This comes mainly from the observation that haloperidol and other neuroleptic drugs that block dopamine receptors reduce the frequency and intensity of tics and vocalizations in TS patients, whereas catecholamine stimulant drugs have the opposite effect. In addition, the absence of premovement potentials prior to the tics indicates that these movements are subcortical in origin (116). Furthermore, recent evidence suggests that there are similarities and differences between the findings for TS and OCD with regard to event-related brain potentials (ERPs) (117). In this study, behavioral parameters and lateralized readiness potential (LRP) confirmed that both groups were well able to initiate motor responses in that both "Go" and "Stop" stimuli elicited an enhanced frontal negative activity in both groups, but in addition, "Stop" stimuli were associated with a frontal shift of the NoGo-Anteriorization (NGA) in the TS group but not in the OCD group.

Since the late 1980s, neuroimaging studies using positron-emission tomography and single photon emission tomography have suggested that the frontal areas and basal ganglia are implicated in the pathogenesis of TS (118–120). Since then, a number of studies have implicated the role of frontostriatal pathways in the pathophysiology of TS (see Ref. 121). Furthermore, a dysfunction in the cortico-striatal-thalamo-cortical pathways (CSTC) circuitry has been implicated not only in TS, but also in OCD (see Ref. 122). There is growing evidence about the role of multiple parallel neuronal circuits involving cortex, basal ganglia, and thalamus in the pathophysiology of TS and OCB (123), and that a failure of inhibition in these circuits may be the cause of inappropriate release of fixed action patterns and OCB (124). It has been proposed that the above-mentioned basal ganglia cortical circuits may be "hyperactive in OCD" as evidenced by the hyperperfusion and increased metabolic changes in the orbitofrontal cortices and basal ganglia in OCD patients (125,126). On the other hand, available literature on perfusion patterns in TS suggests hypoperfusion rather than increased blood flow (see Ref. 127).

Features of OCD may also be seen in patients with basal ganglia and monoaminergic disorders. Animal studies (128) reveal that monkeys with globus pallidus lesions exhibit ritual-like behaviors. It has also been suggested (129,130) that OCD, at least in some patients, may be due to basal ganglia dysfunction, while other findings support evidence of involvement of the caudate nucleus (131). Within monozygotic twins discordant for TS severity, differences in D_2 dopamine receptor binding in the head of the caudate nucleus predicted differences in phenotypic severity, but this relation was not observed in putamen (92). Further evidence for the link is from the writings by Williams et al. (132), who described a patient with a compulsive movement disorder with cavitation of the caudate nucleus. Furthermore, Bonnet (133) studied the neurochemistry and anatomical substrates of vocalizations, blinking, and tics in TS and concluded that the cingulum was the possible anatomical site for TS. This is one of the two areas of the brain destroyed when psychosurgery is employed in the most severe and intractable cases of OCD, which usually brings on a dramatic improvement in symptoms (134).

With regard to neurochemistry, while dopamine is implicated in TS, serotonin is thought to be the major neurotransmitter involved in OCD. This stems primarily from the results of treatment studies of OCD involving selective serotonin-reuptake inhibitor (SSRI) drugs. However, results from both recent treatment and pharmacological challenge studies do not exclude the possibility of dopamine abnormalities in OCD and serotonin abnormalities in TS (see Ref. 135). Furthermore, there is growing evidence to suggest the existence of anatomic and functional interactions between 5-hydroxytryptamine (5-HT) and dopaminergic systems, especially in the basal ganglia areas (136). 5-HT neurons are believed to maintain a tonic inhibitory influence on dopaminergic function in some regions of the brain, especially the midbrain and brainstem projections to the forebrain (137). Thus the neuroanatomic hypothesis that the basal ganglia and its orbitofrontal connections may form the neuronal circuit which subserves TS and OCB, and the available evidence about the interaction between 5-HT and dopamine, are compatible with the role of the above structures and neurotransmitters in the pathophysiology of TS spectrum OCB. Better understanding of the neurochemical abnormalities in TS and OCD has led to better pharmacological treatment approaches in TS + OCD (for review, see Ref. 135).

To summarize, despite differences in the effectiveness of pharmacological treatment in the two disorders that suggest that dopamine is the major neurotransmitter in TS and serotonin is that involved in OCD, other observations from animal studies, the association of OCD with secondary Tourettism, and the effectiveness of combined treatment methods suggest that the tics, vocalizations, and OCD in TS patients and their relatives may be products of common neurophysiological disturbances. The striatum and limbic system receive extensive projections from both dopamine and serotonin transmitter systems, and disturbances in these parts of the brain could be responsible for dopamine-mediated tics and vocalizations and serotonin-mediated obsessions and compulsions in these patients. In this regard, the findings of a recent study of whole-blood serotonin in TS and OCD are noteworthy (138). The biochemical data of this study suggest that in tic + OCD and in tic-free OCD patients 5-HT dysregulation plays a role, but not necessarily in pure TS. Serotonergic dysregulation within tic + OCD and tic-free OCD were noted to be distinct, suggesting differences in underlying pathophysiology.

Obsessive-Compulsive Disorder and Tourette's Syndrome Conclusions

The evidence presented suggests that TS and OCD have genetic and phenomenological overlaps with similar pathophysiological and neurochemical abnormalities. The phenotype of the anticipated TS gene(s) may be expressed as a spectrum of symptoms with chronic multiple tics or TS alone at one end and OCD at the other. This TS-associated OCD appears to represent a separate subcategory of the DSM-IV-defined OCD, indicating that OCD in its entirety may be composed of a heterogeneous group of conditions of different etiology. If so, it would be necessary to reevaluate both the classification and treatment of OCD. In this regard, it is interesting to note the findings of the recent Johns Hopkins OCD family study, which concluded that tic disorders constitute an alternative expression of the familial OCD phenotype (139). Future studies are needed to confirm these conclusions, and the results from both the ongoing genetic linkage studies and other family studies are eagerly awaited (see Ref. 140).

In conclusion, therefore, it would appear that at least some types of OCD are an integral part of TS. In this context, it is interesting to note that Janet (69) in 1903, in his treatise *Les Obsessions et la Psychiasthenie*, described three stages of psychasthenic illness: the first was the "psychasthenic state"; the second was "forced agitations," which included motor tics; and the third was obsessions and compulsions (141).

SELF-INJURIOUS BEHAVIOR

Self-injurious behavior is a dramatic but poorly studied phenomenon, and successful treatments of it remain elusive (142). SIB, which may be categorized by both the type of patient and the clinical context in which it occurs, is being recognized in more and more disorders and, as a result, may lead to further understanding of these disorders and their pathophysiology.

Self-injurious behavior is self-inflicted, nonaccidental injurious behavior, which is variously referred to as self-mutilation, self-injury, self-destructive behavior, and deliberate self-harm. It is seen in patients with a variety of disorders, including TS. In DSM-IV, impulsive SIB among nonpsychotic, intellectually normal individuals is acknowledged as an impulse disorder in its own right (5), and several authors have documented their patients' symptoms suggesting that there is a specific and impulsive SIB syndrome (143–145).

Thumb sucking, lip chewing, tongue rolling, and bruxism are common behaviors found in normal children, probably because of their soothing effect (146), and in some cultures can take the form of recognized rituals (see Ref. 147 for review). In most cases, however, SIB is indicative of psychopathology or physical illness. Occasionally, repeated factitious injury may result in a Munchausen-type syndrome (148).

Self-Injurious Behavior and Tourette's Syndrome

In his original paper in 1885, Gilles de la Tourette (6) described two patients with TS who injured themselves. The first was a 24-year-old man who had many movements of his head and neck (6):

> His mouth opens wide; when it closes again one can hear the teeth of both jaws gnashing violently. Quite often his tongue is caught between them and abruptly seized and lacerated; it is moreover all covered in scars: on one occasion a piece was completely transacted and detached; there is still on its undersurface a wound of one centimeter wide and fairly deep.

The other patient was a 14-year-old boy who "sometimes opened and shut his mouth with some force and abruptness so that his lower lip was bitten so as to draw blood" (6). As has already been mentioned, Dr. Samuel Johnson also had SIB and TS.

A number of other case reports of SIB in TS patients have subsequently appeared, including accounts of picking compulsively at sores (16), punching of the abdomen (149), lip biting resulting in swollen and lacerated sores, filing of teeth with a nail file (150), slapping of the mouth and torso, kicking the opposite leg, tongue biting (151), head banging (152), tongue or cheek biting (153,154), pummeling of the head and chest (29), repeated digging of the forefinger into the hollow of the cheek (155), eye damage (156) resulting in blindness (154), tooth extraction (157), and two cases of unspecified self-mutilation that disappeared following treatment with haloperidol (158). In one large study of 145 patients, hitting (oneself or others) was the second most frequent complex movement, making up 35% of a total of 252 complex movements found in 106 patients (8).

Several studies have specifically investigated SIB in the context of TS (see Ref. 159). Moldofsky et al. (160) examined 15 patients with TS and found that 8 had SIB, the patients biting their lips, cheeks, or tongues or striking themselves. Van Woert et al. (161) described a patient who had typical symptoms of TS, but who also had lip- and tongue-biting behavior which resulted in ulceration. This prompted them to inquire further into SIB in TS by mailing a questionnaire to members of the U.S. Tourette Syndrome Association (TSA). One hundred eleven questionnaires were completed by either the patients or their parents, and 49 (43%) reported SIB, of which the most common were head banging, biting of the tongue, cheeks, lips, and extremities, and self-hitting.

Nee et al. (28) studied 50 patients with TS and specifically investigated SIB. Patients were categorized as having SIB if they had either a history or physical evidence of directed self-harming action. Twenty-four individuals (48%) were classified as having SIB. Examples included repeatedly and forcefully pushing a sharpened pencil into the ear canal, pressing vigorously on the eyeball, persistent biting of the lips to the point of drawing blood and causing difficulty with healing, and placing fingers on a hot stove, resulting in painful, serious burning. Stefl (30) mailed a questionnaire to 555 affiliates of the TSA of Ohio. Of the 431 completed questionnaires returned, 34% admitted to SIB.

In their epidemiological study, Caine et al. (53) detected 41 TS subjects among over 142,000 pupils enrolled in the public and private schools of Monroe County in New York. Seven of the 41 (17%) had SIB, including hitting themselves, touching hot objects, repetitive lip biting, scab pulling, or repetitively sticking pins under the skin.

Robertson et al. (147) studied 90 patients fulfilling DSM-III criteria (50) for TS (the first Queen Square cohort). Thirty patients (33%) (18 males, 12 females) admitted to SIB. Twenty-three types of SIB were reported, including head banging, body punching or slapping, head or face punching or slapping, banging of the body against a hard object, poking sharp objects into the body, scratching parts of the body, and putting the hands through a window. Among the other single types of SIB were putting the head through a window, pinching of the face, dislodging of teeth due to excess grinding, knees hitting the chin, scraping a leg against hard or rough surfaces, poking the umbilicus with the forefinger, violent head shaking, attempting to dislocate joints, purposely walking into obstacles with the intention of injury, reckless driving with the specific aim of being injured, and, finally, two eye injuries: pressing hard on the eyeballs and sticking a fork into the eye. Fourteen of the patients showed more than one type of SIB. None caused tissue damage that necessitated protective devices, although several who punched themselves had severe bruising, while others bled from injuries that, at times, required medical intervention in the acute situation. One patient who hit his head persistently developed a cyst as a result and had to have it removed surgically. Thirteen of

14 head bangers had CT brain scans, and 2 showed cavum septum pellucidum cavities. Only these 2 scans of the total of 73 scans performed were abnormal, which is statistically significant. Of the total group of 90 TS patients, 54 adults completed psychiatric rating scales, including the Hostility and Direction of Hostility Questionnaire (HDHQ) and the LOI. Results indicated that TS patients had scores much higher than those of normal control populations and that SIB was significantly related to all aspects of hostility and obsessionality in that the SIB patients obtained significantly higher scores on the rating scales than did those subjects without such behavior. In addition, patients with SIB were more anxious and neurotic and had more general psychopathology. In the total group of 90 patients, SIB was significantly related to the cumulative number of motor tics and tics of the legs (i.e., the severity of TS motor symptoms) and a past psychiatric history. No relationships with other demographic or motor or other aspects of TS emerged. Patients who had a history of head banging gave a history of having had to attend a special school, being aggressive toward other people, and experiencing a greater number of motor tics than those without head banging. There were no other differences between those with or without head banging with regard to demographic data or TS symptoms. Patients who had exhibited head banging rated themselves as significantly more psychiatrically disturbed, with depression, criticism of others, and neurosis (147). Robertson et al. (147) also reported four additional TS patients who had severe SIB resulting in serious eye injuries. They were all refractory to treatment, and one died as a result of severe head shaking while another required psychosurgery.

In the second Queen Square cohort (Eapen et al., submitted for publication; 162), 148 TS patients were studied. Sixty-four (43.5%) admitted to having SIB. Examples of SIB in the second cohort were similar to those in the first cohort, and, once again, head banging was the most common (30; 46.9%) followed by dangerous touching of hot objects (36; 26.1%). Hitting themselves and lacerating were followed by various biting maneuvers.

Robertson and Gourdie (56) studied a British pedigree spanning six generations that was multiply affected by TS. Of 122 members identified, 85 were individually examined and 50 were diagnosed as being affected by tics (cases), of which 48 were mild. Cases and noncases could be distinguished on the basis of echophenomena, OCB, and the trait score of the LOI and SIB. Similar findings were noted in a subgroup analysis of 91 adults from the second Queen Square cohort (162), where SIB was found to be positively correlated with OCB in the patient as well as the presence of coprophenomena, echophenomena, aggression, and attention-deficit/hyperactivity disorder (ADHD). With regard to scores on psychopathology rating scales, SIB was found to be associated with HDHQ sum of hostility, trait score on the Spielberger State Trait Anxiety Inventory, and Eysenck neuroticism (162).

In another study by Hebebrand et al. (163), TS patients were found to have obsessions concerning harming self or others, intrusive nonsense words, music or sounds, thoughts about something bad (fire, death, illness) happening, and compulsions such as checking, excessive washing, and tooth brushing, cleaning rituals, counting, and hoarding or collecting things. Thus the incidence of SIB in the TS cohorts is much higher than in general and psychiatric populations, being found in 17% (53), 33% (147), 34% (30), 43% (161), 44% (162), 48% (28), and 53% (160) of TS individuals. In an international multisite database of 3500 TS patients (61), 14% (range 4–43%) were found to have comorbid SIB with significant predominance of females over males. Anger control problems, sleep difficulties, coprolalia, and SIB were noted to be higher in individuals with comorbidity. Although severity of TS symptomatology was related to SIB in one large cohort (55), the finding of SIB in both TS pedigree (56) and epidemiological (53) settings suggests that SIB may be found in TS individuals of even mild to moderate severity.

Shentoub and Soulairac (164) observed SIB to be a fairly frequent occurrence in 9–17% of normal infants up to the age of 2 years at a child-care center. In psychiatric populations, several studies have addressed the question of the frequency of SIB. Thus all the inpatients of a large psychiatric hospital were screened for SIB and 4% were found to have such behavior: males, although apt to make more violent attacks upon themselves, self-mutilated less than females (165). In another study by Hassanyeh (166) in an adult psychiatric hospital, patients who inflicted lacerations to themselves represented just under 1% of both admission and long-stay patients. Others (167) suggest that SIB by laceration in a general, psychiatric population occurs in about 4%. On the other hand, SIB among mentally retarded people occurs between 7% and 9% of such individuals, increasing to 14–19% of institutionalized retarded children and occurring in as many as 40% of institutionalized psychotic children (168). In which other conditions is SIB found, and what are the links, if any, between those disorders and TS? As has been said, some types of SIB are found in normal children and may be accepted as ritual in some cultures (see Ref. 147 for review), but in most cases, SIB is associated with psychopathology.

Self-Injurious Behavior and the Lesch–Nyhan Syndrome

Self-injurious behavior resulting in mutilative lesions has been described in a variety of conditions, but perhaps the paradigm is the Lesch–Nyhan syndrome (LNS), which is due to a deficiency of hypoxanthine–guanine phosphoribosyltransferase (HGPT) (169). LNS is an X-linked recessive disorder of purine metabolism that affects only males, with increased excretion of urinary uric acid and characterized by hypotonia, spasticity, chorea, athetosis, dystonia, dysarthria, dysphagia, mental and growth retardation, hyperuricemia, and nephrolithiasis. The most striking behavioral characteristic of LNS is destructive biting of the fingers and lips. It has also been documented that LNS patients are aggressive in a bizarre compulsive way, often using profanities (170–173). Decreased levels of homovanillic acid (174) and 3-methoxy-4-hydroxy phenylethylene (175) have been reported in the CSF of LNS patients, indicating reduced dopamine and norepinephrine turnover. High concentrations of 5-hydroxyindole acetic acid (175) in the CSF have also been reported, suggesting increased serotonin turnover. These findings provide support for the presence of abnormal central monoamine metabolism in LNS and are consistent with the changes found in autopsy of brains of LNS patients (176). Since the early descriptions, numerous authors have reported on SIB in the syndrome. Most note the lip and finger biting but have also found biting of the tongue, poking of the eyes and nose, and head banging (177–180). A specific mutation of the HGPT located in the q26–28 region of the X chromosome has been identified in LNS (181).

An early report of raised serum uric acid in three patients with TS (182), a suggestion of similarities between the SIB encountered in LNS and TS (183), and the control by L-5-hydroxytryptophan of SIB in LNS (184) and in one patient with TS (185) set the stage for studies into purine and serotonin metabolism in TS. Moldofsky et al. (160) found normal serum uric acid and adenine and HGPT in a group of 15 TS patients, of whom over half had SIB. Van Woert et al. (185) confirmed normal activities of HGPT in fresh erythrocytes in TS patients compared to controls, but reported less stable HGPT from the hemolysates of patients compared to controls; in addition, the hemolysates of TS patients that had the most abnormal patterns were from cases who exhibited severe SIB. The authors therefore suggested that TS was a disorder of purine metabolism. This suggestion has not, to date, received wide support. Robertson et al. (147,162) measured serum uric acid in some of the TS patients in the first two Queen Square cohorts, and in all, the values were normal. Specifically, in the second cohort, serum uric acid was measured in 80 TS patients and was found to be normal in 78 (162). In addition, the type of SIB encountered in most TS cohorts is not similar to the type seen in LNS.

Self-Injurious Behavior, Tourette's Syndrome, and Intelligence

Self-injurious behavior occurs frequently in the mentally retarded or learning-disabled, occurring in some 3.5–40% of such individuals (142,186–188). In addition, it has been pointed out that outward-directed aggression is common among the mentally retarded and frequently coexists with SIB that is usually stereotypic and repetitive (142). In one study of TS patients with SIB that addressed this issue, there was no association with intelligence. The mean full-scale IQ of that cohort of patients on the Wechsler Intelligence Scales was 99.7 (SD 15.2) (147). However, the type of SIB seen in that TS cohort was similar to the type seen in mentally retarded populations, which can include face rubbing resulting in broken facial skin and bleeding, head-to-object banging, hand-to-hand punching and slapping, face scratching, skin picking, hand biting, lip chewing, and eye gouging (189). Among the mentally retarded, most studies have shown that SIB is more common in the more profoundly handicapped and is positively associated with the length of institutionalization (189). Of added importance is that in one study (190), TS in the setting of mental retardation was not associated with SIB.

Another specific disorder associated with mental retardation is de Lange's syndrome (191) in which patients have a characteristic facial appearance. SIB in this condition takes a variety of forms, including types seen in TS, such as self-scratching and head and face slapping, present in about half the patients with the syndrome (189,191–194). None of the patients in the cohort of Robertson et al. (147) had this particular diagnosis.

Self-Injurious Behavior, Tourette's Syndrome, and Neuroacanthocytosis

An important differential diagnosis to consider when SIB occurs in the setting of a movement disorder such as TS is neuroacanthocytosis (195–198). The disorder usually presents in the third or fourth decade of life with orofacial dyskinesias that may include tics such as tongue protrusion, grimacing, and involuntary sucking and lip movements. Other movements also occur, e.g., excessive blinking and jerking of arms, legs, head, and trunk; chorea of hands and legs; finger snapping; and dystonic movements. There is generalized wasting of limbs, weakness, and hypotonic dysarthria. Vocalizations are common and include sucking noises, explosive sounds, and echolalia (195–198). SIB resulting from smacking movements (196) occurs, and injuries incurred from tongue, lip, and cheek biting are characteristic (195,198). In the disorder, approximately 5–15% of the erythrocytes are acanthocytes (196). The diagnosis is confirmed by the characteristic blood picture and thus distinguished from TS. The majority of patients in one large TS cohort had blood investigated for the presence of acanthocytes, and none of them received the diagnosis (147).

Self-Injurious Behavior, Tourette's Syndrome, and Schizophrenia

A wide variety of SIB is seen in such psychotic disorders as schizophrenia (199–201). Of interest in the context of this discussion is that severe eye injuries, including enucleation, occur much more often in schizophrenia than in any other disorder, and the majority of SIB, and specifically these eye injuries, seem to be in response to psychotic experiences, frequently of a religious nature (142,202–208). Four TS patients have been documented to have severe SIB resulting in eye injuries (147). Psychosis is rare in TS patients (209,163) and is mainly associated with mental retardation (209a,210). More specifically, no patients were psychotic in the large TS cohort in which SIB was common and the eye injuries were documented (147).

Self-Injurious Behavior, Tourette's Syndrome, and Depression

Patients with depressive illness also exhibit SIB, some similar to those seen in TS, including head banging (211) and, in the case of psychotically depressed patients, eye injuries such as enucleation (164). In some studies, all adult patients in large TS cohorts completed the Beck Depression Inventory (BDI) (212) and the depression subscale of the CCEI (213), and no associations were found between depression scores on either rating scale and the presence of SIB (147). However, in the second Queen Square cohort, analyses of the scores obtained on the above scales in 90 adult TS patients revealed that SIB was associated with depression scores (162).

Self-Injurious Behavior, Tourette's Syndrome, and Autism

It has been suggested that etiological factors underlying autism, a pervasive developmental disorder, may contribute to a vulnerability to express a tic disorder (214). In fact, Baron-Cohen et al. (215,216) recently reported a much higher than expected rate of TS in two screened samples of individuals with autism. SIB, regarded as "secondary self-stimulation," is found in 37–40% of children with autism. The most common forms are biting of the wrist or the back of the hand, head banging, self-scratching, self-hitting, self-pinching, and hair pulling (217). The head punching and banging may often be ritualistic and can result in wheals, hematomas, and frontal bossing (218). The compulsive nature of the SIB seen in this autistic population is similar to that seen in TS, but no patients in one large TS study had a diagnosis of autism (147).

Self-Injurious Behavior, Tourette's Syndrome, Personality, and Personality Disorders

Self-injurious behavior can also occur in people with personality disorders; this is most commonly manifested as wrist slashing or cutting of various parts of the body including the forearms, antecubital fossi, abdomen, and thighs (199,201,219,220). It has been suggested that, of the patients with personality disorders who slash their wrists, those with the borderline personality are particularly liable to this form of behavior (200,221). As has been said, self-inflicted eye injuries are rare outside the setting of psychosis, but there has been one case report of a young man who repeatedly injured his left eye and who was diagnosed as suffering from borderline personality disorder (222). SIB is so common in patients with this diagnosis that DSM-III (50) onward included self-destructive acts, including SIB, among the diagnostic criteria for borderline personality disorder.

It is of interest in this context that adult TS patients in the first two Queen Square cohorts completed the Borderline Syndrome Index (BSI) (223), a rating scale purporting to measure aspects of the borderline personality, and those with SIB had very significantly higher scores on this particular instrument (147,162). However, wrist cutting was not typical of the patients' SIB. SIB exhibited by individuals with personality and character disorders is characterized by several fairly consistent features, and five stages of the SIB act have been described by Leibenluft et al. (224). These are as follows: 1) the precipitating event (e.g., the loss of a significant relationship), 2) escalation of the dysphoria, 3) attempts to forestall the SIB, 4) SIB, and 5) the aftermath, such as relief from tension (224). These specific stages of the SIB act have not yet been studied in the setting of TS, and it is suggested that such precise description of the SIB will help elucidate its etiology in TS.

Are any types of personality overrepresented in SIB populations, and, more specifically, is there a relationship between SIB and, in particular, obsessionality? Using standardized rating scales, several studies have assessed aspects of psychopathology in people who injure themselves. In one, McKerracher et al. (225) used the CCEI on female psychopaths who indulged in SIB and found that those who mutilated themselves scored significantly higher on obsessional, phobic, and somatic items, the obsessional scores being the most discriminative between the subjects ($n = 13$) and a control population ($n = 8$). The total score was also significantly higher in the mutilators. The Eysenck Personality Inventory (EPI) was also administered to the two groups, but no significant differences in neuroticism, extraversion, or lie scores were found.

Gardner and Gardner (226) studied 22 nonpsychotic female habitual self-cutters and compared them with nonpsychotic controls who did not indulge in SIB, also using the CCEI and the obsessionality section of the Tavistock Inventory (TI). The mean CCEI scores for all the subscales of the CCEI (with the exception of the hysteria subscale) were higher for the cutters than the controls. The only subscale on which the cutters scored significantly higher than the controls was on the obsessional subscale, which was mirrored by a significantly higher score on the obsessionality section of the TI. Morgan et al. (227) also gave the CCEI to a cohort of 368 patients who engaged in SIB; there were high scores with respect to anxiety, previous SIB, and a history of visiting a general practitioner for "nerves." Gardner and Gardner (226) also examined repeated self-cutters using the CCEI and found that the obsessionality scores were significantly higher than in a control sample. Obsessional illness per se is not associated with SIB, although compulsive lip biting in a person of normal intelligence has been reported (228). In summary, however, it seems that obsessionality is associated with SIB, although it should be noted that scores of obsessionality as measured by rating scales are increased by depression (229).

It is also debated whether self-injurious behaviors are obsessions, compulsions, or impulsions. In a recent study using factor analysis, Cath et al. (230) identified three factors: an impulsive factor related to TS, a compulsive factor related to OCD, and an obsessive factor related to tic-free OCD. They observed that aggressive repetitive thoughts, contamination worries, and washing behaviors were more frequently experienced by tic-free OCD, while mental play (defined by these authors as repetitive seemingly useless thoughts or images, mostly not unpleasant in nature, and intended as a pastime), echophenomena, touching, and SIB were reported more frequently by TS, and that OCD individuals with tics were intermediate being closer to tic-free OCD. These investigators in another report (231) noted that TS + OCD patients reported more Tourette-related impulsions such as mental play, echophenomena, and impulsive or self-injurious behaviors than patients with OCD (no tics).

Bennun (232) assessed 20 mutilators, depressives, and controls, matched for age, sex, and marital status, using the BDI and the HDHQ. With regard to total hostility, mutilators scored significantly higher than depressives, who in turn scored significantly higher than controls. The assessment of intropunitive hostility revealed no significant difference between the two clinical groups, with both being significantly different from the controls. However, acting out hostility was significantly more common among self-mutilators. Hostility, as with obsessionality, is increased by depression (233).

The results of the study of SIB in TS by Robertson et al. (147) compare favorably with those of these previous investigations, in that significantly and specifically high obsessionality, hostility, and general psychopathology (as judged by subscales and total score of the CCEI, as well as, in their cohort, the BSI scores) were found to be associated with SIB.

Personality problems may have their origins in deprived early childhood, and major separations, family violence, and physical or sexual abuse during childhood have been shown to correlate with SIB later in life (234–237). Furthermore, in a TS clinic population, Robertson et al. (238) noted that TS patients had significantly more personality disorders, anxiety, depression, and obsessionality than controls.

Other Causes of Self-Injurious Behavior

Some sensory neuropathies may lead to unintentional oral SIB, including trigeminal sensory loss from any cause, and, for example, syringobulbia and anesthesia dolorosa and the congenital sensory neuropathy associated with anhidrosis (see Ref. 147). None of the patients in the TS cohort of Robertson et al. (147) showed any evidence of a sensory neuropathy. Although rare, case reports of SIB are found in several other conditions, including epilepsy, alcoholism, drug (e.g., LSD) abuse, unspecific organic or toxic psychosis, acute reactive psychosis, Addison's disease, Huntington's disease, hysteria, Prader–Willi syndrome, and Klinefelter's syndromes (see Ref. 147). Although some TS patients abused alcohol or drugs in one cohort (147), none of the other diagnoses was made.

Head Banging, Self-Injurious Behavior, and Tourette's Syndrome

Head banging was one of the most common forms of SIB in both Queen Square cohorts. CT scans were performed on 73 of 90 TS patients, and the only two abnormalities encountered were cavum septum pellucidum cavities, both in subjects who exhibited repetitive head banging; both abnormal scans, in addition, showed ventricular enlargement (147). In a review by Robertson (209), the vast majority of TS patients' scans were normal. Cavum septum pellucidum cavities are normal occurrences during fetal life (239,240) and, at autopsy in a large series of premature births, the incidence was found to be 100% (240). The incidence decreases with age and has been reported to be 12% in children aged 6 months to 16 years (240) and 30% in children of unspecified age (241), but in adults, the incidence has been found in only 0.9% of adult autopsies (241) and between 0.1% and 0.4% in pneumoencephalographic (PEG) studies on adult neurological patients (242,243). In one TS population (147), the incidence was found to be much greater. In the first Queen Square cohort of 73 who had CT scans, the incidence was 2.7%, but when only the head bangers were taken into account, the incidence rose to 15%. This may well be relevant in the light of the literature on the incidence of such cavities in boxers, where it has been found to occur in between 56% and 60% in PEG and air-encephalographic studies (244–246) and as high as 92% in postmortem studies (247). In addition, some 3% of nonboxers in the same investigation had a penetrated cavum, compared to 77% of the boxers; however, in 5 of the 15 nonboxers showing the abnormality, there was firm clinical or neuropathological evidence of past head injury (247). It would appear therefore that the anomaly can be either developmental (a normal occurrence) or acquired (due to head injury), and in TS patients, the latter mechanism is proposed (147).

The Biochemistry of Self-Injurious Behavior in Tourette's Syndrome

When investigating the relationship between two disorders such as SIB and TS, one should examine the possible etiological theories, and indeed, it seems that there are some possible biochemical links between SIB and TS. A biochemical basis of TS has been suggested for some time, and the dopaminergic system has received the most support as being abnormal (114). It is therefore of interest that not only has the dopaminergic system been implicated in the LNS (175,248), but, in addition, several studies and reviews have implicated dopaminergic systems in SIB in both animal experiments and human studies (249–252).

Neuropeptides have also received much attention in the SIB literature. Corbett and Campbell (250), in a review, noted possible links between endorphins, which are probably neuromodulators with a central analgesic action, and the clinical observations in stereotyped SIB. Others (167) have also suggested the role of β-endorphins in SIB. In 10 patients with a DSM-III diagnosis of borderline personality disorder who habitually mutilated themselves, Coid et al. (253) found significantly raised mean plasma metenkephalin concentrations compared to those of healthy controls. However, no differences were found in the levels of corticotrophin, N-lipotropin, or c-lipotropin (β-endorphin). In addition, the raised levels of metenkephalin appeared to depend on the severity of the patients' symptoms and how recently they had mutilated themselves. Sandman et al. (254) showed that patients with SIB and stereotypy have elevated O-endorphin plasma levels when compared to those of controls. It is of interest in this context that patients with SIB have been successfully treated with the opiate antagonists naloxone (255) and naltrexone (256–265), suggesting that these medications, by affecting regulation of the endorphin/enkephalin systems, may be able to alter SIB. It is of special interest therefore that both overactivity (266) and underactivity (267) of the endogenous opioid system have been postulated in TS, which may reflect either different phases of the disease or the existence of different subgroups among patients with TS. Furthermore, it has been suggested that, while the motor tics of TS possibly reflect neuronal denervation of striatal dopaminergic neurons, SIB may represent opioid denervation with alterations in opioid receptor sensitivity involving striato-limbic hypothalamic circuits (268). Along this line, deregulation of hypothalamic dopamine and opioid activity has been suggested as the pathophysiological mechanism of SIB in TS (269). Muller-Vahl et al. (270) demonstrated an increase in dopamine transporter activity in a study of 12 TS and 9 control subjects using SPECT and ^{123}1-labeled 2beta-carbomethoxy-3beta-(4-iodophenyl) tropane (^{123}1-beta-CIT). They found significantly higher striatal activity ratios in TS than in controls and also an association between binding ratios and SIB and lack of impulse control.

In addition, a postmortem examination of a patient with TS showed a total absence of dynorphin-like (DLI)-positive woolly fibers in the dorsal part of the external segment of the globus pallidus; the ventral pallidum exhibited very few DLI-positive fibers (271). The patient was a 57-year-old man with a history of TS since the age of 5. He was not a typical TS patient in that he took an overdose of methylphenidate at the age of 36, and at the age of 38, his treatment had included 14 unilateral right-sided electroconvulsive therapy treatments and a variety of neuroleptic agents; he also engaged in severe SIB. At age 52, a hypernephroma was discovered, and although it was surgically removed, it may well have had nonmetastatic cerebral effects. Nevertheless, the striking immunohistochemical findings of decreased DLI fibers in the striatum suggested that it constitutes a distinct pathological change in the brain in TS (270). This study has been replicated and similar results were found in six TS patients (Haber et al., presented at the Second World Tourette Symposium, Boston, 1991).

Kurlan et al. (272) reported a significant reduction in TS tic symptomatology in a controlled trial of naloxone and placebo, confirming previous case reports (273). Moreover, several case reports of exacerbation of TS symptomatology by jogging (274) and withdrawal of chronic opiate therapy have been documented (275–277), giving further support to the involvement of the opioid system in TS. Similarly, Dillon (278) reported a 7-year-old boy with TS, pervasive developmental disorder, borderline mental retardation, and history of SIB who was treated for 21 months with clonidine transdermal patches (0.1–0.5 mg weekly), and when clonidine was withdrawn over 4 weeks, the patient developed multiple self-destructive behaviors involving the theme of suffocation.

Although pain is not generally recognized as a symptom of tic disorders, three types of pain complaints have been described in the context of TS (279). One is musculoskeletal pain produced by repeated performance of a tic; the second is pain during voluntary efforts to suppress their tics; and the third involves patients who obtain relief from tics while experiencing pain. The latter group might deliberately provoke pain to obtain its benefit (279).

Interestingly, abnormalities of serotonin have been demonstrated in both TS (114) and LNS (176). In light of animal data that have tied aggression to serotonergic depletion and the suggestion that SIB represents a form of aggression, Mizuno and Yugari (184) successfully gave 5-hydroxytryptophan to four patients with SIB and LNS. Seven subsequent studies have shown only two successes. Coccaro et al. (280), however, showed that patients with SIB and personality disorders had abnormal neuroendocrine challenge tests measuring serotonergic activity, while Lopez Ibor and Lopez Ibor Alino (281) found low CSF 5-HIAA in SIB patients with major depressive disorder. Another basis for consideration of a role for the serotonin system in SIB is the similarity of some of its features to those of OCD. Three early clinical studies specifically reported severe eye SIB occurring in patients with OCD (226,282, 283). In addition, Yaryura-Tobias and Neziroglu (284) suggested a compulsive mutilatory syndrome that possibly involved the hypothalamus/serotonergic pathways. Thereafter, studies employing the LOI, the TI, and the CCEI reported that patients with SIB scored significantly higher on obsessional scores than a control population (226,227). The results of studies by Robertson et al. (147,162) compare favorably with these previous investigations in that significantly and specifically high obsessionality was found to be associated with SIB. Furthermore, studies have reported successful treatment of OC-SIB with drugs that have preferential action on serotonin, such as the serotonin-specific tricyclic antidepressant, clomipramine (283), and the SSRI, fluoxetine (285).

Self-Injurious Behavior and Tourette's Syndrome: Conclusions

Self-injurious behavior is encountered in various clinical syndromes, including TS (286). Taking the review of the literature into account, it would appear that SIB in TS may well be underreported to date, as those studies addressing the subject specifically have found a substantial proportion of patients exhibiting such behavior. Results suggest, in addition, that the clinical correlates of SIB are the severity of TS symptoms and psychopathology, the latter being assessed by standardized rating scales. In particular, TS patients with SIB and self-mutilators in other studies scored highly on obsessionality and hostility measures. This is particularly interesting in that several studies (see Ref. 287) have also found links between obsessionality and hostility in TS patients and coprophenomena and echophenomena, the core features of TS. Thus SIB may be part of the syndrome in some patients, which would fit in with the suggestion that TS may well be a heterogeneous condition (288,289). It must also be acknowledged at this point that these patients probably reflect the more severe end of the spectrum; associated behaviors of TS are generally seen only in physician-referred patients, not in self- or media-referred subjects in epidemiological studies (53). Thus clinic patients represent the severe end of the clinical severity scale. However, the finding of SIB in the TS pedigree study of Robertson and Gourdie (56) suggests that SIB may at times be part and parcel of even milder forms of TS.

The types of SIB in TS patients were, in general, not typical of those encountered in patients with LNS, neuroacanthocytosis, schizophrenia, depression, or personality disorders, but were nonspecific and somewhat similar to those found in mentally retarded (learning-disabled) populations. Of importance is the fact that the patients were of average intelligence. There are, however, difficulties in comparing the results of studies investigating SIB, as there are many varying definitions of such behavior (189,232,290). In the majority of cases of deliberate SIB, the more usual means is ingestion of toxic substances or drugs (291); such cases were not included in most studies. Several patients did incur serious injuries, perhaps exemplified by blindness, cavum septum pellucidum cavities, and death. With regard to a biochemical substrate for TS patients with SIB, the most likely areas implicated appear to be the dopaminergic, serotonergic, and endogenous opioid systems.

Management of Self-Injurious Behavior in Tourette's Syndrome

Another question to be addressed is management. Clinical experience has shown that this can be very difficult at times. Because SIB in one cohort (147) was related to both severity of TS symptoms and psychopathology, one possibility is that with treatment of the manifestations of TS, the SIB may itself disappear and/or be reduced as a consequence. In addition to medication, in some patients, various behavior techniques—such as tracking (self-recording), a combination of different reinforcements (vicarious learning) and response-chain interruption procedures, operant self-control procedures, and aversion treatment—have all been used successfully to treat SIB (217, 292–294).

How, therefore, does one treat the SIB encountered in TS? It should be said that the area has not been investigated and the methods that have been successfully documented in the literature are mainly in the form of isolated case reports. Based on biochemical abnormalities that have been suggested in both TS and SIB, we suggest that the following agents be used alone or in combination: dopamine antagonists, SSRIs, clonidine, naloxone and naltrexone (295), lithium, and β-blockers (296,297). Finally, psychosurgery must be borne in mind as a life-saving treatment in the most severe cases (298). Clearly, further studies investigating SIB in TS need to be conducted to validate/replicate results and explore areas that were beyond the scope of previous investigations.

GENERAL DISCUSSION AND OVERALL CONCLUSIONS

Tourette's syndrome is a complex disorder that has been referred to as both impulsive and compulsive and that seems to be related in several ways to OCD and, in some cases, is associated with SIB. What are the links, if any, between TS, OCD, and SIB? It has been shown (vide supra) that abnormalities of dopamine and serotonin have both been implicated in the pathophysiology of TS, OCD, and SIB. Are there any other disorders that share characteristics and these similarities in neurochemistry?

Trichotillomania was first described by Hallopeau (299) in 1889 as a form of alopecia resulting from excessive hair pulling and may thus represent a form of SIB. In DSM-IV (5), this condition is recognized as a disorder of impulse control, and in this context, there are reports of successful treatment with lithium (300). Furthermore, Swedo et al. (301) have suggested that trichotillomania is related to OCD and serotonergic abnormalities, and there are now several reports of successful treatment of the disorder with SSRIs (301–305). It has also been documented that there is an increased rate of OCD in the families of trichotillomania patients (306). With respect to SIB, there have been reports of comorbidity of trichotillomania and SIB (307). Like trichotillomania, TS has also been argued to be a disorder of both impulse control (308) and a variant of OCD (vide supra). To date and to the best of our knowledge, however, there are few documented cases of TS and trichotillomania and no studies of dopamine abnormalities in trichotillomania. One such international collaborative study is underway. Further studies into the families and treatment of these disorders (TS, OCD, SIB, and trichotillomania) may shed light on their interrelationships, pathophysiology, and, indeed, classification.

Onychophagia, or severe nail biting, may be regarded as a form of SIB. It has recently been shown, in a single case study by Lipinski (309) and a double-blind study by Leonard et al. (310), to respond to clomipramine in a manner significantly superior to that with desipramine. Thus onychophagia may well be another disorder that has been classified as one of impulse control, but because of its response to the SSRIs, it may well be related to the OCD spectrum of disorders and therefore serotonin-related. Once again, no cases of onychophagia and TS or onychophagia and dopamine disturbances have been documented to the best of our knowledge.

Serotonergic mechanisms seem to be involved in at least some types of SIB, and it is in this context that it is interesting that SIB has also been reported in association with eating disorders in which 5-HT is being implicated as well (311). There are a few isolated reports of TS and eating disorders (312–314). In addition, Comings (315) argues that the TS gene is very common, being found in between 5% and 20% of the general population. Comings also suggests that the gene is responsible for many disorders including such eating disorders as compulsive not-eating (anorexia nervosa) or compulsive eating followed by vomiting (bulimia) (315). Other neurotransmitters have also been invoked as abnormal in TS. Thus the dopaminergic and opiate systems have received support as being abnormal both in TS and in SIB.

Aggression is fairly common in severe TS patients, and SIB may be considered introverted aggression. It is suggested that this aspect of psychopathology may be treated with the SSRIs. Psychosurgery has been used in TS with severe SIB (298), TS with OCD (316), and pure OCD (134). A case of TS with SIB was reported by Haber et al. (271), who found low dynorphin in the globus pallidum. Perhaps in these cases, histological samples after surgery or postmortem could provide further clues.

We suggest that TS is a heterogeneous condition with a core symptomatology that is uniform and genetically determined (motor and vocal tics), but with a pattern of associated symptoms that, although classic, are variable (coprolalia, echophenomena, paliphenomena, OCD, SIB, ADHD, etc.) and are likely to be the result of a variety of genetic and environmental factors in predisposed individuals. In this regard, it is also to be noted that anger problems, sleep difficulties, coprolalia, and SIB seem to be more commonly encountered in TS individuals with comorbidity (88). A recent factor analysis study of 29 tic symptoms in 85 TS probands found 4 factors: 1) aggressive phenomena, 2) purely motor and phonic tic symptoms, 3) compulsive phenomena, and 4) tapping and absence of grunting, and the authors suggested that three of these factors may indicate presence of heritable components of the TS phenotype (317). It has also been reported that familial factors contribute significantly to OC symptom dimension phenotypes in TS families; this familial contribution could be genetic or environmental (318). The exact genetic mechanisms involved in TS are as yet unclear. While most would agree that it is an inherited disorder, the possibility of genetic heterogeneity ought to be considered. It seems that OCD, likewise, is heterogeneous in both clinical presentation and etiology (319,320), with one subtype linked to TS. Finally, it is suggested that SIB is a heterogeneous condition and that SIB in the context of TS may, in some cases, represent a complex tic, in others an impulsion, and in still others a compulsion. Further studies into the genetics, phenomenology, neurobiology, and treatment of SIB, OCD, and TS will unravel this complex relationship further and may well lead to further classification of these disorders.

REFERENCES

1. Itard JMG. Memoire sur quelques fonctions involuntaires des appareils de la locomotion de la prehension et de la voix. Arch Gen Med 1825; 8:385–407.
2. McHenry LC Jr. Samuel Johnson's tics and gesticulations. J Hist Med 1967; 22:152–168.
3. Murray TJ. Dr. Samuel Johnson's movement disorders. Br Med J 1979; i:1610–1614.
4. Boswell J. The Life of Samuel Johnson LLD. London: George Routledge & Sons, 1867.
5. American Psychiatric Association. Diagnostic and Statistical Manual of Mental Disorders. 4th ed. Washington, DC: American Psychiatric Publishing, 1994.
6. Gilles de la Tourette G. Etude sur une affection nerveuse caracterisee par de l'incoordination motrice accompagnee d'echolalie et de copralalie. Arch Neurol 1885; 9:19–42, 158–200.
7. Stevens H. The syndrome of Gilles de la Tourette and its treatment. Med Ann DC 1964; 33:277–279.

8. Shapiro AK, Shapiro E, Bruun RD, Sweet RD. Gilles de la Tourette Syndrome. New York: Raven Press, 1978.
9. Hoogduin K. On the diagnosis of obsessive-compulsive disorder. Am J Psychother 1986; 40:36–51.
10. Gilles de la Tourette G. La maladie des tics convulsifs. Sem Med 1899; 19:153–156.
11. Guinon G. Sur la maladie des tics convulsifs. Rev Med 1886; 6:50–80.
12. Grasset J. Lecons sur un cas de maladie des tics et un cas de tremblement singulier de la tete et des membres gauches. Arch Neurol 1890; 20:27–45, 187–211.
13. Robertson MM, Reinstein DZ. Convulsive tic disorder: Georges Gilles de la Tourette, Guinon and Grasset on the phenomenology and psychopathology of Gilles de la Tourette Syndrome. Behav Neurol 1991; 4:29–56.
14. Meige H, Feindel E. Tics and Their Treatment. In: Wilson SAK, ed. London: Sidney Appleton, 1907.
15. Wilson SAK. Tics and allied conditions. J Neurol Psychopathol 1927; 8:93–109.
16. Ascher E. Psychodynamic consideration in Gilles de la Tourette's disease (maladie des tics): With a report of five cases and discussion of the literature. Am J Psychiatry 1948; 105:267–276.
17. Bockner S. Gilles de la Tourette's disease. J Ment Sci 1959; 105:1078–1081.
18. Zausmer DM. The treatment of tics in childhood: A review and follow-up study. Arch Dis Child 1954; 29:537–542.
19. Torup E. A follow-up study of children with tics. Acta Paediatr Scand 1962; 51:261–268.
20. Kelman DH. Gilles de la Tourette's disease in children: A review of the literature. J Child Psychol Psychiatry 1965; 6:219–226.
21. Fernando SJM. Gilles de la Tourette's syndrome: A report on four cases and a review of published case reports. Br J Psychiatry 1967; 113:607–617.
22. Corbett JA, Matthews AM, Connell PH. Tics and Gilles de la Tourette's syndrome: A follow-up study and critical review. Br J Psychiatry 1969; 115:1229–1241.
23. Comings DE, Comings BG. Tourette syndrome: Clinical and psychological aspects of 250 cases. Am J Hum Genet 1985; 37:435–450.
24. Abuzzahab FE, Anderson FO. Gilles de la Tourette's syndrome. Minn Med 1973; 56:492–496.
25. Asam A. A follow-up study of Tourette syndrome. In: Friedhoff AJ, Chase TN, eds. Gilles de la Tourette Syndrome. Advances in Neurology. Vol. 35. New York: Raven Press, 1982.
26. Hagin RA, Beecher R, Pagano G, et al. Effects of Tourette syndrome on learning. In: Friedhoff AJ, Chase TN, eds. Gilles de la Tourette Syndrome. Advances in Neurology. Vol. 35. New York: Raven Press, 1982.
27. Montgomery MA, Clayton PJ, Friedhoff AJ. Psychiatric illness in Tourette syndrome patients and first-degree relatives. In: Friedhoff AJ, Chase TN, eds. Gilles de la Tourette Syndrome. Advances in Neurology. Vol. 35. New York: Raven Press, 1982.

28. Nee LE, Caine ED, Polinsky RJ, Eldridge R, Ebert MH. Gilles de la Tourette syndrome: Clinical and family study of 50 cases. Ann Neurol 1980; 7:41–49.
29. Morphew JA, Sim M. Gilles de la Tourette's syndrome: a clinical and psychopathological study. Br J Med Psychol 1969; 42:293–301.
30. Stefl ME. Mental health needs associated with Tourette syndrome. Am J Publ Health 1984; 74:1310–1313.
31. Yaryura-Tobias JA, Neziroglu F, Howard S, et al. Clinical aspects of Gilles de la Tourette syndrome. J Orthomol Psychiatry 1981; 10:263–268.
32. Shapiro AK, Shapiro E, Wayne H, Clarkin J. The psychopathology of Gilles de la Tourette's syndrome. Am J Psychiatry 1972; 129:87–94.
33. Shapiro E, Shapiro AK, Clarkin J. Clinical psychological testing in Tourette's syndrome. J Pers Assess 1974; 38:464–478.
34. Shapiro AK, Shapiro ES. Tourette syndrome: History and present status. In: Friedhoff AJ, Chase TN, eds. Gilles de la Tourette Syndrome. Advances in Neurology. Vol. 35. New York: Raven Press, 1982:17–23.
35. Roth WF, Luton FH. The mental health program in Tennessee. Am J Psychiatry 1942; 99:662–675.
36. Bebbington P. The Prevalence of OCD in the Community. Current Approaches: "Obsessive Compulsive Disorder." Duphar Med Relat 1990; 7–19.
37. Vazquez-Barquero J-L, Diez-Manrique JF, Pena C, Aldana J, Samaniego-Rodriguez C, Menendez Arango J, Mirapeix C. A community mental health survey in Cantabria: A general description of morbidity. Psychol Med 1987; 17:227–242.
38. Myers JK, Weissman MM, Tischler GL, Holzer CE, Leaf PJ, Orvaschel H, Anthony JC, Boyd JH, Burke JD, Kramer M, Stolzman R. Six month prevalence of psychiatric disorders in three communities: 1980–1982. Arch Gen Psychiatry 1984; 41:959–967.
39. Robins LN, Helzer JE, Weissman MM, Orvaschel H, Gruenberg E, Burke JD, Regier DA. Lifetime prevalence of specific disorders in three sites. Arch Gen Psychiatry 1984; 41:949–958.
40. Karno M, Hough RL, Burnham MA, Escobar JI, Timbers DM, Santana F, Boyd JH. Lifetime prevalence of specific psychiatric disorders among Mexican Americans and non-Hispanic whites in Los Angeles. Arch Gen Psychiatry 1987; 44:695–701.
41. Burnham MA, Hough RL, Escobar JI, Karno M, Timbers DM, Telles CA, Locke BZ. Six month prevalence of specific psychiatric disorders among Mexican Americans and non-Hispanic whites in Los Angeles. Arch Gen Psychiatry 1987; 44:687–694.
42. Blazer D, George LK, Landerman R, Pennybacker M, Melville ML, Woodbury M, Manton KG, Jordan K, Locke B. Psychiatric disorders: A rural/urban comparison. Arch Gen Psychiatry 1985; 42:651–656.
43. Canino GJ, Bird HR, Shrout PE, Rubio-Stipec M, Bravo M, Martinez R, Sesman M, Guevara LM. The prevalence of specific psychiatric disorders in Puerto Rico. Arch Gen Psychiatry 1987; 44:727–735.

44. Bland RC, Newman SC, Orn H. Epidemiology of psychiatric disorders in Edmonton. Acta Psychiatr Scand 1988; 77(suppl 338).
45. Reiger DA, Boyd JH, Burke JD, Rae DS, Myers JK, Kramer M, Robins LN, George LK, Karno M, Locke BZ. One month prevalence of mental disorders in the United States. Arch Gen Psychiatry 1988; 45:977–986.
46. Weissman MM, Leaf PJ, Tischler GL, Blazer DG, Karno M, Bruce ML, Florio MP. Affective disorders in five United States communities. Psychol Med 1988; 18:141–154.
47. Oakley-Browne MA, Joyce PR, Wells JE, Bushnell JA, Hornblow AR. Christchurch Psychiatric Epidemiology Study, part 1: Six month and other period prevalences of specific psychiatric disorders. Aust N Z J Psychiatry 1989; 23:315–326.
48. Wells JE, Bushnell JA, Hornblow AR, Joyce PR, Oakley-Browne MA. Christchurch Psychiatric Epidemiology Study: Methodology and lifetime prevalence for specific psychiatric disorders. Aust N Z J Psychiatry 1989; 23:327–340.
49. Hwu HG, Yeh EK, Chang LY. Prevalence of psychiatric disorders in Taiwan defined by the Chinese Diagnostic Interview Schedule. Acta Psychiatr Scand 1989; 79:136–147.
50. American Psychiatric AssociationDiagnostic and Statistical Manual of Mental Disorders. 3d ed. Washington, DC: American Psychiatric Publishing, 1980.
51. Leckman JF, Zhang H, Alsobrook JP, Pauls DL. Symptom dimensions in obsessive compulsive disorder: Toward quantitative phenotypes. Am J Med Genet 2001; 105:28–30.
52. Frankel M, Cummings JL, Robertson MM, et al. Obsessions and compulsions in Gilles de la Tourette's syndrome. Neurology 1986; 36:378–382.
53. Caine ED, McBride MC, Chiverton P, Bamford KA, Rediess S, Shiao J. Tourette syndrome in Monroe County school children. Neurology 1988; 38:472–475.
54. Van de Wetering BJM, Cohen AP, Minderaa RB, et al. Het Syndroom van Gilles de la Tourette: Klinische Bevindigen. Ned Tijdschr Geneeskd 1988; 132:21–25.
55. Robertson MM, Trimble MR, Lees AJ. The psychopathology of the Gilles de la Tourette syndrome: A phenomenological analysis. Br J Psychiatry 1988; 152: 383–390.
56. Robertson MM, Gourdie A. Familial Tourette's syndrome in a large British pedigree: Associated psychopathology, severity and potential for linkage analysis. Br J Psychiatry 1990; 156:515–521.
57. Robertson MM, Trimble MR. Gilles de la Tourette syndrome in the Middle East: Report of a cohort and a multiply affected large pedigree. Br J Psychiatry 1991; 158:416–419.
58. Robertson MM, Verrill M, Mercer M, et al. Tourette's syndrome in New Zealand: A postal survey. Br J Psychiatry 1994; 164:263–266.
59. Pauls DL, Alsobrook JP II, Goodman W, et al. A family study of obsessive compulsive disorder. Am J Psychiatry 1995; 152:76–84.

60. Comings DE, Comings BG. A controlled study of Tourette syndrome, I–VII. Am J Hum Genet 1987; 41:701–866.
61. Robertson MM, Channon S, Baker J, et al. The psychopathology of Gilles de la Tourette Syndrome: A controlled study. Br J Psychiatry 1993; 162:114–117.
62. Robertson MM, Banerjee S, Fox-Hiley PJ, et al. Personality disorder and psychopathology in Tourette's syndrome: A controlled study. Br J Psychiatry 1997; 171:283–286.
63. Zohar AH, Pauls DL, Ratzoni G, et al. Obsessive-compulsive disorder with and without tics in an epidemiological sample of adolescents. Am J Psychiatry 1997; 154(2):274–276.
64. Freeman RD, Fast DK, Burd L, Kerbeshian J, Robertson MM, Sandor P. An international perspective on Tourette syndrome: Selected findings from 3,500 individuals in 22 countries. Dev Med Child Neurol 2000; 42(7):436–447.
65. Rasmussen SA, Tsuang MT. Clinical characteristics and family history in DSM-III obsessive-compulsive disorder. Am J Psychiatry 1986; 143:317–322.
66. Pitman RK, Green RC, Jenike MA, Mesulam MM. Clinical comparison of Tourette's disorder and obsessive-compulsive disorder. Am J Psychiatry 1987; 144:1166–1171.
67. Rapoport JL. The neurology of obsessive-compulsive disorder. J Am Med Assoc 1988; 260:2888–2890.
68. Pitman RK, Jenike MA. Coprolalia in obsessive-compulsive disorder: A missing link. J Nerv Ment Dis 1988; 176:311–313.
69. Janet P. Les obsessions et la Psychiasthenie. Vol. 1. Paris: Felix Alcan, 1903.
70. Cummings JL, Frankel M. Gilles de la Tourette syndrome and the neurological basis of obsessions and compulsions. Biol Psychiatry 1985; 20:1117–1126.
71. Eapen V, Robertson MM, Alsobrook JP II, Pauls DL. Obsessive compulsive symptoms in Gilles de la Tourette Syndrome and obsessive compulsive disorder: Differences by diagnosis and family history. Am J Med Genet 1997; 74:432–438.
72. Muller N, Putz A, Kathmann N, et al. Characteristics of obsessive-compulsive symptoms in Tourette's syndrome, obsessive-compulsive disorder, and Parkinson's disease. Psychiatry Res 1997; 70(2):105–114.
73. Santangelo SL, Pauls DL, Goldstein JM, et al. Tourette's syndrome: What are the influences of gender and comorbid obsessive-compulsive disorder? J Am Acad Child Adolesc Psych 1994; 33:795–804.
74. de Groot C, Janus M, Bornstein RM. Clinical predictors of psychopathology in children and adolescents with Tourette syndrome. J Psychiatr Res 1995; 29(1):59–70.
75. Kurlan R, Daragjati C, Como PG, et al. Non-obscene complex socially inappropriate behavior in Tourette's syndrome. J Neuropsychiatry Clin Neurosci 1996; 8:311–317.
76. George MS, Trimble MR, Ring HA, et al. Obsessions in obsessive compulsive disorder with and without Gilles de la Tourette's syndrome. Am J Psychiatry 1993; 150:93–96.

77. Iida J, Sakiyama S, Iwasaka H, Hirao F, et al. The clinical features of Tourette's disorder with obsessive-compulsive symptoms. Psychiatry Clin Neurosci 1996; 50(4):185–189.
78. Holzer JC, Goodman WK, McDougle CJ, et al. Obsessive compulsive disorder with and without a chronic tic disorder: A comparison of symptoms in 70 patients. Br J Psychiatry 1994; 164:469–473.
79. Cath DC, Spinhoven P, van Woerkom TC, van de Wetering BJ, Hoogduin CA, Landman AD, Roos RA, Rooijmans HG. Gilles de la Tourette's syndrome with and without obsessive-compulsive disorder compared with obsessive-compulsive disorder without tics: Which symptoms discriminate? J Nerv Ment Dis 2001; 189(4):219–228.
80. Petter T, Richter MA, Sandor P. Clinical features distinguishing patients with Tourette's syndrome and obsessive compulsive disorder from patients with obsessive compulsive disorder without tics. J Clin Psychiatry 1998; 59:456–459.
81. Rasmussen SA, Eisen JL. The epidemiology and differential diagnosis of obsessive compulsive disorder. J Clin Psychiatry 1994; 55(10):5–10.
82. McElroy SL, Phillips KA, Keck PE. Obsessive compulsive spectrum disorder. J Clin Psychiatry 1994; 55(10):33–51.
83. Shapiro AK, Shapiro E. Evaluation of the reported association of obsessive compulsive symptoms or disorder with Tourette's disorder. Compr Psychiatry 1992; 33:152–165.
84. Leckman JF, Walker WK, Goodman WK, et al. 'Just right' perceptions associated with compulsive behaviors in Tourette's syndrome. Am J Psychiatry 1994; 151:675–680.
85. Miguel EC, Coffey BJ, Baer L, et al. Phenomenology of intentional repetitive behaviours in obsessive compulsive disorder and Tourette's disorder. J Clin Psychiatry 1995; 56:246–255.
86. Miguel EC, Baer L, Coffey BJ, et al. Phenomenological differences appearing with repetitive behaviours in obsessive compulsive disorder and Gilles de la Tourette's syndrome. Br J Psychiatry 1997; 170:140–145.
87. Baer L. Factor analysis of symptom subtypes of obsessive compulsive disorder and their relation to personality and tic disorders. J Clin Psychiatry 1994; 55(3):18–23.
88. Ellison RM. Gilles de la Tourette syndrome. Med J Aust 1964; 1:153–155.
89. Jenkins RL, Ashby HB. Gilles de la Tourette syndrome in identical twins. Arch Neurol 1983; 40:249–251.
90. Segal NL, Dysken MW, Bouchard TJ Jr, Pedersen NL, Eckert ED, Heston LL. Tourette's disorder in a set of reared apart triplets: Genetic and environmental influences. Am J Psychiatry 1990; 147:196–199.
91. Price RA, Kidd KK, Cohen DJ, et al. A twin study of Tourette syndrome. Arch Gen Psychiatry 1985; 42:815–820.
92. Wolf SS, Jones DW, Knable MB, Gorey JG, Lee KS, Hyde TM, Coppola R, Weinberger DR. Tourette syndrome: Prediction of phenotypic variation in monozygotic twins by caudate nucleus D2 receptor binding. Science 1996; 273(5279):1225–1227.

93. Kidd KK, Pauls DL. Genetic hypotheses for Tourette syndrome. In: Friedhoff AJ, Chase TN, eds. Gilles de la Tourette Syndrome. Advances in Neurology. Vol. 35. New York: Raven Press, 1982:243–249.
94. Pauls DL, Towbin KE, Leckman JF, et al. Gilles de la Tourette's syndrome and obsessive compulsive disorder. Arch Gen Psychiatry 1986; 43:1180–1182.
95. Pauls DL, Leckman J, Towbin KE, et al. A possible genetic relationship exists between Tourette's syndrome and obsessive-compulsive disorder. Psychopharmacol Bull 1986; 22:730–733.
96. Pauls DL, Raymond CL, Robertson M. The genetics of obsessive compulsive disorders: A review. In: Zohar Y, Ramussen S, eds. Psychobiological Aspects of Obsessive Compulsive Disorder. New York: Wiley, 1989.
97. Pauls DL, Raymond CL, Hurst CR, Rasmussen S, Goodman W, Leckman JF. Transmission of obsessive compulsive disorder and associated behaviors. Proceedings of the 43rd Meeting of the Society of Biological Psychiatry, Montreal, Canada.
98. Lenane MC, Swedo SE, Leonard H, Pauls DL, Sceery W, Rapoport JL. Psychiatric disorders in first degree relatives of children and adolescents with obsessive compulsive disorders. J Am Acad Child Adolesc Psychiatry 1990; 29(3):407–412.
99. Nestadt G, Samuels J, Riddle M, et al. A family study of obsessive compulsive disorder. Arch Gen Psychiatry 2000; 57(4):358–363.
100. Pauls DL. The genetics of obsessive compulsive disorder and Gilles de la Tourette syndrome. Psychiatr Clin North Am 1992; 15(4):759–766.
101. Lenane MC, Swedo SE, Leonard H, et al. Psychiatric disorders in first degree relatives of children and adolescents with obsessive compulsive disorder. J Am Acad Child Adolesc Psychiatry 1990; 29:407–412.
102. Riddle MA, Scahill L, King R, et al. Obsessive compulsive disorder in children and adolescents: Phenomenology and family history. J Am Acad Child Adolesc Psychiatry 1990; 29:766–772.
103. Bellodi L, Sciuto G, Diaferia G, et al. Psychiatric disorders in the families of patients with obsessive compulsive disorder. Psychiatr Res 1992; 42:111–120.
104. Pauls DL, Raymond CL, Stevenson JE, et al. A family study of Gilles de la Tourette syndrome. Am J Hum Genet 1991; 48:154–163.
105. Black DW, Noyes R Jr, Goldstein RB, et al. A family study of obsessive compulsive disorder. Arch Gen Psychiatry 1992; 49:362–368.
106. Leonard HL, Lenane MC, Swedo SE, et al. Tics and Tourette's disorder: A 2- to 7 year follow-up of 54 obsessive-compulsive children. Am J Psychiatry 1992; 149:1244–1251.
107. Rapoport JL, Leonard HL, Swedo SE, et al. Obsessive compulsive disorder in children and adolescents: Issues in management. J Clin Psychiatry 1993; 54:27–29.
108. Cavallini MC, Pasquale L, Bellodi L, et al. Complex segregation analysis for obsessive compulsive disorder and related disorders. Am J Med Genet 1999; 88(1):38–43.

109. Lichter DG, Dmochowski J, Jackson LA, et al. Influence of family history on clinical expression of Tourette's syndrome. Neurology 1999; 52:308–316.
110. Pauls DL, Van de Wetering B. The genetics of tics and related disorders. In: Robertson MM, Eapen V, eds. Movement and Allied Disorders in Childhood. New York: John Wiley and Sons, 1995:13–30.
111. Pauls DL, Leckman JF. The inheritance of Gilles de la Tourette's syndrome and associated behaviours: Evidence for autosomal dominant transmission. N Engl J Med 1986; 315:993–997.
112. Eapen V, Pauls DL, Robertson MM. Evidence for autosomal dominant transmission in Gilles de la Tourette syndrome—United Kingdom cohort. Br J Psychiatry 1993; 162:593–596.
113. Alsobrook JP, Pauls DL. The genetics of Tourette syndrome. Neurol Clin 1997; 381–393.
114. Caine ED. Gilles de la Tourette's syndrome: A review of clinical and research studies and consideration of future directions for investigation. Arch Neurol 1985; 42:393–397.
115. Alexander GE. Functional neuroanatomy of the basal ganglia. In: Robertson MM, Eapen V, eds. Movement and Allied Disorders in Childhood. New York: John Wiley and Sons, 1995:13–30.
116. Obeso JA, Rothwell JC, Marsden CD. The neurophysiology of Tourette's syndrome. In: Friedhoff AJ, Chase TN, eds. Gilles de la Tourette Syndrome. Advances in Neurology. Vol. 35. New York: Raven Press, 1982:105–114.
117. Johannes S, Wieringa BM, Mantey M, Nager W, Rada D, Muller-Vahl KR, Emrich HM, Dengler R, Munte TF, Dietrich D. Altered inhibition of motor responses in Tourette syndrome and obsessive-compulsive disorder. Acta Neurol Scand 2001; 104(1):36–43.
118. Chase TN, Foster NL, Fedio P, et al. Gilles de la Tourette syndrome: Studies with the fluorine-18-labelled fluorodeoxyglucose positron emission tomographic method. Ann Neurol 1984; 15(suppl):S175.
119. Chase TN, Geoffrey V, Gillespie M, et al. Structural and functional studies of Gilles de la Tourette syndrome. Rev Neurol (Paris) 1986; 142:851–855.
120. Hall M, Costa DC, Shields J, Heavens J, Robertson M, Ell PJ. Brain perfusion patterns with 99Tcm-HMPAO/SPECT in patients with Gilles de la Tourette syndrome: Short report. Nucl Med 1990; Suppl 27:243–245.
121. Federicksen KA, Cutting LE, Kates WR, et al. Disproportionate increases of white matter in right frontal lobe in Tourette syndrome. Neurology 2002; 58:85–89.
122. Rauch SL, Whalen PJ, Curran T, Shin LM, Coffey BJ, Savage CR, McInerney SC, Baer L, Jenike MA. Probing striato-thalamic function in obsessive-compulsive disorder and Tourette syndrome using neuroimaging methods. Adv Neurol 2001; 85:207–224.
123. King RA, Scahill L. Obsessive-compulsive disorder in children and adolescents. In: Robertson MM, Eapen V, eds. Movement and Allied Disorders in Childhood. New York: John Wiley and Sons, 1995:43–56.

124. Insel TR. Toward a neuroanatomy of obsessive-compulsive disorder. Arch Gen Psychiatry 1992; 49:739–744.
125. Swedo SE, Leonard HL. Childhood movement disorders and obsessive compulsive disorder. J Clin Psychiatry 1994; 55(3):32–37.
126. Rubin RT, Villanueva-Meyer J, Ananth J, et al. Regional xenon 133 cerebral blood flow and cerebral technetium 99m HMPAO uptake in unmedicated patients with obsessive compulsive disorder and matched normal control subjects. Arch Gen Psychiatry 1992; 49:695–702.
127. Eapen V, Yakeley J, Robertson MM. Gilles de la Tourette syndrome and obsessive compulsive disorder. In: Fogel BS, Schiffer RB, Rao M, eds. Neuropsychiatry. 2nd ed. Baltimore: Lippincott Williams and Wilkins. In press.
128. McLean P. Effects of lesions of the globus pallidus on species typical display behaviour in squirrel monkeys. Brain Res 1978; 149:175–196.
129. Laplane D, Widlocher D, Pillon B, et al. Compulsive behaviour of the obsessional type with bilateral circumscribed pallidostriatal necrosis (encephalopathy following a wasp sting). Rev Neurol (Paris) 1981; 137:269–276.
130. Swedo SE, Rapoport JL, Cheslow DL. High prevalence of obsessive-compulsive symptoms in patients with Sydenham's chorea. Am J Psychiatry 1989; 146:246–249.
131. Luxenberg JS, Swedo SE, Flament MF, et al. Neuroanatomical abnormalities in obsessive-compulsive disorder. Am J Psychiatry 1988; 145:1089–1093.
132. Williams AC, Owen C, Heath DA. A compulsive movement disorder with cavitation of caudate nucleus. J Neurol Neurosurg Psychiatry 1988; 51:447–448.
133. Bonnet KA. Neurobiological dissection of Tourette syndrome: A neurochemical focus on a human neuroanatomical model. In: Friedhoff AJ, Chase TN, eds. Gilles de la Tourette Syndrome. Advances in Neurology. Vol. 35. New York: Raven Press, 1982:77–82.
134. Bird JM, Crow CD. Psychosurgery in obsessional-compulsive disorder: Old techniques and new data: current approaches. Obsessive Compulsive Disorder. Duphar Med Relat 1990:82–92.
135. Eapen V, Robertson MM. Tourette syndrome and co-morbid obsessive compulsive disorder: Therapeutic interventions. CNS Drugs 2000; 13(3):278–281.
136. Graybiel AM. Neurotransmitters and neuromodulators in the basal ganglia. Trends Neurosci 1990; 13:244–254.
137. George MS. Obsessive compulsive disorder: New perspectives in clinical practice. Int Clin Psychopharmacol 1991; 6(3):57–68.
138. Cath DC, Spinhoven P, Landman AD, van Kempen GM. Psychopathology and personality characteristics in relation to blood serotonin in Tourette's syndrome and obsessive-compulsive disorder. J Psychopharmacol 2001; 15(2): 111–119.
139. Grados MA, Riddle MA, Samuels JF, Liang KY, Hoehn-Saric R, Bienvenu OJ, Walkup JT, Song D, Nestadt G. The familial phenotype of obsessive-compulsive disorder in relation to tic disorders: The Hopkins OCD family study. Biol Psychiatry 2001; 50(8):559–565.
140. The TSA International Consortium for Genetics. A complete genome screen in

sib pairs affected by Gilles de la Tourette syndrome. Am J Hum Genet 1999; 65:1428–1436.

141. Pitman RK. Pierre Janet on obsessive compulsive disorder (1903). Arch Gen Psychiatry 1987; 44:226–232.
142. Winchel RM, Stanley MS. Self-injurious behavior: A review of the behavior and biology of self-mutilation. Am J Psychiatry 1991; 148:306–317.
143. Siomopoulos V. Repeated self-cutting: An impulse neurosis. Am J Psychother 1974; 28:85–94.
144. Pattison EM, Kahan J. The deliberate self-harm syndrome. Am J Psychiatry 1983; 140:867–872.
145. Favazza AR. Bodies Under Seige. Baltimore: Johns Hopkins University Press, 1987.
146. Jankovic J. Orofacial and other self-mutilations. Adv Neurol 1988; 49:365–381.
147. Robertson MM, Trimble MR, Lees AJ. Self-injurious behaviour and the Gilles de la Tourette syndrome: A clinical study and review of the literature. Psychol Med 1989; 19:611–625.
148. Meadow R. Munchausen syndrome by proxy. Arch Dis Child 1982; 57:92–98.
149. Dunlap JR. A case of Gilles de la Tourette's disease (Maladie des tics): a study of the intrafamily dynamics. Nerv Ment Dis 1960; 130:340–344.
150. Bruun RD. Gilles de la Tourette's syndrome: An overview of clinical experience. J Am Acad Child Psychiatry 1984; 23:126–133.
151. Eisenberg L, Ascher E, Kanner L. A clinical study of Gilles de la Tourette's disease (maladie des tics) in children. Am J Psychiatry 1959; 115:715–726.
152. Eldridge R, Sweet R, Lake CR, Shapiro AK. Gilles de la Tourette's syndrome: Clinical, genetic, psychologic, and biochemical aspects in 21 selected families. Neurology 1977; 27:115–124.
153. Eriksson B, Persson T. Gilles de la Tourette's syndrome: Two cases with an organic brain injury. Br J Psychiatry 1969; 115:315–353.
154. Stevens A Jr, Blachly PH. Successful treatment of the maladie des tics. Am J Dis Child 1966; 112:541–545.
155. Obendorf CP. Simple tic mechanism. J Am Med Assoc 1916; 16:99–100.
156. Eisenhauer GL, Woody RC. Self-mutilation and Tourette's disorder. J Child Neurol 1987; 2:265–267.
157. Woody RC, Eisenhauer G. Tooth extraction as a form of self-mutilation in Tourette's disorder. South Med J 1986; 79:1466.
158. Lieh Mak F, Chung SY, Lee P, Chen S. Tourette syndrome in the Chinese: A follow up of fifteen cases. Adv Neurol 1982; 35:281–284.
159. Robertson MM. Self-injurious behavior and Tourette syndrome. Adv Neurol 1992; 58:105–114.
160. Moldofsky H, Tullis C, Lamon R. Multiple tics syndrome (Gilles de la Tourette's syndrome). J Nerv Ment Dis 1974; 15:282–292.
161. Van Woert MH, Jutkowitz R, Rosenbaum D, Bowers MB. Gilles de la Tourette's syndrome: Biochemical approaches. In: Yahr MD, ed. The Basal Ganglia. New York: Raven Press, 1976.

162. Eapen V, Fox-Hiley P, Banerjee S, Robertson MM. Tourette syndrome: A clinical and psychopathological analysis in an adult UK cohort. Submitted for publication.
163. Hebebrand J, Klug B, Fimmers R, et al. Rates for the disorders and obsessive compulsive symptomatology in families of children and adolescents with Gilles de la Tourette syndrome. J Psychiatr Res 1997; 31(5):519–530.
164. Shentoub SA, Soulairac A. L'Enfant Automutilateur. Psychiatr Enfant 1961; 3:119.
165. Phillips RH, Alkan M. Recurrent self-mutilation. Psychiatr Q 1961; 35:424–431.
166. Hassanyeh F. Self-mutilation in psychiatric inpatients. Br J Clin Soc Psychiatry 1985; 3:27–29.
167. Fairburn A, Hassanyeh F. Self mutilation. Practitioner 1981; 225:1498–1499.
168. Barron J, Sandman CA. Relationship of sedative-hypnotic response to self-injurious behavior and stereotypy by mentally retarded clients. Am J Ment Defic 1983; 88:177–186.
169. Kelley WN. Hypoxanthine-guanine phosphoribosyltransferase deficiency in the Lesch–Nyhan syndrome and gout. Fed Proc 1968; 27:1047–1052.
170. Lesch M, Nyhan WL. A familial disorder of uric acid metabolism and central nervous system function. Am J Med 1964; 36:561–570.
171. Nyhan WL. Introduction: Clinical and genetic features. Fed Proc 1968; 27: 1027–1033.
172. Nyhan WL. Clinical features of the Lesch–Nyhan syndrome. Arch Intern Med 1972; 130:186–192.
173. Nyhan WL. The Lesch–Nyhan syndrome. Dev Med Child Neurol 1978; 20:376.
174. Silverstein F, Smith CB, Johnston MV. Effect of clonidine on platelet alpha 2-adrenoreceptors and plasma norepinephrine of children with Tourette syndrome. Dev Med Child Neurol 1985; 27:793–799.
175. Jankovic J, Caskey TC, Stout T, Butler IJ. Lesch–Nyhan syndrome: A study of motor behavior and cerebrospinal fluid neurotransmitters. Ann Neurol 1988; 23:466–469.
176. Lloyd KG, Hornykiewics O, Davidson L, Shannak K, Farley I, Goldstein M, Shibuya M, Kelley WN, Fox IH. Biochemical evidence of dysfunction of brain neurotransmitters in the Lesch–Nyhan syndrome. N Engl J Med 1981; 305: 1106–1111.
177. Shear CS, Nyhan WL, Kirman BH, Stern J. Self-mutilative behavior as a feature of the de Lange syndrome. J Pediatr 1971; 78:506–509.
178. Gilbert S, Spellacy E, Watts RWE. Problems in the behavioural treatment of self-injury in the Lesch–Nyhan syndrome. Dev Med Child Neurol 1979; 21:795–800.
179. Scully C. The orofacial manifestations of the Lesch–Nyhan syndrome. Int J Oral Surg 1981; 10:380–383.
180. Christie R, Bay C, Kaufman IA, Bakay B, Borden M, Nyhan WL. Lesch–Nyhan disease: Clinical experience with nineteen patients. Dev Med Child Neurol 1982; 24:293–306.

181. Gibbs RA, Caskcy CT. Identification and localization of mutations at the Lesch Nyhan locus by ribonuclease A cleavage. Science 1987; 236:303–307.
182. Pfeiffer CC, Ilie Y, Nichols RE, Sugerman AA. The serum urate level reflects degree of stress. J Clin Pharmacol 1969; 9:384–392.
183. Seegmiller JE. In discussion, Hoefnagel D, Seminars on Lesch–Nyhan syndrome (summary). Fed Proc 1968; 27:1046.
184. Mizuno T, Yugari Y. Prophylactic effect of L-5-hydroxytryptophan on self-mutilation in the Lesch–Nyhan syndrome. Neuropaediatrics 1975; 6:13–23.
185. Van Woert MH, Yip LC, Balis ME. Purine phosphoribosyltransferases in Gilles de la Tourette syndrome. N Engl J Med 1977; 297:210–212.
186. Reid AH, Ballinger BR, Heather BB. Behavioural syndromes identified by cluster analysis in a sample of 100 severely and profoundly retarded adults. Psychol Med 1978; 8:399–412.
187. Matin MA, Rundle AT. Physiological and psychiatric investigations into a group of mentally handicapped subjects with self-injurious behaviour. J Ment Defic Res 1980; 24:77–85.
188. Buitelaar JK. Self-injurious behaviour in retarded children: Clinical phenomena and biological mechanisms. Acta Paedopsychiatr 1993; 56(2):105–111.
189. Murphy GH. Self-injurious behaviour in the mentally handicapped: An update. Newsl Assoc Child Psychol Psychiatry 1985; 7:2–11.
190. Goldney RD, Simpson IG. Female genital self mutilation, dysorexia and the hysterical personality: The Caenis syndrome. Can Psychiatr Assoc J 1975; 20: 435–441.
191. Singh NN, Pulman RM. Self-injury in the De Lange syndrome. J Ment Defic Res 1979; 23:79–81.
192. Bryson Y, Sakati N, Nyhan WL, Fish CH. Self-mutilative behavior in the Cornelia de Lange syndrome. Am J Ment Defic 1971; 76:319–324.
193. Johnson HG, Ekman P, Friesen W. A behavioural phenotype in the de Lange syndrome. Pediatr Res 1976; 10:843–850.
194. Fadel KM. Self-mutilation. Psychiatr Pract 1985; 4:19–26.
195. Critchley EMR, Clark DB, Wikler A. Acanthocytosis and neurological disorder without betalipoproteinemia. Arch Neurol 1968; 18:134–140.
196. Bird TD, Cederbaum S, Valpey RW, Stalil WL. Familial degeneration of the basal ganglia with acanthocytosis: A clinical, neuropathological, and neurochemical study. Ann Neurol 1978; 3:253–258.
197. Kito S, Itoga E, Hiroshige Y, Matsumoto N, Miwa S. A pedigree of amyotrophic chorea with acanthocytosis. Arch Neurol 1980; 37:514–517.
198. Sakai T, Mawatari S, Twashita H, Goto I, Kuroiwa Y. Choreoacanthocytosis: Clues to clinical diagnosis. Arch Neurol 1981; 38:335–338.
199. Graff H, Mallin R. The syndrome of the wrist cutter. Am J Psychiatry 1967; 124:36–42.
200. Rinzler C, Shapiro DA. Wrist-cutting and suicide. J Mt Sinai Hosp NY 1968; 25:485–488.
201. Rosenthal RJ, Rinzler C, Walshe R, Klausner E. Wrist cutting syndrome: The meaning of a gesture. Am J Psychiatry 1972; 128:47–52.

202. Crowder JE, Gross CA, Heiser JF, Crowder AM. Self-mutilation of the eye. J Clin Psychiatry 1979; 40:420–423.
203. Tapper CM, Bland RCM, Danyluk L. Self-inflicted eye injuries and self-inflicted blindness. J Nerv Ment Dis 1979; 167:311–314.
204. Arons BS. Self-mutilation: Clinical examples and reflections. Am J Psychother 1981; 35:550–557.
205. Stannard K, Leonard T, Holder G, Shilling J. Oedipism reviewed: As case of bilateral ocular self-mutilation. Br J Ophthalmol 1984; 68:276–280.
206. Rogers T, Pullen I. Self-inflicted eye injuries. Br J Psychiatry 1987; 151:691–693.
207. Rosen DH, Hoffman AM. Focal suicide: Self-enucleation by two young psychotic individuals. Am J Psychiatry 1972; 128:1009–1011.
208. MacLean G, Robertson BM. Self-enucleation and psychosis. Arch Gen Psychiatry 1976; 33:242–249.
209. Robertson MM. The Gilles de la Tourette syndrome: The current status. Br J Psychiatry 1989; 154:147–169.
209a. Golden GS, Greenhill L. Tourette syndrome in mentally retarded children. Ment Retard. Arch Gen Psychiatry 1989; 19:17.
210. Reid AH. Gilles de la Tourette syndrome in mental handicap. J Ment Defic Res 1984; 28:81–83.
211. Yesavage JA. Direct and indirect hostility and self-destructive behaviour by hospitalized depressives. Acta Psychiatr Scand 1983; 68:345–350.
212. Beck AT, Ward CH, Mendelson M, Mock J, Erbaugh J. An inventory for measuring depression. Arch Gen Psychiatry 1961; 4:561–571.
213. Crown S, Crisp AH. A short clinical diagnostic self-rating scale for psychoneurotic patients: The Middlesex Hospital Questionnaire (MHQ). Br J Psychiatry 1966; 122:917–923.
214. Leckman JF, Cohen DJ. Descriptive and diagnostic classification of tic disorders. In: Cohen DJ, Bruun RD, Leckman JF, eds. Tourette's Syndrome and Tic Disorders: Clinical Understanding and Treatment. New York: Wiley, 1990: 3–19.
215. Baron-Cohen S, Mortimore C, Moriarty J, Izaguirre J, Robertson M. The prevalence of Gilles de la Tourette's syndrome in children and adolescents with autism. J Child Psychol Psychiatry 1999; 40(2):213–218.
216. Baron-Cohen S, Scahill VL, Izaguirre J, Hornsey H, Robertson MM. The prevalence of Gilles de la Tourette syndrome in children and adolescents with autism: a large scale study. Psychol Med 1999; 29(5):1151–1159.
217. Zealley AK. Mental Handicap. Companion to Psychiatric Studies. 3d ed. Edinburgh: Churchill-Livingstone, 1983:386.
218. Kinnell HG. 'Addiction' to a strait jacket: A case report of treatment of self-injurious behaviour in an autistic child. J Ment Defic Res 1983; 28:77–79.
219. Virkkunen M. Self-mutilation and anti-social personality disorder. Acta Psychiatr Scand 1976; 54:347–352.
220. Bach-Y-Rita G. Habitual violence and self-mutilation. Am J Psychiatry 1974; 131:1018–1020.

221. Schaffer CB, Carroll J, Abramowitz SI. Self-mutilation and the borderline personality. J Nerv Ment Dis 1982; 170:468–473.
222. Griffin N, Webb MGT, Parker RR. A case of self-inflicted eye injuries. J Nerv Ment Dis 1982; 170:53–56.
223. Conte HR, Plutchik R, Karsau TB, Jerrett IL. A self-report borderline scale: Discriminative validity and preliminary norms. J Nerv Ment Dis 1980; 168:428–435.
224. Leibenluft E, Gardner DL, Cowdry RW. The inner experience of the borderline self-mutilator. J Pers Disord 1987, 1317–1324.
225. McKerracher DW, Loughnane T, Watson RA. Self-mutilation in female psychopaths. Br J Psychiatry 1968; 114:829–832.
226. Gardner AR, Gardner AJ. Self-mutilation, obsessionality and narcissism. Br J Psychiatry 1975; 127:127–132.
227. Morgan HG, Burns-Cox CJ, Pocock H, Pottle S. Deliberate self-harm: Clinical and socioeconomic characteristics of 368 patients. Br J Psychiatry 1975; 127: 564–574.
228. Lyon LS. A behavioural treatment of compulsive lip-biting. J Behav Ther Exp Psychiatry 1983; 14:275–276.
229. Kendell RE, Discipio WJ. Eysenck personality scores of patients with depressive illness. Br J Psychiatry 1968; 114:767–770.
230. Cath DC, Spinhoven P, Hoogduin CA, Landman AD, van Woerkom TC, van de Wetering BJ, Roos RA, Rooijmans HG. Repetitive behaviors in Tourette's syndrome and OCD with and without tics: What are the differences? Psychiatry Res 2001; 101(2):171–185.
231. Cath DC, Spinhoven P, van de Wetering BJ, Hoogduin CA, Landman AD, van Woerkom TC, Roos RA, Rooijmans HG. The relationship between types and severity of repetitive behaviors in Gilles de la Tourette's disorder and obsessive-compulsive disorder. J Clin Psychiatry 2000; 61(7):505–513.
232. Bennun I. Depression and hostility in self-mutilation. Suicide Life-Threat Behav 1983; 13:71–84.
233. Phillip AE. Psychometric changes associated with response to drug treatment. Br J Soc Clin Psychol 1971; 10:138–143.
234. Grunebaum HU, Klerman GL. Wrist slashing. Am J Psychiatry 1967; 124:527–534.
235. Roy A. Self mutilation. Br J Med Psychol 1978; 51:201–203.
236. Green AH. Self-destructive behavior in battered children. Am J Psychiatry 1978; 135:579–582.
237. Carroll J, Schaffer C, Spensley J, Abramowitz SI. Family experiences of self-mutilating patients. Am J Psychiatry 1980; 137:852–853.
238. Robertson MM, Banerjee S, Fox-Hiley PJ, et al. Personality disorder and psychopathology in Tourette's syndrome: A controlled study. Br J Psychiatry 1997; 171:283–286.
239. Bruyn GW. Agenesis septi pellucidi, cavum septi pellucidi, cavum vergae and cavum veli interpositi. In: Vinken PJ, Bruyn GW, eds. Handbook of Clinical Neurology. Vol. 30. Amsterdam: Elsevier/North Holland 1977:299–336.

240. Shaw CM, Alvord EC. Cava septi pellucidi et vergae: Their normal and pathological states. Brain 1969; 92:213–224.
241. Swenson O. Nature and occurrence of the cavum septi pellucidi. Arch Pathol 1944; 37:119–123.
242. Bonitz G. Sur klinische-diagnostischen Bedeutung des erweiterten und komkumizierenden cavum septi pellucidi. Nervenarzt 1969; 40:121–128.
243. Sonntag I, Nadjmi M, Lajosi F, Fuchs G. Anlagebedingte Gehirnanomalien der Mittellinie. Nervenarzt 1971; 42:531–539.
244. Isherwood I, Mawdsley C, Ferguson FR. Pneumoencephalographic changes in boxers. Acta Radiol 1966; 5:654–661.
245. Johnson J. Organic psychosyndromes due to boxing. Br J Psychiatry 1969; 115:45–53.
246. Spillane JD. Five boxers. Br Med J 1962; ii:1205–1210.
247. Corsellis JAN, Bruton CJ, Freeman-Browne D. The aftermath of boxing. Psychol Med 1973; 3:270–303.
248. Casas-Bruge M, Almenar C, Grau IM, Jane J, Herrerea-Marschitz M, Ungerstedt V. Dopaminergic receptor supersensitivity in self-mutilatory behaviour of Lesch–Nyhan disease. Lancet 1985; i:991.
249. Jones IH, Barraclough BM. Auto-mutilation in animals and its relevance to self-injury in man. Acta Psychiatr Scand 1978; 58:40–47.
250. Corbett JA, Campbell HJ. Causes of severe self-injurious behavior. In: Mittler P, De Jong JM, eds. Mental Retardation: New Horizons. Biomedical Aspects. Vol. 11. Baltimore: University Park Press, 1980:285–292.
251. Gorea E, Lombard MC. The possible participation of a dopaminergic-system in mutilating behaviour in rats with forelimb deafferentiation. Neurosci Lett 1984; 48:75–80.
252. Breese GR, Criswell HE, Duncan GE, Mueller RA. Dopamine deficiency in self-injurious behavior. Psychopharmacol Bull 1989; 25:353–357.
253. Coid JM, Allolio B, Rees LH. Raised plasma metenkephalin in patients who habitually mutilate themselves. Lancet 1983; ii:545–546.
254. Sandman CA, Barron JL, Chicz-DeMet A, DeMet EM. Plasma B-endorphin levels in patients with self-injurious behavior and stereotypy. Am J Ment Retard 1990; 95:84–92.
255. Richardson HS, Zaleski WA. Naloxone and self-mutilation. Biol Psychiatry 1983; 18:99–101.
256. Herman BH, Hammock MK, Arthur-Smith A, Egan J, Chatoor I, Werner A, Zelnik N. Naltrexone decreases self-injurious behaviour. Ann Neurol 1987; 77:550–552.
257. Herman BH, Hammock MK, Egan J, Arthur-Smith A, Chatoor I, Werner A. Role for opioid peptides in self-injurious behavior: Dissociation from autonomic nervous system functioning. Dev Pharmacol Ther 1989; 12:81–89.
258. Barrett RP, Feinstein C, Hole WT. Effects of naloxone and naltrexone on self-injury: A double-blind, placebo-controlled analysis. Am J Ment Retard 1989; 93:644–651.

259. Lienemann J, Walker FD. Reversal of self-abusive behavior with naltrexone. J Clin Psychopharmacol 1989; 9:448–449.
260. Lienemann J, Walker FD. Naltrexone for treatment of self-injury. Am J Psychiatry 1989; 146:1639–1640.
261. Smith KC, Pittelkow MR. Naltrexone for neurotic excoriations. J Am Acad Dermatol 1989; 20:860–861.
262. Kars H, Broekema W, Glaudemans-Van Gelderen I, Verhoeven WMA, van Ree JM. Naltrexone attenuates self-injurious behavior in mentally retarded subjects. Biol Psychiatry 1990; 27:741–746.
263. Sandman CA, Barron JL, Colman H. An orally administered opiate blocker, naltrexone, attenuates self-injurious behavior. Am J Ment Retard 1990; 95:93–102.
264. Sandyk R, Iacono RP, Allender J. Naloxone ameliorates compulsive touching behavior and tics in Tourette's syndrome. Ann Neurol 1986; 20:437.
265. Sandyk R, Iacono RP, Crinnian C, Bamford CR, Consroe PF. Effects of naltrexone in Tourette's syndrome. Ann Neurol 1986; 20:437.
266. Sandyk R. The effects of naloxone in Tourette's syndrome. Ann Neurol 1985; 18:367–368.
267. Gillman MA, Sandyk R. Opiatergic and dopaminergic function and Lesch–Nyhan syndrome. Am J Psychiatry 1985; 142:1226.
268. Sandyk R. Opioid neuronal denervation in Gilles de la Tourette syndrome. Int J Neurosci 1987; 35(1–2):95–98.
269. Sandyk R, Bamford CR. Deregulation of hypothalamic dopamine and opioid activity and the pathophysiology of self-mutilatory behavior in Tourette's syndrome. J Clin Psychopharmacol 1987; 7(5):367.
270. Muller-Vahl KR, Berding G, Brucke T, et al. Dopamine transporter binding in Gilles de la Tourette syndrome. J Neurol 2000; 247(7):514–520.
271. Haber SN, Kowall NW, Vonsattel JP, et al. Gilles de la Tourette's syndrome: A postmortem neuropathological and immunohistochemical study. J Neurol Sci 1986; 75:225–241.
272. Kurlan R, Majumdar L, Deeley C, Mudholkar GS, Plumb S, Como PG. A controlled trial of propoxyphene and naltrexone in Tourette's syndrome. Ann Neurol 1991; 30(1):19–23.
273. Gadoth N, Gordon CR, Streifler J. Naloxone in Gilles de la Tourette's syndrome. Ann Neurol 1987; 21:415.
274. Jacome DE. Jogging and Tourette's disorder. Am J Psychiatry 1987; 144(8): 1100–1101.
275. Lichter D, Manjumdar L, Kurlan R. Opiate withdrawal unmasks Tourette's syndrome. Clin Neuropharmacol 1988; 11:559–564.
276. Walters AS, Hening W, Chokroverty S. Letter to the editor. Mov Disord 1990; 5:89–91.
277. Bruun R, Kurlan R. Opiate therapy and self-harming behavior in Tourette's syndrome. Mov Disord 1991; 6:184–185.
278. Dillon JE. Self-injurious behaviour associated with clonidine withdrawal in a child with Tourette's disorder. J Child Neurol 1990; 5(4):308–310.

279. Riley DE, Lang AE. Pain in Gilles de la Tourette syndrome and related tic disorders. Can J Neurol Sci 1989; 16(4):439–441.
280. Coccaro EF, Siever LJ, Klar HM, et al. Serotonergic studies in patients with affective and personality disorders. Arch Gen Psychiatry 1989; 46:587–599.
281. Lopez Ibor JJ, Lopez Ibor Alino JM. The pharmacological treatment of obsessive neurosis, anorexia nervosa, delusions of reference and the Klein Levin syndrome. Arch Fam Med 1971; 20:2–10.
282. Stinnett JL, Hollender MH. Compulsive self-mutilation. J Nerv Ment Dis 1970; 150:371–375.
283. Primeau F, Fontaine R. Obsessive disorder with self-mutilation: A subgroup responsive to pharmacotherapy. Can J Psychiatry 1987; 32:699–701.
284. Yaryura-Tobias JA, Neziroglu F. Compulsions, aggression, and self-mutilation: A hypothalamic disorder? Orthomol Psychiatry 1978; 7:114–117.
285. Hollander E, Fay M, Cohen B, Campeas R, Gorman JM, Liebowitz MR. Serotonergic and noradrenergic sensitivity in obsessive-compulsive disorder: Behavioral findings. Am J Psychiatry 1988; 148:1015–1017.
286. Robertson MM. Tourette syndrome, associated conditions and the complexities of treatment. Brain 2000; 123:425–462.
287. Robertson MM. Self-Injurious behavior and Tourette syndrome. Adv Neurol 1992; 58:105–114.
288. Lees AJ, Robertson MM, Trimble MR. A clinical study of Gilles de la Tourette syndrome in the United Kingdom. J Neurol Neurosurg Psychiatry 1984; 47:1–8.
289. Robertson M, Evans K, Robins A, et al. Abnormalities of copper in Gilles de la Tourette syndrome. Biol Psychiatry 1987; 22:968–978.
290. Corbett J. Aversion for the treatment of self-injurious behaviour. J Ment Defic Res 1975; 19:79–95.
291. Odejide AO, Williams AO, Ohaeri JU, Ikusean BA. The epidemiology of deliberate self-harm: The Ibadan experience. Br J Psychiatry 1986; 149:734–737.
292. Sanchez V. Behavioural treatment of chronic hair pulling in a two year old. J Behav Ther Exp Psychiatry 1979; 10:241–245.
293. Cordle CH, Long CG. The use of operant self-control procedures in the treatment of compulsive hair-pulling. J Behav Ther Exp Psychiatry 1980; 11:127–130.
294. Bayer CA. Self-monitoring and mild aversion treatment of trichotillomania. J Behav Ther Exp Psychiatry 1972; 3:139–141.
295. Konicki PE, Schulz S. Rationale for clinical trials of opiate antagonists in treating patients with personality disorders and self-injurious behaviour. Psychopharmacol Bull 1989; 25:556–563.
296. Luchins DJ, Dojka D. Lithium and propranolol in aggression and self-injurious behaviour in the mentally retarded. Psychopharmacol Bull 1989; 25:372–375.
297. Ruedrich SL, Grush L, Wilson J. Beta adrenergic blocking medications for aggressive self-injurious mentally retarded persons. Am J Ment Retard 1990; 95:110–119.

298. Robertson M, Doran M, Trimble MR, Lees AJ. The treatment of Gilles de la Tourette syndrome by limbic leucotomy. J Neurol Neurosurg Psychiatry 1990; 53:691–694.
299. Hallopeau M. Alopecie par grattage (trichomanie ou trichotillomanie). Ann Dermatol Venereol 1889; 10:440–441.
300. Christenson GA, Popkin MK, Mackenzie TB, Realmuto GM. Lithium treatment of chronic hair pulling. J Clin Psychiatry 1991; 52:116–120.
301. Swedo SE, Leonard HL, Rapoport JL, Lenane MC, Goldberger EL, Cheslow DL. A double-blind comparison of clomipramine and desipramine in the treatment of trichotillomania (hair pulling). N Engl J Med 1989; 321:497–501.
302. George MS, Brewerton TD, Cochrane C. Trichotillomania (hair pulling). N Engl J Med 1990; 322:470–471.
303. Dech B, Budow L. The use of fluoxetine in an adolescent with Prader–Willi syndrome. J Am Acad Child Adolesc Psychiatry 1991; 30:298–302.
304. Pollard CA, Ibe O, Krojanker DN, Kitchen AD, Bronson SS, Flynn TM. Clomipramine treatment of trichotillomania: A follow-up report on four cases. J Clin Psychiatry 1991; 52:128–130.
305. Walsh KH, McDougle CJ. Trichotillomania. Presentation, diagnosis and therapy. Am J Clin Dermatol 2001; 2(5):327–333.
306. Lenane MC, Swedo SE, Rapoport JL, et al. Rates of obsessive compulsive disorder in first degree relatives of patients with trichotillomania: A research note. J Child Psychol Psychiatry 1992; 33(5):925–933.
307. Adam BS, Kashani JH. Trichotillomania in children and adolescents: Review of literature and case report. Child Psychiatry Hum Dev 1990; 20:159–168.
308. Comings DE, Comings BG. A controlled study of Tourette syndrome I–VII. Am J Hum Genet 1987; 41:701–866.
309. Lipinski JF. Clomipramine in the treatment of self-mutilating behaviors. N Engl J Med 1991; 324:1441.
310. Leonard HL, Lenane MC, Swedo SE, Rettew DC, Rapoport JL. A double-blind comparison of clomipramine and desipramine treatment of severe onychophagia (nail biting). Arch Gen Psychiatry 1991; 48(10):922–927.
311. Jacobs BW, Isaacs S. Pre-pubertal anorexia nervosa: A retrospective controlled study. J Child Psychol Psychiatry 1986; 27:237–250.
312. Annibali JA, Kales JD, Tan TL. Anorexia nervosa in a young man with Tourette's syndrome. J Clin Psychiatry 1986; 47:324–326.
313. Larocca FEE. Gilles de la Tourette's (the movement disorder): The association of a case of anorexia nervosa in a boy. Int J Eat Disord 1984; 3:89–93.
314. Guarda AS, Treasure J, Robertson MM. Eating disorders and Tourette syndrome: A case series of comorbidity and associated obsessive compulsive symptomatology. CNS Spectr 1999; 4(2):77–86.
315. Comings DE. Tourette Syndrome and Human Behavior. Duarte, CA: Hope Press, 1990.
316. Kurlan R, Kersun J, Ballantine HT Jr, Caine ED. Neurosurgical treatment of severe obsessive compulsive disorder associated with Tourette's syndrome. Mov Disord 1990; 5:152–155.

317. Alsobrook JP II, Pauls DL. A factor analysis of tic symptoms in Gilles de la Tourette's syndrome. Am J Psychiatry 2002; 159:291–296.
318. Leckman JF, Pauls DL, Zhang H, et al. Obsessive-compulsive symptom dimensions in affected sibling pairs diagnosed with Gilles de la Tourette syndrome. Am J Med Genet. In press.
319. Nestadt G, Samuels JF, Riddle MA, et al. Obsessive compulsive disorder: Defining the phenotype. J Clin Psychiatry 2002; 63(suppl. 6):5–7.
320. Pato MT, Pato CN, Pauls DL. Recent findings in the genetics of OCD. J Clin Psychiatry 2002; 63(suppl. 6):30–33.

5

New Directions in the Treatment of Comorbid Attention Deficit Hyperactivity Disorder and Tourette's Syndrome

Donna R. Palumbo

University of Rochester School of Medicine and Dentistry
Rochester, New York, U.S.A.

INTRODUCTION

Attention deficit hyperactivity disorder (ADHD) is a common neurodevelopmental syndrome with symptom onset typically by age 7, and often symptoms are evident between the ages of 3 and 5 years. Prevalence rates for ADHD vary depending on methodology. However, the majority of studies report prevalence rates of 3–6% within a school-aged population, but those receiving treatment are at the lower end of the prevalence rate (1).

Tourette's syndrome (TS) is also common, occurring in 1–3% of school-age children (2–4). For the majority of these children, tics are accompanied by a comorbid psychiatric condition with symptom severity warranting treatment. In fact, most children with TS may not require medication to manage tics, but rather medications to manage their comorbid conditions, which can be more impairing than the tics themselves. It is estimated that 50–75% of children with TS will have comorbid ADHD (5,6). The high rate of comorbidity between ADHD and TS is hypothesized to involve shared pathophysiology of basal ganglia circuitry (7–9).

The diagnosis and effective treatment of ADHD in a child with TS can be critical to their academic, social, and interpersonal functioning. The school performance of a child with TS may be impaired by various combinations of several problems, but associated ADHD appears to be the most important contributing factor (6). In a recent study of social and emotional adjustment in 72 children with TS, tic severity and frequency was not associated with social, behavioral, or emotional functioning even after controlling for the effects of medication. However, ADHD diagnosis was found to be highly correlated with those outcomes (10).

The Diagnosis of Attention Deficit Hyperactivity Disorder

Attention deficit hyperactivity disorder is primarily characterized by two groups of core symptoms: (1) inattention and (2) hyperactive and impulsive behaviors. These symptoms represent disturbances in the spheres of cognition and motor functioning. Currently, the DSM-IV (11) categorizes ADHD into three major subtypes: (1) Predominantly Inattentive Type (Table 1), (2) Predominantly Hyperactive/Impulsive Type (Table 2), and (3) Combined Type. Combined Type is the most common with about 60% of children with ADHD having symptoms of both inattention and hyperactivity/impulsivity. More boys than girls tend to have predominantly Hyperactive/Impulsive Type and more girls than boys tend to have predominantly Inattentive Type. Because the Inattentive Type is a disruption of cognitive function that may not always be evident in overt behavior, girls tend to be underdiagnosed or diagnosed at a later age than boys. However, in TS, there may be a higher rate of Inattentive-Type ADHD in both genders than is seen in primary ADHD.

Table 1 DSM-IV Criteria: Symptoms Necessary for Inattentive Subtype of ADHD

Carelessness
Difficulty sustaining attention during activity
Trouble following through
Avoids tasks requiring sustained mental effort
Difficulty organizing
Loses important items
Easily distracted
Forgetful in daily activities
Does not appear to be listening when spoken to directly

Manifestation of the following symptoms occurs often. Must have six or more symptoms for a period of 6 months to a degree that is maladaptive and inconsistent with developmental level.

Table 2 DSM-IV Criteria: Symptoms Necessary for Hyperactive/Impulsive Subtype of ADHD

Hyperactivity
Squirms and fidgets
Cannot stay seated
Runs/climbs excessively
On the go/driven by a motor
Talks excessively
Cannot perform leisure activities quietly
Impulsivity
Blurts out answer
Cannot wait turn
Intrusive/interrupts others

Manifestation of the following symptoms occurs often. Must have six or more symptoms for a period of 6 months to a degree that is maladaptive and inconsistent with developmental level.

In addition to meeting symptom-specific criteria, children must also meet impairment criteria for ADHD to be a valid diagnosis.

The diagnosis of ADHD is made based on history, observation, and medical evaluation. Tools that are useful in obtaining observational data include teacher and parent rating scales of childhood behaviors, including those associated with ADHD. Most commonly used are the Conners Parent (CPRS) and Teacher (CTRS) Rating Scales (12).

In children with TS, excluding other comorbid conditions that can also disrupt attention is critical. Because obsessive compulsive disorder (OCD) is also highly comorbid with TS, this is an important differential to consider. Children with OCD may have attentional problems because of their obsessions, which can result in internal preoccupation and lack of appropriate attention to external stimuli. Similarly, children who suppress their tics may experience attentional problems simply because of the extent of mental energy they expend focusing on tic suppression, leaving little in reserve for focusing on other task. Anxiety disorders, depression, and other psychiatric problems can also result in "pseudo-ADHD" symptoms; that is, symptoms that mimic ADHD, wherein the etiology is not ADHD but another disorder. The differential of attentional dysfunction is critical to the effective treatment of the symptoms, because management significantly differs depending on the underlying cause. In many TS cases, ADHD co-occurs with OCD or other mood and anxiety disorders, and multiple modes of treatment are necessary.

Treatment Issues

The most effective treatment of ADHD is multimodal, and includes medication, academic accommodations, and behavioral interventions. The recent MTA study (13) demonstrated that when a multimodal approach to ADHD treatment was implemented, 68% of the subjects attained "normalized" behavior. While behavioral therapy alone may not be fully effective in controlling ADHD symptoms in the majority of cases, behavioral treatments are a powerful adjunct to medication management.

Medication management remains the mainstay of current treatment for ADHD, especially because behavioral specialists are simply not available in many communities. In this chapter, both medication options and psychosocial interventions will be discussed.

PHARMACOTHERAPIES

The Stimulant Controversy

In the past, treatment of ADHD in children with TS has been highly controversial. However, current research demonstrating safety and efficacy of stimulant therapy in this population is shedding empirical light on this issue. While stimulant medications are the mainstay of treatment for children with ADHD and methylphenidate (MPH) is the most commonly used stimulant (14), the controversy over using stimulants in children with TS began decades ago, based largely on observational data. Stimulant use has been associated with a reported worsening of tics in many children with TS (15). However, some have argued that the natural history of the disorders, with ADHD symptoms typically appearing before tics, led to a mistaken causal association between stimulant use for treatment of ADHD and tic expression. It was postulated then that in most cases, tics would have occurred even without stimulant use. In addition, others argued that the observed worsening of tics in TS patients treated with stimulants may actually be a result of the natural waxing and waning course of tics. These disparate views led to an ongoing controversy in the field.

The earliest reports of a possible causative role for MPH in precipitating or exacerbating tics occurred during the 1970s, with reported increased risk estimated at 10–53% (16,17). This led to the Food and Drug Administration (FDA) issuing a "black box" warning contraindicating the use of stimulant medications in TS patients or even in children with ADHD who have a family history of tics or TS. In general practice, clinicians have largely adopted this recommendation.

The early data regarding stimulant-induced tics were mainly observational or anecdotal with little empirical evidence to support the findings. For example, between 1974 and 1977, MPH was cited as the cause of tics in 25% of a total of 256 cases of children with ADHD and special-education needs (18). However, data from our own epidemiological study of tics in a school-based population revealed a rate of 23.4% in a special-education population (n = 341) independent of medication status (19). Even in the regular education population, tic rates were higher than previously reported (18.5%; n = 1,255). A mainstream school epidemiological study conducted in the U.K., where stimulant use is quite rare, reported similar prevalence rates (2). Thus tic rates in children have been grossly underestimated and higher tic rates seem to have been falsely correlated with MPH use.

Conversely, several researchers reported that stimulant therapy can be highly effective for treating ADHD in children with TS and that the potential benefits may outweigh the possible disadvantage of tic exacerbation. In the 1980s, retrospective studies by some clinicians led to reports that stimulants are well tolerated by many patients with tic disorders (20,21). Following these reports was a study by Price et al. (22) in which they followed six pairs of monozygotic twins with TS who were discordant for stimulant treatment. They found no clear relationship between the onset of tics and stimulant use. Interestingly, the stimulant-treated twins had a tendency toward lower tic severity in the long term.

The first clinical trial reported was a four-case, single-blind comparison of the effects of MPH in patients with ADHD and a tic disorder (23), in which suppression of tics was reported. Law and Schachar (24) reported a random assignment crossover study between MPH and placebo in 91 children with ADHD with and without comorbid tics. They found no significant difference between the placebo and MPH groups in tic development and exacerbations. Gadow et al. (25) followed with a double-blind study in which robust dose-related improvement in ADHD symptoms was demonstrated, with subtle increases in motor tic frequency on one measure, and no differences in tic frequency and severity across 12 other measures. They followed with another well-designed study of 29 subjects with mild to moderate TS and ADHD who were treated for 2 years with MPH and concluded that treatment with MPH does not result in long-term exacerbation of vocal or motor tics (26). Data from a double-blind, placebo-controlled study comparing both MPH and dextroamphetamine in subjects with severe TS and ADHD yielded interesting results. While about 21% of the subjects in the MPH arm experienced a transient increase in tics, these diminished over time in the majority of children. However, tic severity increased in 25% of the dextroamphetamine group, and only 1 child out of 20 demonstrated any waning of tic severity over time (27). Thus we have some evidence that tics may respond differentially to the type of stimulant, with amphetamine-based compounds being more problematic than MPH.

In 1996, the Treatment of ADHD in Children with Tourette's Syndrome (TACT) clinical trial was initiated (6). This was a multicenter, double-blind, placebo-controlled, parallel groups, 2 × 2 factorial design investigation of MPH and clonidine, used alone or in combination, for the treatment of ADHD in children with a comorbid chronic tic disorder. The study was designed to assess the efficacy of the study medications for the symptoms of ADHD and their influence on tic severity, as well as to obtain further data regarding the safety of MPH and clonidine, particularly when combined. This was the first large-scale study of either MPH or clonidine, as well as the combination, in this population. A double-blind observation period of 16 weeks was employed in this trial, which is longer than the observation period in almost all prior studies. The results of this study demonstrated MPH to be effective for the symptoms of ADHD in this population, with the magnitude of the effect of MPH on ADHD comparable to that found in many studies of MPH-responsiveness in primary ADHD with a similar dosage level (average 26 mg/day). Surprisingly, the study demonstrated that not only was MPH not associated with a worsening of tics but that tic severity lessened at all measured time points during MPH therapy. Thus these results indicate that prior concerns that MPH worsens tics and that the drug should be avoided in patients with tics or a family history of such do not hold for most patients. Recently, additional scientific data has supported the observation that use of MPH to treat ADHD in children with TS is safe and effective and, in general, does not lead to tic exacerbation. If tic exacerbation does occur, it tends to be transient and tics return to baseline without having to discontinue treatment.

As a result of this growing body of research, the NIH consensus statement on ADHD reports minimal risk of tic development with stimulant use (28). However, despite the overwhelming scientific data to the contrary, to date the FDA has refused to critically examine this evidence and the "black box" warning to avoid treatment in children with tics remains on most stimulants.

With the advent of long-acting MPH products, stimulant treatment choices for children with ADHD and tics have expanded. Long-acting MPH products have the advantage of fewer side effects owing to eliminating the peaks and troughs in plasma levels found with short-acting MPH and minimizing "rebound" phenomena (29). While no empirical data is yet available, it is our experience that long-acting MPH treatments are better tolerated in children with TS and ADHD than short-acting MPH treatments and are the treatment of choice for many of our TS clinic patients. Data we presented from the pivotal trials of OROS-MPH ("Concerta") (30), an osmotically releasing MPH product that provides about 12 hr of effective treatment in one dose, demonstrate little effect on tics (31). In these studies, Concerta was well tolerated in children with a preexisting tic disorder. Only 40 out of 407 children (9.8%) in the long-term, open-label study experienced tics, with those children who had a history of tics reporting a similar number of tic episodes (1.57) to those children with no history of tics. The majority of tic episodes experienced were mild or moderate in intensity and severe tics were an extremely rare occurrence. Only 2% of children ($n = 8$) discontinued treatment because of tics during the long-term, open-label study. The percentage of children experiencing tics each month during the first 12 mo of the open-label study remained constant (~5%).

Newer long-acting stimulants include Metadate CD, Ritalin LA, and Adderall XR. Metadate CD and Ritalin LA are both MPH products that utilize a beaded delivery system that provides about 8 hr of effective treatment in one dose and can be sprinkled. Adderall XR is an amphetamine-based compound that also has a beaded delivery system, can be sprinkled, and provides about 12 hr of effective treatment with one dose. Of all the long-acting stimulants, Adderall XR has the greatest side-effect profile. Focalin is a shorter-acting MPH product in which the L-isomer has been removed and only has the D-isomer retained. Therefore fewer side effects are reported with Focalin with similar rates of efficacy as seen with other stimulants. In the future, an MPH patch will become available for continuous release of MPH for up to 24 hr. See Table 3 for stimulant type and dosing information.

Alpha-Agonists

Because of the pharmacological controversies of using stimulants in TS patients, alternative medications have been investigated. The alpha-agonists are most commonly used, mainly clonidine and guanfacine. Both are imidazoline derivatives and act primarily as agonists at presynaptic α_2-noradrenergic receptors. Based on the hypothesis that ADHD is pathophysiologically related to an overactive noradrenergic system (32–35), it is reasonable to suggest that the alpha-agonists may be beneficial in managing ADHD in children with TS. They have the added benefit of offering some tic suppression as well, and several studies have reported that clonidine is an effective tic-suppressing medication (6,36–38). Some authors also reported that clonidine was even more beneficial for associated behavior problems, including ADHD and aggressive and oppositional behavior (39). However, early, small-scale, double-blind studies yielded inconsistent results regarding the efficacy of clonidine for tics and ADHD in children with TS (39,40). Clonidine use also became controversial when, in 1995, three cases of sudden death in children receiving combined treatment with MPH and clonidine were reported. While the authors of the two papers discussing these cases concluded that there was no convincing evidence of any dangerous interaction between the drugs (41,42), both authors decried the need for controlled clinical trials of safety and efficacy for this drug combination in children with ADHD. The previously cited TACT trial (6) addressed these issues in a large-scale study of clonidine, MP, and the combination of both for treatment. In this study, the greatest magnitude of effect on ADHD symptoms was found in the combination treatment. However, clonidine alone was found to significantly

Table 3 Dosing Information for Stimulants

Brand name	Generic name	How supplied	Daily dose (mg)	Duration of action (hr
Ritalin	Methylphenidate HCI	Tablets: 5, 10, and 20 mg	2.5–60	4
Ritalin SR	Methylphenidate HCI, sustained release	Tablets: 20 mg	20–60	8
Ritalin LA	Methylphenidate, extended release	Capsules: 20, 30, and 40 mg Can be sprinkled	20–60	8
Focalin	D-methylphenidate	Tablets: 2.5, 5, and 10 mg	2.5–20	4
Metadate ER	Methylphenidate, extended release	Capsules: 10 and 20 mg	10–60	6
Metadate CD	Methylphenidate, controlled delivery	Capsules: 20 mg Can be sprinkled	20–60	9
Concerta	OROS-methylphenidate	Capsules: 18, 27, 36, and 54 mg	18–72	12
Adderall	D-,L-amphetamine	Tablets: 5, 10, 20, and 30 mg Can be sprinkled	2.5–60	6
Adderal XR	D-,L-amphetamine, extended release	Capsules: 5, 10, 15, 20, 25, and 30 mg Can be sprinkled	5–30	12
Dexedrine	Dextroamphetamine	Tablets: 5 mg	2.5–40	4
Dexedrine Spansule	Dextroamphetamine, sustained release	Capsules: 5, 10, and 15 mg	5–40	8
Cylert	Pemoline	Tablets: 18.75, 37.5, and 75 mg Chewable tablets: 37.5 mg	18.75–112.5	12

improve ADHD symptoms and appeared to have the greatest effect on impulsivity and hyperactivity based on item analysis of the Conners Rating Scales. Clonidine also lessened tics. Importantly, there were no serious safety concerns that emerged for patients in the clonidine or combination treatment arms, in which all subjects received periodic ECGs.

Clonidine should be started as a single bedtime dose (0.05 mg) and carefully titrated over a period of 2–4 weeks, as this minimizes side effects, particularly sedation. The medication is given in two to four divided doses per day. The onset of action of clonidine may be delayed for 8–12 weeks. The total daily dose of clonidine ranges from 0.05 to 0.6 mg/day.

Guanfacine has emerged as a popular treatment choice for children with TS and ADHD. Similar to clonidine, it is thought to dampen tics while improving ADHD symptoms, but with a lower rate of sedation than with clonidine. In addition, dosing is less frequent; thus guanfacine use is more convenient. Three open-label studies of guanfacine, with a total of 36 subjects, have been reported (43–45). These studies showed promising results for tic reduction, but not for ADHD symptoms. Scahill et al. (46) demonstrated reduction of tics in a double-blind, placebo-controlled, 8-week trial of guanfacine in 34 children with tic disorders and comorbid ADHD. Tic severity decreased by 31%, but there was no significant difference between the placebo and treatment groups on reduction of ADHD symptoms as measured by the hyperactivity index of the Conners Parent Questionnaire. Both groups demonstrated a reduction in ADHD symptoms. On a continuous performance test, the treatment group demonstrated a significant improvement in performance. Therefore guanfacine may be effective at improving the more cognitive components of ADHD, but not very effective at reducing the overt behavioral symptoms. In a double-blind, placebo-controlled crossover comparing guanfacine to dextroamphetamine for the treatment of ADHD in a small adult sample, similar rates of efficacy were reported for guanfacine as dextroamphetamine (47). However, dextroamphetamine was preferred by the subjects, who reported it increased "motivation," whereas guanfacine did not. Large studies will be necessary to further determine guanfacine's efficacy in a comorbid TS/ADHD population. Guanfacine daily doses range from 0.5 to 4 mg/day, given at bedtime or twice daily.

Antidepressants

Because both the dopaminergic and noradrenergic systems have been implicated in the pathophysiology of ADHD, antidepressants have long been of interest in its treatment. Tricyclics have been considered second-line agents for the treatment of ADHD. However, in children with TS and ADHD, their use is limited because of reported effects on tics. As with stimulants, contradictory findings have been reported of tic precipitation (48), exacerbation (49–51), improvement (52,53), and neutral effects (54,55). Spencer et al. (56) examined the efficacy of nortriptyline in children with ADHD and a comorbid tic disorder. This was an open-label study of 12 male children in which improvement of ADHD and decreased tic severity was reported over a 19-mo follow-up period. The same group also investigated open-label desipramine treatment in 33 children with ADHD and comorbid tic disorders and obtained similar results (57). All of these studies are limited in that they were either case reports or not well-controlled. Given the concerns regarding side effects of tricyclics, including sudden death, and reduced efficacy for ADHD in comparison to stimulants, the use of tricyclics in this population has been waning, but may be of benefit in children with a comorbid mood disorder.

Buproprion, which affects dopaminergic and noradrenergic mechanisms, has also been touted as a second-line agent to treat ADHD. A single-blind trial (58) demonstrated moderate to marked improvement in global behavioral measures in a small sample of children who were diagnosed with ADHD or conduct disorder. Conners et al. (59) demonstrated efficacy in a 6-week, randomized, double-blind, parallel group, placebo controlled study of 109 children diagnosed with ADHD. They found significant benefits but at effect sizes lower than those found in stimulant studies. A small, double-blind study ($n = 15$) of children and adolescents with ADHD compared buproprion with methylphenidate and found comparable efficacy on ADHD and global ratings (60). However, this study employed a crossover design with a brief, 2-week washout, which makes interpreting these results problematic. Two small, adult ADHD treatment studies (61,62) demonstrated significant improvement in ADHD symptoms. However, a randomized, double-blind, parallel-group comparison of buproprion to methylphenidate in 30 adults with ADHD did not demonstrate statistically significant improvement on rating scale measures (63). In adult ADHD populations, comorbidity with anxiety and depression is quite high, and measured improvement in ADHD ratings may be secondary to improvement in comorbid symptoms rather than improvement in core ADHD symptoms per se. However, in patients with TS and ADHD, an additional concern is tic exacerbation as reported by Spencer et al. (64) in four patients treated with buproprion, with immediate amelioration upon discontinuation of treatment. Dosing ranges from 300 to 450 mg/day. Problematic with buproprion treatment is delayed onset of action, taking 4–6 weeks to achieve therapeutic levels.

Deprenyl, an MAO-B inhibitor, has been demonstrated in reduce ADHD symptoms in two small studies of children with TS and comorbid ADHD. Jankovic (65) reported significant improvement of ADHD symptoms without tic exacerbation in 26 of 29 children treated in an open-label study. Feigin et al. (66), in a double-blind, placebo-controlled crossover study of 24 children and adolescents with ADHD and comorbid TS, found marginal improvement in ADHD symptoms and tic severity. However, larger studies were not conducted. Buspirone is another medication that demonstrated efficacy in an open-label trial of ADHD children (67), but a large-scale, placebo-controlled, double-blind study was terminated because of lack of effect.

Selective serotonin-reuptake inhibitors (SSRIs) have not yet been studied in this population, nor is their any hypothetical reason to believe they would improve core ADHD symptoms or tics (68). In fact, some agents such as venlafaxine, fluoxetine, and sertraline are associated with behavioral activation and can aggravate symptoms of ADHD (69).

Antipsychotics

In general, although antipsychotic medications are indicated for the treatment of tics, they are generally not used for the treatment of ADHD. In many children with comorbid ADHD and TS, when both tic suppression and control of ADHD are warranted, combination therapy with a stimulant and an alpha-agonist is typically first-line treatment. However, in cases where both tics and ADHD are severe, the combination of a low-dose atypical antipsychotic and a stimulant can be beneficial. Risperidone has been found to be well-tolerated and effective in reducing tics in a double-blind study of 41 adults with TS (70) and has also been found to reduce more severe behavior (e.g., aggression) in a childhood ADHD population (71). In our TS clinic population, risperidone is the most frequently used atypical antipsychotic. Open-label trials of olanzapine (72,73) in children with TS and comorbid ADHD have demonstrated a significant decrease in tic severity, but no effect was found on comorbid ADHD symptoms. Similar findings in TS samples have been reported for ziprasidone (74), pergolide (75), and remoxipride (76).

Novel Agents

Atomoxetine is a nonstimulant medication recently approved by the FDA to treat ADHD. Its mechanism of action is believed to be via blockade of the presynaptic norepinephrine transporter. An open-label trial in children with ADHD demonstrated safety and efficacy, with significant improvement in core ADHD symptoms (77). In a randomized, placebo-controlled trial of atomoxetine in 297 children diagnosed with ADHD, results similarly showed it was safe and well tolerated, with significant improvement in ADHD symptoms as well as improved family and social functioning (78). One problem with atomoxetine is delay of onset of action, requiring 2–4 weeks of therapy before optimal therapeutic responses are achieved. Also, combination treatment with SSRIs must be approached very cautiously. Multicenter trials to assess safety and efficacy of atomoxetine in children with ADHD and comorbid tic disorders are currently underway. For now, atomoxetine's effect on tics is unknown, although it is not expected to have tic-suppressing effects.

Modafanil is an atypical stimulant therapy chemically unrelated to other stimulants. It has been approved for treatment of narcolepsy and has gained some attention as a treatment for ADHD. However, data remains very limited regarding the efficacy of Modafanil in ADHD. Small sample sizes and open-label studies have characterized the studies thus far. Rugino and Copley

(79) recently reported an open-label study in 11 children with ADHD over a 4-week time period. Unblinded ratings showed only modest improvement in the ADHD rating-scale measures. Thus far, the rationale for choosing Modafanil over traditional stimulants for the treatment of children with TS and ADHD has not been established.

Nicotinic agents have been studied in both ADHD and TS populations with varying results. One of the first reports suggesting that nicotine may be useful in treating ADHD was by Levin et al. (80). In a small adult ADHD population, they used active and placebo nicotine patches to demonstrate overall clinical global ratings improvement in the treatment phase. They followed up with an open study of chronic nicotine use and obtained similar results (81). However, neither study demonstrated improvement in core ADHD symptoms as measured by ADHD rating scales. Dursun et al. (82) reported reduction of tics in TS patients treated with nicotine patches in an open study, and Silver et al. (83) reported potentiation of haloperidol with nicotine in a TS population; however, side effects limit chronic use of nicotine. In an 8-week, double-blind, placebo-controlled study of mecamylamine (a selective nicotinic receptor agonist) in 61 children and adolescents with TS, results did not support the drug as a therapy for TS. The authors concluded nicotinic agents are best suited as an adjunct to neuroleptic treatment to suppress tics. Therefore there is scant data to support the use of nicotinic agents to treat comorbid ADHD in a TS population.

Donepezil, which blocks acetylcholinesterase in the central nervous system (CNS), has been tried in patients with comorbid ADHD and TS but not in controlled clinical trials. There are anecdotal reports of improved cognitive functioning in children with a variety of neurodevelopmental syndromes when treated with donepezil. Case reports suggest usefulness as a nonstimulant treatment option (84). Wilens et al. (85) reported a series of five cases in which donepezil was used as adjunctive treatment for ADHD youth, with demonstrated improvement in behavior and functioning. The potential cognitive-enhancing role of cholinergic agents suggests that there may be a treatment effect on executive functioning, which is often impaired in children with TS and ADHD, rather than on the primary symptoms. However, lacking controlled clinical trials, the true effects of this medication on TS and ADHD symptoms and associated cognitive dysfunction are yet to be determined.

PSYCHOSOCIAL TREATMENTS

The most effective treatment of ADHD is multimodal, and includes medication, academic accommodations, and behavioral interventions (13). In the MTA trial, when psychosocial treatment was combined with medication management, children required lower doses of stimulants to achieve normalization of behavior and a higher percentage of children achieved normalization (68%). In children with comorbid TS and ADHD, these interventions are critical in helping the child achieve normal social, academic, and interpersonal skills.

Specific psychosocial techniques have been empirically demonstrated to be effective in reducing core behavioral difficulties in children with ADHD. These are (1) parent training, (2) classroom management, (3) social skills training, and (4) academic skills training.

Parent training focuses on behavior within the family. Parents are taught to implement behavioral strategies to help manage their child's ADHD behaviors. Structured parent training programs such as the COPE program (86) have empirically demonstrated reduction of inappropriate behaviors. Initially, parents attend weekly sessions with a therapist that can last from 8 to 16 weeks. After the initial training period, support and contact with the therapist continues as long as necessary. Often, during major developmental transitions or life stressors, maintenance sessions and relapse prevention sessions are required. Classroom management involves collaboration between teachers and parents to target and reduce inappropriate behaviors. Classroom behaviors are identified and a "Daily Report Card" (DRC) is developed that serves to monitor and change identified behaviors (Fig. 1) (87).

The DRC also serves as a means of communication between parents and teachers. Rewards are determined for acceptable behavior and consequences applied for unacceptable behavior. The rewards and consequences are applied both in school and at home so that there is consistent reinforcement for desired behaviors. If the correct rewards have been identified, this is a highly motivating and effective technique that is easily implemented.

Social skills training occurs in a group setting, and teaches children to improve interactions with peers, resolve conflicts, and manage anger appropriately. The focus is on developing social and behavioral competencies, decreasing aggression, and building self-esteem. Initially, sessions are weekly for anywhere from 8 to 16 weeks, with follow-up programs for generalization of skills and relapse prevention. These are often integrated with the parent and teacher interventions.

Academic skills training targets overall skills necessary for academic success and helps children improve organizational strategies and study habits. Often, this can be achieved via the school system, with a teacher's aid or resource teacher working with the student. While not all of these interventions are available in all communities, the implementation of any of these can significantly improve treatment outcomes.

Under the Individuals with Disabilities Education Act of 1992, children with TS and ADHD are eligible for special classroom accommodations. For many of these children, simple accommodations such as testing modifications, reduced homework load, preferential seating, and a safe place to release tics can significantly improve academic functioning. A significant percentage

Sample Daily Report Card

Child's Name: ______________________ Date: ______________

	Special	Language Arts	Math	Reading	SS/Science
Follows class rules with no more than 3 rule violations per period.	Y N	Y N	Y N	Y N	Y N
Completes assignments within the designated time.	Y N	Y N	Y N	Y N	Y N
Completes assignments at 80% accuracy.	Y N	Y N	Y N	Y N	Y N
Complies with teacher requests. (no more than 3 instances of noncompliance per period)	Y N	Y N	Y N	Y N	Y N
No more than 3 instances of teasing per period.	Y N	Y N	Y N	Y N	Y N

OTHER

Follows lunch rules.	Y	N
Follows recess rules.	Y	N

Total Number of Yeses ____________
Total Number of Noes ____________
Percentage ____________

Teacher's Initials:_______
Comments:

Figure 1 Sample "report card" for monitoring behaviors.

of children with TS will have a comorbid learning disability (88) and testing to identify the specific learning disorder is necessary. For those children, and depending on the type and extent of the disorder, additional school-based accommodations may be necessary, including specialized placements. One of the most common forms of learning problems in children with TS and comorbid ADHD is executive dysfunction, which affects planning, organization, and sequencing skills. Handwriting is often differentially affected as well. All of these problems must be taken into consideration during academic planning. Individualized educational accommodations are also necessary and implemented via the school system with a professional working in conjunction with the schools and the practitioner, parents and school must work together to find the school setting best suited to the child's individual needs.

CONCLUSIONS

The treatment of children with TS and comorbid ADHD requires multimodal therapy for optimal outcome. Medication, psychosocial interventions, and academic accommodations are all integral components of treatment. Previous recommendations to avoid the use of stimulants in children with tics appears unwarranted based on current research findings, particularly for MPH. The alpha-agonists, notably clonidine, have proven to be safe and effective in this population. In our TS clinic population, the vast majority of children with comorbid ADHD are treated with stimulants with good response and few side effects. Often, this is in combination with an alpha-agonist for tic suppression. In severe cases, we augment stimulant therapy with an atypical antipsychotic. There is little other empirical data to support the use of alternate agents, although the antidepressants and most notably buproprion, have been widely used in this population. Novel agents that are currently under investigation hold promise as future treatment options.

ACKNOWLEDGMENT

I thank Lauma Pirvics for completing library searches and Donna LaDonna for preparation of the manuscript.

REFERENCES

1. Goldman LS, Genel M, Bezman RJ, Slanetz PJ. Diagnosis and treatment of attention-deficit/hyperactivity disorder in children and adolescents. Council on Scientific Affairs. American Medical Association. JAMA 1998; 279(14):1100–1107.
2. Mason A, Banerjee S, Eapen V, Zeitlin H, Robertson M. The prevalence of Tourette syndrome in a mainstream school population. Dev Med Child Neurol 1998; 40:292–296.

3. Comings D, Himes J, Comings B. An epidemiologic study of Tourette's syndrome in a single school district. J Clin Psychiatry 1990; 51:463–469.
4. Kurlan R, Whitmore D, Irvine C, Mcdermott M, Como P. Tourette's syndrome in a special education population: a pilot study involving a single school district. Neurol Clin 1994; 44:699–702.
5. Comings D, Comings B. Tourette syndrome: clinical and psychological aspects of 250 cases. Am J Hum Genet 1985; 35:435–450.
6. Kurlan R, Como P, Miller B, Palumbo D, Deeley C, Andresen E, et al. The behavioral spectrum of tic disorders: a community-based study. Neurol Clin 2002; 59:414–420.
7. Sheppard D, Bradshaw J, Purcell R, Pantelis C. Tourette's and comorbid syndromes: obsessive compulsive and attention deficit hyperactivity disorder. Clin Psychol Rev 1999; 19:531–552.
8. Palumbo DR, Maughan A, Kurlan R. Hypothesis III: Tourette's syndrome is only one of several causes of a developmental basal ganglia syndrome. Arch Neurol 1997; 54:475–483.
9. Mink J. Basal ganglia dysfunction in Tourette's syndrome: a new hypothesis. Ped Neurol 2001; 25:190–198.
10. Carter A, O'Connell D, Schultz R, Scahill L, Leckman J, Pauls D. Social and emotional adjustment in children affected with Gilles de la Tourette's syndrome: associations with ADHD and family functioning. J Child Psychol Psychiatry 2000; 41(2):215–223.
11. American Psychiatric Association. Diagnostic and Statistical Manual of Mental Disorders. 4th ed. Washington, DC: American Psychiatric Press, 1994.
12. Conners C. Manual For Conners Rating Scales. Toronto: Multi-Health Systems, 1990.
13. Group MC. 14-Month randomized clinical trial of treatment strategies for attention-deficit/hyperactivity disorder. Arch Gen Psychiatry 1999; 56:1073–1086.
14. Safer D, Krager J. A survey of medication treatment for hyperactive-inattentive students. JAMA 1988; 260:2256–2258.
15. Lowe T, Cohen T, Detlor J, Kremenitzer M, Shaywitz B. Stimulant medications precipitate Tourette's syndrome. JAMA 1982; 247:1729–1731.
16. Denckla M, Bemporad J, Mackay M. Tics following methylphenidate administration: a report of 20 cases. JAMA 1976; 235:1349–1351.
17. Golden G. Gilles de la Tourette's syndrome following methylphenidate administration. Dev Med Child Neurol 1974; 16:76–78.
18. Tanner C, Goldman S. Epidemiology of Tourette syndrome. Neurol Clin 1997; 15:395–402.
19. Kurlan R, Mcdermott M, Deeley C, Como P, Brower C, Eapen S, et al. Prevalence of tics in school children and association with placement in special education. Neurology 2001; 57:1383–1388.
20. Erenberg G, Cruse R, Rothner A. Gilles de la Tourette's syndrome: effects of stimulant drugs. Neurology 1985; 35:1246–1251.
21. Shapiro A, Shapiro E. Do stimulants provoke, cause, or exacerbate tics and Tourette's syndrome? Compr Psychiatry 1981; 22:265–273.
22. Price R, Leckman J, Pauls D, Cohen D, Cohen D, Kidd K. Gilles de la Tourette's

syndrome tics and central nervous system stimulants in twin and non-twins. Neurology 1986; 36:232–237.
23. Sverd J, Gadow K, Paolicelli L. Methylphenidate treatment of attention deficit disorder in boys with Tourette's syndrome. J Am Acad Child Adolesc Psych 1989; 28:574–579.
24. Law S, Schachar R. Do typical clinical doses of methylphenidate cause tics in children treated for attention-deficit hyperactivity disorder? J Am Child Adolesc Psychiatry 1999; 38(3):944–951.
25. Gadow K, Sverd J, Sprafkin J, Nolan E, Eznor S. Efficacy of methylphenidate for attention deficit hyperactivity disorder in children with tic disorder. Arch Gen Psychiatry 1995; 52:444–455.
26. Gadow K, Sverd J, Sprafkin J, Nolan E, Grossman S. Long-term methylphenidate therapy in children with comorbid attention-deficit hyperactivity disorder and chronic multiple tic disorder. Arch Gen Psychiatry 1999; 56:330–336.
27. Castellanos F, Giedd J, Elia J, Marsh W, Ritchie G, Hamburger S, et al. Controlled stimulant treatment of ADHD and comorbid Tourette's syndrome: effects of stimulant and dose. J Am Assoc Child Adolesc Psychiatry 1997; 36:589–596.
28. Statement NC. Diagnosis and treatment of attention deficit hyperactivity disorder (ADHD). 1998: NIH Consensus Statement. 1998:1–37.
29. Swanson J, Connor D, Cantwell D. Combining methylphenidate and clonidine: ill-advised. J Am Acad Child Adolesc Psych 1999; 38:617–619.
30. Group CAS. Initiating concerta (OROS MPH HCI) Qd in children with attention-deficit hyperactivity disorder. J Clin Res 2000; 3:59–76.
31. Palumbo D, on behalf of the Concerta Study Group. ADHD treatment with concerta MPH: effects on tics. 49th Annual Meeting of the American Academy of Child and Adolescent Psychiatry. San Francisco Oct 22–27, 2002. Poster.
32. Zametkin A, Rapoport J. Neurobiology of attention deficit disorder with hyperactivity: where have we come in 50 years? J Am Acad Child Adolesc Psych 1987; 26:676–686.
33. Svensson T, Bunney B, Aghajanian G. Inhibition of both noradrenergic agonist clonidine. Brain Res 1975; 92:291–306.
34. Steere J, Arnsten A. The alpha$_2$-noradrenergic agonist guanfacine improves delayed response performance and calms behavior in young monkeys: relevance to attention-deficit disorder. Soc Neurosci Abstr 1994; 20:831.
35. Arnsten A, Steere J, Hunt R. The contribution of alpha 2-noradrenergic mechanisms of prefrontal cortical cognitive function. Potential significance for attention-deficit hyperactivity disorder. Arch Gen Psychiatry 1996; 53:448–455.
36. Hunt R, Capper L, O'Connell D. Clonidine in child and adolescent psychiatry. J Child Adolesc Psychiatry 1990; 1:87–102.
37. Leckman J, Hardin M, Riddle M, Stevenson J, et al. Clonidine treatment of Gilles de la Tourette's syndrome. Arch Gen Psychiatry 1991; 48:324–326.
38. Goetz C, Tanner C, Wilson R, Carroll V, Como P, Shannon K. Clonidine and Gilles de la Tourette syndrome: double-blind study using objective rating methods. Ann Neurol 1987; 21:307–310.
39. Singer H, Brown J, Quaskey S, Rosenberg L, Mellits E, Denckla M. The treatment of attention-deficit hyperactivity disorder in Tourette's syndrome: a

double-blind placebo controlled study with clonidine and desipramine. Pediatrics 1995; 95:74–81.
40. Hunt R, Minderaa R, Cohen D. Clonidine benefits for children with attention deficit disorder and hyperactivity: report of a double-blind placebo-crossover therapeutic trial. J Am Acad Child Adolesc Psych 1985; 24:617–629.
41. Swanson J, Flockhart D, Udrea D, Cantwell D, Conner D, Williams L. Clonidine in the treatment of ADHD: questions about safety and efficacy. J Adolesc Psychopharmacol 1995; 5:301–304.
42. Popper C. Combining methylphenidate and clonidine: news reports about sudden death. J Child Adolesc Psychopharmacol 1995; 5:157–166.
43. Chappell P, Riddle M, Scahill L, Lynch K, Schultz R, Arnsten A, et al. Guanfacine treatment of comorbid attention-deficit hyperactivity disorder and Tourette's syndrome: preliminary clinical experience. Am Acad Child Adolesc Psych 1995; 34:1140–1146.
44. Horrigan J, Barnhill L. Guanfacine for treatment of attention-deficit hyperactivity disorder in boys. J Child Adolesc Psychopharmacol 1995; 5:215–222.
45. Hunt R, Arnsten A, Asbell M. An open trial of guanfacine in the treatment of attention deficit hyperactivity disorder. J Am Acad Child Adolesc Psych 1995; 34:50–54.
46. Scahill L, Chappell P, Kim Y, Schultz R, Katsovich L, Shepherd E, et al. A placebo-controlled study of guanfacine in the treatment of children with tic disorders and attention deficit hyperactivity disorder. Am Psychiatr Assoc 2001; 158:1067–1074.
47. Taylor F, Russo J. Comparing guanfacine and dextroamphetamine for the treatment of adult attention-deficit/hyperactivity disorder. J Clin Psychopharmacol 2001; 21:223–228.
48. Parraga H, Cochran M. Emergence of motor and vocal tics during imipramine administration in two children. J Child Adolesc Psychopharmacol 1992; 3:227–234.
49. Fras I, Karlage J. The use of methylphenidate and imipramine in Gilles de la Tourette's disease in children. Am J Psychiatry 1977; 134:195–197.
50. Fras I. Gilles de la Tourette's syndrome: effects of tricyclic antidepressants. NY State J Med 1978; 78:1230–1232.
51. Abuzzahab F, Anderson F. Gilles de la Tourette: international registry. Minn Med 1973; 56:492.
52. Messiha F, Knopp W. A study of endogenous dopamine metabolism in Gilles de la Tourette disease. Dis Nerv Syst 1976; 37:470–475.
53. Sandyk R, Bamford C. Beneficial effects of imipramine on Tourette's syndrome. Int J Neurosci 1988; 39:27–29.
54. Dillon D, Salzman I, Schulsinger D. The use of imipramine in Tourette's syndrome and attention deficit disorder: case report. J Clin Psychiatry 1985; 46:348–349.
55. Sverd J, Curley A, Jandorf L, Volkersz L. Behavior disorder and attention deficits in boys with Tourette syndrome. J Am Acad Child Adolesc Psych 1988; 27:413–417.
56. Spencer T, Biederman J, Wilens T, Steingard R, et al. Nortriptyline treatment of children with attention deficit hyperactivity disorder and tic disorder or Tourette's syndrome. J Am Acad Child Adolesc Psych 1993; 32:205–210.

57. Spencer T, Biederman J, Kerman K, Steingard R, et al. Desipramine treatment of children with attention deficit hyperactivity disorder and tic disorder or Tourette's syndrome. J Am Acad Child Adolesc Psych 1993; 32:354–360.
58. Simeon JG, Ferguson H, Van Wyck Fleet J. Bupropion effects in attention deficit and conduct disorders. Can J Psychiatry 1986; 31:581–585.
59. Conners K, Casat C, Gualtien T, Weller E, Reader M, Reiss A, et al. Bupropion hydrochloride in attention deficit disorder with hyperactivity. Am Acad Child Adolesc Psych 1996; 35:1314–1321.
60. Barrickman L, Perry P, Allen A, Kuperman S, Arndt S, Herrmann K, et al. Bupropion versus methylphenidate in the treatment of attention-deficit hyperactivity disorder. Am Acad Child Adolesc Psych 1995; 34:649–657.
61. Wender P, Reimherr FW. Bupropion treatment of attention-deficit hyperactivity disorder in adults. Am J Psychiatry 1990; 147:1018–1020.
62. Wilens T, Spencer T, Biederman J, Girard K, Doyle R, Prince J, et al. A controlled clinical trial of bupropion for attention deficit hyperactivity disorder in adults. Am Psychiatr Assoc 2001; 158:282–288.
63. Kuperman S, Perry P, Gaffney G, Lund B, Bever-Stille K, Arndnt S, et al. Bupropion SR vs. methylphenidate vs. placebo for attention deficit hyperactivity disorder in adults. Ann Clin Psychiatry 2001; 1:129–134.
64. Spencer T, Biederman J, Steingard R, Wilens T. Bupropion exacerbates tics in children with attention deficit hyperactivity disorder and Tourette's disorder. J Am Acad Child Adolesc Psych 1993; 32:211–214.
65. Jankovic J. Deprenyl in attention deficit associated with Tourette's syndrome. Arch Neurol 1993; 50:286–288.
66. Feigin A, Kurlan R, Mcdermott M, Beach J, Dimitsopulos T, Brower C, et al. A controlled trial of deprenyl in children with Tourette's syndrome and attention deficit hyperactivity disorder. Am Acad Neurol 1996; 46:965–968.
67. Malhotra S, Santosh P. Mrcpsych. An open clinical trial of buspirone in children with attention deficit/hyperactivity disorder. Am Acad Child Adolesc Psych 1998; 37:364–371.
68. Emslie G, Walkup J, Pliszka S, Ernst M. Nontricyclic antidepressants: current trends in children and adolescents. Am Acad Child Adolesc Psych 1999; 39:517–528.
69. Olvera R, Pliszka S, Luh J, Tantum R. An open trial of venlafaxine in the treatment of attention-deficit/hyperactivity disorder in children and adolescents. J Child Adolesc Psychopharmacol 1996; 6:241–250.
70. Bruggeman R, Van Der Linden C, Buitelaar J, Gericke G, Hawkridge S, Temlett J. Risperidone versus pimozide in Tourette's disorder: a comparative double-blind parallel-group study. J Clin Psychiatry 2001; 62:50–56.
71. Bramble D, Cosgrove P. Parental assessments of the efficacy of risperidone in attention deficit hyperactivity disorder. Clin Child Psychol Psychiatry 2002; 7:225–233.
72. Budman C, Gayer A, Lesser M, Shi Q, Bruun R. An open-label study of the treatment efficacy of olanzapine for Tourette's disorder. J Clin Psychiatry 2001; 62:290–294.
73. Stamenkovic M, Schindler S, Saschauer H, Dezwaan M, Willinger U, Kasper S. Effective open-label treatment of Tourette's disorder with olanzapine. Int Clin Psychopharmacol 2000; 12:23–28.

74. Sallee F, Kurlan R, Goetz C, Singer H, Scahill L, Law G, et al. Ziprasidone treatment of children and adolescents with Tourette's syndrome: a pilot study. Am Acad Child Adolesc Psych 2000; 39:292–299.
75. Gilbert D, Sethuraman G, Sine L, Peters S, Sallee F. Tourette's syndrome improvement with pergolide in a randomized double-blind, crossover study. Am Acad Neurol 2000; 54:1310–1315.
76. Buitelaar J, Choen-Kettenis P, Vlutters H, Westenberg H, et al. Remoxipride in adolescents with Tourette's syndrome: an open pilot study. J Child Adolesc Psychopharmacol 1996; 5(2):121–128.
77. Spencer T, Beiderman J, Heiligenstein J, Wilens T, Faries D, Prince J, et al. An open-label, dose-ranging study of atomoxetine in children with attention deficit hyperactivity disorder. J Child Adolesc Psychopharmacol 2001; 11:251–265.
78. Michelson D, Faries D, Wernicke J, Kelsey D, Kendrick K, Sallee F, et al. Atomoxetine in the treatment of children and adolescents with attention-deficit/hyperactivity disorder: a randomized, placebo-controlled, dose-response study. Pediatrics 2001; 108:E83.
79. Rugino T, Copley T. Effects of modafinil in children with attention-deficit/hyperactivity disorder: an open-label study. Am Acad Child Adolesc Psych 2001; 40:230–235.
80. Levine E, Conners C, Sparrow E, Hinton S, Erhardt D, Meck W, et al. Nicotine effects on adults with attention-deficit/hyperactivity disorder. Psychopharmacology 1996; 123:55–63.
81. Levin E, Conners C, Silva D, Canu W, March J. Effects of chronic nicotine and methylphenidate in adults with attention deficit/hyperactivity disorder. Exp Clin Psychopharmacol 2001; 9:83–90.
82. Dursun S, Reveley M. Differential effects of transdermal nicotine on microstructured analyses of tics in Tourette's syndrome: an open study. Psychol Med 1997; 27:483–487.
83. Silver A, Shytle R, Philipp M, Wilkinson B, Mcconville B, Sanberg P. Transdermal nicotine and haloperidol in Tourette's disorder: a double-blind placebo-controlled study. J Clin Psychiatry 2001; 62:707–714.
84. Hoopes S. Donepezil for Tourette's disorder and ADHD. J Clin Psychopharmacol 1999; 19:381–382.
85. Wilens TE, Biederman J, Wong J, Spencer TJ, Prince JB. Adjunctive donepezil in attention deficit hyperactivity youth: case series. J Child Adolesc Psychopharmacol 2000; 10(3):217–222.
86. Cunningham C. Improving availability, utilization, and cost efficacy of parent training programs for children with disruptive behavior disorders. In: Peters R, Mcmahon R, eds. Preventing Childhood Disorders, Substance Abuse, and Delinquency: Banff International Behavioral Science Series. 1996:374.
87. Atkins M, Pelham W, Licht M. The development and validation of objective classroom measures for conduct and attention deficit disorders. Advances in Behavioral Assessment of Children and Families. Greenwich, CT: JAI Press, 1988:3–33.
88. Kurlan R, Fett K, Parry K, Como P. School problems in Tourette's syndrome. Ann Neurol 1991; 30:275–276.

6

Anxiety and Other Comorbid Emotional Disorders

Barbara J. Coffey
New York University Child Study Center
New York, New York, U.S.A.

Deborah Frisone
McLean Hospital
Belmont, Massachusetts, U.S.A.

Loren Gianini
Massachusetts General Hospital
Cambridge, Massachusetts, U.S.A.

INTRODUCTION: TOURETTE'S DISORDER AND EMOTIONAL COMORBIDITY

Anxiety, mood, and other emotional symptoms have been described in patients with Tourette's disorder (TD) for many years. In 1899, in "La Maladie des Tics Convulsif," the first scientific paper on behavioral and emotional aspects of Tourette's syndrome, de la Tourette described "fears, phobias, and arithmomania" in his original report on nine cases (1). In *Studies on Hysteria*, Freud described facial tics and nervousness in Frau Emmy Von N, who may have had TD, and, in 1907, in *Tics and Their Treatment*, Meige and Feindel described a patient with Tourette's disorder who probably had both obsessive–compulsive disorder (OCD) and depression (2,2a).

In recent years, there has been increasing recognition of the clinical and scientific significance of comorbid emotional and behavioral disorders in TD

(3–15). Although the majority of studies on comorbidity in TD have focused on OCD and attention-deficit/hyperactivity disorder (ADHD) (16–20), the extant literature suggests that other anxiety and mood disorders may also complicate the course of TD in clinically referred patients (16,21–26). This is not surprising, given that both ADHD and OCD are frequently comorbid with mood and other anxiety disorders (23,27–30). However, there have been few rigorous studies of mood and non-OCD anxiety disorders in clinically referred individuals with TD.

The prevalence of comorbid mood and anxiety symptoms and disorders is reported to be rather high in clinical settings, particularly in specialty clinics (24,31,32). This observation could derive from several potential sources, including ascertainment bias that individuals who seek specialty clinical evaluation are likely to be more severely afflicted and meet criteria for more than one disorder compared those who do not seek specialty evaluation. However, a recent study by our group suggests that this may not be the case, and that comorbid disorders are highly prevalent in youth with TD, even in general child and adolescent psychiatry settings.

Subjects were all consecutively referred children and adolescents meeting DSM-III-R diagnostic criteria for TD on structured diagnostic interviews ascertained through a specialized TD clinic ($n = 103$) and a general pediatric psychopharmacology clinic ($n = 92$) within the same academic medical center (Tables 1 and 2). Although specialized in pediatric psychopharmacology, the latter program was not a tertiary care service because approximately half of the referrals had not been evaluated or treated before. All children in both programs were comprehensively evaluated using the same assessment battery that included the Children's Schedule for Affective Disorders and Schizophrenia for School-Age Children—Epidemiological Version (K-SADS-E)

Table 1 Clinical and Demographic Characteristics of Nonspecialized and Specialized Clinic Patients with TD

	Nonspecialized clinic patients ($n = 92$)		Specialized clinic patients ($n = 103$)		Overall significance
	Mean	SD	Mean	SD	p
Current age	10.8	3.23	10.8	3.62	0.89
Socio-economic status (SES)	2.0	1.13	2.2	1.24	0.42
Past GAF	47.9	7.50	48.6	7.57	0.54
Current GAF	51.3	7.32	51.9	6.52	0.55
Gender (% male)	82	90	83	80	0.06

Table 2 Tic Characteristics of Nonspecialized and Specialized Clinic Patients with TD

	Nonspecialized clinic patients (n = 92)		Specialized clinic patients (n = 103)		Overall significance
	Mean	SD	Mean	SD	p
TD impairment (worst ever) (1 = mild; 2 = moderate; 3 = severe)	1.7	0.73	2.2	0.79	0.000
TD impairment (current) (1 = mild; 2 = moderate; 3 = severe)	1.5	0.70	1.7	0.75	0.031
Duration of TD (years)	4.3	3.53	5.3	3.69	0.053
Onset of TD (years)	6.0	2.79	5.5	2.68	0.22
	n	%	n	%	p
Psychiatric hospitalization	13	14	15	14	0.93
Current TD	76	83	101	98	0.000

(33). Subjects from the TD specialty and the general pediatric psychopharmacology clinic ascertainment sources could not be differentiated with regard to past (global assessment of functioning, GAF: 48.6 ± 7.6 vs. 47.9 ± 7.5, ns) or current (GAF: 51.9 ± 6.5 vs. 51.3 ± 7.3, ns) interpersonal functioning, current severity of TD (1.7± 0.75 vs. 1.5 ± 0.7, ns), mean age of onset of TD (5.5 ± 2.7 vs. 6.0 ± 2.8 years, ns), or duration of TD (5.3 ± 3.7 vs. 4.3 ± 3.5 years, ns). However, small but statistically significant differences were observed in the rate of current TD (98% vs. 83% respectively; $p < 0.005$) and lifetime tic severity (2.2 ± 0.8 vs. 1.7± 0.73, $p < 0.005$) which were higher in the TD specialty clinic patients (Table 3).

Lifetime rates of psychiatric comorbidity were overwhelmingly high in youth with TD irrespective of ascertainment source, and rates of individual psychiatric comorbid disorders were almost identical in the two ascertainment groups. The most prevalent comorbid disorder in each clinical setting was ADHD (72% and 84%, ns). However, notable in this study were high lifetime rates of major mood disorders (57% and 60%, ns) and non-OCD anxiety disorders (40% and 35%, ns), which were overall more prevalent than lifetime rates for OCD (36% and 21%, ns).

Children and adolescents who met criteria for TD on structured diagnostic interviews shared very similar clinical correlates, irrespective of their ascertainment source through specialized or nonspecialized TD pro-

Table 3 Comorbidity of TD Subjects by Ascertainment Site

	Nonspecialized clinic patients (n = 92)		Specialized clinic patients (n = 103)		Overall significance
Diagnosis	n	%	n	%	p
Pure (noncomorbid) TD	2	2	5	5	0.31
Mood disorders					
Major depressive disorder	45	49	56	54	0.49
Any bipolar disorder	20	22	16	16	0.24
Dysthymia	9	10	4	4	0.09
Any mood disorder	55	60	59	57	0.65
Anxiety disorders					
Panic disorder	10	11	15	15	0.45
Agoraphobia	21	23	27	26	0.61
Social phobia	15	16	5	5	0.008
Simple phobia	25	27	30	30	0.73
OCD	19	21	37	36	0.021
Overanxious disorder	29	32	32	32	0.97
Separation anxiety	22	24	39	39	0.028
Multiple (2+) anxiety disorders (not OCD)	32	35	41	40	0.47

grams. Overall rates of mood and non-OCD anxiety disorders were high (34).

ANXIETY DISORDERS AND TD

A bidirectional relationship between TD and OCD is apparent in most clinically referred patient cohorts (16,35,36). Obsessive–compulsive symptoms or OCD has been reported in 20–60% of Tourette's patients (37); patients with OCD have about a 7% lifetime risk of TD (28) and 20% risk of tics (29). Family studies indicate that OCD is found at a higher rate in close relatives of individuals with TD than in controls, independent of OCD symptoms in the proband, which further supports this bidirectional relationship (19,38,39).

TD and OCD share many common features, including a waxing and waning course, repetitive behaviors and complex movements or rituals, preoccupation with sexual and aggressive themes, and partially voluntary suppression of symptoms with subsequent buildup of inner tension. In addition, previous studies have suggested that patients with TD plus OCD have higher levels of disability than those without comorbid OCD (3,6,9, 23,40).

In contrast, although comorbidity with OCD has long been recognized as associated with a more severe TD phenotype (6,18,41–43), very little is known about the role of non-OCD anxiety disorders in TD patients. However, non-OCD anxiety disorders may be more frequent in TD patients than in the general population, and encompass a wide range of conditions that can also be associated with significant morbidity and dysfunction (21,23,44,45).

Investigators have described elevated rates of trait anxiety, phobias, panic attacks, and generalized anxiety disorder in TD patients (17,44). Although Comings and Comings (17) reported that there was no correlation between the number of tics and phobias in his study of TD and anxiety, fear of crowds and of being alone significantly differentiated TD severity groups (mild, moderate, and severe). In a study of 47 children with ADHD and chronic tics dichotomized by tic severity, Nolan et al. (46) reported that rates of separation anxiety and overanxious disorder were higher in the groups with more severe tics. Pitman et al. (23) studied 16 adult patients with TD, 16 with OCD, and 16 controls, and reported that both the TD and OCD groups had high rates of generalized anxiety disorder compared to controls. In several studies, Robertson et al. (44,47) reported elevated rates of anxiety symptoms (both obsessive–compulsive and non-OCD) in adults with TD in a clinical sample, compared to normal controls. Similarly, Cath et al. (48) reported elevated rates of anxiety symptoms on the Spielberger State–Trait Anxiety Inventory in a clinical sample of adults with TD compared to normal controls.

In a recent study of a clinical sample of 190 children with Tourette's disorder, non-OCD anxiety disorders, in general, and separation anxiety disorder, in particular, were highly associated with tic severity. In this study, 190 subjects evaluated in a TD specialty clinic were divided into Mild/ Moderate and Severe tic severity groups. No meaningful differences in age of onset of TD (5.7 ± 2.6 and 5.9 ± 3.0 years) or duration of TD were noted when controlling for age. As expected, the severe TD group had more impairment in psychosocial functioning as indicated by lower GAF scores (past 44.5 ± 6.4 vs. 49.8 ± 7.5, $p < 0.001$; current 48.3 ± 5.9 vs. 53.0 ± 6.9, $p < 0.001$).

Psychiatric comorbidity was overwhelmingly present irrespective of tic severity status (94.8% for Mild/Moderate TD and 100% for Severe TD) (Table 4). Examination of comorbidity with anxiety disorders revealed that although OCD was overrepresented among the Severe TD cases, the difference failed to reach threshold for statistical significance (42% vs. 25% for Severe and Mild/Moderate TD, respectively, $p < 0.02$). However, with the

Table 4 Comorbidity by TD Severity of Sample with Mild/Moderate vs. Severe TD (n = 190)

	Mild/moderate TD (n = 134)		Severe TD (n = 56)		Significance (χ^2)
Diagnosis	n	%	n	%	p
Any comorbidity	127	94.8	56	100	0.08
Mood disorders					
Major depressive disorder	66	49.3	33	58.9	0.22
Bipolar disorder	19	14.2	16	28.6	0.02
Dysthymia	9	6.7	4	7.1	0.92
Any mood disorder	75	56.0	36	64.3	0.29
Anxiety disorders					
Panic disorder	12	9.0	13	23.2	0.01
Agoraphobia	25	19.0	22	39.3	0.001
Social phobia	14	10.5	6	10.7	0.97
Simple phobia	34	25.6	21	38.2	0.08
OCD	33	24.8	23	41.8	0.02
Overanxious disorder	36	27.1	25	45.5	0.01
Separation anxiety	32	24.2	28	50.9	0.001
Any anxiety disorder	71	53.0	39	69.6	0.03
Multiple (≥2) anxiety disorders	43	32.3	30	53.6	0.01

exception of social and simple phobia, all other anxiety disorders were significantly overrepresented among Severe TD subjects including panic disorder (23% vs. 9%, $p < 0.01$), agoraphobia (39% vs. 19%, $p < 0.01$), separation anxiety disorder (51% vs. 24%, $p < 0.001$), and overanxious disorder (46% vs. 27%, $p < 0.01$). It is noteworthy that separation anxiety disorder was the disorder that most robustly predicted high tic severity, even when controlling for the presence of OCD or other anxiety disorders (OR 2.98, $p < 0.001$). These findings revealed the importance of non-OCD anxiety disorders as risk factors for tic severity in children with TD.

Because in this sample patients with OCD had a greater likelihood of non-OCD anxiety disorders, it is possible that OCD could be a modulator of tic severity. Although OCD is frequently comorbid with other anxiety disorders (28,49,50), these findings suggested that specific associations exist between tic severity and non-OCD anxiety disorders that are not accounted for by the presence of OCD alone.

Evidence that anxiety may contribute to tic severity is supported in the frequent exacerbation of tics that occur in children with TD before return to school, and in the tic ameliorative effects of the high-potency benzodiazepine anxiolytic, clonazepam (51,52). The α-adrenergic agonist, clonidine, and tricyclic antidepressants such as desipramine may also ameliorate tics through their putative anxiolytic effects (53–58). Considering the documented anxiogenic effects of neuroleptics in TD patients (59–61), it is possible to speculate that increased doses of neuroleptics during periods of tic exacerbation may render the patient more susceptible to anxiety, and thus more likely to experience increased tics.

In addition, it is also possible that anxiety-associated hyperarousal could result in central nervous system noradrenergic spikes that may disrupt or hypersensitize cortico-striatal–thalamic–cortical (CSTC) circuits postulated to be involved in the production of tics (16,62–65).

MOOD DISORDERS AND TD

Patients with TD have been reported to score higher than normal controls on psychopathology ratings for depression (44). Robertson et al. administered three standardized self-reports of psychopathology (Leyton Obsessional Inventory, Beck Depression Inventory, and Spielberger State–Trait Anxiety Inventory) to 22 adults with TD, 19 with major depression (MD), and 21 normal controls. Results indicated that the groups with TD and MD scored significantly higher than the comparison group on all measures, although scores on the depression scale were lower in the TD than in the MD group (44). Comings (66) and Comings and Comings (67) reported on the Diagnostic Interview Schedule for mood disorders that 23% of the TD patients had a clinically significant score as compared to 2% of the control group (66,67). Pitman et al. (23) studied 16 patients with TD, 16 with OCD, and 16 controls, and reported that both the TD and OCD groups had high rates of unipolar depressive disorders. In a study of personality disorders in TD, Robertson et al. (44,47) reported significantly elevated rates of depressive symptoms on the Beck Depression Rating Scale in adults in a clinical sample, compared to normal controls. Similarly, Cath et al. (48) reported elevated rates of depressive symptoms on the Montgomery–Asberg Depression Rating Scale in a clinical sample of adults with TD, compared to normal controls.

Interestingly, high rates of bipolar disorder have been reported in clinical samples of patients with TD. Kerbeshian et al. (68) reported that bipolar disorder was overrepresented in a community sample of Tourette's disorder patients. Similarly, Berthier and Campos (69) reported a high lifetime prevalence for general psychopathology in 90 selected adult TD patients seen on a neurology service, and that 30 (33%) met criteria for bipolar disorder. More recently, in a study of clinically referred youth with TD, our team reported high rates of mood disorders and a significant association between mood disorders and overall illness morbidity as measured by the need for psychiatric hospitalization (Tables 5 and 6). Subjects were 156 consecutively referred children and adolescents (ages 5–20 years) with TD ascertained through an outpatient pediatric psychopharmacology program at a major academic medical center. All subjects were comprehensively evaluated with a clinical interview by a child and adolescent psychiatrist and an assessment battery that included K-SADS-E (33).

Nineteen (12%) of the 156 children and adolescents with TD required psychiatric hospitalization. Although tic severity was marginally significant as a predictor of psychiatric hospitalization ($p < 0.05$), major depression ($p < 0.016$) and bipolar disorder ($p < 0.001$) were robust predictors of psychiatric hospitalization, even after adjusting for all other variables. In addition to psychiatric hospitalization, results were also evaluated using GAF score as a binary variable with GAF < 50 as the dependent measure in a multiple logistic regression. This analysis confirmed that when GAF score < 50 was the outcome variable, the strongest predictor variables remained bipolar disorder ($p < 0.001$) and major depression ($p < 0.001$) (26).

The high prevalence rate for bipolar disorder in children with severe tics is both novel and intriguing. Although the diagnosis of childhood mania

Table 5 Demographic and Clinical Characteristics of TD Illness ($n = 156$)

	No hospitalization ($n = 137$)		Past hospitalization ($n = 19$)		Significance (χ^2)
	Mean	SD	Mean	SD	p
Current age	10.5	3.0	14.4	3.2	0.001
SES	2.1	1.1	2.5	1.5	ns
Past GAF	51.0	6.1	37.9	6.4	0.001
Current GAF	53.7	5.7	44.7	8.3	0.001
	n	%	n	%	
Gender (% male)	112	82.4	16	84.2	ns
TD duration	4.5	3.2	6.9	4.7	0.0058
TD impairment (worst ever)[a]					0.007
Mild	52.0	38.5	2.0	11.1	
Moderate	52.0	38.5	6.0	33.3	
Severe	31.0	23.0	10.0	55.6	

[a] $p = 0.003$ between mild and severe.

Table 6 Comorbidity of Hospitalized vs. Nonhospitalized TD Subjects (n = 156)

	No hospitalization (n = 137)		Past hospitalization (n = 19)		Significance
Diagnosis	n	%	n	%	p
Mood disorders					
Major depressive disorder	59	43.4	17	89.5	0.001
Bipolar disorder	13	9.6	11	57.9	0.001
Dysthymia	10	7.4	0	0	ns
Any mood disorder	68	50	18	94.7	0.001
Anxiety disorders					
Panic disorder	14	10.3	7	36.8	0.002
Agoraphobia	30	22.4	6	31.6	ns
Social phobia	15	11.1	4	21.1	ns
Simple phobia	43	31.9	4	21.1	ns
OCD	30	22.1	10	52.6	0.004
Overanxious disorder	36	26.7	11	61.1	0.003
Separation anxiety	36	26.9	9	50	0.044
Multiple (2+) anxiety disorders (not OCD)	47	34.8	10	52.6	ns
Any anxiety disorder	77	56.6	13	68.4	ns

remains controversial, recent studies document that it can be reliably made when using structured diagnostic interview methodology (70). Interestingly, the rate of comorbid bipolar disorder observed in this sample of youth with TD is consistent with findings reported in adults with TD (68). In addition, because severe affective dysregulation, often manifested by temper outbursts and aggression, is characteristic of juvenile bipolar disorder (71,70), it is possible that the explosive outbursts ("rage attacks") recently reported in a substantial minority of youth with TD (3) may be a manifestation of undiagnosed bipolar disorder.

ETIOLOGY OF THE RELATIONSHIP BETWEEN TOURETTE'S SYNDROME AND EMOTIONAL DISORDERS

Anxiety and mood disorders observed in clinically referred youth with TD may result from several factors. It is possible that there may be an etiologic association between TD and emotional disorders at a rate higher than chance. Recently developed neurobiological models support theoretical relationships between movement and emotion, primarily through contiguous pathways in the basal ganglia, thalamus, and cortex (4,16,72–74). Motor, vocal, behavioral, cognitive, and emotional dysfunction may represent manifestations of an underlying core disinhibition problem in patients with TD (16).

In addition, adjustment to living with a chronic and potentially socially impairing illness is likely to result in a variety of emotional reactions and self-esteem vulnerabilities. Repeated experiences of demoralization, sadness, social anxiety, and inhibition could render the child more vulnerable to adjustment disorders with mixed anxiety and/or depressive features or more chronic and recurrent syndromes. Some studies have reported that children with TD have difficulty with peer relations and social skills, which could lead to subsequent emotional reactions including anxiety and depression (75). Finally, neuroleptic treatment, often used to ameliorate tics, has been reported to be associated with dysphoria, depression, and separation anxiety symptoms (61,76,77).

Whatever the etiology, in clinical settings, emotional symptoms are very common and may often be more problematic to the patient than the tics. These symptoms and disorders need to be comprehensively identified and differentiated from tics because they will require specific intervention and treatment.

DIAGNOSTIC EVALUATION OF COMORBID EMOTIONAL DISORDERS

Diagnostic evaluation in clinical samples of youth with TD should include a comprehensive assessment of the entire emotional comorbidity spectrum, including OCD, non-OCD anxiety disorders, and mood disorders. Structured or semistructured diagnostic interviews, such as the Diagnostic Interview Schedule for Children (DISC) or the K-SADS, can supplement multiaxial DSM-IV classification. These diagnostic instruments can facilitate the evaluation of these disorders, in that they can provide both lifetime and current history and thus avoid errors of omission. If use of a structured or semistructured diagnostic instrument is not feasible, then systematic psychiatric assessment of emotional symptoms using formal diagnostic criteria, such as the fourth edition of the American Psychiatric Association's *Diagnostic and Statistical Manual of Mental Disorders* (78), is recommended.

Rating instruments can provide quantitative measures of tic severity, such as frequency and intensity. Standardized rating scales such as the Yale Global Tic Severity Scale (Y-GTSS) rate tics-related impairment (79). Specific rating scales for OCD (the Children's Yale-Brown Obsessive–Compulsive Scale or C-YBOCS), anxiety, and mood disorders are also recommended (80).

Quantitative measures of nontic features can be helpful in the prioritization of target symptoms for treatment.

TREATMENT CONSIDERATIONS

For patients with clinically significant comorbid emotional symptoms or disorders, treatment should tailored to the specific diagnostic category or symptoms of most concern. Education regarding the nature of the comorbid disorder, parent guidance, referral to support groups, and ongoing monitoring are essential for all patients and their families. Children with very few mood and anxiety symptoms and/or mild tics may need only supportive monitoring, or brief supportive therapy.

Those youth with emotional disorders of clinical concern should be treated, regardless of tic severity. Multimodal treatment of TD plus the mood or anxiety disorder are indicated, combining pharmacological agents and individual and/or family therapy. Often a combination of medication with cognitive or behaviorally oriented therapy is helpful. Parent guidance and support are essential. Monotherapy with a "broad-spectrum" agent, if feasible, is recommended as the initial pharmacological approach. Selection of one agent that is likely to address as many of the primary symptoms as possible is a reasonable starting point. For example, for a child with TD plus OCD or depression, in which anxiety or depressive symptoms are causing the most distress or impairment, monotherapy with a selective serotonin-reuptake inhibitor (SSRI) is recommended as a first-line approach. A child with comorbid TD and early-onset bipolar disorder is a candidate for first-line treatment with an atypical neuroleptic such as risperidone, olanzapine, or ziprasidone. Both the tics and major mood disorder are likely to respond to the atypical neuroleptic.

Often, clinically referred youth with TD meet criteria for several comorbid psychiatric disorders of clinical significance such as ADHD, OCD, and major depression. In this situation, patients may require the simultaneous use of more than one medication to ameliorate both tics and emotional symptoms. This approach, described as "targeted combined pharmacotherapy," involves the careful, judicious use of more than one medication simultaneously. The combined use of risperidone and fluoxetine would be an example of a combination used to treat both tics and obsessive–compulsive disorder. This approach should be carefully monitored and periodically reevaluated because both tics and emotional symptoms wax and wane.

Medication trials should be initiated by the introduction of one medication at a time, especially if targeted combined pharmacotherapy is necessary. The primary goal of treatment should be an adequate trial of each agent in terms of dosage and duration. For the majority of patients, medication should be initiated at a low (usually subtherapeutic) dose and gradually titrated upward. Therapeutic effects and side effects should be closely monitored, especially when more than one agent is administered simultaneously. Medication interactions, especially through the P450 cytochrome oxidase liver enzyme system, may be more likely when targeted combined pharmacotherapy is used, especially with the use of selective serotonin reuptake inhibitors.

The decision as to the duration of medication trials will depend on a variety of factors including efficacy, adverse effects, potential for long-term toxicity, and the natural history of the patient's individual course. Converging evidence suggests that tics may diminish over time, as the child moves into adolescence; however, long-term follow-up studies of the course of mood and anxiety disorders in the context of TD are lacking (81–83).

Children and adolescents with TD and comorbid emotional disorders may also be candidates for nonpharmacological intervention. Cognitive behavioral approaches are indicated for OCD and can be used for non-OCD anxiety disorders such as separation anxiety disorder and specific phobias. Cognitive–behavioral and interpersonal or supportive therapy can be helpful for mood disorders.

SUMMARY

In summary, emotional symptoms are very common in clinically referred children and adolescents with TD. Although the etiology of the relationship between TD and mood and non-OCD anxiety disorders is not known, it is possible that there are neurobiological, familial, and psychosocial stressors/life event factors that contribute multifactorially to the clinical picture. Emotional disorders such as anxiety and depression may be more problematic to the patient than the tics, with regard to overall illness severity and the potential for adverse outcomes such as school and social failure. The emotional symptoms and comorbid mood and anxiety disorders must be comprehensively identified and differentiated from tics because they will require specific intervention and treatment. More studies of the course, treatment, and outcome of mood and anxiety disorders in TD patients are needed.

REFERENCES

1. de la Tourette G. La maladie des tics convulsifs. Sem Med 1899; 19:153–156.
2. Breur J, Freud S. The Standard Edition: Studies on Hysteria. Vol. 2. (1883–1895). Frau Emmy von N. 48–105. London: Hogarth Press.

2a. Meige H, Feindel E. Tics and Their Treatment. New York: William Wood, 1907.
3. Bruun R, Budman C. The course and prognosis of Tourette syndrome. In: Jankovic J, ed. Tourette Syndrome. Neurologic Clinics. Vol. 15. Philadelphia: WB Saunders, 1997:291–298.
4. Cohen DJ, Friedhoff AJ, Leckman JF, Chase TN. Tourette syndrome. Extending basic research to clinical care [review]. Adv Neurol 1992; 58:341–362.
5. Comings DE, Comings BG. A controlled study of Tourette syndrome: II. Conduct. Am J Hum Genet 1987; 41:742–760.
6. Comings DE, Comings BG. A controlled study of Tourette syndrome: IV. Obsessions, compulsions, and schizoid behaviors. Am J Hum Genet 1987; 41:782–803.
7. Kerbeshian JBL, Klug Marilyn. Comorbid Tourette's disorder and bipolar disorder: an etiologic perspective. Am J Psychiatry 1995; 152(11):1646–1651.
8. Leckman JF, Pauls DL, Peterson BS, Riddle MA, Anderson GM, Cohen DJ. Pathogenesis of Tourette syndrome. Clues from the clinical phenotype and natural history [review]. Adv Neurol 1992; 58:15–24.
9. Leonard HL, Swedo SE, Rapoport JL, et al. Tourette syndrome and obsessive–compulsive disorder [review]. Adv Neurol 1992; 58:83–93.
10. Nolan E, Sverd J, Gadow K, Sprafkin J, Ezor S. Associated psychopathology in children with both ADHD and chronic tic disorder. J Am Acad Child Adolesc Psychiatry 1996; 35:1622–1630.
11. Park S, Como PG, Cui L, Kurlan R. The early course of the Tourette's syndrome clinical spectrum. Neurology 1993; 43:1712–1715.
12. Riddle MA, Leckman JF, Hardin MT, Anderson GM, Cohen DJ. Fluoxetine treatment of obsessions and compulsions in patients with Tourette's syndrome [letter]. Am J Psychiatry 1988; 145:1173–1174.
13. Spencer T, Biederman J, Harding M, Wilens T, Faraone S. The relationship between tic disorders and Tourette's syndrome revisited. J Am Acad Child Adolesc Psychiatry 1995; 34:1133–1139.
14. Sverd J. Tourette syndrome and autistic disorder: a significant relationship. Am J Med Genet 1991; 39:173–179.
15. Swedo SE, Leonard HL. Childhood movement disorders and obsessive compulsive disorder. J Clin Psychiatry 1994; 55:32–37.
16. Cohen DJ, Leckman JF. Developmental psychopathology and neurobiology of Tourette's syndrome [review]. J Am Acad Child Adolesc Psychiatry 1994; 33:2–15.
17. Comings DE, Comings BG. A controlled study of Tourette syndrome: III. Phobias and panic attacks. Am J Hum Genet 1987d; 41:761–781.
18. de Groot C, Bornstein R, Spetie L, Burriss BA. The course of tics in Tourette's syndrome: a 5-year follow-up study. Ann Clin Psychiatry 1994; 6:227–233.
19. Pauls DL. The genetics of obsessive compulsive disorder and Gilles de la Tourette's syndrome [review]. Psychiatr Clin North Am 1992; 15:759–766.
20. Swedo S, Rapoport J, Leonard H. Obsessive compulsive disorder in children and adolescents. Arch Gen Psychiatry 1989; 46:335.
21. Coffey B, Frazier J, Chen S. Comorbidity, Tourette syndrome, and anxiety disorders [review]. Adv Neurol 1992; 58:95–104.

22. Comings DE, Comings BG. A controlled study of Tourette syndrome: I. Attention-deficit disorder, learning disorders, and school problems. Am J Hum Genet 1987; 41:701–741.
23. Pitman RK, Green RC, Jenike MA, Mesulam MM. Clinical comparison of Tourette's disorder and obsessive–compulsive disorder. Am J Psychiatry 1987; 144:1166–1171.
24. Robertson MM, Channon S, Baker J, Flynn D. The psychopathology of Gilles de la Tourette's syndrome: a controlled study. Br J Psychiatry 1993; 162:114–117.
25. Coffey B, Biederman J, Geller D, et al. Anxiety disorders and tic severity in juveniles with Tourette's disorder. J Am Acad Child Adolesc Psychiatry 2000; 39:562–568.
26. Coffey B, Biederman J, Geller D, et al. Distinguishing illness severity from tic severity in children and adolescents with Tourette's Disorder. J Am Acad Child Adolesc Psychiatry 2000; 39:556–561.
27. Leonard H, Swedo S, Rapoport J. Treatment of childhood obsessive compulsive disorder with clomipramine and desmethylimipramine: a double blind crossover comparison. Psychopharmacol Bull 1988; 24:93–95.
28. Rasmussen SA, Eisen JL. Epidemiology and clinical features of obsessive–compulsive disorder. In: Jenike M, Baer L, Minichiello W, eds. Obsessive Compulsive Disorder: Theory and Management. Chicago: Year Book Medical Publishers, 1990:10.
29. Swedo S, Rapoport J, Leonard H, et al. Obsessive Compulsive Disorder in children and adolescents. Arch Gen Psychiatry 1989; 46:335.
30. Swedo S, Leonard H, Rapoport J. Childhood onset obsessive compulsive disorder. In: Jenike MA, Baer L, Minichiello WA, eds. Obsessive–Compulsive Disorders: Theory and Management. Boston: Mosby Year Book, 1990:28–38.
31. Stefl ME. Mental health needs associated with Tourette syndrome. Am J Public Health 1984; 74:1310–1313.
32. Singer HS, Rosenberg LA. Development of behavioral and emotional problems in Tourette syndrome. Pediatr Neurol 1989; 5:41–44.
33. Orvaschel H, Puig-Antich J. Schedule for Affective Disorders and Schizophrenia for School-Age Children: Epidemiologic 4th Version. Ft. Lauderdale: Nova University, Center for Psychological Study, 1987.
34. Coffey B, Biederman J, Spencer T, Geller D, Faraone S, Bellordre C. Informativeness of structured diagnostic interviews in the identification of Tourette's disorder in referred youth. J Nerv Ment Dis 2000; 188:583–588.
35. Frankel M, Cummings JL, Robertson MM, Trimble MR, Hill MA, Benson DF. Obsessions and compulsions in Gilles de la Tourette's syndrome. Neurology 1986; 36:378–382.
36. Comings DE, Comings BG. A controlled study of Tourette syndrome: IV. Obsessions, compulsions, and schizoid behaviors. Am J Hum Genet 1987; 41:782–803.
37. Grad LR, Pelcovits D, Olson M, Matthews M, Grad G. Obsessive–compulsive symptomatology in children with Tourette's Syndrome. J Am Acad Child Adolesc Psychiatry 1987; 26:69–73.

38. Pauls DL, Hurst CR, Kruger SD, Leckman JF, Kidd KK, Cohen DJ. Gilles de la Tourette's syndrome and attention deficit disorder with hyperactivity. Evidence against a genetic relationship. Arch Gen Psychiatry 1986; 43:1177–1179.
39. Pauls DL, Raymond CL, Stevenson JM, Leckman JF. A family study of Gilles de la Tourette syndrome. Am J Hum Genet 1991; 48:154–163.
40. Coffey B, Miguel E, Biederman J, Baer L, Rauch S, O'Sullivan R, Savage C, Phillips K, Borgman A, Green-Leibovitz M, Moore E, Park K, Jenike M. Tourette's Disorder with and without Obsessive Compulsive Disorder: are they different? J Nerv Ment Dis 1998; 186:201–206.
41. Bornstein RA. Neuropsychological correlates of obsessive characteristics in Tourette syndrome. J Neuropsychiatry Clin Neurosci 1991; 3:157–162.
42. Kurlan R, Como PG, Deeley C, McDermott M, McDermott MP. A pilot controlled study of fluoxetine for obsessive–compulsive symptoms in children with Tourette's syndrome. Clin Neuropharmacol 1993; 16:167–172.
43. Marcus D, Kurlan R. Tics and its disorders. Neurol Clin 2001; 19:735–758.
44. Robertson MM, Channon S, Baker J, Flynn D. The psychopathology of Gilles de la Tourette's syndrome. A controlled study. Br J Psychiatry 1993; 162:114–117.
45. Comings DE, Comings BG. A controlled study of Tourette syndrome: III. Phobias and panic attacks. Am J Hum Genet 1987; 41:761–781.
46. Nolan E, Sverd J, Gadow K, Sprafkin J, Ezor S. Associated psychopathology in children with both ADHD and chronic tic disorder. J Am Acad Child Adolesc Psychiatry 1996; 35:1622–1630.
47. Robertson M, Banerjee S, Fox Hiley P, Tannoch C. Personality disorders and psychopathology in Tourette's Syndrome: a controlled study. Br J Psychiatry 1997; 171:283–286.
48. Cath D, Spinhoven P, Hoogduin C, et al. Repetitive behaviors in Tourette's Syndrome and OCD with and without tics: what are the differences? Psychiatry Res 2001; 101:171–185.
49. Leonard H, Swedo S, Rapoport J. Treatment of childhood obsessive compulsive disorder with clomipramine and desmethylimipramine; a double blind crossover comparison. Psychopharmacol Bull 1988; 24:93–95.
50. Steingard R, Dillon-Stout D. Tourette's syndrome and obsessive compulsive disorder. Clinical aspects [review]. Psychiatr Clin North Am 1992; 15:849–860.
51. Borison RL, Ang L, Chang S, Dysken M, Comaty JE, Davis JM. New pharmacological approaches in the treatment of Tourette syndrome. Adv Neurol 1982; 35:377–382.
52. Goetz CG. Clonidine and clonazepam in Tourette syndrome [review]. Adv Neurol 1992; 58:245–251.
53. Goetz CG, Tanner CM, Wilson RS, Carroll VS, Como PG, Shannon KM. Clonidine and Gilles de la Tourette's syndrome: double-blind study using objective rating methods. Ann Neurol 1987a; 21:307–310.
54. Leckman JF, Cohen DJ, Detlor J, Young JG, Harcherik D, Shaywitz BA. Clonidine in the treatment of Tourette syndrome: a review of data. Adv Neurol 1982; 35:391–401.

55. Leckman JF, Hardin MT, Riddle MA, Stevenson J, Ort SI, Cohen DJ. Clonidine treatment of Gilles de la Tourette's syndrome. Arch Gen Psychiatry 1991; 48:324–328.
56. Singer H, Brown J, Quaskey S, Rosenberg L, Mellits D, Denckla M. The treatment of attention-deficit hyperactivity disorder in Tourette's syndrome: a double blind placebo controlled study with clonidine and desipramine. Pediatrics 1995; 95:74–81.
57. Spencer T, Biederman J, Kerman K, Steingard R, Wilens T. Desipramine treatment of children with attention deficit hyperactivity disorder and tic disorder or Tourette's syndrome. J Am Acad Child Adolesc Psychiatry 1993; 32:354–360.
58. Bruun RD. Clonidine treatment of Tourette syndrome. Adv Neurol 1982a; 35:403–405.
59. Bruun RD. Dysphoric phenomena associated with haloperidol treatment of Tourette syndrome. Adv Neurol 1982b; 35:433–436.
60. Bruun RD. Subtle and underrecognized side effects of neuroleptic treatment in children with Tourette's disorder. Am J Psychiatry 1988; 145:621–624.
61. Linet LS. Tourette syndrome, pimozide, and school phobia: the neuroleptic separation. Am J Psychiatry 1985; 142:613–615.
62. Peterson B, Riddle MA, Cohen DJ, et al. Reduced basal ganglia volumes in Tourette's syndrome using three-dimensional reconstruction techniques from magnetic resonance images. Neurology 1993; 43:941–949.
63. Riddle MA, Leckman JF, Anderson GM, et al. Plasma MHPG: within- and across-day stability in children and adults with Tourette's syndrome. Biol Psychiatry 1988a; 24:391–398.
64. Riddle MA, Leckman JF, Anderson GM, et al. Tourette's syndrome: clinical and neurochemical correlates. J Am Acad Child Adolesc Psychiatry 1988b; 27: 409–412.
65. Singer HS, Hahn IH, Krowiak E, Nelson E, Moran T. Tourette's syndrome: a neurochemical analysis of postmortem cortical brain tissue. Ann Neurol 1990; 27:443–446.
66. Comings BDAC. A controlled study of Tourette Syndrome: V. Depression and mania. Am J Hum Genet 1987; 41:804–821.
67. Comings DE, Comings BG. A controlled family history study of Tourette's syndrome: III. Affective and other disorders. J Clin Psychiatry 1990; 51:288–291.
68. Kerbeshian J, Burd L, Klug M. Comorbid Tourette's disorder and bipolar disorder: an etiologic perspective. Am J Psychiatry 1995; 152:1646–1651.
69. Berthier MLJK, Campos VM. Bipolar disorder in adult patients with Tourette's syndrome: a clinical study. Biol Psychiatry 1998; 43:364–370.
70. Biederman J, Faraone S, Mick E, et al. Attention-deficit hyperactivity disorder and juvenile mania: an overlooked comorbidity? J Am Acad Child Adolesc Psychiatry 1996; 35:997–1008.
71. Wozniak J, Biederman J, Kiely K, et al. Mania-like symptoms suggestive of childhood onset bipolar disorder in clinically referred children. J Am Acad Child Adolesc Psychiatry 1995; 34:867–876.
72. Demeter S. Structural imaging in Tourette syndrome [review]. Adv Neurol 1992; 58:201–206.

73. Singer HS, Walkup JT. Tourette syndrome and other tic disorders. Diagnosis, pathophysiology, and treatment [review]. Medicine 1991; 70:15–32.
74. Wolf SJ, Jones DW, Knable M, Gorey J, Lee KS, Hyde T, Coppola R, Weinberger D. Tourette syndrome: prediction of phenotypic variation in monozygotic twins by caudate nucleus D2 receptor binding. Science 1996; 1225–1227.
75. Stokes A, Bawden HN, Camfield PR, Backman JE, Dooley JM. Peer problems in Tourette's disorder. Pediatrics 1991; 87:936–942.
76. Bruun RD. Subtle and underrecognized side effects of neuroleptic treatment in children with Tourette's disorder. Am J Psychiatry 1988; 145:621–624.
77. Mikkelsen EJ, Detlor J, Cohen DJ. School avoidance and social phobia triggered by haloperidol in patients with Tourette's disorder. Am J Psychiatry 1981; 138:1572–1576.
78. American Psychiatric Association. Diagnostic and Statistical Manual of Mental Disorders. 4th ed. Washington, DC: American Psychiatric Press, Inc., 1994.
79. Leckman JF, Riddle MA, Hardin MT, et al. The Yale Global Tic Severity Scale: initial testing of a clinician-rated scale of tic severity. J Am Acad Child Adolesc Psychiatry 1989; 28:566–573.
80. Goodman WK, Price LH, Rasmussen SA, Mazure C, Delgado P, Heninger GR, Charney DS. The Yale-Brown Obsessive Compulsive Scale: II. Validity. Arch Gen Psychiatry 1989; 46:1012–1016.
81. Leckman J, Zhang H, Vitale A, et al. Course of tic severity in Tourette's syndrome: the first two decades. Pediatrics 1998; 102:14–19.
82. Coffey B, Biederman J, Geller D, et al. The course of Tourette's disorder: a literature review. Harv Rev Psychiatry 2000; 8:192–198.
83. Burd LK, Klug A, Benz B. Long-term follow-up of an epidemiologically defined cohort of patients with Tourette syndrome. J Child Neurol 2001; 16:431–437.

7

Aggressive Symptoms and Tourette's Syndrome

Cathy L. Budman
New York University School of Medicine
New York
and North Shore University Hospital
Manhasset, New York, U.S.A.

Lori Rockmore
Mount Sinai School of Medicine
New York, New York, U.S.A.

Ruth Dowling Bruun
New York University School of Medicine
Westhampton Beach, New York, U.S.A.

OVERVIEW

Aggressive symptoms encompass heterogeneous behaviors, ranging from milder temper tantrums and recurrent verbal aggression to self-injurious behaviors, serious physical assault, and destruction of objects. Aggressive symptoms in Tourette's syndrome (TS) are common in clinical settings where approximately 25–70% of TS patients report anger control problems, irritability, and recurrent behavioral outbursts (1–6). In a descriptive study of 3500 individuals with TS surveyed worldwide using a multisite, international database, 37% reported a history of anger control problems and 25% described current problems with anger control (4). An uncontrolled clinical study of

64 TS patients in Japan reported aggressiveness and impulsivity in 48%, self-injurious behaviors in 20.3%, and domestic violence in nearly 11% (7).

Aggressive symptoms in TS are common in community samples as well (8,9). In a community survey conducted by the Tourette Syndrome Foundation of Canada among the 446 respondents aged 6–78 years, 21.4% of children and 15% of adults reported problems with aggression and 30% of children and 19% of adults reported problems with temper control (5). A community-based survey in Sweden of 58 children identified with TS aged 5–15 years revealed that 35% of these children were considered by their teachers to have major problems secondary to a variety of aggressive symptoms including repeated verbal aggression, physical aggression, or destructive tendencies (10).

However, the high rates of psychiatric comorbidity in most TS samples (11), medication-induced behavioral toxicity or side effects (12,13), misdiagnosis (14), as well as varying definitions of the TS phenotype (15) have made it difficult to untangle the association between aggressive behaviors and TS. Furthermore, the lack of valid constructs of circumscribed behavioral domains and of standardized measures with interrater reliability using multiple informants to assess these phenomenologically and etiologically complex symptoms has limited many previous studies (16,17). Not withstanding such challenges, the study of aggressive symptoms in TS is of both practical and heuristic interest. When present, aggressive symptoms are a leading cause of morbidity in TS, often resulting in psychiatric hospitalization, residential placement, and severe family distress (18–22). In addition, the study of aggressive symptoms in TS, which are likely to be influenced by environmental, genetic, immunomodulatory, and/or neuroendocrine regulatory factors, may contribute to our understanding of the mechanisms that facilitate or inhibit self-regulation. This chapter will review significant current concepts in the understanding and treatment of aggression and will attempt to examine how theses findings may relate to aggressive symptoms in TS.

Developmental Considerations

The "terrible twos" are considered a normal developmental phase in children characterized by aggressive behaviors such as temper tantrums and noncompliance with adult requests. Typical temper tantrums among preschoolers include throwing oneself on the floor, kicking, screaming, and holding one's breath (23). Among 800 children aged 3–12 attending a general pediatric outpatient clinic in India, 182 (22.8%) were found to have temper tantrums, most commonly in children 3–5 years (75.3%) and least commonly in children aged 9–12 years (3.9%) (24). In this study, temper tantrums were approximately three times more common in boys than girls and more likely to be accompanied by a history of postnatal trauma, seizure disorder, tics, hyperkinesis, enuresis, head banging, and sleep disturbances.

By the time children enter elementary school, most have developed the capacity to tolerate frustration, delay impulses and gratification, inhibit aggressive urges, and follow rules (25,26). The acquisition of self-regulatory skills in physiological, emotional, and behavioral domains represents important maturational milestones; the absence or incompetence of such functioning has profound implications for psychosocial adaptation. Externalizing behavior problems, such as developmentally inappropriate symptoms of aggression and impulsivity, are among the most common forms of childhood maladaption leading to increased risks for academic failure, family conflict, rejection by peers, and low educational, social, and occupational attainment (27). Externalizing symptoms that can be identified in the toddler and preschool years often persist into middle childhood and adolescence (28,29).

While the ability to delay gratification and inhibit impulses improves as children get older, even controlling for age, self-regulation appears correlated with the capacity to focus one's attention and engage with the environment (30,31).

Based on studies in adults and adolescents, it has been proposed that underarousal of the autonomic nervous system, as manifested by low resting heart rate and/or low heart rate variability, reflects a lack of such focus/engagement with the environment and is a core characteristic of aggressive behavior (32,33). However, few studies examining the correlation between resting heart rate and aggression have been conducted on very young children and existing studies report conflicting results (34–36).

In contrast, high heart rate variability as measured by resting respiratory sinus arrhythmia (RSA) appears to be a consistent index of normal emotional reactivity and attentional ability in infants and young children (34,37–40). Preliminary studies show a relationship between externalizing symptoms and lowered heart rate variability in 2-year-old children, 11-year-old boys, and in adolescent boys (34,42,43). Changing heart rate variability in response to external stress may also be an important marker for the ability to effectively allocate attention for problem solving. The observed suppression of RSA in situations where coping and emotional regulation are demanded may reflect physiological mechanisms that facilitate complex responses involved in the regulation of attention and behavior. Failure to suppress RSA under such circumstances may be related to dysregulated behavior and aggression (34,35). Clearly, more studies are needed to investigate how physiological underregulation relates with aggression and whether such underregulation is relevant to the excessive stress reactivity associated with TS.

Disinhibited or increased motoric activity is a common feature of many externalizing behaviors and appears to be a strong predictor of both acute and chronic aggression. In a longitudinal study of trajectories of physical aggression in boys aged 6–15 years, high levels of motoric hyperactivity and oppositional behaviors assessed in kindergarten were demonstrated to be the most powerful predictors of a "high aggression" developmental course; individually, these risk factors increased the risk of aggression by about a factor of 3, but in combination, the risk was increased by more than ninefold (45). This risk may be particularly relevant for children with TS who demonstrate significant motoric hyperactivity preceding the onset of repetitive, involuntary movements ("tics") during early childhood.

In addition to regulating movement, accomplishing goal-directed activities requires the ability to flexibly sustain, shift, and sequence attention. Cognitive control, in contrast to impulsivity, requires the filtering out of irrelevant environmental information and the inhibition of inappropriate psychomotor responses. Emotional regulation, characterized by the amplification, attenuation, or maintenance of a particular emotional state, is an important component of cognitive control. Diminished cognitive control and capacity for goal-directed activities are cardinal symptoms of several neuropsychiatric conditions, including depression. Studies of depressed adults show that self-rumination (i.e., inability to shift focus) tends to exacerbate and prolong depressed moods, whereas the ability to divert attention to something other than the negative mood is an adaptive strategy for reducing tension and anxiety (46–48). Impaired refocusing of one's attention (e.g., due to obsessional thinking or rumination) appears to exacerbate angry states, whereas the ability to engage in activities that are highly absorbing and entertaining can reduce angry states (49,50). Therefore the child who is unable to refocus attention, whether from physiological or meta-cognitive disruptions, is more vulnerable to sustained negative affective states and may be more likely to resort to tantrums or explosive outbursts than his/her nonaggressive counterparts (34).

Problems in attention modulation, development of self-regulation, and behavioral inhibition emerge early in life and demonstrate consistency over time and context (51). Persistent problems in self-regulation manifest in a variety of common childhood psychiatric disorders frequently comorbid with TS, including mood disorders (MD), obsessive-compulsive disorder (OCD), attention-deficit/hyperactivity disorder (ADHD), oppositional defiant disorder (ODD), and conduct disorder (CD).

Types of Aggression

Research methodologies developed for the quantitative study of animal aggression have identified several neuroanatomically and neurophysiologically distinct subtypes (52–55). *Predatory aggression* is characterized by interspecies, offensive behaviors leading to the most efficient elimination of a targeted victim (56). *Intermale aggression* represents intraspecies aggression among males that is typically nonlethal and has the aim of establishing a dominance hierarchy for access to females and food (57). *Territorial aggression*, both intraspecies and interspecies in nature, involves aggression used to define and defend spaces that are also connected with reproductive and food resources and may result in annihilation of the perceived intruder (58). *Maternal aggression* and *fear-induced aggression* are protective aggressive behaviors provoked by perceived threats to the animal's offspring or self (59). *Irritable aggression* encompasses reactive aggressive responses to noxious sensory intrusions such as excessive noise, uncomfortable changes in ambient temperature, starvation, or painful stimuli (59). *Instrumental aggression* includes aggressive behaviors that are learned and reinforced by applying experimental manipulations (60).

The putative existence of similar subtypes of aggression in children has been suggested from clinical studies using observation, laboratory paradigms, and statistical analyses of behavioral characteristics. These subtypes include the following: *hostile* vs. *instrumental* (61), *overt* vs. *covert* (62), *reactive* vs. *proactive* (63), *defensive* vs. *offensive* (64), *affective* vs. *predatory* (65), and *impulsive* vs. *controlled* (66).

Based on levels of physiological arousal, two types of aggressive behaviors, *reactive* and *proactive*, have been defined in children (67). Reactive aggression is characterized by high physiological arousal, disinhibition, and affective instability, whereas proactive aggression (also referred to in the literature as *controlled* or *nonimpulsive aggression*) is accompanied by low levels of physiological arousal and is calculated to attain a specific goal. Examples of proactive aggression reported in TS clinic populations include conduct problems such as bullying, stealing, or cruelty to animals (9,68,69). Symptoms of reactive aggression in TS would include temper outbursts and "rage attacks" (18,70).

Several instruments have been applied to the study of aggressive behaviors in children. Using modified DSM-IV diagnostic criteria for intermittent explosive disorder, the Rage Screen and Questionnaire assesses the presence and characteristics of explosive outbursts in children with TS; however, psychometric data for this screen are not currently available (Budman et al., in press). The Overt Aggression Scale, an observational scale, is designed for use in adults in inpatient settings and can be used to quantify aggression in children (71,72). Scales with items aimed at capturing predatory/proactive and affective/reactive aspects of aggression attempt to address the problem of delineating aggression subtypes (63,65). Several teacher rating scales such as the Teacher's Report Form (TRF) (73), Inattention/Overactivity With Aggression (IOWA) Conners (74), and the New York Teacher

Rating Scale (75) rate the frequency of certain aggressive behaviors. The recently developed Children's Aggression Scale–Parent Version (CAS-P) shows promise as an instrument that assesses a broad range of factors including severity, frequency, pervasiveness, and diversity of aggression while less confounded by other nonaggressive disruptive behaviors and may be of particular value as a research tool (76).

Genetics and Aggression

In contrast to many personality traits, aggression shows no consistent pattern of genetic influence (77). Genetic effects appear to be more relevant to aggression in children and adults but explain little of the variance observed in adolescent aggression (78). While some studies have shown that genetic effects account for approximately 50% of the variance in aggression (79), others have reported insignificant differences between monozygotic (MZ) and dizygotic (DZ) twins when compared using standardized measures of aggressive behavior (80). However, in a study of 182 pairs of male MZ twins and 118 pairs of male DZ twins, Seroczynski et al. (81) found that impulsivity and irritable aggression share more overlapping genetic and environmental influences.

Polymorphisms in genes that regulate the activity of neuromodulators or in genes that code for structural components of relevant brain networks are likely to contribute to individual differences in susceptibility to aggression. There is some evidence that regulatory polymorphism of the monoamine oxidase A gene may be associated with variability in aggression, impulsivity, and central nervous system serotonergic responses (82). Preliminary data also suggest that an allele for tryptophan hydroxylase (TPH) polymorphisms may be associated with suicide attempts in violent offenders and with impulsive aggression in personality-disordered patients (83,84). Studies using both animal models and humans show that alterations in the genes that regulate serotonergic function play an important role in impulsive aggression (85).

Both factor and segregation analyses using data gathered on 128 full siblings and their 54 sets of parents collected by the Tourette Syndrome Association International Consortium for Genetics Affected Sibling Pair Study report that the particular OC symptom dimension characterized by aggressive, sexual, and religious obsessions and checking compulsions is highly heritable (86). Preliminary evidence suggests that susceptibility to explosive outbursts in TS may also be heritable (Matthews, personal communication, 2002).

Neural Substrates of Aggression

The regulation of aggressive behaviors involves a diversity of multiply interacting neurotransmitters including norepinephrine (NE), dopamine

(DA), and serotonin (5-HT). DA, along with opiate, androgen, and adrenocorticotrophin regulatory systems, appear to facilitate expression of sexual behavior and aggression, whereas 5-HT and NE modulate inhibitory responses (87). Disturbances of central serotonergic function have been linked with externally directed aggression and impulsivity in both animal models and humans (88–90).

Earlier studies of depressed adult patients who had committed violent suicidal acts showed low cerebrospinal fluid (CSF) levels of the serotonin metabolite 5-hydroxyindoleacetic acid (5-HIAA) (91). More recent studies have demonstrated low CSF 5-HIAA in adult criminal offenders and armed forces personnel with a history of violence (92).

Abnormal central 5-HT physiology in aggression is also suggested by challenge studies using the 5-HT agonist D-fenfluramine. Normally, D-fenfluramine leads to an increase in prolactin, but this hormone response is blunted in adults with borderline personality disorder and impulsive aggression; the degree of impulsive aggression appears inversely correlated with the prolactin response (93). These results have been replicated using D-fenfluramine in adult patients with impulsive–aggressive personality disorders, using D-fenfluramine in combination with a serotonin antagonist in normal controls, as well as in clinical studies using the direct 5-HT_{2c} agonist metachlorophenylpiperazine (m-CPP) (94–96).

While a relationship between central 5-HT and aggression has been consistently demonstrated in adults, studies in children with disruptive disorders have yielded more conflicting data. A study of children with juvenile-onset obsessive-compulsive disorder and disruptive behaviors indicated an inverse association between 5-HT function and measures of conduct disorder (97). Similarly, in a sample of 6- to 17-year-old boys with disruptive behavior disorders, levels of CSF 5-HIAA were found to be inversely correlated with ratings of aggressive behavior (98). In contrast, a study in 6- to 12-year-old boys with attention-deficit/hyperactivity disorder (ADHD) reported a positive correlation between CSF 5-HIAA and aggression (99), and a study of 15 prepubertal and 8 adolescent males with disruptive behavior found no association between the prolactin response to fenfluramine challenge and measures of aggression (100). After failing to replicate their earlier findings of an enhanced prolactin response to fenfluramine in 10 aggressive boys compared with 15 nonaggressive boys aged 7–11 years with ADHD (101), Halperin et al. combined their original sample with a replication sample to yield a total of 50 children who were then divided into younger (mean age 7.93) and older (mean age 10.08) subgroups. Their analysis suggested that younger aggressive children (i.e., <9.1 years old) had a significantly greater prolactin response to fenfluramine challenge when compared with their nonaggressive counterparts, but no such difference existed in the older age group, implying that aggressive children may undergo different developmental trajectories in 5-HT function (102). While these clinical studies are intriguing, their results must be interpreted cautiously since most did not fully evaluate the potentially confounding variables of additional psychiatric comorbidity and/or medication exposure/side effects.

Disruption of the hypothalamic–pituitary–adrenal (HPA) axis manifested by abnormal cortisol secretion has been reported in association with aggression in violent adult offenders and in aggressive boys with disruptive behavior disorders (103–105). In a study of 38 clinic-referred boys aged 7–12 years with aggression, low salivary cortisol levels were associated with the persistent and early onset of aggression (106). A study of 52 girls aged 15–17 years with conduct disorder compared with 41 normal controls also reported low cortisol levels (107) which is significant given that typically normal females have even higher basal and reactive levels of cortisol than do normal males (108). Among 20 children aged 7–12 years with oppositional defiant disorder or conduct disorder, a challenge experiment using the 5-HT_{2B} and 5-HT_{2d} receptor agonist sumatriptan demonstrated significantly higher peak levels of growth hormone and an absence of the usual cortisol response in comparison with the control group (109).

Animal studies suggest that centrally acting arginine vasopressin (AVP) plays a facilitatory role in aggressive behavior, putatively by its interactions with the serotonin system (110). AVP-containing neurons in the suprachiasmatic and paraventricular nuclei project to limbic areas, including the hippocampus and amygdala, and also play a role in memory acquisition and retrieval (111). There are sexual differences in the density and projections of AVP reactive neurons, which are more numerous in males and sensitive to testosterone (112). Such dimorphism may also contribute to the higher frequency of aggressive behaviors in males compared with females. A potential role for dimorphic extrahypothalmic AVP projections in mediating tic symptoms in TS has been preliminary investigated (113) and may also relate to aggressive symptoms in this disorder.

A study measuring CSF AVP in 26 aggressive adults with personality disorders supports a role for central AVP in enhancing aggressive behavior (114). Although no attempts were made to assess concurrent symptoms of aggression, elevated levels of CSF AVP have been reported in both child and adult OCD patients (115,116). In contrast, in matched samples aged 13–60 years, similar concentrations of CSF AVP were found when 29 patients with OCD, 23 patients with TS, and 31 normal controls were compared (117). While this study also did not evaluate impulsive aggressive symptoms, an increase in oxytocin levels in a subset of patients with OCD independently identified as being without a personal or family history of tic disorders was found that was highly statistically significant (117). CSF oxytocin level was also correlated with current severity of OCD (117). These data emphasize the importance of studying biologically homogenous patient samples since most previous neurophysiological studies of aggression have neglected potentially significant confounding variables such as tic-related and OCD-related status.

NEUROANATOMY AND NEUROIMAGING IN AGGRESSION

Symptoms of aggression may result from a variety of organic etiologies. In a study of 286 cases of explosive rage, Elliot (118) found that 102 patients had developed the condition following a specific brain insult such as closed-head injury, viral encephalitis, stroke, and Huntington's chorea and 184 had a history of explosive outbursts during childhood. A recent study of 145 adults examined 3–12 months after the onset of stroke showed that inability to control anger and aggression occurred in nearly one-third of all poststroke patients and was closely related to motor dysfunction, dysarthria, emotional incontinence, and lesions affection the frontal–lenticulocapsular–pontine base areas (119). Of note, poststroke emotional incontinence and explosive aggression tended to co-occur and shared similar lesion distribution (119). It has been well established clinically and experimentally that lesions in regions of the orbital frontal cortex (OFC) or prefrontal cortex (PFC) produce clinical presentations characterized by aggression and impulsivity (120,121). Specifically, damage to the orbitofrontal cortex appears associated with the greatest risk of reactive aggression (122). Interestingly, this region has also been implicated in obsessive-compulsive disorder and in shifting attentional sets (123). Neuroimaging studies in normal subjects suggest that part of the usual automatic regulatory response that controls the intensity of expressed anger involves activation in the left OFC, anterior cingulate cortex (ACC), and anterior temporal poles bilaterally (124).

Recent structural and functional neuroimaging studies of aggression provide converging evidence implicating abnormal prefrontal and subcortical brain networks (125). Specifically, a circuit encompassing several regions of the PFC, amygdala, hippocampus, hypothalamus, ACC, insular cortex, ventral striatum, and other interconnected structures has been implicated in emotion regulation and cognitive control (126).

The PFC is also a region with a high density of serotonin type-2 receptors that develops more slowly than other brain areas, reaching maturation only late in adolescence (127). Enhanced serotonergic neurotransmission in this region is associated with improved capacity to inhibit impulsive aggression. The acquisition of self-regulatory mechanisms, which emerge and improve gradually during childhood, is believed closely related to the maturation of the PFC. Consequently, processes that interfere with normal

PFC maturation can be expected to be associated with a variety of disinhibited behaviors including aggression.

Using functional MRI (fMRI) to compare normal children aged 8–12 with young adults aged 19–33, Bunge et al. (128) demonstrated an association between immature cognitive control (i.e., decreased capacity to filter out irrelevant environmental information and to inhibit inappropriate responses) in children and an inability to recruit certain PFC regions. Activation of the right ventrolateral PFC during tasks that require subjects to withhold or stop responding, suppress interference from irrelevant stimuli, or shift cognitive sets characteristic of adult response inhibition circuitry did not occur in younger children.

Impulsive aggression has been associated with frontotemporal abnormalities in studies using magnetic resonance imaging (MRI). In a study of 10 violent male psychiatric inpatients with heterogeneous diagnoses including personality disorder and schizophrenia, 6 showed mesial temporal atrophy (129). A quantitative MRI study of patients with temporal lobe epilepsy and affective-impulsive aggression showed amygdala atrophy or periamygdaloid lesions more frequently than in controls (130). A structural MRI study of 21 men from the community diagnosed with aggression and antisocial personality disorder showed an 11% reduction in prefrontal gray matter volume in the absence of discernable brain lesions when compared with 34 healthy subjects, 26 subjects with substance dependence, and 21 psychiatric controls (131).

Metabolic abnormalities in the PFC have been demonstrated in adults with impulsive aggression using positron emission tomography (PET) (132–134). An early PET study of violent male psychiatric inpatients demonstrated decreased cerebral blood flow to the temporal cortex in all cases; two subjects also showed decreased flow to their frontal lobes (135). An inverse relationship between life history of impulsive aggression and regional cerebral glucose metabolism in the orbitofrontal cortex was reported in a PET study of 17 patients with personality disorders (136). In a study of 41 murderers who pled not guilty by reason of insanity compared with 41 normal controls, reduced glucose metabolism in the bilateral prefrontal cortex, the posterior parietal cortex, and the corpus callosum was demonstrated in the experimental subjects. Abnormal asymmetries of activity (left hemisphere lower than right) were found in the amygdala, thalamus, and media temporal gyrus including the hippocampus (137).

In a study of murderers who were dichotomously classified as either impulsive or predatory, the affective, impulsive murderers showed reductions in the lateral PFC metabolism compared with both controls and the predatory group. Increased metabolic rates in subcortical regions of the right hemisphere including the hippocampus, amygdala, thalamus, and midbrain were detected in the impulsive murderers compared with controls and predatory murderers. Prefrontal functioning was reduced in affective murderers compared with control and comparison groups, while subcortical functioning was increased (137). These authors proposed that depending upon the presence of social triggers and early stressful environmental circumstances, increased right hemisphere subcortical activity could predispose individuals to violent behavior.

A single photon emission computerized tomography (SPECT) study of 40 adults with a history of impulsive aggression compared with 40 nonaggressive psychiatric controls showed decreased activity in the prefrontal cortex, increased activity in the anteromedial frontal lobes, increased activity in the left basal ganglia or limbic system or both, and focal left temporal lobe abnormalities (138).

Abnormal metabolism in both cortical and subcortical structures also occurs in subjects with TS and explosive rage. A recent 18-fluorodeoxyglucose PET resting-state study of 12 unmedicated adults with TS that compared seven subjects with rage to five subjects without rage showed left frontal hypometabolism, bilateral caudate hypometabolism more significantly right-sided, left thalamus, and bilateral cerebellum hypermetabolism (Budman et al., unpublished).

Neuroimaging studies have also implicated abnormal serotonin activity in patients with impulsive aggression. Blunted responses to fenfluramine challenge in orbitofrontal, adjacent ventral, medial, and cingulate cortical regions were shown when six impulsive aggressive patients with personality disorders were compared with five control subjects (139). Soloff et al. (140) report a greater response to serotonergic challenge in the orbital and medial prefrontal cortex of control subjects compared with borderline personality disorder subjects. Regional metabolic activity in response to the serotonergic stimulus m-CPP was examined in 13 subjects with impulsive aggression and 13 normal controls using PET. Unlike normal subjects, patients with impulsive aggression did not show activation specifically in the left anteromedial orbital cortex in response to m-CPP. The normally activated anterior cingulate was deactivated in these patients, and in contrast, the posterior cingulate was activated in patients and deactivated in controls. Such data suggest that decreased activation of the inhibitory response to a serotonergic stimulus may be associated with impaired modulation of aggressive impulses (141).

In summary, increasing evidence suggests that impulsive aggression may be due to an impaired capacity for regulating and controlling aggressive impulses generated from subcortical structures due to deficient prefrontal regulation, and that abnormal serotonin activity is likely to play an important role in this pathophysiology. It is possible that a reduction in the normal neurodevelopmental processes of hemispheric specialization may lead to reduced functional lateralization with less regulation of the right hemisphere by left hemisphere inhibitory processes, thereby contributing to the expression of violence in predisposed individuals. For example, in animal models, rats who are stressed early in life are right-hemisphere-dominant for mice killing, but severing the corpus callosum in these rats leads to increased muricide, indicating that the left hemisphere acts to inhibit the right-hemisphere-mediated killing via an intact corpus callosum (142). Since abnormalities of both subcortical and cortical structures as well as disturbed serotonin function are believed to be associated with TS, it is reasonable to hypothesize that at least some aggressive behaviors in TS may have an underlying neural basis.

Psychiatric Comorbidities and Aggression in TS

Using the current psychiatric nosology of DSM-IV-TR, aggression appears in several psychopathological diagnostic categories including paranoid schizophrenia, mental disorders due to a general medical condition, intermittent explosive disorder, and antisocial and borderline personality disorders (143). Aggression is also a common symptom in psychiatric disorders of childhood such as ADHD, conduct disorder, and pervasive developmental disorder (PDD) (144). Impulsive, irritable aggressive behaviors or "affective storms" frequently occur in children suffering from underlying mood disorders, particularly mania (145–147). Specific aggressive symptoms such as "anger attacks" have been reported to occur at increased frequency in patients with primary diagnoses of affective disorders and/or anxiety disorders (148,149). Since both community-based and clinical studies reveal significant rates of OCD, ADHD, separation anxiety, overanxious disorder simple phobia, social phobia, agoraphobia, mania, major depression, and oppositional defiant behaviors in children with tics or TS, the confounding variable of psychiatric comorbidities poses one of the most daunting obstacles to the study of aggressive symptoms in this disorder (150,151).

An exploratory clinical study of 90 patients with Tourette's syndrome revealed a significant association of aggression, hostility, and obsessionality with copro- and echo-phenomena and with a family history of tics or TS (152). While some investigations suggest that aggressive symptoms may be related to tic severity (153,154), other studies have failed to find this relationship and instead implicate an association between aggressive symptoms in TS and psychiatry comorbidity (155). An association between psychiatric comorbidity and explosive outbursts or "rage attacks" in children with TS has been demonstrated in both uncontrolled and controlled clinical studies (2,18,156). A pilot study of 12 children with TS presenting with explosive outbursts revealed the presence of comorbid OCD and ADHD in all cases (18). A subsequent study comparing 37 children with rage attacks and TS to 31 children with TS without rage attacks revealed higher frequencies of ADHD, OCD, and ODD in the rage group, who also had a higher total number of current comorbid psychiatric diagnoses compared with their control counterparts. The two groups did not differ with respect to tic type or tic severity, however (2). In a study of aggressive behavior in 33 unmedicated children with TS and 6 healthy control subjects, Stephens and Sandor (156) also showed that children with TS and comorbid ADHD or OCD are at increased risk for developing aggressive behavior compared with children with TS alone. Budman et al. (unpublished) recently examined clinical predictors of explosive outbursts in children with TS by comparing 48 children with rage attacks and TS to 65 children with TS without rage attacks using structured measures that assessed both lifetime and current psychiatric comorbidities. Again, no differences between the two groups in terms of tic types or severity were evident, but a current diagnosis of major depression, depression NOS, bipolar type I, ADHD combined type, ODD and OCD (but not non-OCD anxiety disorders), and past history of OCD or ODD were all significant predictors of rage attacks in TS. In addition, children with TS and rage attacks were also more likely to be using mood stabilizers, selective serotonin-reuptake inhibitors, or other antidepressants than their control counterparts and had families that were perceived as more "controlling." Descriptive data compiled from a large international database also suggest that individuals with TS alone have a low frequency of anger control problems; the highest prevalence of such symptoms occurred in individuals with TS and comorbid ADHD and OCD (4).

Attention-deficit/hyperactivity disorder, itself a common child psychiatric disorder, often co-occurs with oppositional defiant and conduct disorders and may account for a significant proportion of disruptive behaviors in TS patients (157–159). Data from controlled studies of patients from a specialty tic clinic showed that children with TS only did not differ from unaffected controls, while the TS + ADHD group scored significantly higher than controls on both parental and teacher ratings of aggression and delinquent behavior (157,158). An earlier onset of ADHD symptoms appears associated with more severe externalizing symptoms including aggression (160).

Attention-deficit/hyperactivity disorder is also often comorbid with affective disorders, and there are extensive data indicating that the risks for aggressive behaviors in adolescents are heightened by underlying mood disorders (161–163). Using rates of hospitalization and global assessment of functioning (GAF) scores as outcome variables, clinical evidence suggests that comorbid mood disorders are most strongly associated with illness morbidity in TS (20).

The presence of multiple psychiatric comorbidities with overlapping symptomatology in most clinical TS samples has made it difficult to delineate causal relationships with aggressive symptoms. Nonetheless, it is evident that TS uncomplicated by comorbid psychiatric disorders does not render increased risk for aggressive symptoms. Therefore the presence of such symptoms should prompt a careful psychiatric evaluation and review of current psychotropic medications.

PHARMACOLOGICAL TREATMENT OF AGGRESSION IN TOURETTE'S SYNDROME

Available data support a dichotomy between "impulsive-affective" and "controlled-predatory" subtypes of aggression that becomes relevant when devising treatment strategies. It is believed that the impulsive-affective subtype of aggression is more likely to respond to pharmacological and psychosocial interventions aimed at decreasing irritability, impulsivity, and arousal, whereas the controlled-predatory subtype of aggression may be more likely to respond to behavioral therapies. Effective management of aggression often necessitates a combination of both pharmacological and nonpharmacological approaches. Nonpharmacological therapies such as psychoeducation, anger management, dialectic behavioral therapy, and relapse prevention therapies can work synergistically with pharmacological treatment.

This section briefly overviews basic principles of the pharmacological management of impulsive aggression since few studies have specifically evaluated treatment of aggressive symptoms in TS. A critical first step in the management of aggressive behaviors in TS is a comprehensive neuropsychiatric evaluation with identification of potentially treatable causes for such symptoms including medication side effects, psychosocial stresses, trauma or abuse, underlying medical problems, and psychiatric comorbidity. When psychiatric disorders are present, a careful assessment of how symptoms impact on daily functioning must be conducted with the patient, his/her family, and school/work personnel so that specific treatment goals can be appropriately defined and prioritized.

A variety of medication classes have been used for the treatment of impulsive aggressive symptoms including 5-HT_{1A} agonists, 5-HT_2 antagonists, selective serotonin-reuptake inhibitors (SSRI), mixed serotonin/norepinephrine reuptake inhibitors, lithium, anticonvulsants, anxiolytics, typical and atypical neuroleptics, α_2 agonists, β-blockers, opiate antagonists, and dopamine agonists (164,165).

Attempts to modulate serotonin neurotransmission have been among the more widely studied approaches to treating impulsive aggression. SSRIs, specifically fluoxetine, fluvoxamine, and sertraline, have been demonstrated to decrease impulsive aggression in patients with borderline personality disorder, depression, and in patients with intermittent explosive disorder

(166,167). Citalopram has shown efficacy in an open-label study for the treatment of children and adolescents with impulsive-affective aggression (168). An open-label study using trazodone, a weak inhibitor of 5-HT reuptake and potent antagonist of 5-HT_{2A} and 5-HT_{2c} receptors for treatment of conduct disorder in hospitalized children, showed overall reductions in aggression and impulsivity (169). Paroxetine decreased both the frequency and severity of rage attacks in an open-label study of children and adults with TS (170).

Mood stabilizers such as carbamazepine, diphenylhydantoin, divalproex sodium, and lithium have yielded promising results in recent placebo-controlled trials of adolescents with explosive outbursts, in children with conduct disorder, and in adult patients with personality disorders and other psychiatric conditions with aggressive symptoms (92,171–175). The potential usefulness of these agents for treatment of aggressive symptoms in TS, however, has not been well studied to date.

Although conventional neuroleptics have been used effectively to reduce aggressive symptoms in both children and adults with various neuropsychiatric disorders, enthusiasm for their use has been tempered by concerns about tardive dyskinesia and other extrapyramidal side effects, prompting exploration of the atypical neuroleptics as potential alternatives with fewer such adverse effects. Atypical neuroleptics such as clozapine, risperidone, ziprasidone, and olanzapine have been shown in controlled studies to reduce aggressive behaviors in a variety of populations (176–184). In a retrospective review of treatment response, risperidone was shown to be as effective as monotherapy for treatment of aggression in children with Tourette's disorder (185).

Convincing data emphasizing the efficacy of stimulants in improving ADHD-associated overt aggression such as irritability, anger outbursts, physical assaults, and other conduct problems in children have been provided by a meta-analysis by Connor et al. (186). However, these investigators reported diminished stimulant treatment efficacy for aggression-related behaviors when comorbid conduct disorder or mental retardation was present. While a comorbid tic disorder appears to have a limited impact on ADHD outcome (187), comorbid ADHD is highly associated with disruptive behavior and functional impairment in children with TS (159). Given the accumulating evidence that psychostimulant medication can be safely used in children with tics, it is important to treat ADHD in children with comorbid ADHD and TS since these children may be at increased risk for aggressive symptoms (188–191). A role for the α_2-adrenergic agonist clonidine, either alone or in combination with psychostimulant for treatment of aggression, is also supported by recent studies in children and may be the treatment of choice for children with comorbid ADHD and tic disorders (191–193). Finally, β-adrenergic agents have been reported to be effective in reducing aggressive symptoms in dementia, ADHD, personality disorders, and traumatic brain injuries (194). Their usefulness in treating aggressive symptoms in TS has not be widely explored to date.

The future study of clinical and genetic subtypes of TS will have important implications for the treatment of associated symptoms including aggression. As environmental, psychosocial, and physiological risk factors are better identified, more comprehensive and effective treatment of aggression in TS will become possible.

CONCLUSION

When present, aggressive symptoms in TS are a leading cause of morbidity. While unlikely to occur at increased frequency in people with TS alone, a variety of aggressive behaviors are commonly encountered in the clinical setting and are frequently associated with specific types and/or combinations of psychiatric comorbidity. Controlled research and longitudinal studies are needed to better understand the relationship, if any, between aggressive symptoms and the underlying tic diathesis. Improved assessment of these phenomenologically and etiologically complex symptoms will ultimately lead to improved, more specific treatments.

The growing scientific and clinical literature on aggression implicates neurobiological factors as playing an important role in the predisposition to and development of aggressive symptoms. Similar factors are likely to be relevant in the pathophysiology of aggressive symptoms in TS and warrant further exploration.

REFERENCES

1. King R, Scahill L. Emotional and behavioral difficulties associated with Tourette syndrome. In: Cohen D, Goetz C, Jankovic J, eds. Tourette Syndrome. Philadelphia, PA: Lippincott Williams and Wilkins, 2001:79–88.
2. Budman C, Bruun R, Park K, Lesser M, Olson M. Explosive outbursts in children with Tourette syndrome. J Am Acad Child Adolesc Psych 2000; 39:1270–1276.
3. Comings D, Comings B. Tourette syndrome: clinical and psychological aspects of 250 cases. Am J Hum Genet 1985; 37(3):435–450.
4. Freeman R, Fast D, Burd L, Kerbeshian J, Robertson M, Sandor P. An international perspective on Tourette syndrome: selected findings from 3500 cases in 22 countries. Dev Med Child 2000; 42:436–447.
5. Wand R, Matazow A, Shady G, Furer P, Staley D. Tourette syndrome: associated symptoms and most disabling features. Neurosci Biobehav Rev 1993; 17:272–275.

6. Santangelo S, Pauls D, Goldstein J. Tourette syndrome: What are the influences of gender and comorbid obsessive compulsive disorder? J Am Acad Child Adolesc Psych 1994; 33:795–804.
7. Kano Y, Ohta M, Nagai Y. Clinical characteristics of Tourette syndrome. Psychiatry Clin Neurosci 1998; 52:51–57.
8. Scahill L, Schwab-Stone M, Merikangas K, Leckman J, Zhang H, Kasl S. Psychosocial and clinical correlates of ADHD in a community sample of school-age children. J Am Acad Child Adolesc Psych 1999; 38:976–984.
9. Stefl M. Mental health needs associated with Tourette syndrome. Am J Publ Health 1984; 74:1310–1313.
10. Kadesjo B, Gillberg C. Tourette's disorder: epidemiology and comorbidity in primary school children. J Am Acad Child Adolesc Psych 2000; 39(5):548–555.
11. Coffey B, Park K. Behavioral and emotional aspects of Tourette syndrome. Neurol Clin 1997; 15:277–289.
12. Bruun R, Budman C. Neuroleptic-induced behavior disorders in patients with Tourette syndrome. In: Richardson M, Haugland G, eds. The Use of Neuroleptics in Children. Washington, DC: American Psychiatric Press, 1996:185–198.
13. Bruun R. Subtle and under-recognized side effects of neuroleptic treatment in children with Tourette's disorder. Am J Psychiatr 1988; 145:621–624.
14. Kompoliti K, Goetz C. Hyperkinetic movement disorders misdiagnosed as tics in Gilles de la Tourette syndrome. Mov Disord 1998; 13(3):477–480.
15. Palumbo D, Maughan A, Kurlan R. Hypothesis III: Tourette syndrome is only one of several causes of a developmental basal ganglia syndrome. Arch Neurol 1997; 34:475–483.
16. Maiuro R. Intermittent explosive disorder. In: Dunner DL, ed. Current Psychiatric Therapy. Philadelphia: Saunders, 1996.
17. Coccaro E, Kavoussi R, Berman M, Lish J. Intermittent explosive disorder-revised: development, reliability, and validity of research criteria. Comp Psychiatr 1998; 39(6):368–376.
18. Budman C, Park K, Olson M, Bruun R. Rage attacks in children and adolescents with Tourette syndrome: a pilot study. J Clin Psychiatry 1998; 59:576–580.
19. Budman C, Feirman L. The relationship of Tourette's syndrome with its psychiatric comorbidities: Is there an overlap? Psych Annals 2000; 31:541–548.
20. Coffey B, Biederman J, Geller B, Spencer T, Frazier J, Cradock K, Magovrevic T. Distinguishing illness severity from tic severity in children and adolescents with Tourette's disorder. J Am Acad Child Adolesc Psych 2000; 39:556–561.
21. Dooley J, Brna P, Gordon K. Parent perceptions of symptoms severity in Tourette's syndrome. Arch Dev Child 1999; 81:440–441.
22. Leckman J, Cohen D, Eds. Tourette's Syndrome: Tics, Obsessions, Compulsions: Developmental Psychopathology and Clinical Care. New York: Wiley, 1999:155–176.
23. Geelard E. Observations on temper tantrums in children. Am J Orthopsychiatr 1945; 15:238–241.
24. Bhatia S, Dhar N, Singhal P, Nigam M, Malik S, Mullick D. Temper tantrums:

prevalence and etiology in a non-referral outpatient setting. Clin Pediatr 1990, 311–315.
25. Tremblay R. The development of aggressive behavior during childhood: What have we learned in the past century? Int J Behav Dev 2000; 24:129–141.
26. Kochanska G, Murray K, Coy K. Inhibitory control as a contributor to conscience in childhood: from toddler to early school age. Child Dev 1997; 68:263–277.
27. Loeber R. Development and risk factors of juvenile antisocial behavior and delinquency. Clin Psychol Rev 1990; 10:1–41.
28. Olson S, Bates J, Sandy J, Lanthier R. Early developmental precursors of externalizing behavior in middle childhood and adolescence. J Abnorm Child Psychol 2000; 28(2):119–133.
29. Campbell S, Pierce E, March C, Ewing L, Szumowski E. Hard-to-manage preschool boys: symptomatic behavior across contexts and time. Child Dev 1994; 65:836–851.
30. Cousens P, Nunn K. Is "self-regulation" a more helpful construct than attention? Clin Child Psychol Psychiatry 1997; 2:27–43.
31. Logue A, Forzano L, Ackerman K. Self-control in children: age, preference for reinforcer amount and delay, and language ability. Learn Motiv 1996; 27:260–277.
32. Raine A. Autonomic nervous system activity and violence. In: Stoff DM, Cairns RB, eds. Aggression and Violence. Mahwah, NJ: Lawrence Erlbaum, 1996:145–168.
33. Raine A, Venables P, Mednick S. Low resting heart rate at age three years predisposes to aggression at age 11 years: Evidence from the Mauritius Child Health Project. J Acad Child Adolesc Psych 1997; 36:1457–1464.
34. Calkins S, Dedmon S. Physiological and behavioral regulation in two-year-old children with aggressive/destructive behavior problems. J Abnorm Child Psychol 2000; 28(2):103–118.
35. Eisenberg N, Fabes R, Guthrie I, Murphy B, Maszk P, Holgren R, Suh K. The relations of regulation and emotionality to problem behavior in elementary school. Dev Psychopathol 1996; 8:141–162.
36. Zahn-Waxler C, Cole P, Welsh J, Fox N. Psychophysiological correlates of empathy and prosocial behaviors in preschool children with behavior problems. Dev Psychopathol 1995; 7:27–48.
37. Richards J, Cameron D. Infant heart rate variability and behavioral developmental status. Infant Behav Dev 1989; 12:45–58.
38. Stifter C, Braungart J. The regulation of negative reactivity in infancy: Function and development. Dev Psychol 1995; 31:448–455.
39. Richards J. Respiratory sinus arrhythmia predicts heart rate and visual responses during visual attention in 14- and 20-week-old infants. Psychophysiology 1985; 22:1010–1019.
40. Stifter C, Fox N. Infant reactivity: Physiological correlates of newborn and 5-month temperament. Dev Psychol 1990; 26:582–588.
41. Suess P, Porges S, Plude D. Cardiac vagal tone and sustained attention in school-age children. Psychophysiology 1994; 31:17–22.

42. Pine D, Wasserman G, Miller L, Coplan J, Bagiella E, Kovelenku P, Myers M, Sloan R. Heart period variability and psychopathology in urban boys at risk for delinquency. Psychophysiology 1998; 35(8):521–529.
43. Mezzacappa E, Tremblay R, Kindlon D, Saul J, Arseneault L, Seguin J, Pihl R, Earls F. Anxiety, antisocial behavior, and heart rate regulation in adolescent males. J Child Psychol Psychiatry 1997; 38:457–469.
44. Porges S, Doussard-Roosevelt J, Portales L, Greenspan S. Infant regulation of the vagal "brake" predicts child behavior problems: A psychobiological model of social behavior. Dev Psychobiol 1996; 29:697–712.
45. Nagin D, Tremblay R. Parental and early childhood predictors of persistent physical aggression in boys from kindergarten to high school. Arch Gen Psychiatry 2001; 58:389–394.
46. Bromberger J, Matthews K. A "feminine" model of vulnerability to depressive symptoms: A longitudinal investigation of middle-aged women. J Pers Soc Psychol 1996; 70:591–598.
47. Thayer R, Newman J, McClain T. Self-regulation of mood: Strategies for changing a bad mood, raising energy, and reducing tension. J Pers Soc Psychol 1994; 67:910–925.
48. Carver C, Scheier M, Weintraub J. Assessing coping strategies: A theoretically based approach. J Pers Soc Psychol 1989; 56:267–283.
49. Rusting C, Nolen-Hoeksema S. Regulation responses to anger: Effects of rumination and distraction on angry mood. J Pers Soc Psychol 1998; 74:790–803.
50. Zillman D. Mood management: Using entertainment to full advantage. In: Donohew L, Sypher H, Higgins E, eds. Communications, Social Cognition, and Affect. Hillsdale, NJ: Erlbaum, 1988:147–171.
51. Block J. Studying personality the long way. In: Funder D, Parke R, Tomlinson-Keasy C, Widaman K, eds. Studying Lives Through Time: Personality and Development. Washington, DC: American Psychological Association, 1993:9–41.
52. Bruin J, van Oyen H, van de Poll N. Behavioral changes following lesions of the orbital prefrontal cortex in male rats. Behav Brain Res 1993; 10:209–232.
53. Eggers M, Flynn J. Effect of electrical stimulation of the amygdala on hypothalamically elicited attack behavior in cats. J Neurophysiol 1963; 26:705–720.
54. Eichelman B. Animal and evolutionary models of impulsive aggression. In: Hollander E, Stein D, eds. Impulsivity and Aggression. Chichester, UK: Wiley, 1995:59–90.
55. Moyer K. A model of aggression with implications for research (proc). Psychopharm Bull 1977; 13(1):14–15.
56. Karlin P. The Norway rat's killing response to the white mouse. Behavior 1956; 10:81–103.
57. Robinson B, Alexander M, Browne G. Dominance reversal resulting from aggressive responses evoked by brain stimulation. Physiol Behav 1969; 4:749–752.
58. Kruk M, van der Poel A, Meehis W, Hermans J, Mostert P, Mos J, Lohman A. Discriminant analysis of the localization of aggression-inducing electrode placements in the hypothalamus of male rats. Brain Res 1983; 260:61–79.

59. Moyer KE. Kinds of aggression and their physiological basis. Commun Behav Biol 1968; 2–65.
60. Ulrich R, Johnson M, Richardson J, Wolff P. The operant conditioning of fighting behaviors in rats. Psychol Records 1963; 13:465–470.
61. Atkins M, Stoff D. Instrumental and hostile aggression in childhood disruptive behavior disorders. J Abnorm Child Psychol 1993; 21:165–178.
62. Loeber R, Schmaling K. Empirical evidence for overt and covert patterns of antisocial conduct problems: A meta-analysis. J Abnorm Child Psychol 1985; 13:337–352.
63. Dodge K, Croie J. Social information-processing factors in reactive and proactive aggression in children's peer groups. J Pers Soc Psychol 1987; 52:1146–1158.
64. Blanchard D. Applicability of models of human aggression. In: Flannelly K, Blanchard R, Blanchard D, eds. Biological Perspectives on Aggression. New York: Alan R, Liss, 1984:49–74.
65. Vitiello B, Behar D, Hunt J, Stoff D, Ricciuti A. Subtyping aggression in children and adolescents. J Neuropsychiatry Clin Neurosci 1990; 2:189–192.
66. Megargee E. Undercontrolled and overcontrolled personality types in extreme antisocial aggression. Psychol Monogr 1966; 60(3).
67. Dodge K. The structure and function of reactive and proactive aggression. In: Pepler D, Rubin K, eds. The Development and Treatment of Childhood Aggression. Hillsdale, NJ: Erlbaum, 1991:201–218.
68. Nee L, Polinsky R, Eldridge R, Ebert M. Gilles de la Tourette syndrome: Clinical and family study of 50 cases. Ann Neurol 1980; 7:41–49.
69. Robertson M, Banerjee S, Fox Hiley P, Tannock C. Personality disorder and psychopathology in Tourette's syndrome: A controlled study. Br J Psychiatry 1997; 171:283–286.
70. Erenberg G, Cruse R, Rothner A. The natural history of Tourette syndrome: A follow-up study. Ann Neurol 1987; 22:383–385.
71. Yudofsky S, Silver J, Jackson W, Endicott J, Williams D. The Overt Aggression Scale for the objective rating of verbal and physical aggression. Am J Psychiatr 1986; 43:35–39.
72. Malone R, Lucbbert J, Pena-Ariet M, Biesecker K, Delaney M. The Overt Aggression Scale in a study of lithium in aggressive conduct disorder. Psychopharmacol Bull 1994; 30:215–218.
73. Achenbach T. Manual for the Teacher's Report Form and 1991 Profile. Burlington: University of Vermont Department of Psychiatry, 1991.
74. Loney J, Milich R. Hyperactivity, inattention, and aggression in clinical practice. In: Walraich M, Routh D, eds. Advances in Developmental and Behavioral Pediatrics. Greenwich, CT: JAE, 1982:113–147.
75. Miller L, Klein R, Piacentini J, Abikoff H, Shah M, Samoila A, Guardini M. The New York Teacher Rating Scale for disruptive and antisocial behavior. J Am Acad Child Adolesc Psych 1995; 34:359–370.
76. Halperin J, McKay K, Newcorn J. Development, reliability, and validity of the Children's Aggression Scale—Parent version. J Am Acad Child Adolesc Psych 2002; 41(3):245–252.

77. Plomin R, Nitz K, Rowe D. Behavioral genetics and aggressive behavior in childhood. In: Lewis M, Miller S, eds. Handbook of Developmental Psychopathology. New York: Plenum Press, 1990:119–134.
78. Lyons M, True W, Eisen S, Goldberg J, Meyer J, Araone S, Eaves L, Tsuang M. Differential heritability of adult and juvenile antisocial traits. Arch Gen Psychiatry 1995; 52:906–915.
79. Rushton J, Fulker D, Neale M, Nias D, Eysendck H. Altruism and aggression: The heritability of individual differences. J Pers Soc Psychol 1986; 50:1192–1198.
80. Plomin R, Foch T, Rowe D. Bobo clown aggression in childhood: Environment, not genes. J Res Pers 1981; 15:331–342.
81. Seroczynski A, Bergeman C, Coccaro E. Etiology of the impulsivity/aggression relationship: Genes or environment? Psychiatry Res 1999; 86:41–52.
82. Mannuck S, Flory J, Ferrell R, Mann J, Muldoon M. A regulatory polymorphism of the monoamine oxidase A gene may be associated with variability in aggression, impulsivity and central nervous system serotonergic responsivity. Psychiatry Res 2000; 95(1):9–23.
83. New A, Gelernter J, Yovell Y. Tryptophan hydroxylase genotype is associated with impulsive–aggression measures: A preliminary study. Am J Med Genet 1998; 81(1):13–17.
84. Nielsen D, Virkkunen M, Lappalainen J, Eggert M, Brown G, Long J, Goldman D, Linnoila M. A tryptophan hydroxylase gene marker for suicidality and alcoholism. Arch Gen Psychiatry 1998; 55(7):593–602.
85. Bjork J, Moeller F, Swann A, Machado M, Hanis D. Serotonin 2a receptor T102C polymorphism and impaired impulse control. Am J Med Genet 2002; 114:336–339.
86. Leckman J, Pauls D, Zhang H, Rosario-Campos M, Katsovich L, Kidd K, Pakstis A, Alsobrook J, Robertson M, McMahon W, Walkup J, van de Wetering B, King, R. Cohen D and the Tourette Syndrome Association International Consortium for Genetics. Am J Med Genet. In press.
87. Coccaro E, Kavoussi R. Neurotransmitter correlates of aggression. In: Stoff D, Cairns R, eds. The Neurobiology of Clinical Aggression. Mahwah, NJ: Lawrence J Erlbaum Associates, 1996:67–85.
88. Higley J, Mehlman P, Taub D, Higley S, Suomi S, Linnoila M, Vickers J. Cerebrospinal fluid monoamine and adrenal correlates of aggression in free-ranging rhesus monkeys. Arch Gen Psychiatry 1992; 49:436–441.
89. Higley J, King S, Hasert M, Champoux M, Suomi S, Linnoila M. Stability of interindividual differences in serotonin function and its relationship to severe aggression and competent social behavior in rhesus macaque females. Neuropsychopharmacology 1996; 4:67–76.
90. Van Goozen S, Matthys W, Cohen-Kettenis P, Wetenberg H, Engeland H. Plasma monoamine metabolites and aggression: Two studies of normal and oppositional defiant children. Eur Neuropsychopharmacol 1999; 9:141–147.
91. Asber M, Traksman L, Thoren P. 5-HIAA in the cerebrospinal fluid. A biochemical suicide predictor. Arch Gen Psychiatry 1976; 33(10):1193–1197.
92. Coccaro E, Siever L. Pathophysiology and treatment of aggression. In: David

K, Charney D, Coyle J, et al., eds. Neuropsychopharmacology: The Fifth Generation of Progress. Philadelphia: Lippincott Williams & Wilkins, 2002:1709–1723.
93. Coccaro E, Siever L, Klar H, Maurer G, Cochrane K, Cooper T, Mohs R, Davis K. Serotonergic studies in patients with affective and personality disorders: Correlates with suicidal and impulsive aggressive behavior. Arch Gen Psychiatry 1989; 46(7):587–599.
94. Coccaro E, Berman M, Kavoussi R, Hauger R. Relationship of prolactin response to D-fenfluramine to behavioral and questionnaire assessments of aggression in personality-disordered men. Biol Psychiatry 1996; 40(3):157–164.
95. Coccaro E, Kavoussi R, Oakes M, Cooper T, Hauger R. 5-HT2a/2c receptor blockade by amersergide fully attenuates prolactin response to D-fenfluramine challenge in physically healthy human subjects. Psychopharmacology 1996; 126(1):24–30.
96. Coccaro E, Kavoussi R, Trestman R, Gabriel S, Cooper T, Siever L. Serotonin function in human subjects: Intercorrelations among central 5-HT indices and aggressiveness. Psychiatry Res 1997; 73(1–2):1–14.
97. Hanna G, Yuwiler A, Coates J. Whole blood serotonin and disruptive behaviors in juvenile obsessive-compulsive disorder. J Am Acad Child Adolesc Psych 1995; 34:28–35.
98. Kruesi M, Rapoport J, Hamburger S, Hibbs E, Potter W, Lenane M, Brown G. Cerebrospinal fluid monoamine metabolites, aggression, and impulsivity in disruptive behavior disorders of children and adolescents. Arch Gen Psychiatry 1990; 47:419–426.
99. Castellanos F, Elia J, Kruesi M, Gulotta C, Mefford I, Potter W, Ritchie G, Rapoport J. Cerebrospinal fluid monoamine metabolites in boys with attention-deficit hyperactivity disorder. Psychiatry Res 1994; 52:305–316.
100. Stoff D, Pasatiempo A, Yeung H, Cooper T, Bridger W, Ravinovich H. Neuroendocrine responses to challenge with DL-fenfluramine and aggression in disruptive behavior disorders of children and adolescents. Psychiatry Res 1992; 43:263–276.
101. Halperin J, Sharma V, Siever L, Schwartz S, Matier K, Wornell G, Newcorn J. Serotonergic function in aggressive and non-aggressive boys with attention-deficit hyperactivity disorder. Am J Psychiatr 1994; 151:243–248.
102. Halperin J, Newcorn J, Schwartz S, Vanshdeep S, Siever L, Koda V, Gabriel S. Age-related changes in the association between serotonergic function and aggression in boys with ADHD. Biol Psychiatry 1997; 41:682–689.
103. Virkkunen M. Urinary free cortisol secretion in habitually violent offenders. Acta Psychiatr Scand 1985; 72:40–44.
104. Van Goozen S, Mattys W, Cohen-Kettenis P, Gispen-de Wied C, Wiegant V, van England H. Salivary cortisol and cardiovascular activity during stress in oppositional defiant disorder boys and normal controls. Biol Psychiatry 1998; 43:532–539.
105. McBurnett K, Lahey B, Capasso L, Loeber R. Aggressive symptoms and

salivary cortisol in clinic-referred boys with conduct disorder. Ann NY Acad Sci 1996; 20:169–178.
106. McBurnett K, Lahey B, Rathouz P, Loeber R. Low salivary cortisol and persistent aggression in boys referred for disruptive behavior. Arch Gen Psychiatry 2000; 58:38–43.
107. Pajer K, Gardner W, Rubin R, Perel J, Neal S. Decrease cortisol levels in adolescent girls with conduct disorder. Arch Gen Psychiatry 2001; 58:297–302.
108. Gallucci W, Baum A, Lave I, Rabin D, Chrousos G, Gold P, Kling M. Sex differences in sensitivity of the hypothalamic–pituitary–adrenal axis. Health Psychol 1993; 12:420–425.
109. Snoek H, Van Goozen S, Matthys C, Singy H, Koppeschaar H, Westenbeg H, Van Engeland H. Serotonergic functioning in children with oppositional defiant disorder. A sumatriptan challenge study. Biol Psychiatry 2002; 15:19–25.
110. Ferris C, Meloni R, Loppel G, Perry K, Fuller R, Delville Y. Vasopressin/serotonin interactions in the anterior hypothalamus control aggressive behavior in golden hamsters. J Neurosci 1997; 17:4331–4340.
111. Buijs R. Intra and extrahypothalmic vasopressin and oxytocin pathways in the rate: Pathways to the limbic system, medulla oblongata and spinal cord. Cell Tissue Res 1978; 252:355–365.
112. Ferris C. Role of vasopressin in aggressive and dominant/subordinate behaviors. In: Pedersen C, Caldwell J, Jirkowski G, Insel T, eds. Oxytocin in Maternal, Sexual and Social Behaviors—Annals of the New York Academy of Sciences. New York: New York Academy of Sciences, 1992:212–226.
113. Peterson B, Leckman J, Scahill L, Naftolin F, Keefe D, Charest J, Cohen D. Hypothesis: steroid hormones and sexual dimorphisms modulate symptoms expression in Tourette's syndrome. Psychoneuroendocrinology 1992; 17:553–563.
114. Coccaro E, Kavoussi R, Hanger R, Cooper T, Ferris C. Cerebrospinal fluid vasopressin levels: Correlates with aggression and serotonin function in personality-disordered subjects. Arch Gen Psychiatry 1998; 55:708–714.
115. Artemus M, Pigott T, Kalogeras K, Demistrack M, Drubbert B, Murphy D, Gold P. Abnormalities in the regulation of vasopressin and corticotrophin releasing factor secretion in obsessive-compulsive disorder. Arch Gen Psychiatry 1992; 49:9–20.
116. Swedo S, Leonard H, Kruesi M, Rettew D, Listwak S, Berrettini W, Stipetic M, Hamburger S, Gold P, Potter W, Rapoport J. Cerebrospinal fluid neurochemistry in children and adolescents with obsessive-compulsive disorder. Arch Gen Psychiatry 1992; 49:29–36.
117. Leckman J, Goodman W, North W, Chappell P, Price L, Pauls D, Anderson G, Riddle M, McSwiggan-Hardin M, McDougle C, Barr L, Cohen D. Elevated cerebrospinal fluid levels of oxytocin in obsessive compulsive disorder: comparison with Tourette's syndrome and healthy controls. Arch Gen Psychiatry 1994; 51:782–792.
118. Elliott F. Neurological findings in adult minimal brain dysfunction and the dyscontrol syndrome. J Nerv Ment Dis 1982; 170:680–687.

119. Kim J, Choi S, Kwon S, Seo Y. Inability to control anger or aggression after stroke. Neurology 2002; 58:1106–1108.
120. Raine A, Buchsbaum M, LaCasse L. Brain abnormalities in murderers indicated by positron emission tomography. Biol Psychiatry 1997; 42:495–508.
121. Anderson S, Bechara A, Dimasio H, Tranel D, Damasio A. Impairment of social and moral behavior related to early damage in human prefrontal cortex. Nat Neurosci 1993; 2:1032–1037.
122. Blari R, Cipolotti L. Impaired social response reversal. A case of 'acquired sociopathy'. Brain 2000; 123:1122–1141.
123. Swedo S, Schapiro M, Grady C. Cerebral glucose metabolism in childhood onset obsessive compulsive disorder. Arch Gen Psychiatry 1989; 46:518–523.
124. Dougherty D, Shin L, Alpert N, Pitman R, Orr S, Lasko M, Macklin M, Fischman A, Raugh S. Anger in healthy men. A PET study using script-driven imagery. Biol Psychiatry 1999; 46:466–472.
125. Bassarath L. Review Paper: Neuroimaging studies of antisocial behavior. Can J Psychiatry 2001; 46:728–732.
126. Davidson R, Putnam K, Larson C. Dysfunction in the neural circuitry of emotion regulation: A possible prelude to violence. Science 2000; 289:591–594.
127. Casey B, Giedd J, Thomas K. Structural and functional brain development and its relation to cognitive development. Biol Psychol 2000; 54:241–257.
128. Bunge S, Dudukovic N, Thomason M, Vaidya C, Gabrieli J. Immature frontal lobe contributions to cognitive control in children: Evidence from MRI. Neuron 2002; 33:301–311.
129. Chesterman L, Taylor P, Cox T, Hill M, Lumsden J. Multiple measures of cerebral state in dangerous mentally disordered inpatients. Crim Behav Ment Health 1994; 4:228–239.
130. van Elst LT, Woermann F, Lemieux L, Thompson P, Trimble M. Affective aggression in patients with temporal lobe epilepsy: A quantitative MRI study of the amygdala. Brain 2000; 23:234–243.
131. Raine A, Lencz T, Bihrle S, LaCasse L, Colletti P. Reduced prefrontal gray matter volume and reduced autonomic activity in antisocial personality disorder. Arch Gen Psychiatry 2000; 57:119–127.
132. Volkow N, Tancredi L, Grant C, Gillespie H. Brain glucose metabolism in violent psychiatrist patients: A preliminary study. Psychiatry Res 1995; 61:243–253.
133. Goyer P, Andreason P, Semple W, Clayton A, King A, Compton-Toth V, et al. Positron emission tomography and personality disorders. Neuropsychopharmacology 1994; 10:21–28.
134. Raine A, Buchsbaum M, Stanley J, Lottenberg S, Abel L, Stoddard J. Selective reductions in prefrontal glucose metabolism in murderers. Biol Psychiatry 1994; 36:365–373.
135. Volkow N, Tancredi L. Neural substrates of violent behavior: A preliminary study with positron emission tomography. Br J Psychiatry 1987; 151:668–673.
136. Goyer P, Andreason P, Semple W, Clayton A, King A, Compton-Toth B,

Schulz S, Cohen R. Positron emission tomography and personality disorders. Neuropyschopharmacology 1994; 10:21–28.
137. Raine A, Meloy J, Bihrle S, Stoddard J, LaCasse L, Buchsbaum M. Reduced prefrontal and increased subcortical brain functioning assessed using positron emission tomography in predatory and affective murderer. Behav Sci Law 1998; 16:319–332.
138. Amen D, Stubblefield M, Carmichael B, Thisted R. Brain SPECT findings and aggressiveness. Ann Clin Psychiatry 1996; 8:129–137.
139. Siever L, Buschsbaum M, New A, Spiegel-Cohen J, Wei T, Hazlett E, Sevin E, Nunn M, Mitropoulou V. D,l-Fenfluramine response in impulsive personality disorder assessed with 18F-deoxyglucose positron emission tomography. Neuropsychopharmacology 1999; 20:413–423.
140. Soloff P, Meltzer C, Greer P, Constantine D, Kelly T. A fenfluramine-activated FDG-PET study of borderline personality disorder. Biol Psychiatry 2000; 47:540–547.
141. New A, Hazlett E, Buschsbaum M, Goodman M, Reynolds D, Mitropoulou V, Sprung L, Shaw R, Koenigsberg H, Platholi J, Silverman J, Siever L. Blunted prefrontal cortical 18-fluorodeoxyglucose positron emission tomography response to meta-chlorophenylpipierazine in impulsive aggression. Arch Gen Psychiatry 2002; 59:621–629.
142. Denenberg V, Gall J, Berrebi A, Yutzey D. Callosal mediation of cortical inhibition in the lateralized rat brain. Brain Res 1986; 397:327–332.
143. American Psychiatric AssociationDiagnostic and Statistical Manual of Mental Disorders. 4th ed. Washington, DC: American Psychiatric Press, 1994.
144. Weller E, Rowan A, Weller R, Elia J. Aggressive behavior associated with attention-deficit/hyperactivity disorder; conduct disorder, and developmental disabilities. J Clin Psychiatry Monogr 1999; 17(2):2–7.
145. Geller B, Luby J. Child and adolescent bipolar disorder: A review of the past 10 years. J Am Acad Child Adolesc Psych 1997; 36:1168–1176.
146. Weller R, Weller E, Tucker S, Fristad M. Mania in prepubertal children: Has it been underdiagnosed? J Affect Disord 1986; 11:151–154.
147. Wozniak J, Biederman J, Keely K. Mania-like symptoms suggestive of childhood-onset bipolar disorder in clinically referred children. J Am Acad Child Adolesc Psych 1995; 34:867–876.
148. Gould R, Ball S, Kaspi S, Otto M, Pollack M, Shekhar A, Fava M. Prevalence and correlates of anger attacks: A two-site study. J Affect Disord 1996; 39:31–38.
149. Rosenbaum J. Anger attacks in depression. J Clin Psychiatry Monogr 1999; 17(2):15–17.
150. Kurlan R, Como P, Miller B, Palumbo D, Deeley C, Andresen E, Eapen S, McDermott M. The behavioral spectrum of tic disorders. A community-based study. Neurology 2002; 59:414–420.
151. Coffey B, Biederman J, Smoller J, Geller D, Sarin P, Schwartz S, Kim GS. Anxiety disorders and tic severity in juveniles with Tourette's disorder. J Am Acad Child Adolesc Psych 2000; 39(5):562–568.

152. Robertson M, Trimble M, Lees A. The psychopathology of the Gilles de la Tourette syndrome. A phenomenological analysis. Br J Psychiatry 1988; 152:383–390.
153. De Groot C, Janus M, Bornstein R. Clinical predictors of psychopathology in children and adolescents with Tourette syndrome. J Psychiatr Res 1995; 29:59–70.
154. Nolan E, Sverd J, Gadow K, Sprafkin J, Ezor S. Associated pathology in children with both ADHD and chronic tic disorder. J Am Acad Child Adolesc Psych 1996; 35:1622–1630.
155. Erenberg G, Cruse R, Rothner A. Tourette syndrome. Clevel Clin Q 1986; 53:127–131.
156. Stephens R, Sandor P. Aggressive behavior in children with Tourette syndrome and comorbid attention-deficit hyperactivity disorder and obsessive compulsive disorder. Can J Psychiatry 1999; 44:1036–1042.
157. Carter A, O'Donnell D, Schultz R, Scahill L, Leckman J, Pauls D. Social and emotional adjustment in children affected with Gilles de la Tourette's syndrome: Associations with ADHD and family functioning. J Child Psychol Psychiatry 2000; 41:215–223.
158. Spencer T, Biederman J, Harding M, O'Donnell D, Wilens T, Faraone S, Coffey B, Geller D. Disentangling the overlap between Tourette's disorder and ADHD. J Child Psychol Psychiatry 1998; 39:1037–1044.
159. Sukhodolsky D, Scahill L, Zhang H, Peterson B, King R, Lombroso P, Katsovich L, Findley D, Leckman J. Disruptive behavior in children with Tourette Syndrome: Association with ADHD comorbidity, tic severity, and functional impairment. J Am Acad Child Adolesc Psych 2003; 42:98–105.
160. Connor D, Edwards G, Fletcher K, Baird J, Barkley R, Steingard R. Correlates of comorbid psychopathology in children with ADHD. J Am Acad Child Adolesc Psych 2003; 42:193–200.
161. Knox M, King C, Hanna G, Logan D, Ghaziuddin N. Aggressive behavior in clinically depressed adolescents. J Am Acad Child Adolesc Psych 2000; 39(5):611–618.
162. McCracken J, Cantwell D, Hanna G. Conduct disorder and depression. In: Koplewicz H, Klass D, eds. Depression in Children and Adolescents. Philadelphia: Harwood Academic Publishers, 1993:121–132.
163. Schubiner H, Scott R, Tzelepis A. Exposure to violence among inner-city youth. J Adolesc Health, 1993:214–219.
164. Campbell M, Gonzales N, Silva R. The pharmacologic treatment of conduct disorders and rage outbursts. Psychiatr Clin North Am 1992; 15(1):69–85.
165. Pallanti S, Baldini Ross N, Friedberg J, Hollander F. Pychobiology of impulse-control disorders not otherwise specified (NOS). In: D'haenen H, den Boer J, Willner P, eds. Biological Psychiatry. New York: John Wiley & Sons, 2000.
166. Coccaro E, Kavoussi R. Fluoxetine and impulsive aggressive behavior in personality-disordered subjects. Arch Gen Psychiatry 1997; 54(12):1081–1088.
167. Feder R. Treatment of intermittent explosive disorder with sertraline in 3 patients. J Clin Psychiatry 1999; 60:195–196.

168. Amenteros J, Lewis J. Citalopram treatment for impulsive aggression in children and adolescents: An open pilot study. J Am Acad Child Adolesc Psych 2002; 159:266–273.
169. Zubieta J, Alessi N. Acute and chronic administration of trazodone in the treatment of disruptive behavior disorders in children. J Clin Psychopharmacol 1992; 12:346–351.
170. Bruun R, Budman C. Paroxetine treatment of episodic rages associated with Tourette's disorder. J Clin Psychiatry 1998; 59:581–584.
171. Campbell M, Adams P, Small A, Kafantaris V, Silva P, Shell J, Perry R, Overall J. Lithium in hospitalized aggressive children with conduct disorder: A double-blind and placebo-controlled study. J Am Acad Child Adolesc Psych 1995; 34:445–453.
172. Donovan S, Stewart J, Nunes E, Quitken F, Parides M, Daniel W, Susser E, Klein D. Divalproex treatment for youth with explosive temper and mood lability: A double-blind, placebo-controlled crossover design. Am J Psychiatry 2000; 157:818–820.
173. Hollander E, Tracy K, Swann A, Coccaro E, McElroy S, Wozniac J, Sommerville K, Nemeroff C. Treatment of impulsive aggression: Efficacy in cluster B personality disorders. Neuropsychopharmacology 2003; 6:1186–1197.
174. Lewin J, Sumners D. Successful treatment of episodic dyscontrol with carbamazepine. Br J Psychiatry 1992; 261–262.
175. Malone R, Delaney M, Luebbert J, Cater J, Campbell M. A double-blind placebo-controlled study of lithium in hospitalized aggressive children and adolescents with conduct disorder. Arch Gen Psychiatry 2000; 57:649–654.
176. Benedetti F, Sforzini L, Colombo C, Maffei C, Smeraldi E. Low-dose clozapine in acute and continuation treatment of severe borderline personality disorder. J Clin Psychiatry 1998; 59:103–107.
177. Chen N, Bedair H, McKay B, Bowers M, Mazure C. Clozapine in the treatment of aggression in an adolescent with autistic disorder (letter). J Clin Psychiatry 2001; 62:479–480.
178. Chengappa K, Vasile J, Levine J, Ulrich R, Baker R, Gopalani A, Schooler N. Clozapine: Its impact on aggressive behavior among patients in a state psychiatric hospital. Schizophr Res 2002; 53:1–6.
179. Findling R, McNamara N, Branicky L, Schluchter M, Lemon E, Blumer J. A double-blind pilot study of risperidone in the treatment of conduct disorder. J Am Acad Child Adolesc Psych 2000; 39:509–516.
180. Krishnamoorthy J, King B. Open-label olanzapine treatment in five preadolescent children. J Child Adolesc Psychopharmacol 1998; 8:107–113.
181. McDougal D, Holmes J, Carlson D, Pelton G, Cohen D, Price L. A double-blind placebo-controlled study of risperidone in adults with autistic disorder and other pervasive developmental disorders. Arch Gen Psychiatry 1998; 55:633–641.
182. McDougle C, Kem D, Posey D. Case series: Use of ziprasidone for maladaptive symptoms in youths with autism. J Am Acad Child Adolesc Psych 2002; 41:921–927.

183. Scheier H. Risperidone for young children with mood disorders and aggressive behavior. J Child Adolesc Psychopharmacol 1998; 8:49–59.
184. Snyder R, Turgay Aman M, Fisman S. Effects of risperidone on conduct and disruptive behavior disorders in children with subaverage IQs. J Am Acad Child Adolesc Psych 2002; 41:1026–1036.
185. Sandor P, Stephens R. Risperidone treatment of aggressive behavior in children with Tourette's syndrome. J Clin Psychopharmacol 2000; 20:710–712.
186. Connor D, Glatt S, Lopez I, Jackson D, Melloni R. Psychopharmacology and Aggression. I. A Meta-analysis of stimulant effects on overt/covert aggression-related behavior in ADHD. J Am Acad Child Adolesc Psych 2002; 41:253–261.
187. Spencer T, Biederman J, Farone S, Mich E, Coffey B, Geller D, Kagan J, Bearnman S, Wilens T. Impact of tic disorders on ADHD outcome across the life cycle: Findings from a large group of adults with and without ADHD. Am J Psychiatry 2001; 158:611–617.
188. Castellanos F, Giedd J, Elia J, Marsh W, Ritchie G, Hamburger S, Rapoport J. Controlled stimulant treatment of ADHD and comorbide Tourette's syndrome: Effects of stimulant and dose. J Am Acad Child Adolesc Psych 1997; 36:589–596.
189. Gadow K, Sverd J, Sprafkin J, Nolan E, Grossman S. Long-term methylphenidate therapy in children with comorbid attention-deficit hyperactivity disorder and chronic multiple tic disorder. Arch Gen Psychiatry 1999; 56:330–336.
190. Nolan E, Gadow K. Children with ADHD and tic disorder and their classmates: Behavioral normalization with methylphenidate. J Am Acad Psychiatry 1997; 36:597–604.
191. The Tourette's Syndrome Study Group. Treatment of ADHD in children with tics. A randomized controlled trial. Neurology 2002; 58:527–536.
192. Connor D, Barkley R, David H. A pilot study of methylphenidate, clonidine, or the combination of ADHD comorbid with aggressive oppositional defiant or conduct disorder.
193. Kemph J, De Vane C, Levin G, et al. Treatment of aggressive children with clonidine: Results of an open pilot study. J Am Acad Child Adolesc Psych 1993; 32:577–581.
194. Haspel T. Beta-blockers and the treatment of aggression. Harv Rev Psychiatry 1995; 23:274–281.

8

Primary Tic Disorders

Gerald Erenberg
Cleveland Clinic Foundation
Cleveland, Ohio, U.S.A.

INTRODUCTION

Tics are the most common form of movement disorder in childhood. It has been estimated that up to 24% of school-age children will experience tics at one time or another (1). Many will experience mild tics that will go undiagnosed because they are considered part of the child's normal pattern of behavior. For many of these children, the tics will be transient and disappear spontaneously after several weeks or months. For others, the tics will persist for prolonged periods of time and become more complex and severe.

Tics are involuntary, sudden, rapid, recurring, purposeless, nonrhythmic, stereotyped motor movements or vocalizations. As is true for many movement disorders, the specific involuntary movement is often more easily recognized than precisely defined. Tics can be described by their anatomical location, frequency, number, intensity, duration, and complexity. They are generally considered involuntary, but may be accompanied by a premonitory sensory urge. Persons with tics often describe the need to perform the action as irresistible, similar to the need to breathe when trying to hold one's breath for as long as possible.

Tics can typically be suppressed for brief periods of time, ranging from seconds to minutes. They increase in frequency and intensity when the person is under any form of mental or physical stress. Alternatively, some persons will manifest their tics in the most obvious way when they are in a relaxed situation, such as quietly watching television. Tics may be reduced or even disappear during sleep. They also tend to be at a low level when the person is placed in a novel or highly structured situation, and this explains why tics are often not seen when the patient is in the doctor's office. When tics are present over long intervals of time, their severity will wax and wane. The specific form of tic may also be triggered by environmental stimuli. The cough that begins when the patient has an upper respiratory infection may continue for long periods as an involuntary vocal tic. New tics may also come about in imitation of a normally occurring event, such as hearing a dog bark.

Table 1 lists the types of tics. Simple motor tics, which are often the initial symptoms of a tic disorder, typically begin with brief bouts of transient tics involving the face or head. There is often a rostral–caudal progression with tics of the face, head, and shoulders appearing earlier and in a higher proportion of patients than motor tics of the limbs or trunk. Simple motor tics are sudden, brief, meaningless movements such as blinking, grimacing, nose-twitching, lip-pouting, neck-jerking, shrugging, and abdominal tensing.

In contrast, complex motor tics are of longer duration, involve contractions of several muscle groups, and appear more purposeful or deliberate. Examples include rolling the eyes upward or from side to side, thrusting out an arm, squatting, hopping, jumping, and writhing. Dystonic posturing, now known to occur in a minority of patients with Tourette's syndrome (TS), can be counted among the complex motor tics. Other complex motor tics include imitating gestures or movements of other people (echopraxia) or making obscene gestures (copropraxia). Under the heading of complex motor tics are movements that seem compulsive and ritualistic, such as smelling an object, touching one's own or someone else's body, and following a complex pattern of walking, such as hopping on every third step. Because there is a known overlap between tic disorders and obsessive–compulsive behaviors, there is now discussion as to whether these events actually represent obsessive–compulsive behaviors and not tic phenomena. In general, complex motor tics are usually not present in the absence of simple motor tics.

Table 1 Types of Tics

Simple motor
Complex motor
Simple vocal (phonic)
Complex vocal (phonic)
Dystonic
Sensory

Vocal tics may occur in isolation, but they generally occur in persons also having motor tics. Vocal tics usually appear after the onset of motor tics and are also classified as simple or complex. There is an extraordinary range of possible vocal symptoms, and virtually any noise or sound has the potential of evolving into a tic. Simple vocal tics include inarticulate noises and sounds such as throat-clearing, sniffing, grunting, coughing, snorting, lip noises, hissing, screaming or shouting, barking, clicking, stammering, and a variety of syllable sounds such as uh, ee, and bu.

Complex vocal tics involve linguistically meaningful words, phrases, or sentences, which may be shouted out at inappropriate times. During conversations, vocal tics may interfere with the smooth flow of speech. Vocal tics may include repeating the sounds or words of another person (echolalia), repeating one's own sounds or words (palilalia), and involuntary use of obscene language (coprolalia). Like motor tics, vocal tics may develop a ritualistic quality, such as the need to repeat a certain phrase a specific number of times or until it has been said in an exactly "correct" manner.

Sensory tics are defined as patterns of recurrent somatic sensations for which patients attempt to obtain relief by producing movements or vocalizations (2). These sensations are uncomfortable and are localized to specific body regions, and the exact area of discomfort leads to the specific movement or vocalization. The movements may particularly resemble the twisting or writhing type of motor tic often described as dystonic. The understanding that such sensory phenomena occur in a large number of persons with tic disorders had led to a currently unresolved debate as to whether tics are truly involuntary.

DIFFERENTIAL DIAGNOSIS

The nomenclature utilized in describing movement disorders is entirely clinical, and no adequate anatomical, biochemical, or physiological classification exists. Tics must be differentiated from other movement disturbances that can occur in childhood (Table 2) (3,4), including myoclonus, tremor, dystonia, chorea, athetosis, spasms, dyskinesias, and mannerisms. In the usual patient, the identification of a tic disorder is straightforward when made in the context of the overall history and examination.

The diagnosis of tics in children with various developmental disorders may be difficult because peculiar motor movements and language distortions are common in mental retardation, autism, or psychosis (4). Children with these disorders often have complex stereotyped movements, compulsive behavior, odd vocalizations, echolalia, echopraxia, or coprolalia. A further confounding factor is introduced when such patients are treated with neu-

Table 2 Movement Disorders

Myoclonus
Tremor
Dystonia
Chorea
Athetosis
Spasms
Dyskinesias
Mannerisms

roleptic drugs, because both persistent and transient TS have been reported following withdrawal of chronic neuroleptics (5,6). It is possible that tics and the manneristic behavior of developmental disorders may represent a common clinical expression of underlying central nervous system dysfunction.

The differentiation between tics and a seizure disorder should rarely be a problem. On occasion, however, the possibility of myoclonic seizures or complex partial seizures with automatisms is raised. Patients with tics retain consciousness when they have their movements, but an electroencephalogram (EEG) should be performed if there is any doubt.

Sydenham's chorea, the neurological manifestation of rheumatic fever, occurs in the same age group that tic disorders do, and these choreiform movements can easily be mistaken for tics. Close attention to the history, examination for the presence of other signs of rheumatic fever, and awareness of the long-term course of Sydenham's chorea should afford a correct diagnosis. Sydenham's chorea leads to the subacute onset of emotional lability and declining school performance coincident with the onset of the involuntary movements. The chorea may occur as the sole manifestation of rheumatic fever, but it may be associated with carditis and arthritis. Even if untreated, Sydenham's chorea is self-limited and spontaneously disappears over several months. Recurrences are possible, but these repeat episodes tend to be years apart.

Another disorder attributed to an immune response to a streptococcal infection has been labeled pediatric autoimmune neuropsychiatric disorder associated with streptococcal infection (PANDAS). This disorder is being investigated as a possible cause of tic and obsessive–compulsive disorder (OCD) and is fully discussed elsewhere in this volume.

Wilson's disease can lead to involuntary movements that are diverse in nature but can mimic tics. The usual patient will begin to manifest neurological symptoms after the age of 10 years. On the other hand, the most common age of onset for tics is between the ages of 5 and 10 years. Persons with

Wilson's disease may have disorders of other systems, including hepatic dysfunction, hemolytic anemia, or dementia and impulsive behavior.

Other disorders that can be confused with a tic disorder include tardive dyskinesia, chronic amphetamine abuse, posthemiplegic chorea, cerebral palsy, Lesch–Nyhan syndrome, heavy metal poisoning, torsion dystonia, the neuroacanthocytosis syndrome, and subacute sclerosing panencephalitis (7). All are rare and, fortunately, have many features that are clinically different from a tic disorder.

THE SPECTRUM OF TIC DISORDERS

Clinical criteria for the diagnosis of tics are defined operationally in the American Psychiatric Association Diagnostic and Statistical Manual of Mental Disorders, Fourth Edition, Revised (DSM-IV-TR) (8). The three disorders under this reading are: (1) Tourette's disorder, (2) chronic motor or vocal tic disorder, and (3) transient tic disorder (Table 3). These categories are based on the types of tics as well as their duration. Certain features are common to all three categories. They all begin before age 18, are more common in males, and include motor and/or vocal (phonic) tics that occur many times a day.

Transient tic disorder, the most common and mildest of the tic disorders, consists of single or multiple motor and/or vocal tics that occur for at least 2 weeks, but for no longer than 12 consecutive months. The most common forms of tics are blinking, facial movements, throat-clearing, or sniffing. By definition, these tics will disappear permanently after being present for less than 1 year.

A chronic tic disorder consists of either motor or vocal tics, but not both, lasting for more than 1 year. This disorder, which is similar to TS, may consist of a single type of tic only, but there may also be a changing pattern of motor or vocal tics. The tics are often less severe and less bothersome than those in TS.

Tourette's disorder is the diagnosis reserved for those persons who have both multiple motor and vocal tics that have been present for more than 1 year. The tics range in severity from mild to severe. Because the diagnosis of TS is based, in part, on the presence of symptoms for more than 1 year, children seen early in their course cannot be diagnosed with certainly until a sufficient period of time has passed.

An alternative classification has been adopted by the Tourette Syndrome Study Group and endorsed by the Tourette Syndrome Association (TSA) (Table 4) (9). This classification divides tic disorders into those that are transient (present for less than 12 months) and those that are chronic (present

Table 3 DSM-IV-TR Classification of Tics

Transient tic disorder

A. Single or multiple motor and/or vocal tics.
B. The tics occur many times a day, nearly every day for at least 4 weeks, but for no longer than 12 consecutive months.
C. No history of Tourette's chronic motor or vocal tic disorder.
D. The onset is before age 18 years.
E. The disturbance is not due to the direct physiological effects of a substance (e.g., stimulants) or a general medical condition (e.g., Huntington's disease or postviral encephalitis).

Chronic motor or vocal tic disorder

A. Single or multiple motor or vocal tics, but not both, have been present at some time during the illness.
B. The tics occur many times a day, nearly every day, or intermittently throughout a period of more than 1 year, and during this period there was never a tic-free period of more than 3 consecutive months.
C. The onset is before age 18 years.
D. The disturbance is not due to the direct physiological effects of a substance (e.g., stimulants) or a general medical condition (e.g., Huntington's disease or postviral encephalitis).

Tourette's disorder

A. Both multiple motor and one or more vocal tics have been present at some time during the illness, although not necessarily concurrently.
B. The tics occur many times a day (usually in bouts), nearly every day or intermittently throughout a period of more than 1 year, and during this period there was never a tic-free period of more than 3 consecutive months.
C. The anatomical location, number, frequency, complexity, and severity of the tics change over time.
D. The onset is before 18 years.
E. The disturbance is not due to the direct physiological effects of a substance (e.g., stimulants) or a general medical condition (e.g., Huntington's disease or postviral encephalitis).

for more than 12 months). The chronic category is subdivided based on whether there is a single tic or multiple tics and on whether they are motor, vocal, or both. The classification further divides tic syndromes into a "definite" category if the tics have been witnessed, a diagnosis "by history" when the tics have been witnessed by a family member and not an examiner, and a "probable" category for persons who fulfill most, but not all, diagnostic criteria.

Table 4 TS Study Group Classification

A-1.	Definite TS
A-2.	TS by history
B-1.	Definite chronic multiple motor or phonic tic disorder
B-2.	Chronic multiple motor or phonic tic disorder by history
C.	Chronic single motor or phonic tic disorder by history
D-1.	Definite transient tic disorder
D-2.	Transient tic disorder by history
E-1.	Definite nonspecific tic disorder
E-2.	Nonspecific tic disorder by history
F.	Definite tic disorder, diagnosis deferred
G.	Probable TS

THE SPECTRUM OF ASSOCIATED BEHAVIORAL CONDITIONS

Although tics may be chronic, they do not lead to any health problems or physical deterioration. At times, however, the motor tics may be severe enough to lead to local pain. Persons with tics do not have a shortened life span.

A patient's emotional life and his tics are deeply intertwined, but it is no longer believed that these emotional factors are the cause of tics. Complex relationships exist between emotions and tics even in persons whose day-to-day behavior is not out of the ordinary. The severity of children's tics often seems to be a barometer of their emotional state. Many will exhibit a worsening of their symptoms at exciting times, such as holidays, birthdays, or the beginning or ending of school.

A variety of associated behavioral and learning difficulties occur in children with tic disorders (10). Associated behavior and learning difficulties can be present in those with mild tics, as well as in those whose involuntary movements are severe. For many persons, the associated behavioral and learning problems cause more difficulties in everyday life than do the tics (11). Even if tic control is achieved, there is not necessarily a corresponding improvement in the other aspects of the disorder.

The most common associated behavioral difficulties in childhood are of the types considered under the heading of attention deficit/hyperactivity disorder (ADHD). Approximately 50% of children with chronic tics will show evidence of this disorder as manifested by shortened attention span, distractibility, impulsiveness, and motor restlessness (10,12,13). The problems with attentional deficits and hyperactivity usually precede the onset of tics. Many children, therefore, have already received medical attention because of concern regarding behavioral problems, even before the tics have emerged. Some researchers have concluded that the genetic abnormality in TS could be expressed as ADHD without tics (12), but others have reasoned that the commonly observed association between ADHD and TS may represent ascertainment bias, in that persons with both problems are much more likely to be seen for medical evaluation (14).

Obsessive–compulsive behaviors are frequent findings in persons with chronic tic disorders (15,16). Approximately 50% of persons with TS have such symptoms, and many of the complex motor and vocal tics could be considered obsessive–compulsive symptoms and not actual tics. As opposed to attentional difficulties, which usually precede tics, obsessive–compulsive behaviors generally occur after the tics have been present for several years. They tend to worsen and may even first occur during adolescence or early adulthood (17). Obsessive–compulsive symptoms range from mild to severe, and their importance can increase at the same time that the tics are becoming less of a problem. Pauls et al. (18) studied the rates of TS, chronic tic disorder, and obsessive–compulsive disorder (OCD) in first-degree relatives of TS probands. They found an increased rate of OCD in a pattern suggesting that OCD may be an alternative expression of the TS gene.

Other problematic behavioral characteristics have also been noted to occur in persons with chronic tic disorders at a level beyond that expected in the general population (Table 5). These can include unusual levels of anxiety, phobias, fearfulness, emotional lability, low frustration tolerance, impulsivity, aggressiveness, poor socialization skills, and low self-esteem. They tend to coexist with attentional difficulties and frequently lead to temper outbursts that may include screaming, hitting, biting, and threatening others. Self-injurious behavior may also occur (19). Comings (20) has further concluded that, in his experience, other possible behavioral manifestations of chronic tic disorders can include conduct disorders, depression, mania, and panic attacks. It is still uncertain as to whether some of these behavioral difficulties are a direct consequence of having a chronic and stigmatizing disorder, are related only to the ADHD, or are alternative manifestations of the TS gene.

Children with chronic tic disorders often have difficulty in school, and many have repeated grades or are in special-education programs (10,21). Their tics may be disruptive and lead to the mistaken belief that the movements or noises are purposeful, intended to disrupt the classroom or to draw negative attention. Some children will react to the emotional burden of having uncontrollable tics by becoming depressed or aggressive. Those with attentional difficulties may perform poorly because of their short attention span, distractibility, and poor organizational skills. Medications used to treat tic disorders may play a role in limiting school progress, but even untreated children may have poor school performance because of the significant amount of mental energy utilized in suppressing their tics when at school.

Table 5 Associated Behavioral Disturbances

Anxiety
Phobias
Fearfulness
Emotional lability
Low frustration tolerance
Impulsivity
Aggressiveness
Poor socialization skills
Low self-esteem
Self injurious behavior

In addition, many children have underlying learning disabilities as well. Although psychoeducational studies have not uncovered any overall impairment of general intellectual functioning, they have identified patterns of specific learning deficits (22,23). These have included abnormal visual–perceptual performance, reduced visual–motor skills, and discrepancies between verbal and performance IQ. Many of the psychoeducational abnormalities that have been reported are also commonly found in children with ADHD. It is not yet known whether the learning disabilities are related to the chronic tic disorder, the often-associated ADHD, or both.

EVALUATION

Diagnosis must be based on the history and physical examination because there are no diagnostic laboratory studies. A complete past medical history is obtained to determine if there has been any medical event that might have led to tics or other neurological disorders. This history should include detailed questioning regarding prenatal events, birth history, head injuries, episodes of encephalitis or meningitis, poisonings, and medication or drug use. In addition, the developmental, behavioral, and academic histories are important. These include a detailed listing of developmental milestones, estimate of cognitive ability, and history of learning problems. Specific questions must be asked about the possibility of attentional problems, mood lability, depression, anxiety, rituals, and obsessive worries and thoughts, as well as potential compulsive actions.

The age of onset of the involuntary movements, their pattern of waxing and waning, and their exact form should be documented. Questions are asked regarding the possibility of associated sensory urges, suppressibility, and factors associated with worsening or improvement. A detailed family history of tics must be obtained, along with information about others in the family who might have a history of attentional problems, hyperactivity, learning problems, obsessive–compulsive behaviors, or any other form of mental health disturbance.

Except for the tics, physical and neurological examinations are normal in persons with TS or any other form of tic disorder, although the presence of soft neurological signs has sometimes been emphasized in the past (24). Soft signs generally reflect the maturity and degree of development of the central nervous system. Unfortunately, every examiner testing for soft neurological signs seems to have developed his own battery, and standards for scoring are not uniformly applied. There is a high incidence of false-positive as well as false-negative findings, and the presence or absence of soft signs is not a reliable or important part of the evaluation of persons with a tic disorder. As tics can be suppressed while the patient is in the office, no tics may be seen during the interview and examination. Nevertheless, the history can be considered reliable if the description is typical for tics, and tics will usually be seen on subsequent visits.

In the usual patient with a tic disorder, laboratory testing is unnecessary. All clinically available tests will be normal in persons with tic disorders, and laboratory testing is needed only when other causes for the involuntary movements must be considered. EEGs are normal, although some reports have described minor, nondiagnostic abnormalities (25,26). An EEG is useful only in cases where the movements could possibly represent myoclonic or complex partial seizures. Computerized tomography (CT) scans and magnetic resonance imaging (MRI) scans are normal in persons with tic disorders (13). The patient with possible Wilson's disease should have serum copper and ceruloplasmin checked, but the best screening test is actually a slit-lamp examination for Kayser–Fleischer rings. Patients suspected of having Sydenham's chorea or PANDAS should have streptococcal antibody determinations and possibly an echocardiogram. Psychological testing does not diagnose TS but it may identify associated conditions such as learning disabilities or attentional deficits.

Several rating instruments are now available for the assessment of tics and their severity (13). These include videotape protocols or clinical impressions derived from either direct examination or historical data. Available scales include the Hopkins Motor and Vocal Tic Scales, Yale Global Tic Severity Scale, and the Shapiro Tourette Syndrome Severity Scale.

EPIDEMIOLOGY AND ETIOLOGY

Although a genetic marker has not yet been identified, recent studies have indicated a genetic etiology for tic disorders (9). All forms of tics are now felt to represent different points along a spectrum, all of which are attributable to an underlying genetic tendency (27). The finding of transient tic disorders, chronic tic disorders, and TS in the same kindred has led to the concept that all these possible forms of tic disorder are part of the same clinical spectrum and a possible expression of the same genetic defect (28). Pauls and Leckman (29) have reported segregation analysis data collected from families, utilizing a study protocol in which all family members are directly interviewed for the presence of tics or associated behaviors. This information indicates that the disorder is inherited in an autosomal dominant pattern with a sex-specific and incomplete pattern that may be expressed as one form of tic or as obsessive–compulsive disorder. Sex differences noted in TS appear to be related to variability in expressivity, with males having more tic syndromes and females having more obsessive–compulsive behaviors without tics.

The genetic abnormality is thought to lead to abnormality of neurotransmitter function. The exact pattern of abnormality has not yet been definitively determined, but studies have focused on possible abnormalities of dopamine, serotonin, catecholamine, acetylcholine, and gamma amino-butyric acid abnormalities (30). Such abnormal neurotransmitter function would lead to abnormal anatomical function in areas thought relevant to tics such as the interplay between the substantia nigra, striatum, thalamus, and frontal lobes (31).

Most theories have centered on the potential role of dopamine abnormalities because dopamine blockers ameliorate the symptoms (30). Studies that have measured cerebrospinal fluid homovanillic acid, the metabolic end product of dopamine metabolism, have shown conflicting results. Many have found decreased levels, leading to the possibility of hypersensitivity of postsynaptic dopamine receptors.

TS and other tic disorders have been reported in all races, ethnic groups, and socioeconomic classes (19). It occurs more frequently in white than black persons. Initial reports revealed a high percentage of patients to be of Ashkenazi Jewish or Eastern European origin (32); more recent studies, however, have shown that the percentage of patients with these backgrounds is not unusually high (10). TS is predominantly a disorder of males—the male/female ratio is 4:1. An accurate lifetime prevalence rate for tic disorders has not been established. A study in Rochester, Minnesota, gave an estimated annual incidence of 0.05/10,000 (33). A study in North Dakota gave prevalence rates of 1.5 and 9.3 per 10,000 for girls and boys, respectively, and 0.22 and 0.77 per 10,000 for adult women and men (34). Following an extensive informational campaign, Caine et al. (35) diagnosed 41 children among 142,636 pupils enrolled in the Monroe County, New York, school system. All studies have underscored the difficulty in finding persons with mild and nonimpairing symptoms and have concluded that the studies available underestimate the number of affected individuals. More recent studies have come up with a very wide range—from 5 cases per 10,000 (36) to 300 per 10,000 (37).

TREATMENT

No cure exists for any of the primary tic disorders. Potential treatments are symptomatic, and there is no evidence that early treatment alters the natural course of the disorder. The spontaneous waxing and waning of symptoms make it particularly difficult to assess any treatment program and to design adequate studies (38).

Decisions about whether and when to treat an individual patient will depend on the degree to which the tics or other symptoms associated with tic disorders interfere with the person's normal development or ability to function productively. If medication treatment is chosen, it is imperative that an initial decision be reached as to which of the symptoms require treatment, because medications which ameliorate tics often do not improve associated behavioral difficulties. In fact, most persons with milder forms of tic disorders may never require medication treatment.

The initial approach to treatment is to fully explain the disorder to the affected person and his family. Virtually all children with chronic tics have, at some time, been accused of voluntarily doing these mysterious acts. Parents and children react to the diagnosis in a manner that reflects their individual personalities, abilities to cope with uncertainty and stress, and availability of social and medical support. The potential associated problems with behavior or learning disabilities must be brought to the attention of school personnel. Appropriate arrangements may be necessary in the classroom to help overcome a child's problems with learning disabilities, poor handwriting skills, or difficulty with taking timed tests.

Improved understanding can be helped through the services provided by the Tourette Syndrome Association (TSA), an active public support group with many regional offices as well as a national one. TSA members will assist in the education of families by speaking with them directly as well as by sharing their publications.

When symptoms are severe enough to require treatment with medication, the decision to start treatment must be agreed on by the child, family, and physician. Dopamine-blocking agents such as haloperidol remain the best-known medications for the treatment of tics. Neuroleptics are able to reduce tics in 45–70% of those treated, but over 50% will complain of side effects (11). Only 25% report significant improvement without any side effects. Haloperidol, pimozide, and fluphenazine are traditional neuroleptic drugs (39,40). Pimozide was found to be a superior neuroleptic agent in one study (41), but no difference was found in another study (42). Newer neuroleptics such as risperodone are being used extensively (43).

All neuroleptic drugs are used clinically in the same manner. The goal is to find the lowest dosage that will lead to significant improvement while minimizing side effects. To accomplish this, medication is begun at very low dosage and slowly titrated upward. There is no evidence that the concomitant use of anticholinergic medications is of any value in minimizing side effects when given on a routine basis. Frequent side effects include sedation, dysphoria, and weight gain. Subtle side effects can include depression, poor school performance, and school phobias (44). Side effects can occur with even low drug dosages in individual patients. The continued use, or even a discontinuation, of these medications can lead to tardive dyskinesia, tardive dystonia, and the withdrawal emergent syndrome (45–47).

The problems associated with the use of neuroleptic agents have led to a search for alternative medications. Clonidine, an α-adrenergic agonist most frequently used for the treatment of hypertension, is relatively free of severe side effects. It is the most commonly used medication for the treatment of tics (48), although reports on the effectiveness of clonidine have varied. Some studies have indicated that up to 62% of treated patients respond favorably (49), but one study found clonidine to be no more effective than placebo (50). Guanfacine is another α-adrenergic agonist that can be used (51).

Another medication found useful in suppressing tics is clonazepam. A variety of other medications have been tried with variable degrees of success. Among those still considered nonstandard treatments are naltrexone, calcium channel blockers, carbamazepine, and nicotine-containing gum.

Many persons will require medication treatment for associated behavioral abnormalities whether or not they require treatment for tics. The relationship between tic disorders and psychostimulant medications has been controversial. The majority of clinicians believe that these agents have the potential for increasing or inducing tics in some, but not all, persons who are already destined to have a tic disorder. The report published by the Tourette Syndrome Study Group indicated that methylphenidate with or without clonidine could safely be given to children with tics (52). Alternative medications for ADHD include clonidine and the tricyclic antidepressants. Obsessive–compulsive behaviors may also require treatment independent of treatment of other aspects of TS. Newer antidepressants such as clomipramine and fluoxetine are effective by leading to changes in the serotonin system, and they have been found effective in many persons with obsessive–compulsive disorder.

LONG-TERM COURSE AND PROGNOSIS

When a child with tics is initially evaluated, it is not possible to offer a definitive prognosis. The tics may be transient or may become chronic, and they may be mild or severe. In addition, there may or may not be associated behavioral and learning difficulties. Individual components of chronic tic disorders may follow opposite courses. Symptoms of attention deficit disorders tend to begin in the preschool years, peak in the early to middle school years, and become less prominent during adolescence. The motor and vocal tics often begin in the early school years and reach their peak during adolescence, after which they may begin to subside. On the other hand, obsessive–compulsive behaviors will most frequently begin in the later school years and then peak during later adolescence or early adulthood.

Because adolescence is a difficult time of life for almost everyone, it is not surprising that many persons with chronic tic disorders will experience great difficulties during this time. Some patients will have an increase in their tic symptomatology during those years, but this is not a universal occurrence. It is equally important to understand that the same tics present at a younger age may become intolerable during adolescence because of social pressures.

In contrast to earlier descriptions that described TS as inevitably being a lifelong disorder, recent studies have found that up to 73% of patients report that their tics had decreased markedly or disappeared as they entered the latter years of adolescence or early adulthood (11,53). There may not, however, be a proportionate improvement in the associated behavioral difficulties. Moreover, some patients will experience an exacerbation of tics during later adulthood, even if there had been a remission during the earlier adult years (54).

The life adjustments of TS patients has not been adequately studied. Certainly, the severity of the tics is not the only factor that predicts a person's long-term adjustment and outcome. Rather, the associated behavior or emotional problems are more likely to determine social adjustment, vocational status, and marital outcome.

REFERENCES

1. Shapiro E, Shapiro AK. Tic disorders. J Am Med Assoc 1981; 245:1583–1585.
2. Kurlan R, Lichter D, Hewitt D. Sensory tics in Tourette's syndrome. Neurology 1989; 39:731–734.
3. Golden GS. Movement disorders in children: Tourette's syndrome. Dev Behav Pediatr 1982; 3:209–216.
4. Fahn S, Erenberg G. Differential diagnosis of tic phenomena: a neurologic perspective. In: Cohen DJ, Bruun RD, Leckman JF, eds. Tourette's Syndrome and Tic Disorders. New York: Wiley, 1988:41–54.

5. Klawans HL, Falk DK, Nausieda PA, Weiner WJ. Gilles de la Tourette syndrome after long-term chlorpromazine therapy. Neurology 1978; 28:1064–1068.
6. Singer WD. Transient Gilles de la Tourette syndrome after chronic neuroleptic withdrawal. Dev Med Child Neurol 1981; 23:518–521.
7. Fahn S. The clinical spectrum of motor tics. Adv Neurol 1982; 35:341–344.
8. Diagnostic and Statistical Manual of Mental Disorders. 4th revised ed. Washington, DC: American Psychiatric Association, 2000:108–113.
9. Kurlan R. Tourette's syndrome: current concepts. Neurology 1989; 39:1625–1630.
10. Erenberg G, Cruse RP, Rothner AD. Tourette syndrome: an analysis of 200 pediatric and adolescent cases. Clevel Clin Q 1986; 53:127–131.
11. Erenberg G, Cruse RP, Rothner AD. The natural history of Tourette syndrome: a follow-up study. Ann Neurol 1987; 22:383–385.
12. Comings DE, Comings BG. A controlled study of Tourette syndrome: I. Attention deficit disorder, learning disorders and school problems. Am J Hum Gen 1987; 41:701–741.
13. Singer HS, Walkup JT. Tourette syndrome and other tic disorders: diagnosis, pathophysiology, and treatment. Medicine 1991; 70:15–32.
14. Pauls DL, Hurst CR, Kruger SD, Leckman JF, Kidd KK, Cohen DJ. Gilles de la Tourette's syndrome and attention deficit disorder with hyperactivity: evidence against a genetic relationship. Arch Gen Psychiatry 1986; 43:1177–1179.
15. Frankel M, Cummings JL, Robertson MM, Trimble MR, Hill MA, Benson DF. Obsessions and compulsions in Gilles de la Tourette's syndrome. Neurology 1986; 36:378–382.
16. Grad LR, Pelcovitz D, Olson M, Matthews M, Grad G. Obsessive compulsive symptomatology in children with Tourette's syndrome. J Am Acad Child Adolesc Psychiatry 1987; 26:69–73.
17. Leckman JF, Cohen DJ. Descriptive and diagnostic classification of tic disorders. In: Cohen DJ, Bruun RD, Leckman JF, eds. Tourette's Syndrome and Tic Disorders. New York: Wiley, 1988:1–19.
18. Pauls DL, Pakstis AJ, Kurlan R, Kidd KK, Leckman JF, Cohen DJ, Kidd JR, Como P, Sparkes R. Segregation and linkage analysis of Tourette's syndrome and related disorders. J Am Acad Child Adolesc Psychiatry 1990; 29:195–203.
19. Robertson MM. The Gilles de la Tourette syndrome: the current status. Br J Psychiatry 1989; 154:147–169.
20. Comings D. Tourette Syndrome and Human Behavior. Duarte, CA: Hope Press, 1990.
21. Kurlan R, McDermott MP, Deeley C, Como PG, Brower C, Eapen S, Andresen EM, Miller B. Prevalence of tics in schoolchildren and association with placement in special education. Neurology 2001; 57:1383–1388.
22. Golden GS. Psychologic and neuropsycholic aspects of Tourette's syndrome. Neurol Clin 1984; 21:91–102.
23. Bornstein RA. Neuropsychological performance in children with Tourette's syndrome. Psychiatry Res 1990; 33:73–81.
24. Sweet RD, Solomon GE, Wayne H, Shapiro E, Shapiro AK. Neurological

features of Gilles de la Tourette's syndrome. J Neurol Neurosurg Psychiatry 1973; 36:1–9.
25. Krumholz A, Singer HS, Neidermeyer E, Burnite R, Harris K, Electrophysiological studies in Tourette's syndrome. Ann Neurol 1983; 14:638–641.
26. Berger Y, Neufeld MY, Korczyn AD. EEG and brain imaging in Gilles de la Tourette syndrome. Neurology 1990; 40(suppl 1):362.
27. Golden GS. Tics and Tourette's: a continuum of symptoms. Ann Neurol 1978; 4:145–148.
28. Kurlan R, Behr J, Medved L, Como P. Transient tic disorder and the spectrum of Tourette's syndrome. Arch Neurol 1988; 45:1200–1201.
29. Pauls DL, Leckman JF. The inheritance of Gilles de la Tourette's syndrome and associated behaviors: evidence for autosomal dominant transmission. N Engl J Med 1986; 315:993–997.
30. Caine ED. Gilles de la Tourette's syndrome. A review of clinical and research studies and consideration of future directions for investigation. Arch Neurol 1985; 42:393–397.
31. Mink JW. Basal ganglia dysfunction in Tourette's syndrome: a new hypothesis. Pediatr Neurol 2001; 25:190–198.
32. Eldridge R, Sweet R, Lake CR, Ziegler M, Shapiro AK. Gilles de la Tourette's syndrome: clinical, genetic, psychologic, and biochemical aspects in 21 selected families. Neurology 1977; 27:115–124.
33. Lucas AR, Beard CM, Rajput AH, Kurland LT. Tourette syndrome in Rochester, Minnesota, 1968–1979. In: Friedhoff AJ, Chase TN, eds. Gilles de la Tourette Syndrome. New York: Raven Press, 1982:267–269.
34. Burd L, Kerbeshian J, Wikenheiser M, Fisher W. Prevalence of Gilles de la Tourette's syndrome in North Dakota adults. Am J Psychiatry 1986; 143:787–788.
35. Caine ED, McBride MC, Chiverton P, Bamford KA, Rediess S. Tourette's syndrome in Monroe County school children. Neurology 1988; 38:472–475.
36. Apter A, Pauls DL, Bleich A, Zohar AH, Kron S, Ratzoni G, Dycian A, Kotler M, Weizman A, Gadot N, et al. An epidemiologic study of Gilles de la Tourette's syndrome in Israel. Arch Gen Psychiatry 1993; 50:734–738.
37. Mason A, Banerjee S, Eapen V, Zeitlin H, Robertson MM. The prevalence of Tourette syndrome in a mainstream school. Dev Med Child Neurology 1998; 40:292–296.
38. Shapiro AK, Shapiro E. Treatment of tic disorders with haloperidol. In: Cohen DJ, Bruun RD, Leckman JF, eds. Tourette's Syndrome and Tic Disorders. New York: Wiley, 1988:268–280.
39. Singer HS, Gammon K, Quaskey S. Haloperidol, fluphenazine and clonidine in Tourette syndrome: controversies in treatment. Pediatr Neurosci 1985–1986; 12:71–74.
40. Shapiro AK, Shapiro E, Fulop G. Pimozide treatment of tic and Tourette disorders. Pediatrics 1987; 79:1032–1039.
41. Sallee FR, Nesbitt L, Jackson C, Sine L, Sethuraman G. Relative efficacy of haloperidol and pimozide in children and adolescents with Tourette's disorder. Am J Psychiatry 1997; 154:1057–1062.

42. Shapiro E, Shapiro AK, Fulop G, Hubbard M, Mandeli J, Nordlie J, Phillips RA. Controlled study of haloperidol, pimozide and placebo for the treatment of Gilles de la Tourette's syndrome. Arch Gen Psychiatry 1989; 46:722–730.
43. Lombroso PJ, Scahill L, King RA, Lynch KA, Chappell PB, et al. Risperidone treatment of children and adolescents with chronic tic disorders: a preliminary report. J Am Acad Child Adolesc Psychiatry 1995; 34:1147–1152.
44. Braun RD. Subtle and underrecognized side effects of neuroleptic treatment in children with Tourette's disorder. Am J Psychiatry 1988; 145:621–624.
45. Golden GS. Tardive dyskinesia in Tourette syndrome. Pediatr Neurol 1985; 1:192–194.
46. Singer HS. Tardive dyskinesia: a concern for the pediatrician. Pediatrics 1986; 77:553–556.
47. Silverstein FS, Johnston MV. Risks of neuroleptic drugs in children. Child Neurol 1987; 2:41–43.
48. Freeman RD, Fast DK, Burd L, Kerbeshian J, Robertson M, Sandor P. An international perspective on Tourette syndrome: selected findings from 3500 individuals in 22 countries. Dev Med Child Neurol 2000; 42:436–447.
49. Leckman JF, Detlor J, Harcherik DF, Ort S, Shaywitz BA, Cohen DJ. Short and long term treatment of Tourette's syndrome with clonidine: a clinical perspective. Neurology 1985; 35:343–351.
50. Goetz CG, Tanner CM, Wilson RS, Carroll VS, Como PG, Shannon KM. Clonidine and Gilles de la Tourette syndrome: double-blind study using objective rating methods. Ann Neurol 1987; 21:307–310.
51. Chappell PB, Riddle MA, Scahill L, Lynch KA, Schultz R, et al. Guanfacine treatment of comorbid attention-deficit hyperactivity disorder and Tourette's syndrome: preliminary clinical experience. J Am Acad Child Adolesc Psychiatry 1995; 34:1140–1146.
52. Co J, The Tourette's Syndrome Study Group. Treatment of ADHD in children with tics. A randomized controlled trial. Neurology 2002; 58:527–536.
53. Leckman JF, Zhang H, Vitale A, et al. Course of tic severity in Tourette's syndrome: the first two decades. Pediatrics 1998; 102:14–19.
54. Klawans HL. Recurrence of childhood multiple tic in late adult life. Arch Neurol 1985; 42:1079–1080.

9

Tics in Other Neurological Disorders

Joseph Jankovic and Carolyn Kwak
Baylor College of Medicine
Houston, Texas, U.S.A.

TIC PHENOMENOLOGY

Recognition of tics is essential not only in the diagnosis of Tourette syndrome (TS), the most common cause of tics, but also in the diagnosis of other neurological disorders in which tics may occur as one clinical manifestation. The current diagnostic criteria for TS exclude other causes of tics (1,2). Because tics may be confused with other hyperkinetic movement disorders, it is imperative that the full spectrum of phenomenology of tics is appreciated. Tics are characterized by abrupt, repetitive movements (motor tics) or sounds (phonic tics), commonly preceded by a premonitory sensation of an urge, tension, discomfort, or other sensory phenomena (3,4). Motor tics may be classified as either (1) simple tics, involving only one group of muscles, or (2) complex tics, which are coordinated, sequenced movements resembling normal motor acts or gestures (5). Simple motor tics are further classified by frequency and duration of the muscle contraction into clonic, dystonic, or tonic. Clonic tics are abrupt, brief, rapid, jerklike movements, such as excessive blinking and other facial twitches or head and neck jerks. Tics involving briefly sustained muscle contractions have been classified as dystonic and tonic tics. Dystonic tics consist of associated twisting or gyrating motions such as oculogyric or rotatory shoulder movements. Tonic tics involve isometric contractions such as abdominal or limb tensing. Blocking tics, manifested by either start hesitation or a sudden interruption in the normal flow of speech, are often associated with isometric contractions of abdominal muscles producing a Valsava maneuver (forcible exhalation against a closed glottis), which results in a sudden interruption and cessation of speech (6).

Complex motor tics involve sequenced movements consisting of a series of simple motor tics, or repetition of learned, yet nonpurposeful motor gestures, which manifest with inappropriate intensity or erratic timing. Complex motor tics may include head shaking, jumping, squatting, or touching. Complex tics may be also associated with self-injurious behaviors such as head banging, picking, poking, scratching, or stabbing. The phenomenology of complex tic disorders may be integrated with compulsive premonitory urges to complete a sequence of tics, irrespective of physical discomfort or harm resulting from the tic. Other complex tics include copropraxia (socially inappropriate gesturing) and echopraxia (mimicking of others' gestures).

Phonic tics, vocal utterances that result from contractions of the nasopharyngeal and oral passageways, are yet another type of motor tic that may be classified as simple or complex. Simple phonic tics include excessive coughing, throat clearing, grunting, guttural sounds, screaming, sniffing, and squealing. Complex phonic tics consist of meaningless repetitive words or phrases, which include coprolalia (involuntary utterances of obscenities or profanities), echolalia (repetition of others' words), and palilalia (repetition of one's own words, specifically the last syllable).

Premonitory sensations are a hallmark of TS, described as an urge to move, increased tension, a need to apply pressure or stretch a muscle, anxiety, or restlessness. A specific sensory phenomenon in TS patients is the "just right" phenomenon, described as an urge to tic until it feels "just right" (7,8). The presence of an involuntary premonitory sensation preceding a volitional motor response (tic) distinguishes tics from other involuntary movements, such as myoclonus and chorea. Various studies report that over 90% of patients with tics experience a preceding sensory phenomenon, which is transiently relieved after the tic is performed (9). Motor tics are also suppressible, to the extent that premonitory sensations are resistible, further supporting the semivoluntary nature of tics. Furthermore, some (10), but not all (11), patients with tics have premovement potentials (Bereitschafts potential) indicative of a voluntary component to some tics. Tics, similar to myoclonus, are among few movement disorders present during all stages of sleep (12,13).

INVOLUNTARY MOVEMENTS IN THE DIFFERENTIAL DIAGNOSIS OF TICS

Chorea

Chorea is described as an involuntary, abrupt, brief, irregular, continuous, dancelike movement that randomly migrates from one body part to the other.

Impersistence of hand grip and tongue protrusion, irregular frontalis muscle contraction, and pendular patellar reflexes are common findings in patients with chorea. The etiology includes infectious [e.g., Sydenham chorea (SC)], neurodegenerative [e.g., Huntington disease (HD), neuroacanthocytosis], drug-induced (e.g., dopamine receptor-blocking drugs, phenytoin), endocrine and metabolic (e.g., hyperthyroidism, hyperglycemia), vascular, autoimmune, and other disease processes.

Dystonia

Dystonia is a movement disorder characterized by patterned, sustained involuntary agonistic and antagonistic muscle contractions, resulting in a gyrating or twisting motion. Dystonic movements may be repetitive or sustained, involving two or more contiguous muscle groups (segmental dystonia) such as the eyes, neck, shoulder, and upper or lower extremities. Dystonic symptoms may also present as rapid, repetitive movements involving a single muscle group. Dystonic symptoms induced by specific actions or positions such as chewing, playing a musical instrument, walking, or writing are termed task-specific action dystonias. Distinct maneuvers or gestures, referred to as "sensory tricks," are used by the patients to correct the abnormal movement or posture. The use of these tricks may mask the dystonia. Primary (idiopathic) focal and segmental dystonias are the most frequently diagnosed, presenting as cranial dystonia (collectively blepharospasm and oromandibular/lingual dystonia), laryngeal dystonia (spasmodic dysphonia), cervical dystonia (spasmodic torticollis), bruxism/trismus, writer's cramp, or other occupational action dystonias. Axial (truncal) distribution in combination with leg dystonia is referred to as generalized dystonia.

Myoclonus

Myoclonus consists of sudden, brief, involuntary jerks that appear to be shocklike. Myoclonus can be produced by either active muscle contraction (positive myoclonus) or inhibition of ongoing muscle activity (negative myoclonus). The involuntary movement may be preceded by a variety of external stimuli such as light, muscle stretch, noise, touch, visual threat, or other startle cues. Myoclonic jerks may also occur spontaneously, without predictable precipitants. The amplitude and frequency of myoclonus may vary between patients and during the course of the day. The amplitude of a myoclonic jerk may range from a small contraction to involvement of the whole body. The frequency may also vary between patients, ranging from continuous single, intermittent jerks to persistent rhythmic contractions. Myoclonus may present as regular movements, occurring approximately one per second (segmental myoclonus such as palatal or spinal myoclonus), or abrupt, nonrhythmic jerks that decrementally wane within a few seconds (oscillatory myoclonus). The distribution of myoclonus may range from focal, segmental, to generalized.

Stereotypy

A stereotypy is characterized by a continuous, patterned, coordinated, repetitive involuntary movement that appears purposeless or ritualistic. Common stereotypies include body rocking, hand clapping, leg bouncing, pacing, self-caressing, and repetitive tongue protrusion. Oro-facial–lingual movements resembling chewing are often a hallmark of tardive stereotypy, the most common manifestation of tardive dyskinesia. In the setting of pervasive developmental disorders (PDDs) such as Asperger syndrome, autism, Rett syndrome, or mental retardation, stereotypies are often considered to be "self-stimulatory" behaviors. Stereotypies are also observed in conditions such as untreated schizophrenia and neuroacanthocytosis. Self-injurious behaviors, often associated with stereotypies, which result in harm to the body, are also observed in various developmental and psychiatric disorders.

IDIOPATHIC AND GENETIC TIC DISORDERS

TS is the most common primary (idiopathic and inherited) tic disorder (Table 1). As discussed elsewhere in this volume, TS is often associated with comorbidities such as attention-deficit/hyperactivity disorder (ADHD) and obsessive–compulsive disorder (OCD) (14,15). Other idiopathic tic disorders, primarily those that do not meet the Tourette Study Group diagnostic criteria for TS, include transient tic disorder (defined by motor tics present for less than 1 year), coexisting primary dystonia, and adult-onset tics. Other idiopathic and inherited conditions that may present with tics besides other movement disorders include primary (idiopathic and genetic) dystonia (16), HD (17,18), neuroacanthocytosis (19,20), Duchenne muscular dystrophy (21), neurodegeneration with brain iron accumulation (NBIA 1) (22), tuberous sclerosis (23), and biochemical abnormalities with low copper (24).

Primary Dystonia

Dystonic movements share clinical features with motor tics in that they may be rapid, patterned, and repetitive (16,25). Motor tics that are at least transiently sustained, defined as "dystonic tics," such as oculogyric tics, blepharospasm, and rotatory movements of the scapula, may be difficult to distinguish from movements typically seen in patients with primary dystonia. However, dystonic tics are frequently preceded by premonitory sensations, and tend to be less patterned (not always involving the same group of

Table 1 Causes of Tics

(I) Primary

(A) Sporadic

- (1) Transient motor *or* phonic tics (<1 year)
- (2) Chronic motor *or* phonic tics (>1 year)
- (3) Adult-onset (recurrent) tics
- (4) Tourette syndrome
- (5) Primary dystonia

(B) Inherited

- (1) Tourette syndrome
- (2) Huntington disease
- (3) Primary dystonia
- (4) Neuroacanthocytosis
- (5) NBIA
- (6) Tuberous sclerosis
- (7) Wilson disease
- (8) Duchenne's muscular dystrophy
- (9) Albright hereditary osteodystrophy
- (10) Factor VIII hemophilia
- (11) Lesch–Nyhan syndrome
- (12) Neurofibromatosis
- (13) Ehlers–Danlos syndrome
- (14) Congenital adrenal hyperplasia
- (15) Phenylketonuria
- (16) Citrullinemia

(II) Secondary

(A) Infections: encephalitis, Creutzfeldt–Jakob disease, neurosyphilis, Sydenham chorea, HIV, HSV, PANDAS, *M. pneumoniae*, Lyme disease

(B) Drugs: amphetamines, methylphenidate, pemoline, levodopa, cocaine, heroin, carbamazepine, phenytoin, phenobarbital, lamotrigine, antipsychotics, and other dopamine receptor-blocking drug (tardive tics, tardive tourettism)

(C) Toxins: carbon monoxide, wasp venom, mercury

(D) Developmental: static encephalopathy, mental retardation syndromes, autistic spectrum disorders (Asperger, Rett syndrome), fetal alcohol syndrome

(E) Chromosomal disorders: Down's syndrome, Kleinfelter's syndrome, XYY karyotype, 47 XXY, Fragile X, Triple X and 9p mosaicism, partial trisomy 16, 9p monosomy, Beckwith–Wiedemann syndrome, X-linked mental retardation (MRX23)

(F) Other: head trauma, stroke, malignancies, neurocutaneous syndromes, schizophrenia, neurodegenerative diseases, anophthalmia, colpocephaly, pseudohemiparesis, paroxysmal stereotypy, psychogenic tics

Table 1 Continued

(III)	*Related manifestations and disorders*
(A)	ADHD/motor restlessness/akathisia
(B)	OCD/self-injurious behaviors/dermatological manifestations
(C)	Stereotypies/habits/mannerisms
(D)	Migraine headache
(E)	Excessive startle
(F)	Jumping Frenchman
(G)	Disinhibitions/rage attacks
(H)	Phobias/generalized anxiety/mood disorders
(I)	Sleep disorders (PLMS, REM sleep disorder, enuresis)
(J)	GI manifestations (retching, reflux, vomiting)
(K)	Ophthalmic manifestations (blepharospasm, oculogyric)

muscles). Both dystonic tics and premonitory sensations are often alleviated by injections of botulinum toxin (26–28).

Motor tics may also coexist in patients with underlying primary dystonias, or in family members of patients with dystonia (16,25,29,30). Stone and Jankovic (16) initially reported coexisting motor tics in nine patients with primary dystonia (blepharospasm and torticollis), which preceded the dystonic symptoms and described similarities and differences between dystonia and dystonic tics (25). Other reports have drawn attention to the possible association of tics and dystonia in the same family, providing additional evidence for a possible etiologic relationship between TS and primary dystonia (29). Dopa-responsive dystonia with mutations in the *GCH1* gene and TS was found in members of a large Danish family (30). Furthermore, the coexistence of focal dystonia and motor tics has been documented in patients with magnetic resonance imaging (MRI) lesions of the basal ganglia following stroke (31).

Huntington Disease

The random, abrupt movements observed in chorea may resemble motor tics. Although chorea has been reported to be suppressible, premonitory sensations frequently associated with tics are not reported by patients with chorea. In patients evaluated in the Movement Disorders Clinic, chorea is most frequently seen in the setting of HD. This autosomal dominant neurodegenerative disorder, caused by expanded CAG repeats in the *huntigtin* gene on chromosome 4, is characterized by chorea, cognitive decline, and behavioral changes. HD patients may also exhibit disinhibitive behaviors, involuntary vocalizations, and obsessive–compulsive features, all of which are typically present as comorbid features in patients with TS. Therefore the diagnosis of HD in TS patients, and vice versus, may be difficult to recognize. Several cases of adult-onset tics such as coughing, facial grimacing, grunting, head jerking, and sniffing have been reported to be the presenting or coexisting features of HD (17,18). Jankovic and Ashizawa reported a 40-year-old man who had onset of depression and involuntary irregular leg movements, which progressed to his whole body at age 31 years, and who, 8 years later, noted persistent sniffing and coughing attributed to "allergies." The patient then developed other motor tics including facial grimacing and head jerking. The patient also had a strong family history of neurodegenerative disorders and involuntary movements. Neurological examination revealed clonic and dystonic tics of head turning and extension, generalized chorea, and a minimental examination score of 20. An MRI scan showed caudate and cortical atrophy, and a DNA analysis detected a mutation in the HD gene, containing 47 CAG repeats. These case studies have highlighted some important clinical clues to differentiating TS-like symptoms from symptoms of HD. Patients with adult-onset TS with a family history of neurodegenerative disorders should be suspects of HD.

Neuroacanthocytosis

The term "neuroacanthocytosis" was first used by Spitz et al. (19) to describe a form of hereditary chorea associated with a variety of neurological abnormalities such as self-mutilatory behaviors including lip and tongue biting (16%), seizures (42%), cognitive changes (63%), dysphagia (47%), dysarthria (74%), personality and psychiatric changes (58%), areflexia (68%), and amyotrophy (16%). Besides motor and phonic tics present in over 40% of the patients, other involuntary movements associated with neuroacanthocytosis include chorea (58%), dystonia (47%), orofacial dyskinesia (53%), parkinsonism (34%), and involuntary vocalizations (47%). Diagnostic findings include evidence of axonal neuropathy, elevated serum creatine kinase without myopathy, and more than 3% acanthocytes on peripheral blood smear. Positive emission tomography (PET) studies showed a 42% reduction of normal [F]dopa uptake in the posterior putamen (32). Neuronal loss and gliosis were evident in the striatum and pallidum, and possibly the anterior horns of the spinal cord, substantia nigra, and thalamus (33). Nigral neuronal loss is more diffuse in neuroacanthocytosis patients compared to that in Parkinson's disease, where it is most prominent in the ventrolateral region (34). A genome-wide scan in 11 families with autosomal recessive pattern of inheritance revealed linkage to chromosome 9q21 (35), and subsequent studies identified homozygous mutations in the *CHAC* (chorea acanthocytosis) gene (36). Analysis of erythrocyte membrane proteins of six patients with neuroacanthocytosis using high-performance liquid chromatography revealed abnormalities in the covalent binding of fatty acids with an increase in palmitic acid and a decrease in stearic acid (37).

NBIA

NBIA, previously termed Hallervorden–Spatz disease, may also present with tics, self-mutilatory behavior, dementia, dystonia, progressive rigidity, and spasticity (22). Case studies have shown that although rare, tics may be a presenting symptom of this neurodegenerative disorder. Severe incapacitation and early death during adolescence or young adulthood with the onset of symptoms during childhood are common, although symptoms may present as adult-onset parkinsonism and dementia. MRI findings in NBIA reveal marked hypointensity surrounded by an area of hyperintensity on T2-weighted images in the globus pallidus internal (GPi) segment ("eye-of-the-tiger" sign) and hypointensity of substantia nigra reticulata (SNr). The central hypointensity correlates with deposition of iron, whereas the surrounding hyperintensity seems to correlate with gliosis and axonal spheroids (38). Linkage analyses initially localized the NBIA gene on 20p12.3-p13 and subsequently 7-bp deletion and various missense mutations were identified in the coding sequence of gene *PANK-2*, which codes for pantothenate kinase (39). Pantothenate kinase is an essential regulatory enzyme in coenzyme A (CoA) biosynthesis. The disorder with the clinical phenotype of NBIA associated with mutations in the *PANK-2* gene is now referred to as pantothenate kinase-associated neurodegeneration (PKAN) (40). Based on an analysis of 123 patients from 98 families with NBIA-1, Hayflick et al. (41) found that "classic Hallervorden–Spatz syndrome" was associated with *PANK-2* mutation in all cases and one third of "atypical" cases had the mutations within the *PANK-2* gene. Those who had the *PANK-2* mutation were more likely to have dysarthria and psychiatric symptoms, and all had the typical "eye-of-a-tiger" abnormality on MRI with a specific pattern of hyperintensity within the hypointense GPi.

Pervasive Developmental Disorders

Behavioral symptoms such as attention deficit, disinhibition, poor impulse control, and obsessive–compulsive features are commonly observed in patients with TS and developmental disorders such as infantile autism, Asperger syndrome, Rett syndrome, mental retardation, and other PDDs (42,43). One study of 41 PDD cases showed 16 patients who initially presented with autism or PDD and later developed TS symptoms (44). Several studies of patients with Asperger syndrome, a type of autistic disorder characterized by impairment in reciprocal social interactions, circumscribed interest in one topic, speech and language impediments, nonverbal communication problems, lack of empathy for others, motor clumsiness, repetitive behavior, and rigid thinking, also reported the co-occurrence of tics (45–48). Ringman and Jankovic (49) observed eight patients with Asperger syndrome who were referred to the Baylor College of Medicine Movement Disorders Clinic with stereotypies. Seven of eight patients were also diagnosed with a tic disorder, six of whom met the diagnostic criteria for TS.

Another autistic disorder associated with a variety of movement disorders including stereotypies, dystonia, and tics is Rett syndrome. Occurring almost exclusively in girls, this disorder usually presents between the ages of 9 months and 3 years, with gradual social withdrawal, psychomotor regression, loss of acquired communication skills, and hand clumsiness that is gradually replaced by stereotypical hand movements, including hand clapping, wringing, clenching, washing, patting, rubbing, picking, and mouthing. Additionally, Rett girls often exhibit body rocking and shifting of weight from one leg to the other. Although most girls with Rett are able to walk, the gait is usually broad-based and ataxic, associated with retropulsion and loss of balance. Other motor disturbances include respiratory dysregulation with episodic hyperventilation and breath holding, bruxism, ocular deviations, dystonia, myoclonus, tics, athetosis, tremor, jerky truncal and gait ataxia, and parkinsonian findings. In a study of 32 Rett patients, ages 30 months to 28 years, we suggested that the occurrence of the different motor disorders seemed to be age-related (50).

The pathophysiological basis of the motor disturbances in Rett syndrome has not been elucidated. MRI studies have shown generalized brain and bilateral caudate atrophy. In a few postmortem examinations of Rett brains, besides marked reduction in both gray matter and white matter volume, particularly involving the caudate nucleus, some studies also found spongy degeneration of cerebral and cerebellar white matter, deposition of lipofuscin, and depigmentation of substantia nigra and locus coeruleus. The various neuropathological findings have been interpreted as a failure in the proper development or maintenance of synaptic connections. The major advance in understanding the biology of Rett syndrome has come with the discovery of a gene that is responsible for most, but not all, cases of the Rett phenotype. Loss-of-function mutations of the X-linked gene encoding methyl–CpG binding protein 2 (*MECP2*) have been found to be responsible for more than 80% of Rett cases (51). A broad range of associated *MECP2* mutations have been described to involve not only girls and women, but also males, including a variety of autistic spectrum disorders such as Angelman syndrome, learning disabilities, mental retardation, and fatal encephalopathy (52). We excluded mutations in the *MECP2* gene in our population of patients with TS (53).

Other Genetic and Chromosomal Disorders

There have been a number of genetic and chromosomal disorders reported to manifest with tics. Disorders of the X chromosome are among the most frequently reported genetic conditions associated with tics. X-linked mental retardation (MRX23) (54), Albright hereditary osteodystrophy (55), Duchenne muscular dystrophy (21), factor VIII hemophilia (56), fragile X syndrome (57,58), Lesch–Nyhan syndrome (59), triple X and 9P mosaicism (60), and 47 XXY karyotype (61) are among these X-linked disorders. Tics observed in other chromosomal disorders include Down syndrome (62,63), Klinefelter syndrome (64), partial trisomy 16 (65), 9p monosomy (66), and tuberous sclerosis (23). Other documented genetic disorders with coexisting tics and TS symptomatology observed in patients at the Baylor College of Medicine Movement Disorders Clinic include congenital adrenal hyperplasia secondary to 21-hydroxylase deficiency, neurofibromatosis, and phenylketonuria (67). Fragile chromosomal sites and breakpoints have also been recently reported in tic case studies (68–73).

SECONDARY TIC DISORDERS

The term "tourettism" has been used to describe TS-like symptoms secondary to some specific cause (74) (Table 2). Besides TS, tics have been reported secondary to numerous causes such as cerebral infarction, infection, head trauma, medication use, and in association with other neurodegenerative disorders (75–85).

Stroke and Other Brain Lesions

One of the strongest arguments in support of the neurological origin of TS is that TS-like disorders ("tourettism") have been well documented with lesions of the basal ganglia (31). Case reports of two boys who suffered a subcortical stroke, both at age 8 years, presented with subsequent onset of hemidystonia, tics, and behavioral comorbidities. Both had right hemisphere strokes involving the basal ganglia at age 8 years and in both, the latency from the stroke to the onset of left hemidystonia was 2 weeks. In addition to ADHD and OCD, both exhibited cranial–cervical motor tics, but no phonic tics. The temporal relationship between the stroke and subsequent TS-like symptoms, as well as the absence of phonic tics and family history of TS symptoms in our patients, argue in favor of a cause-and-effect relationship and against a simple coincidental occurrence of a stroke and idiopathic TS. Three additional reports have described individual cases of TS-like symptoms secondary to vascular lesions (86). In one report, a 43-year-old man developed motor tics after a four-artery angiography (82). Although neuroimaging was not avail-

Table 2 Acquired Tics/Comorbid Behaviors Secondary to Brain Lesions

Study/case report	Lesion site	Etiology	Symptom
Berthier et al. (107)	Midbrain, infrathalamic, thalamic, striatum	Hypoxic–ischemic necrosis	TS, Asperger
Kwak and Jankovic (31)	Right putamen and caudate, right middle cerebral artery, basal ganglia	Infarction, migrainous ischemic stroke	Tics, hemidystonia, ADHD, OCD
Melling et al. (142)	Facial nerve VII	Vascular compression by anterior, inferior cerebellar artery	Facial tic
Demirkol et al. (92)	Bilateral, symmetrical globus pallidus "tiger's eye" lesion	Unknown	Tics, ADHD, OCD
Hugo et al. (89)	Temporal and frontal lobes	Hypoperfusion and compensatory hyperperfusion	OCD
Rodrigo et al. (87)	Bilateral globus pallidus	Carbon monoxide poisoning, infarction	OCD
Berthier et al. (90)	Frontal and temporal lobes, cingulate, caudate	Tumor (lipoma, hygroma, angioma, hamartoma, tuberous sclerosis), arachnoid cyst, postencephalitic hydrocephalus, head trauma, infarction	OCD
Peterson et al. (93)	Ventral striatum, corpus collosum, thalamus, midbrain	Malignancy	Tics, OCD, with temporal progression of tics and OCD with tumor progression
Simpson and Baldwin (88)	Right inferior parietal	Infarction	OCD
Swoboda and Jenike (86)	Right posterior frontal, right internal carotid occlusion	Infarction	OCD
Max et al. (91)	Frontal and temporal lobe lesions	Head trauma	OCD
Ward (84)	Fronto-parietal lobe, left frontal, lacunar infarcts in right superior cerebellar peduncle and left basal ganglia	Infarction, tumor	Transient feelings of compulsion

able when the case was first reported, a vascular lesion in the basal ganglia was suspected to be responsible for subsequent tics including tongue clicking and protrusion, eye closure, sniffing, frowning, and numerous other motor tics as well as palilalia. Neurobehavioral changes were not reported in this patient. Masso and Obeso (83) described a 66-year-old man with postanoxic hemiballism and concomitant onset of coprolalia, but without motor or phonic tics. Both the hemiballism and coprolalia improved with tetrabenazine. More recently, Ward (84) reported on a 62-year-old woman with acute onset of dysphasia and a subsequent suppressible "urge" to shake her right arm. A computed tomography (CT) scan showed lacunar infarcts in the right superior cerebellar peduncle and left basal ganglia.

Although idiopathic OCD is usually not associated with any identifiable, anatomic lesion (85), several cases of secondary OCD have been documented (86–95). Acquired obsessive–compulsive symptoms have been reported secondary to infarction of inferior parietal lobe (89), posterior frontal lobe (86), both globus pallidi (75), and both caudate nuclei (96). Several documented cases of acquired OCD associated with cerebral malignancy, trauma, or perfusion abnormalities have been attributed to lesions involving the frontal, parietal, and temporal lobes, and cingulate areas (90,93). There is now a substantial body of evidence implicating basal ganglia dysfunction in the pathogenesis of OCD (97–99). In a study of patients with bilateral basal ganglia lesions secondary to trauma, anoxic and toxic encephalopathy, stereotyped behaviors, and obsessive–compulsive behaviors were seen in many of these patients after the reported injuries (97). We and others have observed patients with Parkinson's disease and atypical parkinsonism who have developed features of OCD, such as obsessions with bowels, compulsive gambling, and other ritualistic behaviors as their disease progresses (98).

Acquired TS symptoms of tics and neurobehavioral comorbidities have been reported secondary to a variety of other lesions, usually involving the basal ganglia (97,100–104). Furthermore, various imaging and biochemical studies provide support for frontal–subcortical involvement in mediating human behavior (105). In TS, the cortico-striatal–thalamic–cortical circuit plays an important role in the pathogenesis of TS and related disorders (106). A dysfunction in the dorsolateral prefrontal circuit, which links Brodmann areas 9 and 10 with the dorsolateral head of the caudate, has been implicated in an impairment of "executive functions" and possibly in ADHD. The lateral orbitofrontal circuit originates in the inferior lateral prefrontal cortex (area 10) and projects to the ventral medial caudate. An abnormality in this circuit is associated with personality changes, mania, disinhibition, and irritability. A recent case report described the coexistence of Asperger syndrome and TS caused by hypoxic necrosis of the midbrain, infrathalamic and thalamic nuclei, and striatum (107). Lastly, the anterior cingulate circuit—which arises in the cingulate gyrus (area 24); receives input from the amygdala, hippocampus, medial orbitofrontal cortex, entorhinal cortex, and perirhinal cortex; and projects to the ventral striatum—has been linked to a variety of behavioral problems including OCD (108).

Head Trauma

Tics following head trauma have been relatively rare. However, reports of patients (age range 3–47 years, mean 23 years) who developed tics after closed-head injuries have been documented in the literature (109–111). Motor tics, including phonic tics, and the new onset of obsessive–compulsive symptoms were present within 2–3 weeks of the head injury. Two patients referred to the Baylor College of Medicine Movement Disorders Clinic had preexisting tics, with marked exacerbation of the motor tics after the traumatic incident, suggesting that these patients may have been predisposed to develop tics.

Infections

Extensive research efforts have been recently made to investigate the role of group A β-hemolytic *Streptococcus* (GABHS) as a possible etiological agent of tics and other TS symptomatology (112–114). SC, TS, ADHD, and OCD have been thought to share anatomic pathology of the basal ganglia and the cortico-striato-thalamo-cortical circuits. Pediatric Autoimmune Neuropsychiatric Disorders Associated with Streptococcal infection (PANDAS) have also been studied with interest by clinicians and scientists because of several reported cases of coexisting SC, TS, and OCD (114).

Postencephalitic tourettism, an encephalitic lethargica pandemic associated with TS symptomatology that occurred between 1916 and 1927 in Europe, is another reported secondary infectious cause of TS (74). Motor tics reported included complex vocalizations of blocking, compulsive shouting (klazomania), echolalia, palilalia, and oculogyric crises (115). Autopsy revealed neurofibrillary tangles and neuronal loss in the globus pallidus, hypothalamus, midbrain tegmentum, periaqueductal gray matter, striatum, and the substantia nigra, which lead scientists to target involvement of these structures in the pathogenesis of TS (116). A recent patient with tourettism manifested as the abrupt onset of facial grimacing and shoulder shrugging following an 8-week viral encephalitis revealed bilateral lesions in the basal ganglia on MRI of the brain. Other forms of viral encephalitis caused by agents including the herpes simplex virus (HSV) (117) and the human immunodeficiency virus (HIV) (118,119) have been reported in the presence of motor and phonic tics. *Mycoplasma pneumoniae* and Lyme infections presenting with tics have also been recently documented (120,121).

Drugs and Toxins

Reported use of certain medications or substances such as amphetamines, cocaine, heroin, methylphenidate, pemoline, levodopa, antidepressants, carbamazepine, phenytoin, phenobarbitol, lamotrigine, and other dopamine-blocking agents (neuroleptics) have been known to induce tics (76,77,122–135). Toxins such as carbon monoxide, wasp venom, and mercury have also been noted to cause tics (132,133). Central nervous system stimulants such as dextroamphetamine, methylphenidate, and pemoline used to treat attention-deficit/hyperactivity disorder have been well recognized to exacerbate or precipitate tics (122–126). Substances such as cocaine and heroin have also been known to exacerbate tics (78,135). Cardoso and Jankovic (78) reported three patients diagnosed with a hyperkinetic movement disorder, whose movements were exacerbated with exposure to cocaine. In one patient, cocaine use caused a recurrence of motor tics in a 22-year-old man with TS who had been in remission until the age of 20 years. Other documented reports support cocaine as a cause of tics, even in patients who are not predisposed to have a tic disorder.

"Tardive tourettism" is the term used to describe tics induced by dopamine-blocking agents (neuroleptics) (127,128). However, tics have been rarely reported as a form of tardive dyskinesia—hyperkinetic involuntary movements that result from the use of dopamine-blocking agents. Tardive stereotypies or vocalizations may also be misrecognized as tics, and often treated with dopamine-blocking drugs, which may exacerbate the tardive syndrome. Tics usually improve with dopamine-blocking drugs, suggesting a hyperdopaminergic state. Inconsistent results have been reported for serotonin reuptake inhibitor as a causative agent of tics (129–131).

MISCELLANEOUS DISORDERS

In addition to the tic disorders reported, other disorders associated with tics may include anophthalmia (136), colpocephaly (137), pseudohemiparesis (138), and tumors involving the basal ganglia and limbic regions (139,140). Tics may also be within the spectrum of psychogenic disorders (141) produced intentionally (factitious disorder) or unintentionally (conversion disorder). Psychogenic tic disorders present as a clinical challenge because of the semivolitional, suggestible, suppressible, and intermittent nature of motors tics. However, psychogenic patients who are unaware of, and fail to provide, a history of comorbid features associated with TS may assist clinicians in distinguishing organic from psychogenic etiology. Furthermore, the presence of premonitory sensations that commonly precede idiopathic tics may be absent or excluded from the history of a patient with psychogenic tics.

CONCLUSION

The aim of this review is to draw attention to the importance of distinguishing motor tics from other movement disorders, and to recognize the broad range of disorders associated with tics. It is noteworthy to emphasize that an association does not necessarily define a cause-and-effect relationship. However, several other disorders that present with coexisting tics may provide insights into pathogenic mechanisms underlying idiopathic tic disorders and TS. An understanding of the phenomenology of tics prepares the clinician in recognizing the spectrum of both semivolitional and involuntary movement disorders.

REFERENCES

1. The Tourette Syndrome Classification Study Group. Definitions and classification of tic disorders. Arch Neurol 1993; 50:1013–1016.
2. American Psychiatric Association. Diagnostic and Statistical Manual of Mental Disorders. 4th ed. Washington, DC: American Psychiatric Press, 1994:100–105.
3. Leckman J, Walker D, Cohen D. Premonitory urges in Tourette's syndrome. Am J Psychiatry 1993; 150:98–102.
4. Leckman J, Peterson B, King R, Scahill L, Cohen D. Phenomenology of tics and natural history of tic disorders. In: Cohen DJ, Jankovic J, Goetz CG, eds. Tourette Syndrome. Advances in Neurology. Vol. 85. Philadelphia: Lippincott, Williams and Wilkins, 2001:1–14.
5. Jankovic J, Fahn S. The phenomenology of tics. Mov Disord 1986; 1:17–26.
6. Jankovic J. Phenomenology and classification of tics. In: Jankovic J, ed. Tourette Syndrome. Neurology Clinics of North America. Vol. 15. Philadelphia: WB Saunders, 1997:267–275.
7. Leckman J, Walker D, Goodman W, et al. "Just right" perceptions associated with compulsive behavior in Tourette's syndrome. Am J Psychiatry 1994; 151:675–680.
8. Karp B, Hallett M. Extracorporeal 'phantom tics' in Tourette's syndrome. Neurology 1996; 46:38–40.
9. Scahill L, Leckman J, Marek K. Sensory phenomenon in Tourette's syndrome. In: Weiner W, Lang A, eds. Behavioral Neurology of Movement Disorders. Advances in Neurology. Vol. 65. New York: Raven Press Ltd., 1995:273–280.
10. Karp B, Porter S, Toro C, Hallett M. Simple motor tics may be preceded by a premotor potential. J Neurol Neurosurg Psychiatry 1996; 61:103–106.
11. Obeso J, Rothwell J, Marsden C. The neurophysiology of Tourette syndrome. Adv Neurol 1982; 35:105–114.
12. Fish D, Sawyers D, Allen P. The effect of sleep on the dyskinetic movements of Parkinson's disease, Gilles de la Tourette syndrome, Huntington's disease, and torsion dystonia. Arch Neurol 1991; 48:210–214.

13. Hanna P, Jankovic J. Sleep and tic disorders. In: Chokroverty S, Hening A, Walters, eds. Sleep and Movement Disorders. Woburn, MA: Butterworth-Heinemann, 2003:464–471.
14. Moll G, Heinrich H. Children with comorbid attention-deficit-hyperactivity disorder and tic disorder: evidence for additive inhibitory deficits with the motor systems. Ann Neurol 2001; 49:393–396.
15. Eapen V, Robertson M, Alsobrook J, Pauls D. Obsessive–compulsive symptoms in Gilles de la Tourette syndrome and obsessive compulsive disorder: differences by diagnosis and family history. Am J Med Genet 1997; 74:432–438.
16. Stone L, Jankovic J. The coexistence of tics and dystonia. Arch Neurol 1991; 48:862–865.
17. Kerbeshian J, Burd L, Leech C, et al. Huntington's disease and childhood onset Tourette syndrome. Am J Med Genet 1991; 39:1–3.
18. Jankovic J, Ashizawa T. Tourettism associated with Huntington's disease. Mov Disord 1995; 10:103–105.
19. Spitz M, Jankovic J, Killian J. Familial tic disorder, parkinsonism, motor neuron disease, and acanthocytosis: a new syndrome. Neurology 1985; 35:366–377.
20. Hardie R, Pullon H, Harding A, et al. Neuroacanthocytosis: a clinical, haematological and pathological study of 19 cases. Brain 1991; 114:13–49.
21. Lewis J, Bertorini T. Duchenne muscular dystrophy and Tourette syndrome. Neurology 1982; 32:329–331.
22. Nardocci N, Rumi V, Combi M, et al. Complex tics, stereotypies, and compulsive behavior as clinical presentation of juvenile progressive dystonia suggestive of Hallervorden–Spatz disease. Mov Disord 1994; 9:369–371.
23. Matthews K. Familial Gilles de La Tourette's syndrome associated with tuberous sclerosis. Tex Med 1981; 77:46–49.
24. Robertson M, Evans K, Robinson A, Trimble M, Lascelles P. Abnormalities of copper in Gilles de la Tourette syndrome. Biol Psychiatry 1987; 22:968–978.
25. Jankovic J, Stone L. Dystonic tics in patients with Tourette's syndrome. Mov Disord 1991; 6:248–252.
26. Jankovic J. Botulinum toxin in the treatment of dystonic tics. Mov Disord 1994; 9:347–349.
27. Kwak C, Hanna P, Jankovic J. Botulinum toxin in the treatment of tics. Arch Neurol 2000; 57:1190–1193.
28. Marras C, Andrews D, Sime E, Lang A. Botulinum toxin for simple motor tics: a randomized, double-blind, controlled clinical trial. Neurology 2001; 56:605–610.
29. Németh A, Mills K, Elston J, et al. Do the same genes predispose to Gilles de la Tourette syndrome and dystonia? Report of a new family and review of the literature. Mov Disord 1999; 14:826–831.
30. Romstad A, Dupont E, Krag-Olsen B, Ostergaard K, Guldberg P, Guttler F. Dopa-responsive dystonia and Tourette syndrome in a large Danish family. Arch Neurol 2003; 60:618–622.
31. Kwak C, Jankovic J. Tourettism and hemidystonia secondary to stroke. Mov Disord 2002; 17:821–825.

32. Brooks D, Ibanez V, Playford E, et al. Presynaptic and postsynaptic striatal dopaminergic function in neuroacanthocytosis: a positron emission tomography study. Ann Neurol 1991; 30:166–171.
33. Rinne J, Daniel S, Scaravilli F. The neuropathological features of neuroacanthocytosis. Mov Disord 1994; 9:297–304.
34. Rinne J, Daniel S, Scaravilli F. Nigral degeneration in neuroacanthocytosis. Neurology 1994; 44:1629–1632.
35. Rubio J, Danek A, Stone C. Chorea-acanthocytosis: genetic linkage to chromosome 9q21. Am J Hum Genet 1997; 61:899–908.
36. Rampoldi L, Danek A, et al. Clinical features and molecular basis of neuroacanthocytosis. J Mol Med 2002; 80:475–491.
37. Sakai T, Antoku Y, Iwashita H, et al. Chorea-acanthocytosis: abnormal composition of covalently bound fatty acids of erythrocyte membrane proteins. Ann Neurol 1991; 21(29):664–669.
38. Taylor T, Litt M, Kramer P, et al. Homozygosity mapping of Hallervorden–Spatz syndrome 20p12.3-p13. Nat Genet 1996; 14:479–481.
39. Zhou B, Westaway S, Levinson B, et al. A novel pantothenate kinase gene (*PANK2*) is defective in Hallervorden–Spatz syndrome. Nat Genet 2001; 28:345–349.
40. Thomas M, Hayflick S, Jankovic J. Clinical heterogeneity of pantothenate kinase-associated neurodegeneration (PKAN). Neurology 2002; 58(suppl 3):A322.
41. Hayflick S, Westaway S, Levinson B, et al. Genetic, clinical, and radiographic delineation of Hallervorden–Spatz syndrome. N Engl J Med 2003; 348:33–40.
42. Kano Y, Ohta M, Nagai Y. Tourette's disorder coupled with infantile autism: a prospective study of two boys. Jpn J Psychiatry 1988; 42:49–57.
43. Sverd J. Tourette's syndrome and autistic disorder: significant relationship. Am J Med Genet 1991; 39:173–179.
44. Comings D, Comings B. Clinical and genetic relationships between autism, pervasive developmental disorder and Tourette syndrome: a study of 19 cases. Am J Med Genet 1991; 39:180–191.
45. Asperger H. Die "Autistischen psychopathen" im kindesalter. Arch Psychiatr Nervenkr 1944; 117:76–136.
46. Szatmari P, Bremner R, Nagy J. Asperger's syndrome: a review of clinical features. Can J Psychiatry 1989; 34:554–559.
47. Gillberg I, Gillberg C. Asperger's syndrome—some epidemiological considerations: a research note. J Child Psychol Psychiatry 1989; 30:631–638.
48. Volkmar F, Klin A, Pauls D. Nosological and genetic aspects of Asperger syndrome. J Autism Dev Disord 1998; 28:457–463.
49. Ringman J, Jankovic J. The occurrence of tics in Asperger syndrome and autistic disorder. J Child Neurol 2000; 15:394–400.
50. Fitzgerald P, Jankovic J, Glaze D, Schultz R, Percy A. Extrapyramidal involvement in Rett's syndrome. Neurology 1990; 40:293–295.
51. Fitzgerald P, Jankovic J, Percy A. Rett syndrome and associated movement disorders. Mov Disord 1990; 5:195–203.

52. Akbarian S. The neurobiology of Rett syndrome. Neuroscientist 2003; 9:57–63.
53. Percy A. Rett syndrome: current status and new vistas. Neurol Clin N Am 2002; 20:1125–1141.
54. Searcy E, Burd L, Kerbeshian J, Stenehjem A, Franceschini L. Asperger's syndrome, X-linked mental retardation and chronic vocal tic disorder. J Child Neurol 2000; 15:699–702.
55. Kerbeshian J, Burd L. Asperger's syndrome and Tourette syndrome: the case of the pinball wizard. Br J Psychiatry 1985; 148:731–736.
56. Bowden D, Rothenberg M. Comprehensive care of a mentally retarded, adolescent hemophiliac with tongue-biting tic. Pediatrics 1969; 43:19–25.
57. Kerbeshian J, Burd L, Martsolf J. Fragile X syndrome associated with Tourette symptomatology in a male with moderate mental retardation and autism. J Dev Behav Pediatr 1984; 5:201–203.
58. Finelli P, Pueschel S, Padre-Mendoza T, et al. Neurological findings in patients with the fragile X syndrome. J Neurol Neurosurg Psychiatry 1985; 48:150–153.
59. Jankovic J, Caskey T, Stout J, et al. Lesch–Nyhan syndrome: a study of motor behavior and CSF monoamine turnover. Ann Neurol 1988; 23:466–469.
60. Singh D, Howe G, Jordan H, et al. Tourette's syndrome in a black woman with associated triple X and 9p mosaicism. J Nat Med Assoc 1982; 74:675–682.
61. Jankovic J. Tics in other neurological disorders. In: Kurlan R, ed. Handbook of Tourette's Syndrome and Related Tic and Behavioral Disorders. New York: Marcel Dekker, 1993:167–182.
62. Barabas G, Wardell B, Sapiro M, et al. Coincident Down's and Tourette's syndromes: three case reports. J Child Neurol 1986; 1:358–360.
63. Karlinsky H, Sandor P, Berg J, et al. Gilles de la Tourette's syndrome in Down's syndrome—a case report. Br J Psychiatry 1986; 148:601–604.
64. Louhivuori K, Jakobson T. Prepubertal Klinefelter syndrome: child psychiatric aspects illustrated by two case reports. Ann Clin Res 1969; 1:134–139.
65. Hebebrand J, Martin M, Korner J, et al. Partial trisomy 16p in an adolescent with autistic disorder and Tourette's syndrome. Am J Med Genet 1994; 54:268–270.
66. Taylor L, Krizman D, Jankovic J, et al. 9p monosomy in a patient with Gilles de la Tourette's syndrome. Neurology 1991; 41:1513–1515.
67. Jankovic J. Differential diagnosis and etiology of tics. In: Cohen D, Jankovic J, Goetz C, eds. Advances in Neurology. Philadelphia: Lippincott, Williams and Wilkins, 2001:15–30.
68. Kerbeshian J, Severud R, Burd L, Larson L. Peek-a-boo fragile site at 16d associated with Tourette syndrome, bipolar disorder, autistic disorder, and mental retardation. Am J Med Genet 2000; 96:69–73.
69. Matsumoto N, David D, Johnson E, Konecki D, Burmester J, Ledbetter D, Weber J. Breakpoint sequences of an 1;8 translocation in a family with Gilles de la Tourette syndrome. Eur J Hum Genet 2000; 8:875–883.
70. Petek E, Windpassinger C, Vincent J, Cheung J, Boright A, Scherer S, Kroisel P, Wagner K. Disruption of a novel gene (*IMMP2L*) by a breakpoint in 7q31 associated with Tourette syndrome. Am J Hum Genet 2001; 68:848–858.

71. Kroisel P, Petek E, Emberger W, Windpassinger C, Wladika W, Wagner K. Candidate region for Gilles de la Tourette syndrome at 7q31. Am J Hum Genet 2001; 101:259–261.
72. Crawford F, Ait-Ghezala G, Morris M, Sutcliffe M, Hauser R, Silver A, Mullan M. Translocation breakpoint in two unrelated Tourette syndrome cases, within a region previously linked to the disorder. Hum Genet 2003; 113:154–161.
73. State M, Greally J, Cuker A, Bowers P, Henegariu O, Morgan T, Gunel M, DiLuna M, King R, Nelson C, Donovan A, Anderson G, Leckman J, Hawkins T, Pauls D, Lifton R, Ward D. Epigenetic abnormalities associated with a chromosome 18 (q21–q22) inversion and a Gilles de la Tourette syndrome phenotype. Proc Natl Acad Sci USA 2003; 100:4684–4689.
74. Sacks O. Acquired tourettism in adult life. In: Friedhoff AJ, Chase TN, eds. Gilles de la Tourette Syndrome. Advances in Neurology. New York: Raven Press, 1982:89–92.
75. Kumar R, Lang A. Tourette syndrome. Secondary tic disorders. Neurol Clin 1997; 15:309–331.
76. Lombroso C. Lamotrigine-induced tourettism. Neurology 1999; 52:1191–1194.
77. Moshe K, Iulian I, Seth K, Eli L, Joseph Z. Clomipramine-induced tourettism in obsessive–compulsive disorder: clinical and theoretical implications. Clin Neuropharmacol 1994; 17:338–343.
78. Cardoso F, Jankovic J. Cocaine related movement disorders. Mov Disord 1993; 8:175–178.
79. Bharucha K, Sethi K. Tardive tourettism after exposure to neuroleptic therapy. Mov Disord 1995; 10:791–793.
80. Collacott R, Ismail I. Tourettism in a patient with Down's Syndrome. J Ment Defic Res 1988; 32:163–166.
81. Keefover R, Privite J. Adult-onset tourettism following closed head injury. J Neuropsychiatry Clin Neurosci 1989; 1:448–449.
82. Bleeker H. Gilles de la Tourette's syndrome with direct evidence of organicity. Psychiatr Clin 1978; 11:147–154.
83. Masso J, Obeso J. Coprolalia associated with hemiballismus: response to tetrabenazine. Clin Neuropharmacol 1985; 8:189–190.
84. Ward C. Transient feelings of compulsion caused by hemispheric lesions: three cases. J Neurol Neurosurg Psychiatry 1988; 51:266–268.
85. Leonard H, Swedo S, Lenane M, Rettew D, Hamburger S, Bartko J, Rapoport J. A 2 to 7 year follow-up study of 54 obsessive–compulsive children and adolescents. Arch Gen Psychiatry 1993; 50:429–439.
86. Swoboda K, Jenike M. Frontal abnormalities in a patient with obsessive–compulsive disorder: the role of structural lesions in obsessive–compulsive behavior. Neurology 1995; 45:2130–2134.
87. Rodrigo P, Adair J, Roberts B, Graeber D. Obsessive–compulsive disorder following bilateral globus pallidus infarction. Biol Psychiatry 1997; 42:410–412.
88. Simpson S, Baldwin B. Neuropsychiatry and SPECT of an acute obsessive–compulsive syndrome patient. Br J Psychiatry 1995; 166:390–392.

89. Hugo F, van Heerden B, Zungu-Dirwayi N, Stein D. Functional brain imaging in obsessive–compulsive disorder secondary to neurological lesions. Depress Anxiety 1999; 10:129–136.
90. Berthier M, Kulisevsky J, Gironell A, Heras J. Obsessive–compulsive disorder associated with brain lesions: clinical phenomenology, cognitive function, and anatomic correlates. Neurology 1996; 47:353–361.
91. Max J, Smith W Jr, Lindgren S, Robin D, Mattheis P, Stierwalt J, Morrisey M. Case study: obsessive–compulsive disorder after severe traumatic brain injury in an adolescent. J Am Acad Child Adolesc Psychiatry 1995; 34:45–49.
92. Demirkol A, Erdem H, Inan L, Yigit A, Guney M. Bilateral globus pallidus lesions in a patient with Tourette syndrome and related disorders. Biol Psychiatry 1999; 46:863–867.
93. Peterson B, Bronen R, Duncan C. Three cases of symptom change in Tourette's syndrome and obsessive–compulsive disorder associated with paediatric cerebral malignancies. J Neurol Neurosurg Psychiatry 1996; 61:497–505.
94. LaPlane D, Levasseur M, Pillon B, DuBois B, Baulac M, Mazoyer B, Tran Dinh S, Sette G, Danze F, Baron JC. Obsessive–compulsive and other behavioral changes with bilateral basal ganglia lesions. A neuropsychological, magnetic resonance imaging and positron tomography study. Brain 1989; 112:699–725.
95. Beckson M, Cummings J. Neuropsychiatric aspects of stroke. Int J Psychiatry Med 1991; 21:1–15.
96. LaPlane D, Levasseur M, Pillon B, DuBois B, Baulac M, Mazoyer B, Tran Dinh S, Sette G, Danze F, Baron J. Obsessive–compulsive and other behavioral changes with bilateral basal ganglia lesions. A neuropsychological, magnetic resonance imaging and positron tomography study. Brain 1989; 112:699–725.
97. Salloway S, Cummings J. Subcortical disease and neuropsychiatric illness. J Neuropsychiatry Clin Neurosci 1994; 6:93–99.
98. Alegret M, Junque C, Valldeoriola F, Vendrell P, Marti M, Tolosa E. Obsessive–compulsive symptoms in Parkinson's disease. J Neurol Neurosurg Psychiatry 2001; 70:394–396.
99. Baxter L Jr. Neuroimaging studies of obsessive compulsive disorder. Psychiatr Clin North Am 1992; 15:871–884.
100. Strub R. Frontal lobe syndrome in a patient with bilateral globus pallidus lesions. Arch Neurol 1989; 46:1024–1027.
101. Trautner R, Cummings J, Read S, Benson D. Idiopathic basal ganglia calcification and organic mood disorder. Am J Psychiatry 1988; 145:350–353.
102. Bejjani B, Damier P, Arnulf I, Thivard L, Bonnet AM, Dormont D, Cornu P, Pidoux B, Samson Y, Agid Y. Transient acute depression induced by high-frequency deep-brain stimulation. N Engl J Med 1999; 340:1476–1480.
103. Steffens D, Helms M, Krishnan K, Burke G. Cerebrovascular disease and depression symptoms in the cardiovascular health study. Stroke 1999; 30:2159–2166.
104. McKee A, Levine D, Kowall N, Richardson E Jr, Peduncular hallucinosis associated with isolated infarction of the substantia nigra pars reticulata. Ann Neurol 1990; 27:500–504.

105. Cummings J. Frontal–subcortical circuits and human behavior. Arch Neurol 1993; 50:873–880.
106. Peterson B. Neuroimaging studies of Tourette syndrome: a decade of progress. In: Cohen D, Jankovic J, Goetz C, eds. Tourette Syndrome. Advances in Neurology. Vol. 85. Philadelphia: Lippincott, Williams and Wilkins, 2001:179–196.
107. Berthier M, Kulisevsky J, Asenjo B, Aparicio J, Lara D. Comorbid Asperger and Tourette syndrome with localized mesencephalic, infrathalamic, thalamic, and striatal damage. Dev Med Child Neurol 2003; 45:207–212.
108. Leckman J, Cohen D, Goetz C, Jankovic J. Tourette syndrome: pieces of the puzzle. In: Cohen D, Jankovic J, Goetz C, eds. Tourette Syndrome. Advances in Neurology. Vol. 85. Philadelphia: Lippincott, Williams and Wilkins, 2001:369–390.
109. Fahn S. A case report of post-traumatic tic syndrome. In: Friedhoff A, Chase T, eds. Gilles de la Tourette Syndrome. New York: Raven Press, 1982:249–250.
110. Singer C, Sanchez-Ramos J, Weiner W. A case of post-traumatic tic disorder. Mov Disord 1989; 4:342–344.
111. Siemers E, Pascuzzi R. Posttraumatic tic disorder. Mov Disord 1990; 5:183.
112. Allen A. Group A streptococcal infections and childhood neuropsychiatric disorders: relationships and therapeutic implications. CNS Drugs 1997; 8:267–275.
113. Kurlan R. Tourette syndrome and PANDAS. Will the relation bear out? Neurology 1998; 50:1530–1534.
114. Dale R, Church A, Cardoso F. Post-streptococcal acute disseminated encephalomyelitis with basal ganglia involvement and auto-reactive antibasal ganglia antibodies. Ann Neurol 2001; 50:588–595.
115. Wolfhart G, Ingvar D, et al. Compulsory shouting (Benedek's "klazomania") associated with oculogyric spasms in chronic epidemic encephalitis. Acta Psychiatr Scand 1961; 36:369–377.
116. Howard R, Lees A. Encephalitis lethargica: a report of four recent cases. Brain 1987; 110:19–33.
117. Northam R, Singer H. Postencephalitic acquired Tourette-like syndrome in a child. Neurology 1991; 41:592–593.
118. Nath A, Jankovic J, Pettigrew L. Movement disorders and AIDS. Neurology 1987; 37:36–41.
119. McDaniel J, Summerville M. Tic disorder associated with encephalopathy in advanced HIV disease. Gen Hosp Psychiatry 1994; 16:298–300.
120. Muller N, Riedel M, Forderreuther S, Blendinger C, Abele-horn M. Tourette's syndrome and *Mycoplasma pneumoniae* infection. Am J Psychiatry 2000; 157:481–482.
121. Riedel M, Straube A, Schwarz M, Wilske B, Muller N. Lyme disease presenting as Tourette's syndrome. Lancet 1998; 351:418–419.
122. Biederman J, Wilens T, Mick E, Spencer T, Faraone SV. Pharmacotherapy of attention-deficit/hyperactivity disorder reduces risk of substance abuse disorder. Pediatrics 1999; 104:e20b.

123. Efron D, Jarman F, Barker M. Side effects of methylphenidate and dextroamphetamine in children with attention deficit hyperactivity disorder: a double-blind, crossover trial. Pediatrics 1997; 100:662–666.
124. Gadow K, Sverd J, Sprafkin J. Long-term methylphenidate therapy in children with comorbid attention-deficit hyperactivity and chronic multiple tic disorder. Arch Gen Psychiatry 1999; 56:330–336.
125. Klein R, Abikoff H, Klass E. Clinical efficacy of methylphenidate in conduct disorder with and without attention deficit hyperactivity disorder. Arch Gen Psychiatry 1997; 54:1073–1080.
126. Kurlan R. Methylphenidate to treat ADHD is not contraindicated in children with tics. Mov Disord 2002; 17:5–6.
127. Bharucha K, Sethi K. Tardive tourettism after exposure to neuroleptic therapy. Mov Disord 1995; 10:791–793.
128. Jankovic J. Tardive syndromes and other drug-induced movement disorders. Clin Neuropharmacol 1995; 18:197–214.
129. Dolberg O, Iancu I, Sasson Y, Zohar J. The pathogenesis and treatment of obsessive–compulsive disorder. Clin Neuropharmacol 1996; 19:129–147.
130. Flament M, Bisserbe J. Pharmacologic treatment of obsessive–compulsive disorder: comparative studies. J Clin Psychiatry 1997; 58(suppl 12):18–22.
131. Grados M, Riddle M. Pharmacologic treatment of childhood obsessive–compulsive disorder: from theory to practice. J Child Psychol 2001; 30:67–79.
132. Pulst S, Walshe T, Romero J. Carbon monoxide poisoning with features of Gilles de la Tourette's syndrome. Arch Neurol 1983; 40:443–444.
133. Li A, Chan M, Leung T, Cheung R, Lam C, Fok T. Mercury intoxication presenting with tics. Arch Dis Child 2000; 83:174–175.
134. Daniels J, Baker D, Norman A. Cocaine-induced tics in untreated Tourette's syndrome. Am J Psychiatry 1996; 153:965.
135. Berthier M, Campos V, Kulisevsky J, Valero J. Heroin and malignant coprolalia in Tourette's syndrome. J Neuropsychiatry Clin Neurosci 2003; 15:116–117.
136. Parraga H, Butterfield P. Tourette's syndrome and anophthalmia in a girl: complex differential diagnosis. Can J Psychiatry 1983; 28:206–209.
137. Shaenboen M, Nigro M, Martocci R. Colpocephaly and Gilles de la Tourette's syndrome. Arch Neurol 1984; 41:1023.
138. Burd L, Kerbeshian J, Fisher W. Pseudohemiparesis and Tourette syndrome. J Child Neurol 1986; 1:369–371.
139. Peterson B, Bronen R, Duncan C. Three cases of Gilles de la Tourette's syndrome and obsessive–compulsive disorder symptom change with paediatric cerebral malignancies. J Neurol Neurosurg Psychiatry 1996; 61:497–505.
140. Liu E, Robertson R, du Plessis A. Basal ganglia germinoma with progressive cerebral hemiatrophy. Pediatr Neurol 1999; 20:312–314.
141. Laplane D, Baulac M, Widlocher D, et al. Pure psychic akinesia with bilateral lesions of basal ganglia. J Neurol Neurosurg Psychiatry 1984; 47:377–385.
142. Melling M, Gorzer H, Benham M, Starkel D, Karimian-Teherani D. Compression by looping and perforation of the facial nerve by the anterior inferior cerebellar artery: a possible cause of facial tic. J Neurol Neurosurg Psychiatry 2001; 71:133–134.

10

Drug-Induced Tics

Karen E. Anderson and William J. Weiner
University of Maryland School of Medicine
Baltimore, Maryland, U.S.A.

INTRODUCTION

Tourette's syndrome (TS) is characterized by the waxing and waning of signs and symptoms as a part of the natural history of the disease. External stressors, medications, and behavioral changes may all influence the expression of motor signs and symptoms in TS. Medication effects on TS may be helpful in elucidating the pathophysiology of the illness because certain mechanisms may be implicated by distinct classes of agents. Effects of stimulants on TS have been widely studied. Stimulants' propensity to exacerbate or even induce symptoms of TS has provided important support for the hypothesis that the dopaminergic (DA) system plays a role in the development of tics. Although stimulants may induce or exacerbate tics in some patients with TS or attention-deficit/hyperactivity disorder (ADHD), not all patients experience this side effect. Stimulants also have effects other than simple potentiation of DA neurotransmission, and DA receptor antagonists are not always effective in management of tics in TS patients. Review of drugs that induce or exacerbate tics suggests that a complex interplay of neurotransmitter systems occurs, and that any effect on tics cannot be understood simply as potentiation of DA neurotransmission. This chapter reviews drug-induced exacerbation of tics in existing TS and drug-induced precipitation of tics.

PSYCHOMOTOR STIMULANTS

Methylphenidate, Pemoline, Amphetamine, and Cocaine

There has been much controversy as to whether stimulants exacerbate tics in patients with TS. Because psychomotor stimulants are the most commonly used and currently the most efficacious medications for treatment of ADHD, this poses a treatment dilemma for clinicians who see patients with TS and concomitant ADHD, which is extremely common. Indeed, some estimates suggest that up to half of all patients with TS also have ADHD (1).

Since the early 1960s, there have been over 60 case reports in the literature of tic disorders that were exacerbated by stimulants (2). In a study of 1520 patients treated with stimulant medications, Denckla et al. (3) found that 1.3% developed new tics or experienced worsening of existing tics. In six studies of whether stimulant treatment worsened preexisting tics, tics were found to increase in 6/45 (13%), 13/25 (54%), 3/14 (21%), 4/20 (20%), 2/6 (33%), and 11/39 (28%) of patients (4–8). Varley et al. (9) found that 8% of children treated with stimulants developed tics in a study of 555 patients with ADHD who were followed for a mean duration of 16 months. In the study, those who developed tics were significantly younger than those who did not. Subjects treated with higher doses of stimulant medication were not found to be more likely to develop tics. The 2002 edition of the Physicians' Desk Reference states that the most widely used stimulant for treatment of ADHD, methylphenidate, is contraindicated in patients with tics or TS.

Conversely, other work has suggested that occurrence and severity of tics are not affected by stimulant use. Lipkin et al. (10) performed a cross-sectional analysis of 122 children from an ADHD clinic cohort, all of whom were treated with stimulants. They found that 9% of subjects had tics or dyskinesias, but no relationship was seen between the presence of tics or dyskinesias and medication dosage, history of tics, age, or family history of tics. Gadow et al. (11) conducted a double-blind, placebo-controlled study of 34 children with tics and ADHD who were treated with three differing doses of methyphenidate and placebo, each for 2 weeks. Efficacy was found for ADHD symptoms, and tics did not worsen. These subjects were then followed in an open-label study of methylphenidate for 2 years, and no medication-related exacerbation of tics was seen, although some individuals did experience worsening of tics during the open-label phase (12). Another double-blind, crossover study of 20 patients with TS and ADHD comparing methylphenidate, dextroamphetamine, and placebo found that higher doses of both stimulants exacerbated tics (13). Low doses of the stimulants did not significantly worsen tics. Most subjects had improvement of ADHD symptoms. Most patients who experienced exacerbation of tics with methylphenidate showed resolution of this adverse effect during the 9-week observation phase. However, among those with dextroamphetamine-induced worsening of tics, only 1 of 20 showed decrease in exacerbation. Seventy percent of the subjects remained on stimulant treatment during the open-label follow-up, which lasted up to 3 years. The authors concluded that most patients in the study had an acceptable side effect profile with respect to tics and derived benefit for their ADHD symptoms during medication treatment. They also commented that methylphenidate was generally better tolerated than dextroamphetamine in this group. Law and Schachar (14) found no evidence that methylphenidate exacerbated tics or precipitated onset of tics at a higher rate than placebo in a study of 91 children with ADHD and mild or moderate tics (patients with TS were excluded from this study). Finally, a recent multicenter, randomized, double-blind, placebo-controlled, clinical trial of methyphenidate and clonidine, alone and in combination, examined effects of these medications in patients with tics and concomitant ADHD (15). Worsening of tics was comparable in groups treated with methylphenidate, clonidine, or placebo (20%, 26%, and 22% reported worsening, respectively). Compared with the placebo group, tic severity was found to decrease in clonidine plus methylphenidate, or clonidine, or methylphenidate. ADHD symptoms improved significantly with both medications, with the most improvement seen in the combination group. The authors concluded that methylphenidate and clonidine are effective for treatment of ADHD in patients with tics, and that there was no evidence in this study to support the theory that methylphenidate worsened tic symptoms. In fact, some case reports have suggested that stimulants improved tic symptoms in some patients (6,8,16).

As was seen in the study by Castellanos et al. (13), there may also be varying effects depending on the stimulant used for treatment. Placebo-controlled studies and clinical reports have suggested that dextroamphetamine may worsen tics whereas methylphenidate has no effect on tic symptoms, and clinical work suggests that pemoline may have adverse effects on tics (17–19). A recent commentary by Kurlan (20) reviewing the above literature also notes the waxing and waning inherent in the natural history of tic disorders that may further cloud the issue.

Cocaine

Cocaine inhibits reuptake of DA, and chronic cocaine abuse may lead to depletion of neuronal DA, and thus to secondary hypersensitivity of postsynaptic DA receptors (21). Thus, it would be expected that cocaine abuse could exacerbate tic symptoms and may cause parkinsonism. Because acute reuptake blockade of DA receptors also occurs with cocaine use, acute exacerbation of tics may additionally occur. There have been several reports of patients with TS whose tic symptoms significantly worsened following cocaine abuse (22–25). Pascual-Leone and Dhuna (22) and Attig et al. (26) also report on three patients without a family history of tics who developed new-onset tics after chronic intranasal or "crack" cocaine abuse. It is possible that, in patients with no underlying neurological disorder and no family history of tics, chronic cocaine use may contribute to development of tics, perhaps via induction of dopaminergic hypersensitivity.

Inferences on the Pathophysiology of TS Based on the Phenomenon of Stimulant-Induced Tics

The pathogenesis of tics is unknown, but because of the treatment responsiveness of some tic patients to haloperidol and other D_2 antagonists, tics are thought to be associated with increases in dopaminergic activity (27). This theory is supported by the observation that levodopa, which increases brain DA concentrations, has been reported to increase tic symptoms in TS (28). Thus, stimulant medications would be expected to exacerbate existing tics and perhaps to precipitate new-onset tics because they act via several mechanisms to increase concentrations of synaptic DA (and other biogenic amines).

Amphetamines exert their main central nervous system effects by the release of biogenic amines from their storage sites. The increase in alertness, anorectic effects, and some of the increases in motor activity seen with their administration are probably modulated by the release of norepinephrine (NE) centrally. Other increases in locomotion and stereotypies (repetitive behaviors with no obvious goals or reinforcers) induced by amphetamines are related to the release of DA from nerve terminals, especially in the neostriatum. Higher doses of amphetamines are required to promote DA release in in vitro studies of postmortem material. With escalating doses, psychosis may occur, perhaps because of the release of 5-hydroxytryptamine (serotonin, 5-HT) and also from the release of DA in the mesolimbic system (29). Methylphenidate has basically the same pharmacological actions as amphetamines (29,30). Pemoline differs structurally from methylphenidate, but has similar pharmacological actions. It has a long half-life, enabling once-a-day dosing.

Cocaine acts peripherally to inhibit DA (and biogenic amines) reuptake at synapses (21,31). Although the temporal profile of action of these agents differs, the immediate euphoric effects produced by an intravenous injection of amphetamine or cocaine cannot be differentiated by experienced users (32). The reinforcing effects, or those that lead to repetitive self-administration in animal studies, are believed to be mediated by the action of these agents on the mesolimbic DA system (33).

Stimulants may not only lead to compulsive self-administration of the drugs, but also to stereotypies in normal animals and humans. In animals, compulsive grooming, chewing, and lip smacking have been observed. In humans, more complex activities such as dismantling watches and other mechanical objects that are in good working order may occur. Other repetitive behaviors include bruxism, nail biting, continuous dressing and undressing, sorting objects, and obsessive housecleaning. Some of these stimulant-induced behaviors are similar to the compulsive behaviors and movements characteristic of TS, and both phenomena may share a common dopaminergic mechanism.

Perhaps the strongest evidence for involvement of the DA system in TS is the therapeutic efficacy of DA receptor antagonists (neuroleptics) in alleviating tics. Haloperidol has long been the drug of choice for management of tics, and is associated with an approximately 70% improvement on global ratings of TS (34). The efficacy of medications for suppression of TS symptoms has been reported to be positively correlated with potency of their competition for [^{3}H] haloperidol binding to dopamine D_2 receptors, but not with potency at inhibiting dopamine-sensitive adenylate cyclase (D_1) receptors (35). Imaging studies, however, suggest that D_2 receptor function is normal in unmedicated TS patients.

Recent postmortem work has found an increased number of dopaminergic carrier uptake sites in the striatum, as well as reduction in the second messenger cyclic AMP and decreases in 5-HT and glutamate in the basal ganglia (36). Study of the biogenic amine concentrations and turnover in cerebral spinal fluid (CSF) provide further support for the hypothesis of dopaminergic dysregulation in TS. Homovanillic acid (HVA) has been found to be decreased in the CSF of some TS patients, relative to controls, suggesting that DA turnover was reduced compared to controls (37–40). 5-Hydroxyindoleacetic acid (5HIAA) was also found to be reduced in 25% of patients (38,39). TS patients who were treated with haloperidol were retapped, and a relative normalization of HVA was seen with clinical improvement (40). The increase in CSF HVA from baseline has been interpreted to be consistent with DA receptor hypersensitivity. The blockade of supersensitive DA receptors by haloperidol would decrease negative feedback inhibition of DA neurons and levels of HVA would rise. Neuroleptics acutely increase HVA levels, but this is transient as opposed to the prolonged increase seen in these studies of TS. However, there are several methodological issues that may confound these results. CSF metabolites of DA, NE, and 5-HT may be affected by many factors, including age of subjects, sex, medical condition of controls, stress, diet, medications, circadian rhythms, and physical activity (41). Friedhoff (42) has hypothesized that D_2 receptors, unlike D_1, are sensitive to "adaptive upregulation." Thus, when the D_2 receptor system is blocked, as occurs with administration of haloperidol, it increases the actual number of receptors, which serves to override the blockade. This does not occur in the D_1 system without chronic blockade. Eye blink rate, which is a proposed surrogate measure of central DA activity, has been found to be elevated in some, but not all, studies in TS (43,44).

Although the DA receptor supersensitivity hypothesis of TS has flaws, it has been a productive model in guiding research and providing a conceptual paradigm for the understanding of clinical phenomena. For example, a small number of patients have developed a syndrome similar to TS following chronic neuroleptic exposure, which may cause functional DA receptor supersensitivity. These patients developed spontaneous vocalizations, verbalization (including coprolalia), and motor tics (45,46). This clinical observation supports the DA supersensitivity hypothesis; it also raises the issue of whether the treatment of tics in TS may occasionally lead to the development of another neurological condition—tardive dyskinesia (47).

ANTICHOLINERGIC AND ANTIHISTAMINERGIC DRUGS

Anticholinergic and antihistaminergic drugs have occasionally been reported to exacerbate tics. Antihistamines and anticholinergics have some degree of structural overlap and activity. Both classes of drugs produce sedation, which one would expect would ameliorate tics, but worsening of tic symptoms has been reported in some patients (48,49). Scopolamine was reported to exacerbate vocal tics but improve motor tics in TS, and this effect was reversed after injection of physostigmine an hour later (50).

Cholinergic and dopaminergic balance in the basal ganglia may be important in other movement disorders such as Parkinson's disease (PD), where loss of dopaminergic inhibition of the striatal interneurons leads to hyperactivity of the cholinergic system (51–53). In fact, anticholinergic medication is beneficial in PD. Sandyk (54) has proposed that both motor symptoms and behavioral changes observed in TS may be associated with increases in central cholinergic activity. Thus, one might expect that cholinergic medications would benefit tics because the DA system is presumed to be hyperactive. However, attempts to improve tics with cholinergic loading (choline chloride, lecithin, and physostigmine) have not been impressive, and physostigmine has been shown to worsen tics (48,50,55–57). Thus, there is no clear role for anticholinergic or antihistaminergic medications in the prevention or treatment of tics.

ANTIDEPRESSANT DRUGS

Patients with TS have a high incidence of comorbid depression and anxiety disorders, and are often treated with anitidepressant medications. As is reviewed below, antidepressant use has been associated with development of tics. Thus, the risk of worsening tics associated with use of these medications is an important consideration when treating these patients for behavioral disturbances.

Selective serotonin-reuptake inhibitors (SSRIs), which are the most commonly prescribed class of medications for depression, anxiety disorders, and several other psychiatric and neurological conditions, have been shown to induce tics in some patients. SSRIs act by blocking neuronal transport of serotonin (58). Secondary effects of SSRIs have not been as carefully characterized as in tricyclics, but this increase in serotonin availability at the synapse stimulates a wide range of postsynaptic receptors (59). Fluoxetine, the first SSRI approved in the United States, was reported to exacerbate tics in a patient with Tourette's syndrome (60), but was found to have no effect on tics in a small, double-blind, placebo-controlled crossover trial (61). Kurlan et al. (62) found in a double-blind, placebo-controlled study that fluoxetine produced mild attenuation of tic severity in TS patients.

There have been variable reports regarding fluvoxamine, another SSRI, which is often used for treatment of OCD and depression. One report found that fluvoxamine precipitated eyelid and nasal tics in a 14-year-old boy (63). Another case report stated that fluvoxamine worsened tics in a patient with Tourette's syndrome (64). Small studies looking at the use of fluvoxamine in Tourette's syndrome found that fluvoxamine produced a nonsignificant amelioration of tics in this condition (65,66). Among the other SSRIs, citalopram was shown to significantly reduce tics in Tourette's syndrome in one small study (65), and there have been, to date, no reports of this agent exacerbating tic symptoms. There is one case report of paroxetine worsening tics in a 12-year-old boy with Tourette's syndrome (67).

Tricyclic antidepressants (TCAs) are also widely used for many psychiatric and neurological conditions. Because of their somewhat diverse mechanism of action, prediction of their effect on tics is problematic. Tricyclics primarily increase biogenic amine activity by blockade of reuptake, but they also act as antagonists at various receptors, including those for muscarinic cholinergic, α_1-adrenergic, and H1 and H2 histaminergic neurotransmitters (58). Given the reports of tricyclics' exacerbation of tics, one might expect they have significant dopaminergic activity. However, this has not been demonstrated. Because they cause significant enhancement of both 5-HT and NE activity by preventing reuptake, the cases where they are seen to exacerbate tics suggest that these neurotransmitters also play a role in the etiology of tics.

Work from the late 1970s studying TS found 17 cases where tic exacerbation occurred with TCAs, and one where tics were reliably shown to improve with TCA treatment (28,68). Of note, in some cases of worsening tic, a TCA was added to a standard neuroleptic, or the patient had previously been on neuroleptic treatment.

However, newer work, including double-blind, placebo-controlled studies, suggests that TCAs may actually improve tics in some patients, including those with TS. Desipramine has been the most studied TCA with respect to tics. In a 6-week, double-blind, placebo-controlled study of 41 children and adolescents with tic disorders including TS, desipramine significantly reduced both ADHD and tic symptoms, compared with placebo (69). The authors comment that the effect of desipramine on tics is most likely because of its inhibition of norepinephrine uptake. Singer et al. (70) studied desipramine compared with clonidine for treatment of tics and ADHD in a three-arm, double-blind, crossover study and found that desipramine had no significant effect on tics, but did significantly improve ADHD symptoms. Case series and record reviews have found that the majority of patients with tics and ADHD either have no change in tic symptoms [in one study (71), six of seven showed no change in tics, and one showed worsening], or show some improvement in tics [80% of 30 children with tics had improvement in ADHD and tics, with response sustained for more than a year (72); Spencer et al. (73) found that 80% of 33 children and adolescents with tic disorders showed improvement in both areas of symptomatology]. There have also been case reports suggesting that desipramine is well tolerated in patients with tics (74).

Clomipramine has also received some study for its effects on tics. In a double-blind, placebo-controlled study, Caine et al. (75) treated six TS patients with clomipramine, desipramine, or placebo for 4-week periods. No benefits were found with either medication, and one patient developed severe exacerbation of TS symptoms. Clomipramine was reported to worsen motor tics in one case with obsessive–compulsive disorder and schizoid personality disorder (76), but a few case reports suggest that clomipramine may alleviate tic symptoms (77–80).

Finally, limited work has been conducted on two other TCAs, nortriptyline and imipramine. Nortriptyline was shown to improve tic symptoms in a chart review of 12 cases of children with tics and ADHD (81). Imipramine was reported to decrease tics in TS in one case, and had no effect on TS symptoms in another (28,82).

One cautionary note should be mentioned. As of this writing, it is recommended that cardiac history be carefully screened for risk factors, including patient and family history of cardiac disease, and cardiac function be monitored closely in children who are treated with TCAs because of reports of increases in heart rate and electrocardiogram (EKG) measures of cardiac conduction times (72). Although most cases have been asymptomatic, there are reports in the literature of sudden death in children with ADHD who have been treated with desipramine (83–85).

One case report suggests that trazodone, a phenylpiperazine antidepressant (58), may help to alleviate tic symptoms (86). Selegiline, a selective monoamine oxidase-B inhibitor—which, unlike monoamine oxidase-A inhibitors, does not require dietary restrictions at standard doses—was studied in an open trial of 29 children with TS and ADHD. Two patients had exacerbation of tics, whereas the rest had no effect on tic symptoms (87). Selegiline has not been approved for use in children. Bupropion, a novel antidepressant with weak dopaminergic activity and some structural similarity to amphetamine, was found to exacerbate tics in four children with Tourette's syndrome (88). To date, there have been no case reports of bupropion improving tics.

Mood Stabilizers

There has been little work examining whether mood stabilizers, such as lithium, have an effect on tics. Because tic severity may increase with mania, differentiating the actual effect of mood stabilizer on tics vs. its effect on the treatment of manic symptoms is problematic. It appears that the effect of lithium on tics may be variable because it has been reported to worsen, ameliorate, or have no effect on TS patients (89–91). Lithium affects central cathecholaminergic and indoleaminergic transmission, but may also cause changes in peripheral neuromuscular response (92).

ANTIEPILEPTIC DRUGS

Carbamazepine, one of the most widely used antiepileptic agents in the United States, has structural similarities to imipramine but produces more sedation in many patients. It has been reported to improve tics in one TS case, and to worsen tics in eight other patients, including one with Huntington's disease and one with Alzheimer's disease, suggesting that preexisting neuropathology may contribute to development of tics (93,94). One patient, who was described as developing tics while on stimulants, experienced further exacerbation of tics when stimulants were discontinued and carbamazepine was initiated. Carbamazepine has also been associated with the development of other movement disorders such as orofacial dyskinesias and dystonia, with some authors suggesting that this may be because of its structural similarity to phenothiazines (95). Because carbamazepine is not commonly used to treat ADHD or TS, little clinical data exist.

Phenytoin has been described in the literature as an agent that carries risk of precipitating many movement disorders, including choreoathetosis, oral–facial or oral–buccal dyskinesias, tremors, and dystonias, although these side effects are reported mainly with toxic blood levels of the medication (96,97). Chorea associated with phenytoin use was seen in a patient with nontoxic medication blood levels (98). A case of TS beginning after phenytoin initiation has also been reported in a patient with no known brain dysfunction who had therapeutic levels of the medication. In this case, a switch to carbamazepine resulted in disappearance of the TS symptoms (99).

Barbiturates would be expected to dampen tics because of their sedative effects. However, just as paradoxical disinhibition and excitement may occur in both adults and children who are given barbiturates (100), they have occasionally been reported to worsen tics. Burd et al. (101) reviewed the records of 129 tic patients and found 13 with concomitant epilepsy. Five of these patients were described as developing tics and behavioral disturbances after administration of barbiturates (phenobarbital in particular).

Lamotrigine, a new broad-spectrum anticonvulsant, has been occasionally reported to cause tics (102). Menezes et al. (103) found that five of 400 children treated with lamotrigine in a pediatric neurology clinic developed tics, an incidence of 1.3%. Four of the patients exhibited motor tics, and one developed mostly vocal tics. In three cases, the tics resolved completely within a month following cessation of the drug; tics reappeared with reintroduction of lamotrigine. Another patient showed gradual improvement over 4 months after stopping the medication, and another had improvement with reduction of dose. Because lamotrigine differs structurally from other anticonvulsants and possesses no significant dopaminergic activity, the authors suggest that its blockade of glutamate transmission may contribute to motor system abnormalities (104) by disrupting the balance between glutamatergic and dopaminergic systems (105). There is little clinical data on the effects of other new anticonvulsants on movement disorders.

Topiramate, which may exert its antiseizure effects partly by potentiation of the inhibitory GABA system (106), was reported to treat tics in two TS patients (107); there are no reports of it exacerbating movement disorders. The structure of topiramate differs from that of other antiepileptic medications, and its exact mechanism is unknown. Its potentiation of GABA activity may partly explain the reduction of tics in some patients (106).

OPIOIDS

Drugs affecting the endogenous opioid system have been reported to influence tic symptoms. An opioid agonist, nitrous oxide, was found to exacerbate TS symptoms. This effect was reversible with administration of the opioid antagonist, naloxone (108). Naloxone, or the longer-acting opiate antagonist naltrexone, has been reported to improve symptoms of TS, but there are also reports of these agents worsening TS (109,110). Because precipitous withdrawal from chronic opioid use has been found, in two cases, to worsen TS, underactivity of the endogenous opioid system may play a role in development of tics (111,112).

There have been few controlled studies addressing the effect on tics of drugs acting on the endogenous opioid system. Kurlan et al. (113) compared the opioid agonist propoxyphene and antagonist naltrexone in a double-blind, placebo-controlled, randomized trial in patients with tics. On subjective reports, patients indicated that they experienced lessening of tics with naltrexone treatment, compared with placebo. Neither medication was reported to worsen tics. However, no significant benefit of either the agonist or antagonist was seen on any objective tic ratings, and the authors were cautious in their interpretation of these results. One other open-label study of naltrexone for TS found no significant improvement in tics or other symptoms of TS (114). In a naloxone study, dose effect of the antagonist was studied in 15 TS patients with randomized dosing levels (115). A dose-response effect was seen, with low doses of naloxone significantly decreasing tics, whereas high doses caused a significant increase.

Despite the fact that clinical studies show little effect of opioid antagonists on TS symptoms, there is evidence that the endogenous opioid system interacts with monoaminergic systems that do have more critical involvement in the pathophysiology of tics (116). Postmortem data in five TS patients demonstrated loss of an endogenous opioid peptide, dynorphin, in the basal ganglia (117,118). Other authors have suggested that TS may be related to underactivity of the endogenous opioid system (119). However, further studies are needed to elucidate the role of the endogenous opioid system in the pathophysiology of TS.

SUMMARY

Tic disorders may begin after treatment with stimulant medications in a small number of patients with ADHD. It is not clear, however, whether these patients would have developed tics even without exposure to stimulants because the comorbidity of tics and ADHD is high. Stimulant medications may exacerbate tics in some TS patients, although given the natural waxing and waning of the illness, this effect is difficult to accurately assess. Newer work suggests that stimulants have less effect on tics in TS than was previously reported, and these medications have proven efficacy in the treatment of ADHD in many patients. The most commonly used stimulant, methylphenidate, may have less propensity to cause or exacerbate tics than some of the others in use (pemoline, D-amphetamine), although more studies are required to fully elucidate this point. A commonly abused illicit stimulant, cocaine, has been found to exacerbate tics in patients with a preexisting condition, and may precipitate tics in some patients. This effect is most likely because of stimulants' effects on the dopaminergic system, although their interaction with other receptor systems may play a role as well. Other psychoactive agents that interact with the monoaminergic system, such as anticholinergics, antihistamines, antidepressants, and antiepileptics, may exacerbate or improve tics, but more data are needed before definite conclusions can be made regarding any of these medications. Opioids may increase or decrease tics, and the role of the endogenous opioid system in tics, in general, and in TS, in particular, is unclear. Although medication effects on alertness or mood may significantly affect tic symptoms in a patient, activation of the central dopaminergic systems is most often associated with exacerbation of tics.

REFERENCES

1. Walkup JT, Kahn S, Schuerholz L, Paik Y-S, Leckman JF, Schultz RT. Phenomenology and natural history of tic-related ADHD and learning disabilities. In: Leckman JF, Cohen DJ, eds. Tourette's Syndrome: Tics, Obsessions, Compulsions: Developmental Psychopathology and Clinical Care. New York: John Wiley, 1999:63–79.
2. Robertson MM, Eapen V. Pharmacologic controversy of CNS stimulants in Gilles de la Tourette's syndrome. Clin Neuropharmacol 1992; 15:408–425.
3. Denckla MB, Bemporad JR, McKay MC. Tics following methylphenidate administration. JAMA 1976; 25:149–151.
4. Golden GS. The effect of CNS stimulants on Tourette's syndrome. Ann Neurol 1977; 2:69–70.
5. Bachman DS. Pemoline-induced Tourette's disorder: a case report. Am J Psychiatry 1981; 138:1116–1117.
6. Shapiro A, Shapiro E. Do stimulants provoke, cause, or exacerbate tics and Tourette's syndrome? Comp Psychiatry 1981; 22:265–273.
7. Rapoport JL, Nee L, Mitchell S, Polinsky MR, Ebert M. Hyperkinetic syndrome and Tourette's syndrome. In: Friedhoff AJ, Chase TN, eds. Gilles de la Tourette's Syndrome. New York: Raven, 1982:423–426.
8. Erenberg G, Cruse RP, Rothner AD. Gilles de la Tourette's syndrome: effects of stimulant drugs. Neurology 1985; 35:1346–1348.
9. Varley CK, Vincent J, Varley P, Calderon R. Emergence of tics in children with attention deficit hyperactivity disorder treated with stimulant medications. Comp Psychiatry 2001; 42(3):228–233.
10. Lipkin P, Goldstein J, Ademan A. Tics and dyskinesias associated with stimulant treatment in attention deficit hyperactivity disorder. Arch Pediatr Adolesc Med 1994; 148:859–861.
11. Gadow KD, Sverd J, Sprafkin J, Nolan EE, Ezor SN. Efficacy of methylphenidate for attention-deficit hyperactivity disorder in children with tic disorder. Arch Gen Psychiatry 1995; 52:444–455.
12. Gadow KD, Sverd J, Sprafkin J, Nolan EE, Grossman S. Long-term methylphenidate therapy in children with comorbid attention-deficit hyperactivity disorder and chronic multiple tic disorder. Arch Gen Psychiatry 1999; 56:330–336.

13. Castellanos FX, Giedd JN, Elia J, Marsh W, Ritchie GF, Hamburger SD, Rapoport JL. Controlled stimulant treatment of ADHD and comorbid Tourette's syndrome: effects of stimulant and dose. J Am Acad Child Adolesc Psychiatry 1997; 36(5):589–596.
14. Law SF, Schachar RJ. Do typical clinical doses of methylphenidate cause tics in children treated for attention-deficit hyperactivity disorder? J Am Child Adolesc Psychiatry 1999; 38(8):944–951.
15. Tourette's Study Group. Treatment of ADHD in children with tics: a randomized controlled trial. Neurology 2002; 58(4):527–536.
16. Price RA, Leckman JF, Pauls DL, Cohen DJ, Kid KK. GTS: tics and CNS stimulants in twins and non-twins. Neurology 1986; 36:232–237.
17. Caine ED, Ludlow CL, Polinsky RJ, Ebert MH. Provocative drug testing in Tourette's syndrome: D- and L-amphetamine and haloperidol. J Am Acad Child Psychiatry 1984; 23:147–152.
18. Meyerhoff JL, Snyder SH. Gilles de la Tourette's disease and minimal brain dysfunction: amphetamine isomers reveal catecholamine correlates in an affected patient. Psychopharmacologia 1973; 29(3):211–220.
19. Feinburg M, Carroll BJ. Effects of dopaminergic agonists and antagonists in Tourette's disease. Arch Gen Psychiatry 1979; 979–985.
20. Kurlan R. Methylphenidate to treat ADHD is not contraindicated in children with tics. Mov Disord 2002; 17(1):5–6.
21. Nunes EV, Rosecan GS. Human neurobiology of cocaine. In: Spitz HD, Rosecan GS, eds. Cocaine Abuse: New Directions in Treatment and Research. New York: Brunner/Mazel, 1987:48–94.
22. Pascual-Leone A, Dhuna A. Cocaine-associated multifocal tics. Neurology 1990; 40:999–1000.
23. Mesulam MM. Cocaine and Tourette's syndrome. N Engl J Med 1986; 315:398.
24. Factor SA, Sanchez-Ramos JR, Weiner WJ. Cocaine and Tourette's syndrome. Ann Neurol 1988; 23:423–424.
25. Daniels J, Baker DG, Norman AB. Cocaine-induced tics in untreated Tourette's Syndrome. Am J Psychiatry 1996; 153:7.
26. Attig E, Amyot R, Botez T. Cocaine-induced chronic tics. J Neurol Neurosurg Psychiatry 1994; 57(9):1143–1144.
27. Leckman JF, Walkup JT, Riddle MA, Towbin KE, Cohen DJ. Tic disorders. In: Meltzer HY, Bunney WE, Coyle JT, eds. Psychopharmacology: The Third Generation of Progress. New York: Raven, 1987:1239–1246.
28. Messiha FA, Knopp W. A study of endogenous dopamine metabolism in Gilles de la Tourette's disease. Dis Nerv Syst 1976; 37:470–473.
29. Hoffman B. Catecholamines, sympathomimetic drugs, and adrenergic receptor antagonists. In: Hardman JG, Limbird LE, Gilman AG, eds. Goodman and Gilman's The Pharmacological Basis of Therapeutics. 10th ed. New York: McGraw-Hill, 2001:215–268.
30. Hunt RD, Mandl L, Lau S, Hughes MC. Neurobiological theories of ADHD and Ritalin. In: Greenhill LL, Osman BB, eds. Ritalin: Theory and Patient Management. New York: Liebert, 1991:267–287.

31. Catterall W, Mackie K. Local anesthetics. In: Hardman JG, Limbird LE, Gilman AG, eds. Goodman and Gilman's The Pharmacological Basis of Therapeutics. 10th ed. New York: McGraw-Hill, 2001:367–384.
32. Fishman MW, Schuster CR. Cocaine self-administration in humans. Fed Proc 1982; 41:137–141.
33. O'Brien CP. Drug addiction and abuse. In: Hardman JG, Limbird LE, Gilman AG, eds. Goodman and Gilman's The Pharmacological Basis of Therapeutics. 10th ed. New York: McGraw-Hill, 2001:621–644.
34. Shapiro AK, Shapiro E. The treatment and etiology of tics and Tourette syndrome. Comp Psychiatry 1981; 22:193–205.
35. Stahl SM, Berger PA. Cholinergic and dopaminergic mechanisms in Tourette's syndrome. Adv Neurol 1982; 35:141–150.
36. Singer HS, Wong DF, Brown JE, Brandt J, Krafft L, Shaya E, Dannals RF, Wagner HN Jr, Positron emission tomography evaluation of dopamine D-2 receptors in adults with Tourette syndrome. Adv Neurol 1992; 58:233–239.
37. Butler IJ, Koslow SH, Seifer WE Jr, Caprioli RM, Singer HS. Biogenic amine metabolism in Tourette's syndrome. Ann Neurol 1979; 6:37–39.
38. Cohen DJ, Shaywitz BA, Caparulo BK, Young JG, Bowers MB Jr, Chronic multiple tics of Gilles de la Tourette's disease: CSF acid monoamine metabolites after probenecid administration. Arch Gen Psychiatry 1978; 2:245–250.
39. Cohen DJ, Shaywitz BA, Young JG, Carbonari CM, Nathanson JA, Lieberman D, Bowers MB Jr, Mass JW. Central biogenic amine metabolism in children with the syndrome of chronic multiple tics of Gilles de la Tourette: norepinephrine, serotonin, and dopamine. J Am Acad Child Psychiatry 1979; 18:320–341.
40. Singer HS, Tune LE, Butler IJ, Zaczek AL, Coyle JT. Clinical symptomatology, CSF neurotransmitter metabolites, and serum haloperidol levels in Tourette's syndrome. Adv Neurol 1982; 35:177–183.
41. Koslow SH, Cross CK. CSF monoamine metabolites in Tourette syndrome and their neuroendocrine implications. Adv Neurol 1982; 35:185–197.
42. Friedhoff AJ. Insights into the pathophysiology and pathogenesis of Gilles de la Tourette syndrome. Rev Neurol (Paris) 1986; 142:860–864.
43. Bonnet KA. Neurobiological dissection of Tourette syndrome: a neurochemical focus on a human neuroanatomical model. Advances in Neurology. Vol. 35. New York: Raven Press, 1982:77–82.
44. Karson CN, Kaufman CA, Shapiro AK, et al. Eye-blink rate in Tourette's syndrome. J Nerv Ment Dis 1985; 173:566–568.
45. Klawans HL, Falk DK, Nausieda PA, Weiner WJ. Gilles de la Tourette syndrome after long-term chlorpromazine therapy. Neurology 1978; 28:1064–1068.
46. Klawans HL, Nausieda PA, Goetz CG, Tannger CM, Weiner WJ. Tourette-like symptoms following chronic neuroleptic therapy. Adv Neurol 1982; 35:415–418.
47. Singh SK, Jankovic J. Tardive dystonia in patients with Tourette's syndrome. Mov Disord 1988; 3:274–279.
48. Shapiro AK, Shapiro E, Sweet RD. Treatment of tics and Tourette syndrome.

In: Barbea A, ed. Disorders of Movement. Lancaster, England: MTP Press, 1981:134–144.
49. Shaffi M. The effects of sympathomimetic and antihistamine agents on chronic motor tics and Tourette's disorder. N Engl J Med 1986; 1129–1228.
50. Tanner CM, Goetz CG, Klawans HL. Cholinergic mechanisms in Tourette syndrome. Neurology 1982; 32:1315–1317.
51. Agid Y, Javoy F, Geyenet P. Effects of surgical and pharmacological manipulation of the dopaminergic nigrostriatal neurons on the activity of the neostriatal cholinergic system in the rat. In: Bossier JR, Hippius H, Pichot P, eds. Neuropsychopharmacology. Amsterdam: Excerpta Medica, 1975:480–486.
52. Javoy-Agid F, Ploska A, Agid Y. Microtopography of TH, CAT, and GAD activity in the substantia nigra and ventral tegmental area of control and parkinsonian human brain. Neurochemistry 1982; 37:1221–1227.
53. Hattori T, Singh VK, McGeer EG, et al. Immunohistochemical localization of choline acetyltransferase containing neostriatal neurons and their relationship with dopaminergic synapses. Brain Res 1976; 102:164–173.
54. Sandyk R. Cholinergic mechanisms in Gilles de la Tourette's syndrome. Int J Neurosci 1995; 81:95–100.
55. Moldovsky H, Sandor P. Lecithin in the treatment of Gilles de la Tourette's syndrome. Am J Psychiatry 1983; 140:1627–1629.
56. Barbeau A. Cholinergic treatment in the Tourette syndrome. N Engl J Med 1980; 302:1310–1311.
57. Polinsky RJ, Ebert MH, Caine ED, Ludlow C, Bassich CJ. Cholinergic treatment in the Tourette syndrome. N Engl J Med 1980; 302:1310.
58. Baldessarini RJ. Drugs and the treatment of psychiatric disorders. Depression and anxiety disorders. In: Hardman JG, Limbird LE, Gilman AG, eds. Goodman and Gilman's The Pharmacological Basis of Therapeutics. 10th ed. New York: McGraw-Hill, 2001:447–483.
59. Azmitia EC, Whitaker-Azmitia PM. Anatomy, cell biology, and plasticity of the serotonergic system. In: Bloom FE, Kupfer DL, eds. Psychopharmacology: The Fourth Generation of Progress. New York: Raven Press, 1995:443–449.
60. Gatto E, Pikielny R, Micheli F. Fluoxetine in Tourette's syndrome. Am J Psychiatry 1994; 151(6):946–947.
61. Scahill L, Riddle MA, King RA, Hardin MT, Rasmusson A, Makuch RW, Leckman JF. Fluoxetine has no marked effect on tic symptoms in patients with Tourette's syndrome: a double-blind placebo-controlled study. J Child Adolesc Psychopharmacol 1997; 7(2):75–85.
62. Kurlan R, Como PG, Deeley C, et al. A pilot controlled study of fluoxetine for obsessive–compulsive symptoms in children with Tourette's syndrome. Clin Neuropharmacol 1993; 16:167–172.
63. Lenti C. Movement disorders associated with fluvoxamine. J Am Acad Child Adolesc Psychiatry 1999; 38(8):942–943.
64. Delgado PL, Goodman WK, Price LH, Heninger GR, Charney DS. Fluvoxamine/pimozide treatment of concurrent Tourette's and obsessive–compulsive disorder. Br J Psychiatry 1990; 157:762–765.

65. Bajo S, Battaglia M, Pegna C, Bellodi L. Citalopram and fluvoxamine in Tourette's disorder. J Am Acad Child Adolesc Psychiatry 1999; 38(3):230–231.
66. George MS, Robertson MM, Costa DC, Ell PJ, Trimble MR, Pilowsky L, Verhoeff MPLG. Dopamine receptor availability in Tourette's syndrome. Psychiatry Res Neuroimaging 1994; 55:193–203.
67. Rueth U, Mayer-Rosa J, Schlamp D, Friesleder FJ. Tourette's syndrome and antidepressant therapy: exacerbation of nervous tics by paroxetine. Z Kinder Jugendpsychiatr Psychother 2000; 28(2):105–108.
68. Fras I. Gilles de la Tourette's syndrome: effects of tricyclic antidepressants. NY State J Med 1978; 78:1230–1232.
69. Spencer T, Biederman J, Coffey B, et al. A double-blind comparison of desipramine and placebo in children and adolescents with chronic tic disorder and comorbid attention-deficit/hyperactivity disorder. Arch Gen Psychiatry 2002; 59:649–656.
70. Singer HS, Brown J, Quaskey S, Rosenberg LA, Mellits ED, Denckla MB. The treatment of attention-deficit hyperactivity disorder in Tourette's syndrome: a double-blind placebo-controlled study with clonidine and desipramine. Pediatrics 1995; 95(1):74–81.
71. Riddle MA, Hardin MT, Cho SC, Woolston JL, Leckman JF. Desipramine treatment of boys with attention-deficit hyperactivity disorder and tics: preliminary clinical experience. J Am Acad Child Adolesc Psychiatry 1988; 27(6):811–814.
72. Biederman J, Baldessarini RJ, Wright V, Knee D, Harmatz JS. A double-blind placebo controlled study of desipramine in the treatment of ADD: I. Efficacy. J Am Acad Child Adolesc Psychiatry 1989; 28(5):777–784.
73. Spencer T, Biederman J, Kerman K, Steingard R, Wilens T. Desipramine treatment of children with attention-deficit hyperactivity disorder and tic disorder or Tourette's syndrome. J Am Acad Child Adolesc Psychiatry 1993; 32:334–360.
74. Hoge SK, Biederman J. A case of Tourette's syndrome with symptoms of attention deficit disorder treated with desipramine. J Clin Psychiatry 1986; 47:478–479.
75. Caine ED, Polinsky RJ, Ebert MH, et al. Trial of chlorimipramine and desipramine for Gilles de la Tourette syndrome. Ann Neurol 1979; 5:305–306.
76. Kotler M, Iancu I, Kindler S, Lepkifker E, Zohar I. Clomipramine-induced Tourettism in obsessive compulsive disorder: clinical and theoretical implications. Clin Neuropharmacol 1994; 17:338–343.
77. Iancu I, Kotler M, Bleich A, Lepkifker E. Clomipramine efficacy for Tourette syndrome and major depression: a case study. Biol Psychiatry 1995; 38:407–409.
78. Ratzoni G, Hermesh H, Brandt N, Lauffer M, Munitz H. Clomipramine efficacy for tics, obsessions, and compulsions in Tourette's syndrome and obsessive–compulsive disorder: a case study. Biol Psychiatry 1990; 27:95–98.
79. Donahoe DH, Meador M, Fortune T, Llorena R. Tourette's syndrome and treatment with clomipramine hydrochloride. WV Med J 1991; 87:468–470.

80. Ciprian J. Three cases of Gilles de la Tourette's syndrome—treatment with chlorimipramine. A preliminary report. J Orthomol Psychiatry 1980; 9:116–120.
81. Spencer T, Biederman J, Steingard R, Wilens T. Bupropion exacerbates tics in children with attention-deficit hyperactivity disorder and Tourette's syndrome. J Am Acad Child Adolesc Psychiatry 1993; 32(1):211–214.
82. Dillon DC, Salzman IJ, Schulsinger DA. The use of imipramine in Tourette's syndrome and attention deficit disorder: case report. J Clin Psychiatry 1985; 46:348–349.
83. Biederman J. Sudden death in children treated with a tricyclic antidepressant. J Am Acad Child Adolesc Psychiatry 1991; 30(3):495–498.
84. Varley CK, McClellan J. Case study: two additional sudden deaths with tricyclic antidepressants. J Am Acad Child Adolesc Psychiatry 1997; 36(3):390–394.
85. Popper CW, Elliott GR. Sudden death and tricyclic antidepressants: clinical considerations for children. J Child Adolesc Psychopharmacol 1990; 1(2):125–132.
86. Borison RL, Arg L, Hamilton WJ, et al. Treatment approaches in Gilles de la Tourette syndrome. Brain Res Bull 1983; 11:205–208.
87. Jankovic J. Deprenyl in attention deficit associated with Tourette's syndrome. Arch Neurol 1993; 50:286–288.
88. Spencer T, Biederman J, Steingard R, Wilens T. Bupropion exacerbates tics in children with attention-deficit hyperactivity disorder and Tourette's syndrome. J Am Acad Child Adolesc Psychiatry 1993; 32(1):211–214.
89. Erickson HM Jr, Goggin JE, Messiha FS. Comparison of lithium and haloperidol in Gilles de la Tourette syndrome. Adv Exp Med Biol 1997; 90: 197–205.
90. Hamra BJ, Dunner FH, Larson C. Remission of tics with lithium therapy: case report. J Clin Psychiatry 1983; 44:73–74.
91. Borison RL, Ang L, Chang S, Dysken M, Comaty JE, Davis JM. New pharmacological approaches in treatment of Tourette syndrome. Adv Neurol 1982; 35:377–382.
92. Waziri R, Davenport R. Lithium effects on neuromuscular transmission in manic patients. Common Psychopharm 1979; 3:121–127.
93. Lutz EG. Alternative drug treatments in Tourette's syndrome. Am J Psychiatry 1977; 134:99–100.
94. Neglia JP, Glaze DG, Zion TE. Tics and vocalizations in children treated with carbamazepine. Pediatrics 1984; 76:841–844.
95. Crosley CJ, Swender PT. Dystonia associated with carbamazepine administration: experience in brain-damaged children. Pediatrics 1979; 63(4):612–615.
96. Nausieda PA, Koller WC, Weiner WJ, Klawans HL. Clinical and experimental studies of phenytoin-induced hyperkinesias. J Neural Transm 1979; 45:291–305.
97. Howrie DL, Crumrine PK. Phenytoin induced movement disorder associated with intravenous administration for status epilepticus. Clin Pediatr 1985; 24:467–469.

98. Shulman LM, Singer C, Weiner WJ. Phenytoin-induced focal chorea. Mov Disord 1996; 11(1):111–114.
99. Drake ME, Cannon PA. Tourette's syndrome precipitated by phenytoin. Clin Pediatr 1985; 24:323.
100. Harvey SC. Hypnotics and sedatives. In: Gilman AG, Goodman LS, Rall TW, Murad F, eds. The Pharmacological Basis of Therapeutics. New York: Macmillan, 1985:339–371.
101. Burd L, Kerbeshian J, Fisher W, Gascon G. Anticonvulsant medications: an iatrogenic cause of tic disorders. Can J Psychiatry 1986; 31:419–423.
102. Lomboso CT. Lamotrigine-induced tourettism. Neurology 1999; 52:1191–1194.
103. Menezes MA, Rho JM, Murphy P, Cheyette S. Lamotrigine-induced tic disorder: report of five pediatric cases. Epilepsia 2000; 41(7):862–867.
104. Leach MJ, Lees G, Riddall DR. Lamotrigine: mechanisms of. In: Levy RH, Mattson RH, Medrum BS, eds. Antiepileptic Drugs. 4th ed. New York: Raven Press, 1995:861–869.
105. Carlsson M, Carlsson A. Interactions between glutamatergic and monoaminergic systems within the basal ganglia—implications for schizophrenia and Parkinson's disease. Trends Neurosci 1990; 13:272–276.
106. Perucca E. A pharmacological and clinical review on topiramate, a new antiepileptic drug. Pharmacol Res 1997; 35:241–256.
107. Abuzzahab FS, Brown V. Control of Tourette's syndrome with topiramate. Am J Psychiatry 2001; 158:6.
108. Gilman MA, Sandyk R. Tourette syndrome: effect of analgesic concentrations of nitrous oxide and naloxone. Br Med J 1984; 288:114.
109. Sandyk R. The effects of naloxone in Tourette's syndrome. Ann Neurol 1985; 18:367–368.
110. Sandyk R. Naloxone withdrawal exacerbates Tourette's syndrome. J Clin Psychopharmacol 1986; 6:559–564.
111. Lichter D, Majumdar L, Kurlan R. Opiate withdrawal unmasks Tourette's action syndrome. Clin Neuropharmacol 1988; 6:559–564.
112. Walters AS, Hening W, Chokroverty S. Letter to the editor. Mov Disord 1990; 5:89–91.
113. Kurlan R, Majumadar L, Deeley C, Mudholkar GS, Plumb S, Como PG. A controlled trial of propoxyphene and naltrexone on patients with Tourette's syndrome. Ann Neurol 1991; 30:19–23.
114. Mueller N, Putz A, Straube A. The opiate system in Gilles de la Tourette syndrome: diverse effects of naltrexone treatment. Eur Psychiatry 1994; 9(1):39–44.
115. van Wattum PJ, Chappell PB, Zelterman D, Schahill LD, Leckman JF. Patterns of response to acute naloxone infusion in Tourette's Syndrome. Mov Disord 2000; 15(6):1252–1254.
116. Gillman MA, Sandyk R. The endogenous opioid system in Gilles de la Tourette's syndrome. Med Hypotheses, 1986, 371–378.
117. Haber SN, Kowall NW, Vonsattel JP, Bird ED, Richardson EP Jr. Gilles de la

Tourette's syndrome: a postmortem neuropathological and immunohistochemical study. J Neurol Sci 1986; 75:225–241.

118. Haber SN, Wolfer D. Basal ganglia peptidergic staining in Tourette's syndrome: a follow up study. In: Chase TN, Friedhoff AJ, Cohen DJ, eds. Tourette's Syndrome: Genetics, Neurobiology and Treatment. Advances in Neurology. Vol. 58. New York: Raven Press, 1992:145–150.
119. Merikangas JR, Merikangas KR, Kopp U, et al. Blood choline and response to clonazepam and haloperidol in Tourette's syndrome. Acta Psychiatr Scand 1985; 72:395–399.

11

Rating Tic Severity

Roger Kurlan and Michael P. McDermott
University of Rochester Medical Center
Rochester, New York, U.S.A.

INTRODUCTION

Both the clinical care of patients with Tourette's syndrome (TS) and research efforts directed toward the disorder demand the availability of specific, reliable, and valid methods for measuring the severity of tics. In the clinical setting, rating instruments are useful to monitor the course of symptoms and to gauge response to therapeutic interventions. In the research arena, the need for accurate tic ratings is perhaps most obvious for the assessment of novel therapies, such as drug trials. Rating instruments, however, are also crucial for a variety of other investigative avenues. The search for specific and sensitive biological markers for TS requires correlation with disease severity. In family genetic studies, measurement of tic severity may prove useful in identifying subjects who represent nongenetic phenocopies (and might express milder symptoms) and those expressing different genotypes. For example, we may be able to differentiate subjects who are heterozygous or homozygous for the TS genetic trait based on symptom severity (1). In addition, while tics have been observed quite commonly in the general childhood population, at present it remains unclear what proportion carry the TS genetic trait. The measurement of tic severity in epidemiological studies of tics may be helpful in clarifying this issue. Accurate characterization of the natural history of TS, including both short-term waxing and waning and long-term course, requires precise measures of severity.

PROBLEMS IN RATING TIC SEVERITY

Although tics are generally visible or audible symptoms, there are a variety of clinical characteristics of TS that make objective quantification difficult. First is the marked clinical heterogeneity of the tic disorder itself (2). Simple motor and vocal tics include a wide array of movements and sounds. The more complicated complex motor tics can take a variety of forms and there are many types of complex vocal tics, including coprolalic and echolalic phenomena. Although most motor tics are rapid and shocklike, some patients experience slow, twisting, or tightening movements resembling dystonia ("dystonic tics"). The localized uncomfortable sensations that may precede or accompany motor or vocal tics have been termed "sensory tics." Tics may occur with a wide spectrum of intensity, ranging from barely noticeable to severely disabling. Thus, in developing a theoretical construct of tic "severity," a wide range of features must be considered, including number of tic types, body distribution, frequency, intensity, suppressibility, complexity, and interference with daily functioning. The complex nature of tics often defies specification and makes subject-to-subject comparisons difficult.

Second, for individual patients, tics characteristically follow a waxing and waning course, with days, weeks, or months of mild severity alternating with periods of intensification. Moreover, there appear to be diurnal and seasonal fluctuations. Shapiro et al. (3) found that 40% of patients report a reduction of symptoms in the morning hours and 19% report that tics are less severe in the summer. This natural fluctuation of symptoms represents a major challenge in assessing efficacy during drug trials and may contribute to false-negative diagnostic assignment in family genetic studies.

Third, patients are usually able to voluntarily suppress tics, for periods ranging from seconds to hours. Thus, since patients often suppress in the presence of a physician, tic severity as measured in the office may not be representative, and since the degree of suppression may differ in different environments (e.g., home, school, church), information from a variety of informants may be required for accurate assessment of symptom severity. These observations suggest that situational stimuli and seasonal and diurnal conditions need to be standardized, or at least specified, when measuring tic severity. Finally, some or all tics may be unrecognized by individuals with TS. For example, in family genetic studies, we have found that approximately 30% of subjects diagnosed by examiners as having tics were completely unaware of their symptoms (4). This observation further supports the need for additional informants, such as a parent or teacher, when measuring tics; however, it is important to recognize that many informants have a limited knowledge of TS and have no experience in making valid severity estimates.

In addition to the complexities of the TS tic disorder, evidence suggests that specific behavioral problems, such as obsessive–compulsive disorder and attention-deficit/hyperactivity disorder, may be part of the TS clinical spectrum (5). Thus, an accurate assessment of TS severity and impact on daily functioning must take into account these behavioral problems as well. The evaluation of behavioral problems associated with TS is addressed in Chapters 4–7 and 12.

STATISTICAL CONSIDERATIONS FOR QUANTITATIVE ASSESSMENT OF TICS

Several important issues need to be considered in the development of an instrument for the quantitative assessment of tics. LaRocca (6), who provides a good overview of considerations for scale development in general, makes the important observation that all too often instruments are constructed and put into use without adequate assessment of properties such as reliability, validity, and sensitivity. The implications of this can be serious. For example, a comparative clinical trial that uses an outcome variable with poor test–retest reliability may be much less powerful in detecting meaningful differences between treatment groups than the same trial using a reliable outcome variable.

Target Population

The first issue that needs to be addressed in developing an instrument to rate tic severity is the definition of the target population for whom the instrument is intended. Strict subject inclusion/exclusion criteria must be established so that a theoretical construct may be formulated (i.e., so that a determination may be made as to which aspects of tic disorder are to be measured by the instrument). In what follows it will be assumed that the target population includes all subjects who satisfy current diagnostic criteria for a tic disorder, such as by DSM-IV.

Theoretical Construct

The difficulties in rating tic severity, as discussed above, make it necessary to consider a wide range of features in order to develop a theoretical construct for tic "severity." The term "theoretical construct" simply refers to the abstract notion of what it means for a tic disorder to be more or less severe. The concept of tic severity encompasses a variety of clinical features, such as number of tic types, body distribution, frequency, intensity, suppressibility, complexity, and interference with daily functioning. The formulated rating instrument should therefore quantify or classify in some fashion each of these features in order to produce observable indicators of the construct.

Quantification of Observable Indicators

Some of the above features of tic disorders, like many aspects of neurological and other diseases, are not directly measurable. Therefore, some method must be devised for assigning numbers as a rating of severity. In general, this quantification can be done using either ordinal or interval measurements. An ordinal scale is one in which the steps of the scale are not necessarily equal. For example, in rating tic intensity as "none," "mild," "moderate," "marked," or "extreme," the difference between "extreme" and "marked" may not be the same as the difference between "moderate" and "mild." The numbers assigned to these categories are therefore arbitrary, except that they should preserve the rank order of the scale. Medians, quartiles, or other percentiles are appropriate descriptive statistics for ordinal variables, whereas means and standard deviations are not, because a sum of ranks that take on arbitrary numerical values is not a meaningful descriptive measure.

Interval measurements, on the other hand, have the characteristic that the difference between, for example, ratings 1 and 2 is the same as the difference between ratings 4 and 5. It is desirable to employ interval measurements whenever possible since standard statistical operations may be performed on such measurements, making their analysis more manageable in general. In addition, valid interval measurements tend to be more sensitive to changes in the underlying latent variable. An ordinal measurement may be considered an interval measurement if the numerical values of the "ranks," or steps of the scale, are chosen so that the differences between successive steps accurately reflect the actual differences in the status of the feature being measured. The assumption that this is approximately true is often made with scales, but it is difficult to verify.

For example, suppose the number of body regions affected by tics is used as a measure of one dimension of tic severity, namely, that of body distribution. If one assumes that being affected in the eyes and mouth is equivalent to, say, being, affected in the arms and legs (i.e., each region is of equal importance), this would then be an ordinal measure. If one further assumes that the difference between zero and two affected regions is the same as the difference between two and four affected regions, this would then be an interval measure.

Another common assumption is that the observable indicator or measurement is linearly related to the latent variable (i.e., the measure of a disease state that cannot be observed directly) that is actually of interest. This is one of the assumptions of the so-called Likert model (7) in the case where the measurement is a composite or sum of several individual scale items. As Miller (8) indicates, one can sometimes investigate such an assumption through natural history studies.

Even if one could successfully quantify the individual features of the theoretical construct for tic severity, it is still a difficult task to develop a means for combining such information to determine whether an individual subject is overall more or less severely affected with tic disorder. For example, one subject may have extremely intense tics in only one region of the body, while another has mild to moderate tics in several regions. Which case should be rated as being more severe? Should some features be weighted more heavily than others? If so, how are these weights to bc choscn? Thcsc issucs are rclated to what is often called the dimensionality of the construct (see below).

Standardization of Testing

After suitable means have been developed for quantifying the observable aspects of the theoretical construct, a standardized format for carrying out the assessments needs to be established before proceeding with statistical evaluation of various properties of the instrument. The manner in which all testing is to be done, such as setting, time of day, order of individual items, and methods for distracting subjects to overcome tic suppression, must be well conceived and consistent in all applications. This is particularly important in rating tic severity since seasonal or environmental effects may have a great impact on the resulting measurements (3). Ideally, the format should be documented in a manual of operations that is considered an integral part of the instrument itself. Finally, the evaluators must be well trained and experienced in the use of the instrument.

Reliability (Reproducibility) of Measurement

A desirable property of any measurement is reproducibility. One aspect of this, commonly referred to as test–retest reliability, concerns repeated measurements made on the same subject by the same rater under the same conditions, where it is assumed that the status of the subject regarding what is being measured has not changed between assessments. Given the characteristic waxing and waning quality of tics, however, this assumption must be carefully considered in the designs of studies that assess the reliability of tic disorder ratings.

The concept of reproducibility of measurement involves modeling the relationship between the unobservable true value of the subject's state and an observed, measured assessment of that state. Let Y denote the observed value of an interval measurement of tic severity for a subject. In general, Y will differ from the (unobservable) true value of the tic severity X because of factors such as misinterpretation of the question being asked, misconception of the subject's condition, and other kinds of measurement error. A simple linear model is commonly used to describe the relationship between Y and X:

$$Y = X + e$$

where, for statistical modeling purposes, the measurement error e is assumed to be normally distributed (with mean 0 and variance F_e^2 independently for each subject. In addition, the true scores X are assumed to be normally distributed with mean Φ and variance F_x^2.

A common but faulty approach for computing test–retest reliability is to use the Pearson, or product–moment, correlation coefficient for two replicate measurements. For example, if tic ratings for five subjects are exactly 10 points higher for the first measurement than for the second, perhaps due to natural fluctuation of symptoms, the Pearson correlation coefficient would be equal to 1, falsely indicating perfect reliability. The problem is that systematic error has occurred and the Pearson correlation coefficient is insensitive to this. It is more a measure of agreement regarding relative standing of the subjects than of equality of the two measurements for each subject.

A better approach for the assessment of test–retest reliability is to use the intraclass correlation coefficient. In the simple linear model above, if it may be assumed that the distribution of e (measurement error) is independent of the value of X (true score), then the variation in the observed scores Y may be decomposed into two components, namely subject-to-subject variation in X and error variability:

$$F_y^2 = F_x^2 + F_e^2$$

The intraclass correlation coefficient is then defined as:

$$R = \frac{F_x^2}{F_x^2 + F_e^2}$$

Note that R may take on values ranging from 0 to 1 and is directly interpretable as the proportion of variability in the observed scores that is due to the subject-to-subject variability in the true scores (i.e., not due to measurement error). It has the desirable characteristic of being sensitive to both systematic and measurement error. The value of R may be estimated from the data by using random effects analysis of variance models (e.g., see Ref. 9).

For nominal or ordinal measurements, test–retest reliability is sometimes measured by the overall proportion of agreement of responses (i.e., the proportion of subjects who had the same response at each of the two assessments). This measure does not take into account the fact that a certain proportion of agreement can be expected on the basis of chance alone. A measure that does correct for chance-expected agreement is the kappa statistic proposed by Cohen (10). A weighted version of this statistic can be used to take into account the relative seriousness of each possible disagreement, assuming that this can be quantified (11). Fleiss and Cohen (12) have shown that weighted kappa can be interpreted as an intraclass correlation coefficient. A thorough discussion of the kappa statistic and its variants can be found in Ref. 13.

Another important aspect of measurement reproducibility is interrater reliability, which concerns repeated measurements made on the same subject under the same conditions by different raters, where it is again assumed that the status of the subject regarding what is being measured has not changed between assessments. If Y is the observed value of an interval measurement on a subject, then the linear model often used to describe the relationship between Y and X, the subject's (unobservable) true score, is:

$$Y = X + r + e$$

where X and e are defined as above and r represents the relative effect (positive or negative) of a randomly selected rater on Y (which is assumed to be normally distributed with mean 0 and variance F_r^2). Under the assumption that the random variables X, r, and e are mutually independent, the variance of a subject's measurement can be decomposed as:

$$F_y^2 = F_x^2 + F_r^2 + F_e^2$$

and the interclass correlation coefficient is then defined as:

$$R = \frac{F_x^2}{F_x^2 + F_r^2 + F_e^2}$$

This measure of interrater agreement takes into account the systematic differences that may occur between raters. For example, one rater may consistently rate tic severity one point lower on a scale than another rater simply due to his or her interpretation of the rating scale. The intraclass correlation coefficient may again be estimated with the use of random effects analysis of variance models (9). If the measurement is either nominal or ordinal, the kappa and weighted-kappa statistics may be used to measure interrater agreement.

There is no universal agreement on what values of R and kappa indicate good reliability, but Fleiss (9) and Landis and Koch (14) recommend that values greater than 0.75 be accepted as indicating excellent reliability. Shrout (15) provides a thoughtful discussion of what constitutes adequate reliability.

The validity of certain assumptions is crucial to proper interpretation of the results of a reliability study. One of these assumptions is that the status of the subject has not changed between replicate measurements. This assumption is often regarded as the most unrealistic in practice, so it is important to have the assessments as close together in time as possible. One method for dealing with this is to videotape the assessments, although this approach can also be problematic. For example, one may perceive the status of the subject in a face-to-face interview quite differently from when observed on a videotape, depending on the quality of the videotape. In addition, it may not be proper to combine data obtained in a direct examination with data obtained from a videotaped interview.

A second assumption is that the instrument does not lend itself to learning or practice effects on the part of the subject. For example, a subject may perform a particular task somewhat differently in a repeated test simply because he or she has performed the task before. One way to control this is to interview the subject once or twice before actually carrying out the reliability study, the rationale being that the subject has become familiar enough with the tasks so that any learning effects may be minimized in subsequent replications. Another approach, commonly used for psychological instruments, is to use alternate forms of the relevant test. Of course, it must be assured that the content of the alternate form is the same as that of the original one. This may be verified with a test–retest reliability study that uses alternate forms of the instrument at each assessment.

The statistical assumptions that are common in making inferences about the intraclass correlation coefficient, namely, those mentioned above for random effects analysis of variance models also need to be verified. Applying a carefully chosen transformation to the observed measurements (e.g., square root or logarithmic) will often help in cases in which these assumptions do not hold. Graphical tools such as scatterplots, histograms, and normal probability plots are useful for detecting departures from the assumptions. A readable discussion of these issues can be found in many standard statistical texts (16,17).

There are other considerations that are absolutely essential for carrying out a reliability study. The subject sample should be representative of the target population. Assessments must be carefully standardized, with the conditions being as similar as possible to those in which the scale will be generally applied. The raters should be well trained in the use of the instrument and should perform all assessments independently of one another, with no discussion of the results or alteration in the manner of assessment taking place until the conclusion of the study. There must be strict adherence to the original protocol.

It is vital to carry out reliability studies before putting the scale to use in a major research study. The reliability of individual items of a scale should be assessed as well as that of composite scores obtained from these items. About 20–40 subjects are usually enough to conduct a reliability study for interval measurements (9,18). However, many more (>100) may be needed for nominal or ordinal measurements, depending on the nature of the variables (19). Still more subjects are required if reliability of these measurements within certain population subgroups is to be documented. The consequences of using an unreliable quantitative variable as an outcome measure in a research study can be quite serious. Fleiss (9) provides a good discussion of some of these consequences.

Construction of Composite Measures

When planning a clinical drug trial for TS, it is necessary to identify some primary measures of tic severity for the purpose of sample size determination and analysis prespecification. Since there are many features (e.g., tic complexity) that should be taken into account in measuring tic severity, and since each feature may be quantified with more than one item (e.g., tic complexity might be rated by assessing such items as purposefulness, degree of social acceptability, and duration), the information from several items and/or features will have to be combined in some fashion to form more global measures of severity. Advantages of this include avoiding the common problem of multiple statistical testing and improving reliability, since well-constructed composite measures are usually more reliable than individual ones (20).

An important initial step in constructing composite measures based on the individual items from an instrument is to assess the instrument's *dimensionality*. If all of the features of TS, as measured by an instrument, were highly correlated, it could be argued that tic severity is a unidimensional concept; that is, it may in reality be adequately described by a single latent variable. It is likely, however, that there are a small number of latent variables, or what may also be called dimensions or factors, that together form the theoretical construct of tic severity. It is often the case that these underlying factors cannot be identified through theoretical considerations alone; rather, empirical evidence may also be necessary for their identification. A common statistical method for evaluating the dimensionality of a scale, or in general a set of variables, is factor analysis (20,21). Principal component analysis and multidimensional scaling are related techniques that can also be used for this purpose (20). The primary goal of factor analysis is data reduction in the sense that it seeks to describe the correlation structure among a large set of variables in terms of relatively few latent variables, or factors. It may help identify a small number of groups of items such that items within each group are highly correlated, but items between groups have relatively low correlations.

Factor analysis is of two basic types, exploratory and confirmatory. Exploratory factor analysis seeks to identify the minimum number of latent variables necessary to adequately explain the correlation structure among the scale items, and to suggest hypotheses concerning what these factors may be and what relationship they may have with the observed items. On the other hand, confirmatory factor analysis seeks to investigate specific hypotheses concerning how many dimensions exist and what these latent factors may actually represent. It also involves modeling the relationships between the observed variables and the factors. For the purpose of developing an instrument for rating tic severity, exploratory factor analysis may be used to reveal the presence of more than one dimension in the instrument, and confirmatory factor analysis may be used for eliminating items that may be noninformative or redundant, and for constructing subscales.

Factor analysis may provide a clue as to how to weight individual items based on how well each correlates with related items representing a common factor. Another approach, useful when the items are measured on completely different scales, is to rescale the items to a common metric before they are combined. One method of standardization is the use of the Z-transformation for constructing composite scores, as employed, for example, by Andres et al. (22) in quantifying deficits in amyotrophic lateral sclerosis. For each item, the mean and standard deviation are determined from a large sample of subjects, perhaps corrected for age or other relevant factors, and an individual's score is transformed by subtracting the mean and dividing by the standard deviation. The transformed score reflects how many standard deviations the subject is from the mean of that particular item. The scores from related items may then be summed to form a composite score. The difficulties with this approach relate to the determination of the mean and standard deviation used in the standardization process. Many subjects would be needed for adequately estimating these quantities, and periodic recalibration may be necessary. Another approach is to standardize with reference to a normal group of subjects, although this would seem to be of limited utility for rating tic severity.

Once a composite score, or a small number of composite scores, has been decided upon, each should be evaluated for internal consistency. This concept is simply the extent to which the items making up a composite score are measuring the same latent factor. The so-called "split-halves" method of assessing internal consistency consists of dividing the items into two equal parts, forming composite scores based on the items in each part, and measuring the correlation between these two composite scores. The Spearman–Brown prophecy formula (23) may then be used to estimate the internal consistency coefficient. A major problem with this method is that the way in which the items are divided is arbitrary, and different divisions may lead to different estimates of internal consistency. The more popular Cronbach's alpha (24), which was actually introduced by Guttman (25), may be thought of as the average of the internal consistencies computed from all possible split halves (26). The value of alpha increases as the number of items and the average correlation between the items increase; therefore, the elimination of weakly correlated items or the addition of strongly correlated items will increase alpha. Like the measures of reliability described earlier, a value of alpha greater than 0.75 may be taken to represent excellent internal consistency.

Validity

The term "validity" may be defined as the extent to which an instrument actually measures the theoretical construct that it purports to measure. However, validity should be interpreted in a broader sense in that a valid measure should also satisfy certain theoretical relationships with variables other than those directly related to the theoretical construct. For example, a measure of tic severity may be expected to bear a close relationship to an assessment of daily functioning, such as the Child Global Assessment Scale (27). There are four types of validity that merit discussion: content validity, criterion validity, construct validity, and convergent/discriminant validity.

Content validity is the extent to which the instrument represents all of the dimensions of the theoretical construct. This type of validity is qualitative in the sense that there are no adequate means for its empirical assessment. Content validity must be subjectively judged by the investigator. Therefore, it is desirable that the theoretical construct be widely accepted by researchers in the field of study, and that all theorized features of this construct be sufficiently quantified by the instrument. A scale for tic severity should include items that adequately measure all the known features of tic disorder that were described earlier. Present scales for rating tic disorder have been criticized mainly because of the lack of content validity (see below).

Criterion validity is the extent to which a measurement is related to another so-called "criterion variable" that is known to be highly related to the latent variable of interest (i.e., an independent measure whose validity has been established). This type of validity may also be called postdictive, concurrent, or predictive validity, depending on whether the scale measurement follows, is contemporaneous with, or precedes the criterion. There are several difficulties with measuring the criterion validity of a measure of tic severity, including possible errors in the validity of the criterion and, more seriously, the lack of existing criterion variables. An example of a criterion variable that has been used in assessing the validity of tic measures is response to tic-suppressing drug treatment (28).

A third type of validity, *construct validity*, is the extent to which observed relationships between various measurements are consistent with the reasoning underlying the theoretical construct (i.e., the extent to which the instrument adequately captures the theoretical construct). Variables that are theorized to be highly correlated should exhibit this correlation; the same is true for variables that are theorized to have no association. For example, items measuring the interference of tics with daily activities should be highly correlated with one another, as well as with an independent measure of daily functioning, such as the Child Global Assessment Scale (27). The establishment of construct validity may involve many steps, each of which may lead to modifications of either the instrument or the construct. These steps may consist of reevaluating content validity and reexamining internal consistency and dimensionality as described earlier.

Construct validity is closely related to *convergent/discriminant validity* (29), which may be assessed if at least two independent measures of each trait or feature of the theoretical construct exist. A typical example of this occurs when subjects have been assessed by at least two raters. For a tic rating scale to have convergent validity, the correlations between the two raters' measures of the same item should be large. Discriminant validity is achieved when the convergent validity correlations for the same item are larger than the correlations between different items, whether or not they are from the same rater. In addition, the correlation pattern of items within each feature should be consistent across all raters.

Good general references regarding the concept of validity include Nunnally (20) and Bollen (30). The latter author describes weaknesses in the traditional approach to validity assessment based on observed correlations and proposes a structural equations approach, which involves modeling the relationships between the latent and observed variables.

AVAILABLE INSTRUMENTS

Only a small number of rating scales for tic severity have been published. Of these, few have undergone systematic assessment of reliability and validity, and most are limited by inadequately described procedures, unstandardized conditions, small sample sizes, and incomplete statistical analyses. Ratings have been based either on examiner observations at the time of a clinical interview or on self-reported information obtained from patients, parents, or teachers.

Examiner Ratings

Examiner-based ratings involve clinical judgments about the severity of tic behaviors after observing the patient and reviewing historical information regarding the patient's progress over a certain time period. The Tourette

Syndrome Severity Scale (TSSS) (Table 1) (3,31), developed by Shapiro and Shapiro for use in a clinical trial of pimozide, includes a composite clinician rating of severity comprising five factors: the degree to which tics are noticeable to others, whether they elicit comments or curiosity, whether other individuals consider the patient odd or bizarre, whether tics interfere with functioning, and whether the patient is incapacitated, homebound, or hospitalized because of tics. Scores for the five items are summed and converted to a qualitative global severity rating. The TSSS is simple to use, appears valid and highly reliable when used by physicians, and provides an overall index of tic severity. However, this scale is limited in that it fails to assess the wide range of tic characteristics.

The Tourette Syndrome Global Scale (TSGS) (Fig. 1) (32) was formulated at Yale and combines various ratings for tic symptoms and social functioning into an overall global score for severity. The section on tic symptoms involves rating frequency (on a scale of 0 to 5) and disruption (on a scale of 1 to 5) for simple motor, complex motor, simple phonic, and complex phonic tics. For each tic category, frequency and disruption scores are multiplied and the products are summed to yield a total severity score. The section on social functioning involves rating behavior (conduct), motor restlessness, school and learning problems, and work and occupational problems, each on a scale of 0 to 25. The tic symptom and social functioning scores are then inserted into a mathematical formula that yields a global score.

Table 1 TS Severity Scale

		Ratings			
Severity rating	Total score sum of ratings	Tics noticeable to others	Tics elicit comments or curiosity	Patient considered odd or bizarre	Tics interfere with functioning
None	0	None present (0)	—	—	—
Very mild	0.5	Very few (0.5)	No (0)	No (0)	No (0)
Mild	1 to <2	Some (1)	No (0)	No (0)	No (0)
Moderate	2 to <4	Most (2)	Yes (1)	No (0)	No (0)
Marked	4 to <6	All (3)	Yes (1)	Possibly (1)	Might (1)
Severe	6–8	All (3)	Yes (1)	Yes (2)	Yes (2)
Very severe[a]	9	All (3)	Yes (1)	Yes (2)	Yes (2)

[a] All of the above in addition to being incapacitated, requiring hospitalization, or remaining at home. See Ref. 33 for a detailed description of the anchor points.
Source: Ref. 31.

NAME____________________ DATE____________ RATER____________

CODE FOR FREQUENCY	FREQUENCY (F)						DISRUPTION (D)					
1 = 1 or less in 5 min 2 = 1 in 2 – 4.9 min 3 = from 1 in 1.9 min to 4 in 1 min 4 = 5 or more in 1 min 5 = virtually uncountable	None	Rarely	Occasionally	Frequently	Almost Always	Always	Camouflaged	Audible or Visible	Some Problem	Impaired	Cannot Function	
SIMPLE MOTOR (SM): Nonpurposeful, tics, jerks and/or movements	0	1	2	3	4	5	1	2	3	4	5	FxD = ___
COMPLEX MOTOR (CM): Purposeful, thoughtful actions (systematic actions), rituals, touching self, others, or objects	0	1	2	3	4	5	1	2	3	4	5	FxD = ___
SIMPLE PHONIC (SP): Nonpurposeful noises, throat clearing, coughing	0	1	2	3	4	5	1	2	3	4	5	FxD = ___
COMPLEX PHONIC (CP): Purposeful, insults, coprolalia, words, distinguishable speech	0	1	2	3	4	5	1	2	3	4	5	FxD = ___

BEHAVIOR (B) (conduct)

0	No problem
5	Subtle problems; normal peer, school, and family relations
10	Some problems, at least one relationship area impaired
15	Clear impairment in more than one area
20	Serious impairment, affects all areas
25	Unacceptable social behavior, constant supervision

MOTOR RESTLESSNESS (MR)

0	Normal movement
5	Adventitial movements visible, no problems
10	Increased motor restlessness, clearly visible, some problem
15	Clear motor restlessness, moderate problem
20	Mostly in motion but occasionally stops, impaired functioning
25	Nonstop motion, clearly cannot function

SCHOOL AND LEARNING PROBLEMS

0	No problem
5	Low grades
10	Should be or in some special classes, or repeated grade
15	All special classes
20	Special School
25	Unable to remain in school, home bound

WORK AND OCCUPATIONAL PROBLEMS

0	No problem
5	Stable job, some difficulty
10	Serious problems
15	Lost lots of jobs
20	Almost never employed
25	Unemployed

((SM + CM)/2 + ((SP + CP)/2) + ((B + MR + SCHOOL OR WORK PROBLEMS) X 2/3) = GLOBAL SCORE

Figure 1 Tourette's Syndrome Global Scale (TSSG). A detailed description of the anchor points is provided

There are several problems with this scale. First, it combines information from completely different dimensions in a manner that does not seem to have any empirical justification. Second, the multiplication of frequency by disruption scores exaggerates small differences in tic severity and also causes the social functioning items to be underweighted (33). In addition, its reliability and validity properties have been documented with only a relatively small number of subjects. Finally, this instrument fails to assess several important tic characteristics, such as number of tic types and complexity.

In an effort to more inclusively measure a wider range of tic features, including number, frequency, intensity, complexity, and interference, investigators at Yale developed the Global Tic Severity Scale (GTSS) (Fig. 2) (33). Examiners rate these characteristics for motor and phonic tics independently and generate a total tic score, an overall impairment rating, and a global severity score. The GTSS also includes a checklist for specific types of motor and phonic tics. This has become the most widely used scale for assessing tic severity in clinical studies.

The Yale group has also formulated a Global Clinical Impression Scale (GCIS) (Table 2) for tics that is a 7-point ordinal scale ranging from "normal" to "extremely severe" for a rating of the impact of TS symptoms on daily functioning (33). Each of the anchor points contains a specific description for

	Number	Frequency	Intensity	Complexity	Interference
A. Motor Tics	_____	_____	_____	_____	_____
	Number	Frequency	Intensity	Complexity	Interference
B. Phonic Tics	_____	_____	_____	_____	_____
	Number	Frequency	Intensity	Complexity	Interference
C. Total for All Tics	_____	_____	_____	_____	_____

D. Global Severity Ratings
Motor Tic Score =
Sum Motor Tics (Number + Frequency + Intensity + Complexity + Interference) = _____

Phonic Tic Score =
Sum Phonic Tics (Number + Frequency + Intensity + Complexity + Interference) = _____

Total Tic Score, (Number + Frequency + Intensity + Complexity + Interference) = _____

Overall TS Impairment Rating = _____
Global Severity (Total Tic score + TS impairment) = _____

Figure 2 Yale Global Tic Severity Scale. A detailed description of the anchor points is provided in the source. (From Ref. 33.)

Table 2 Global Clinical Impression Scale (Based on All Available Information Concerning Adverse Impact of Clearly Defined Tic Behaviors)

Normal	No tic symptoms.
Borderline	Questionable tic symptoms. Does not satisfy criteria for a diagnosis of a definite chronic tic disorder.
Moderate	Tic symptoms cause some problems in some areas of functioning and are noticeable to some people some of the time.
Marked	Tic symptoms cause clear problems in more than one area of functioning. Tics are usually frequent and quite noticeable in most situations most of the time.
Severe	Tic symptoms cause significant impairment in primary social role such that functioning in "usual" settings is impossible or in serious jeopardy.
Extremely severe	Tic symptoms are incapacitating and/or have caused serious personal injury.

Source: Ref. 33.

rating of severity. The statistical properties of this scale, however, have apparently not been evaluated.

A second approach for examiner ratings involves the use of patient videotape sessions performed under standardized conditions. For the scale of Goetz and colleagues (28), patients are videotaped in three settings: seated quietly with the examiner in the room, reading aloud with the examiner in the room, and seated quietly with no examiner in the room. Following a review of the videotape, an examiner assesses body regions involved with motor tics, rates motor and vocal tic severity (based on a 0–5 scale), and performs a count of motor and vocal tics. This rating approach was used in a clinical trial assessing the efficacy of clonidine in TS (34), but it is limited by a lack of established content validity. Despite the known minute-to-minute variability and sensitivity to environmental settings of tics, it has been shown that high levels of reliability can be achieved using videotape ratings (3,28). These methods, however, require suitable technical equipment and may be cumbersome.

Self- and Parental Reporting Instruments

Self- and parental reporting scales include a series of structured questions for which the patient or parent chooses the most appropriate response. This approach has been most helpful for large-scale epidemiological and family genetic studies, and it has also proven useful for longitudinal assessment of

Name of patient ______________________ ID#__________________

Date______________________________

Rate each symptom by putting the appropriate number in the box each day. (Use the reverse side for any detailed comments.)

0 = Not at all or symptom-free.	3 = Very much.	Rater:
1 = Just a little.	4 = Extreme.	ε Parent ε Father
2 = Pretty much.	5 = Almost always.	ε Mother ε Other

Date	Mon	Tue	Wed	Thu	Fri	Sat	Sun	
SIMPLE MOTOR								
1. Eyeblinking								Sum of 1 – 11 MON–SUN
2. Other facial tics								
3. Head jerks								
4. Shoulder jerks								#of Symptoms 1–11 MON–SUN
5. Arm movements								
6. Finger or hand movements								
7. Stomach jerks								
8. Kicking leg movements								
9. Tense parts of body								
10. Other:								
11. Other:								
COMPLEX MOTOR								
12. Touching part of body								Sum of 12–22 MON–SUN
13. Touching other people								
14. Touching objects								
15. Can't start actions								# of Symptoms 12–22 MON–SUN
16. Hurts self								
17. Finger or hand tapping								
18. Hopping								
19. Picks at things (clothing, etc.)								
20. Copropraxia								
21. Other:								
22. Other:								
SIMPLE PHONIC								
23. Noises								Sum of 23–28 MON–SUN
24. Grunting								
25. Throat clearing								# of Symptoms 23–28 MON–SUN
26. Coughing								
27. Other:								
28. Other:								
COMPLEX PHONIC								
29. Words								SUM of 29–35 MON–SUN
30. Repeats own words/sentences								
31. Repeats others' speech								# of Symptoms 29–35 MON–SUN
32. Coprolalia (obscene words)								
33. Insults (lack of inhibition)								
34. Other:								
35. Other:								
BEHAVIOR								
36. Argumentative								SUM of 36–41 MON–SUN
37. Poor frustration tolerance								
38. Anger, temper fits								# of Symptoms 36–41 MON–SUN
39. Provocative								
40. Other:								
41. Other:								

Figure 3 Tourette Syndrome Symptom List (TSSL).

the natural course of illness and response to specific therapies. Designed to elicit a patient's detailed medical history for an epidemiological study, the 35-page Tourette Syndrome Questionnaire (TSQ) (35) has questions categorized under the following headings: Patient Personal Data Inventory, General Medical History, History of Tourette Symptomatology, Treatment History, Family History, Prenatal and Birth History, and Developmental History. Another parent and/or self-report instrument was formulated for a needs assessment survey conducted for the Tourette Syndrome Association of Ohio (36). The Tourette Syndrome Symptom List (TSSL) (Fig. 3) (8,37) was created at Yale to assist parents in making daily or weekly ratings of tic severity. Specific tic types (e.g., blinking, grunting) are rated on a 0–5 severity scale daily in a diary format. Ratings can be summed to provide a weekly measurement of tic severity and number of symptoms. In addition, ratings for behavior problems (e.g., anger, argumentativeness) are included. This instrument has been used in monitoring the longitudinal course of TS and in measuring changes during drug trials (38). Self-reporting instruments have a variety of potential limitations, including rater noncompliance, observer bias, and lack of rater expertise.

FUTURE DIRECTIONS

The Tourette Syndrome Association organized a meeting of clinicians and investigators to review the state of rating scales for the disorder. There was a consensus that available instruments were inadequate for current and future research activities. Therefore, the group set out to develop a consensus rating instrument, to be named the "Unified Tic Rating Scale" (UTRS), which would serve to minimize errors in measurement, ensure comparability of results, and provide uniformity in interpretation of results (3). The authors of the UTRS reviewed available rating instruments, adopted and modified some items, and formulated several new items. Although still in development, as presently conceived the UTRS is divided into two sections. The "Historical Ratings" section is based on information provided by the patient and/or other informants and includes assessments of average tic severity for the preceding week. A variety of tic characteristics, such as body distribution, number of types, intensity, and interference, are rated based on the historical information. In the "Examiner Ratings" section, the clinician rates similar tic characteristics based on observations made during completion of the historical ratings section. The UTRS also contains appendices with ratings for attention-deficit/hyperactivity disorder, obsessive–compulsive disorder, and global functioning impairment that assess the overall impact of all aspects of the illness, including tics, medication side effects, behavioral dysfunction, and social disturbances.

A variety of methodological issues must be addressed in the final formulation and testing of the UTRS. Standardized videotape vignettes of a group of tic-disorder patients have been prepared in order to field-test a version of the scale among a large group of clinicians. Properties such as test–retest and interrater reliability, dimensionality, internal consistency, and validity of the instrument will have to be thoroughly investigated, which may lead to further refinements of the scale, or even of the theoretical construct of tic disorder itself.

Once the instrument is finalized, several other issues will need to be addressed before it can be put to use in a major clinical trial. Several relevant composite measures, as constructed from the scale, will need to undergo thorough evaluation. Those that are most clinically relevant and are thought to be most sensitive to changes in the underlying disease process should be considered for use as primary outcome variables in future clinical studies. A natural history study or a pilot study, for example, an open-label trial of tic-suppressing drug therapy, may be helpful in determining which measures to use. In order to determine the sample size required for a therapeutic trial, one must not only have an idea of the smallest, clinically meaningful therapeutic effect, but also an idea of the variability of the primary outcome variable. If this measure is a change from baseline status, it will be particularly important to have an idea of the magnitude of the variability of these changes over time. A natural history or pilot study would be invaluable in this context.

Finally, it will be important to examine the data that have been collected for the existence of certain subgroups that seem to be either mildly or severely affected with tic disorder. This process may lead to new ideas regarding inclusion/exclusion criteria in future clinical studies. In addition, the identification of important stratification variables, for example, age, gender, and known hereditary transmission, would be very beneficial in the design of such studies.

ACKNOWLEDGMENT

This work was supported by the Tourette Syndrome Association (Bayside, New York).

REFERENCES

1. Comings DE, Comings BG, Knell E. Hypothesis: homozygosity in Tourette syndrome. Am J Med Genet 1989; 34:413–421.
2. Kurlan R. Tourette's syndrome: current concepts. Neurology 1989; 39:1625–1630.

3. Shapiro AK, Shapiro ES, Young JG, Feinberg TE. Gilles de la Tourette Syndrome. 2d ed. New York: Raven Press, 1988:451–480.
4. Kurlan R, Behr J, Medved L, Shoulson 1, Pauls D, Kidd KK. Severity of Tourette's syndrome in one large kindred: implication for determination of disease prevalence rate. Arch Neurol 1987; 44:268–269.
5. Kurlan R. What is the clinical spectrum of Tourette's syndrome? Curr Opin Neurol Neurosurg 1988; 1:294–298.
6. LaRocca NO. Statistical and methodologic considerations in scale construction. In: Munsat TL, ed. Quantification of Neurologic Deficit. Boston: Butterworths, 1989:49–67.
7. Likert R. A technique for the development of attitude scales. Educ Psychol Meas 1952; 12:313–315.
8. Miller JP. Statistical considerations for quantitative techniques in clinical neurology. In: Munsat TL, ed. Quantification of Neurologic Deficit. Boston: Butterworths, 1989:69–83.
9. Fleiss JL. The Design and Analysis of Clinical Experiments. New York: Wiley, 1986.
10. Cohen J. A coefficient of agreement for nominal scales. Educ Psychol Meas 1960; 20:37–46.
11. Cohen J. Weighted kappa: nominal scale agreement with provision for scaled disagreement or partial credit. Psychol Bull 1968; 70:213–220.
12. Fleiss JL, Cohen J. The equivalence of weighted kappa and the intraclass correlation coefficient as measures of reliability. Educ Psychol Meas 1973; 33:613–619.
13. Fleiss JL. Statistical Methods for Rates and Proportions. 2d ed. New York: Wiley, 1981.
14. Landis JR, Koch GG. The measurement of observer agreement for categorical data. Biometrics 1977; 33:159–174.
15. Shrout PE. Measurement reliability and agreement in psychiatry. Stat Methods Med Res 1998; 7:301–317.
16. Snedecor GW, Cochran WG. Statistical Methods. 7th ed. Ames: Iowa State University Press, 1980.
17. Neter J, Wasserman W, Kutner MH. Applied Linear Statistical Models. 3rd ed. Boston: Irwin, 1990.
18. Donner A, Eliasziw M. Sample size requirements for reliability studies. Stat Med 1987; 6:441–448.
19. Cantor AB. Sample size calculations for Cohen's kappa. Psychol Methods 1996; 1:150–155.
20. Nunnally JC. Psychometric Theory. New York: McGraw-Hill, 1978.
21. Cureton EE, D'Agostino RB. Factor Analysis: An Applied Approach. Hillsdale, NJ: Lawrence Erlbaum Associates, 1983.
22. Andres PL, Thibodeau LM, Finison LJ, Munsat TL. Quantitative assessment of neuromuscular deficit in ALS. Neurol Clin 1987; 5:125–141.
23. Spearman C. Correlation calculated from faulty data. Br J Psychol 1910; 3:271–295.

24. Cronbach LJ. Coefficient alpha and the internal structure of tests. Psychometrika 1951; 16:297–334.
25. Guttman L. A basis for analyzing test–retest reliability. Psychometrika 1945; 10:255–282.
26. Lord FM, Novick MR. Statistical Theories of Mental Test Scores. Reading, MA: Addison-Wesley, 1968.
27. Shaffer D, Gould MS, Brasic J, Ambrosini P, Fisher P, Bird H, Aluwahlia S. A children's global assessment scale (CGAS). Arch Gen Psychiatry 1983; 40:1228–1231.
28. Goetz CG, Tanner CM, Wilson RS, Shannon KM. A rating scale for Gilles de la Tourette's syndrome: description, reliability and validity data. Neurology 1987; 37:1542–1544.
29. Campbell D, Fiske D. Convergent and discriminant validation by the multitrait–multimethod matrix. Psychol Bull 1959; 56:81–105.
30. Bollen KA. Structural Equations with Latent Variables. New York: Wiley, 1989.
31. Shapiro AK, Shapiro E. Controlled study of pimozide vs. placebo in Tourette's syndrome. J Am Acad Child Psychiatry 1984; 23:161–173.
32. Harcherik DF, Leckman JF, Detlor J, Cohen DJ. A new instrument for clinical studies of Tourette's syndrome. J Am Acad Child Psychiatry 1984; 23:153–160.
33. Leckman JF, Towbin KE, Ort SI, Cohen DJ. Clinical assessment of tic disorder severity. In: Cohen DJ, Bruun RD, Leckman JF, eds. Tourette's Syndrome and Tic Disorders. New York: Wiley, 1988:55–78.
34. Goetz CG, Tanner CM, Wilson RS, Carroll VS, Como PG, Shannon KM. Clonidine and Gilles de la Tourette's syndrome: double-blind study using objective rating methods. Ann Neurol 1987; 21:307–310.
35. Jagger J, Prusoff BA, Cohen DJ, Kidd KK, Carbonari CM, John K. The etiology of Tourette's syndrome: a pilot study. Schizophr Bull 1982; 8:267–278.
36. Stefl ME. The Ohio Tourette Study. School of Planning, University of Cincinnati, 1983.
37. Cohen DJ, Leckman JF, Shaywitz BA. The Tourette syndrome and other tics. In: Shaffer D, Ehrhardt AA, Greenwill L, eds. The Clinical Guide to Child Psychiatry. New York: Free Press, 1984:3–28.
38. Cohen DJ, Detlor J, Young G, Shaywitz BA. Clonidine ameliorates Gilles de la Tourette syndrome. Arch Gen Psychiatry 1980; 37:1350–1357.

12

Neuropsychological Function in Tourette's Syndrome

Peter G. Como
University of Rochester School of Medicine and Dentistry
Rochester, New York, U.S.A.

INTRODUCTION

Tourette's syndrome (TS) is now recognized as a common neuropsychiatric disorder with a spectrum of neurological, behavioral, and cognitive features. There has been a considerable amount of debate over the past two decades regarding whether or not TS patients demonstrate intellectual deficits, specific learning disabilities (LDs), or specific neuropsychological deficits (1). There does appear to be general consensus that specific cognitive and learning deficits are present in TS and occur in a significant percentage of patients, suggesting that early and accurate assessment of these deficits is critical. Neuropsychological and psychoeducational testing is useful for identifying these specific deficits, particularly in TS children who may be more vulnerable to poor school performance, academic failure, and delayed psychosocial development. Early educational intervention for TS patients with learning disabilities and/or specific neuropsychological impairment can improve the quality of their education and enhance academic achievement.

Despite the usefulness of neuropsychological testing for identifying specific cognitive and learning deficits in TS, studies have been hampered by numerous methodological problems. Several early studies had relatively small sample sizes and focused primarily on intelligence testing and one or two additional tasks, which, at that time, were felt to be sensitive for detecting so-called "organicity" or brain dysfunction. Other methodological shortcomings of early neuropsychological research in TS included lack of consistent of neuropsychological test measures, tendency to compare TS samples to normative data instead of age-matched and education-matched normal controls, and, perhaps most importantly, the failure to control for the presence of attention deficit hyperactivity disorder (ADHD) or obsessive–compulsive disorder (OCD), which are now well known to be comorbid behavioral conditions in TS. This is important as patients with ADHD and OCD have specific patterns of neuropsychological findings, many of which overlap with those observed in TS. There is also consistent evidence indicating that both OCD and ADHD clearly have an impact on cognitive and academic functions (2–4). In addition, many neuropsychological studies utilized subjects drawn from TS specialty or mental health clinics rather than epidemiologically ascertained samples. The latter has been problematic as clinic-referred cases tend to represent more severely impaired patient populations (1).

Recent studies have attempted to focus on identifying specific neuropsychological deficits in TS, notably visuomotor integration deficits, motor skill impairment, and executive function (EF) impairment, which are believed to parallel motor deficit (e.g., tics) and may share a common pathobiology (5).

This chapter will review studies of intellectual ability, and examine the controversy regarding the presence and types of LDs, and the patterns of specific neuropsychological impairment felt to be associated with TS.

INTELLECTUAL ABILITY

The majority of studies that assessed intellectual function in TS individuals dating back to the early studies of Shapiro et al. (6,7) indicate that the general intellectual ability of individuals with TS does not differ significantly from that observed in the general population. Moreover, individuals ascertained from epidemiological studies and diagnosed with TS demonstrated a normally distributed range of intelligence quotient (IQ) scores (8). By contrast, below-average IQ scores have been reported in some clinical samples of children diagnosed with TS (9). However, these studies failed to control for the presence of comorbid ADHD, OCD, or learning problems, all of which can substantially lower the intelligence quotient (10–12). However, when clinic samples of TS children without these comorbid conditions are examined, IQ test scores remained normally distributed (13).

Despite the general findings of normally distributed IQ scores in TS, many studies have consistently reported significant differences between verbal and nonverbal abilities in this population. Differences between verbal IQ (VIQ) and performance IQ (PIQ) scores are generally thought to have clinical utility, notably with respect to laterality of cerebral hemispheric dysfunction.

A discrepancy of 15 points or greater between the VIQ and PIQ is considered statistically significant (14), although it remains controversial whether or not this difference is clinically significant (15) as most individuals display relative strengths in one of these domains. This likely represents an older concept of lateralized hemisphere dysfunction based upon large differences in verbal and nonverbal abilities, which prevailed prior to the development of more sensitive and specific neuropsychological tests. Finding of a VIQ ≥ PIQ of 15 points may be suggestive of greater dominant hemisphere or verbal dysfunction, whereas a PIQ ≥ VIQ of 15 points might indicate nondominant hemisphere or visuospatial dysfunction.

Early studies of intellectual ability in TS, prior to the advent of detailed neuropsychological testing, yielded inconsistent results. Some studies found that TS patients as a group have lower PIQ scores suggestive of greater difficulty in visuomotor and visual–perceptual tasks (7,16). Shapiro et al. (7), in their cumulative study of 173 TS patients, found that 40% of patients had a VIQ ≥ PIQ discrepancy of 15 points or more. However, this result has not been reliably replicated in other large samples, or when TS patients with ADHD are excluded (17). In studies that excluded TS patients with ADHD, the percentage of individuals with a 15-point or greater VIQ–PIQ difference was reduced considerably to approximately 10%, which is similar to the population estimates for the Wechsler Intelligence Scale for Children, 3rd Edition (14), one of the most commonly used IQ tests. Despite these methodological shortcomings, there appears to be some agreement that a percentage of TS patients demonstrates a VIQ ≥ PIQ difference of some magnitude, suggesting that individuals with TS may indeed have greater difficulty on tasks of visuomotor speed, visuomotor integration, and perceptual function. Evidence supporting these specific cognitive deficits are reviewed in more detail below.

In summary, there does not appear to be compelling evidence to suggest that persons with TS have lowered intellectual ability and the range of IQ test scores in nonclinical samples is normally distributed. Controversy remains regarding whether TS patients have a significant discrepancy between verbal and performance IQ. This may be largely due to the failure by the majority of studies to control for the presence the common comorbid features of TS such as ADHD, OCD, a primary learning disability, or other psychiatric problems such as depression.

LEARNING DISABILITIES

A specific learning disability in an individual is present when there is a substantial statistical discrepancy between standardized scores of academic achievement and the individual IQ score. For example, a child with average intelligence (e.g., IQ score within the 90–109 range) who tests out in the severely impaired range on a standardized spelling task may likely have a specific spelling disability, or possibly a more general verbal learning disability. The most common type of LD in the general population is a reading disability (18).

A variety of learning disabilities have been described in clinical samples of TS patients; however, the lack of control for TS-related and other psychiatric comorbidities (e.g., ADHD, OCD, depression, conduct disorder, etc.) has made it difficult to identify the learning problems specifically associated with TS (5). There are no long-term outcome studies of the learning patterns in persons with TS. Evidence for specific learning disabilities in TS, based upon stringent diagnostic criteria, have yielded inconsistent findings. Prominent learning and school problems in persons with TS are often highly correlated with the presence of ADHD and not necessarily related to TS itself. In two separate epidemiological studies (19,20), the prevalence of definite or probable tics in students enrolled in full-time special education was considerably higher than the prevalence of tics in students in regular classes. Although these studies demonstrated a higher-than-expected rate of special education placement among children with TS or tics, the reasons for special education placement remain unclear. The reasons for poor school performance in some children with TS may be related to an LD, or it could be a manifestation of behavioral and emotional difficulties, ADHD, or other neuropsychological dysfunction for which children with TS are at increased risk (21–24).

Estimates of the true frequency of learning disabilities in TS have also been hampered by methodological problems, most notably the use of survey and retrospective chart review. Nonetheless, both Erenberg et al. (25) and Abwender et al. (26) found the incidence of learning disabilities to be about 22% in TS children and adolescents. However, neither of these studies specified the nature of the LD. Consistent with previous reports, ADHD but not OCD was a significant predictor of school problems. Children with TS plus ADHD had an almost fourfold increased risk for academic difficulty, compared to those children with TS alone.

Smaller studies of LD in TS that utilized more accurate and stringent diagnostic criteria for LDs (e.g., discrepancy between standardized achievement testing and IQ test score) have provided some clues regarding the prevalence and type of LDs in TS. Hagin et al. (27) observed difficulties with math and written language in a small sample of 10 TS children. Other studies using less stringent diagnostic criteria have reported similar academic deficiencies, notably in arithmetic, reading, spelling, and handwriting (16,28–30). Several other studies using achievement tests of reading, math, and spelling have consistently reported a higher prevalence of deficiency in mathematics in TS children and adolescents (16,31,32). Although these studies found consistent weakness in arithmetic skills relative to other academic abilities, they did not specifically assess for the presence of true LDs using the more rigid diagnostic criteria. Burd et al. (33) assessed the frequency and type of LD in their review of the records of 42 children with TS between the ages of 7 and 18 years using a 1.5 standard deviation (SD) discrepancy score between IQ and achievement testing to indicate the presence of a LD. They reported that 51% of their sample met criteria for a specific LD. Similar to other studies, a math LD was the most common, followed by spelling and reading disabilities. The authors acknowledged that a major limitation of their findings was an ascertainment bias in that their TS clinic focuses on more severely impaired patients. Schuerholz et al. (34) recruited 65 children with TS between the ages of 6 and 14 years for a series of studies on the pathobiology of learning disabilities. Using standardized tests of psychoeducational achievement and a regression-based discrepancy formula of 1.5 SD, they reported an overall frequency of any LD in TS of 23%, consistent with the data reported by Abwender et al. (26) and Erenberg et al. (25), which relied exclusively upon retrospective chart review and survey findings, respectively. Of interest, LDs were only present in TS children diagnosed with comorbid ADHD. The most common LDs in their sample were math and written language, consistent with previous studies. Although these findings appear to suggest a higher-than-expected prevalence of learning disabilities in TS, these estimates are actually similar to the reported population base rates of LDs, estimated at between 15% and 20% (18,35), suggesting that the presence of a specific learning disability in TS is not higher than would be expected in the general population. Schultz et al. (5) evaluated the likelihood of a reading, spelling, or math LD in TS in a case-by-case manner, using both an absolute cutoff of a standard score and the usual 1.5 SD discrepancy definition. A lower range (e.g., 4–16%) of the TS sample met at least one criterion for a specific LD and these individuals had similar types of LDs reported in previous studies. The results of this study, using a more refined technique for designating the presence of LD, suggest that prevalence of LD in TS may actually be lower than originally reported.

In summary, the accumulated literature on LDs in TS suggests that there is an increased risk for school-related problems, but the nature of these problems is clearly multifactorial. The presence of ADHD appears to be the primary factor contributing to learning problems or academic failure in school-age children with TS. The exact prevalence of learning disabilities in TS remains unclear; however, by using very strict diagnostic criteria and standardized tests of academic achievement, the prevalence of LDs in TS may be as high as 20%–25%, although evidence exists that this may reflect an overestimate (5). Moreover, the prevalence of LDs in TS appears similar to the population base rates of LDs, with the primary difference being the type of learning disability observed. Deficiencies in arithmetic and written language skills appear to be the more common type of learning problem in TS compared to reading disabilities, which are more prevalent in the general population. Reliable estimates of the prevalence of these specific LDs in TS must await more rigorously controlled studies that include epidemiologically ascertained samples that use stringent criteria for making the diagnosis of a learning disability.

NEUROPSYCHOLOGICAL DEFICITS

Neuropsychological studies of TS date back to the early 1970s and typically consisted of single case reports or studies with very small sample sizes. The use of more comprehensive neuropsychological test batteries, which often take several to administer and assess a broad array of cognitive functions, has yielded somewhat inconsistent results in TS patient samples. Similar to studies of intellectual ability and learning disabilities, many of these neuropsychological studies failed to control for the presence of comorbid ADHD and OCD in their study design. In addition, these studies also failed to control for the presence of waxing and waning tics, which can potentially interfere with fine motor tasks or timed tasks. However, the failure to control for either ADHD or OCD may actually be less serious given that individuals with either of these behavioral conditions demonstrate patterns of neuropsychological test performance that are similar in many aspects to that observed in controlled studies of TS. This overlapping pattern of neuropsychological deficits among ADHD, OCD, and TS suggests the possibility of common neurobiological substrates (i.e., fronto-striatal circuitry) in the pathogenesis of cognitive dysfunction among these neurobehavioral disorders (36–41).

Despite the methodological limitations of many neuropsychological studies, specific cognitive deficits have been consistently reported in a variety of child and adolescent TS populations. In general, the accumulated neuropsychological literature suggests that the most commonly observed deficits occur on tasks of copying simple and complex geometric designs (often referred to as visuomotor integration ability), tasks of fine motor skill, tasks of visuospatial and visuoperceptual ability, and impairment of so-called EF. EF covers a broad domain of cognitive abilities and behavioral functions, including mental tracking, sustained attention, working memory, planning and organization, goal-directed behavior, cognitive flexibility (e.g., problem solving, set maintenance), and impulse control and self-regulation. EF has been suggested to be largely associated with frontal lobe function and its extensive connections to basal ganglia structures (42).

Visuomotor Integration Ability

The recent excellent review of neuropsychological function in TS by Schultz et al. (5) summarizes the visuomotor integration deficits in TS. In their comprehensive review, 10 of 12 studies of visuomotor integration ability comprising 308 TS patients with a mean age of approximately 10 years found evidence of either a group deficit based upon comparison to normative data, or group differences when normal controls were used. The most common tasks of visuomotor integration included copying tasks of simple and complex geometric designs. The TS samples performed about 1 SD below age norms despite evidence of average intellectual ability. A more difficult copying test, the Rey Complex Figure (RCF), was used in five studies. Whereas copying of simple geometric figures relies primarily on the integration of visuoperceptual and fine motor skills, performance on the RCF also assesses EF, notably planning and organization skills. Unfortunately, with the exception of three studies, the presence of ADHD was not controlled for. In two of the three studies that divided TS samples based upon the presence of ADHD, the TS sample without comorbid ADHD scored significantly higher on the RCF (indicative of better performance) than those with TS plus ADHD (34,43), suggesting that either EF impairment or ADHD may be contributing, in part, to the visuomotor integration deficit characteristic of TS. However, the study by Schultz et al. (21) found no differences on the RCF between TS patients with and without ADHD despite using several different scoring systems, raising some doubts regarding the role of EF in the visuomotor integration deficits observed in TS. Thus, it is possible that ADHD, a condition strongly associated with deficits in EF, may better account for the visuomotor integration deficit in TS.

In summary, there appears to be consistent evidence for a deficit of about 1 SD below age norm in simple visuomotor integration ability in TS. There is inconsistent evidence of copying deficits in TS populations when the EF demands are high. Unfortunately, this deficit has also been consistently observed in children with primary ADHD (44,45), suggesting that it might be the ADHD component and not TS per se that is responsible for the observed deficits in visuomotor integration.

Fine Motor Skill

The literature on deficits in fine motor coordination in TS is equally compelling. However, the magnitude of the deficit may be less pronounced and appears to range from 0.5 to 1.0 SD below age norms (5). A major limiting factor of studies of fine motor skill in TS is the trend to compare results from specific TS samples to normative data rather than age-matched and sex-matched normal control samples, thus limiting the validity of the findings. Nevertheless, studies to date have found consistent evidence of motor skill weakness in TS. The largest series of studies to date has been completed by Yeates and Bornstein (12) and Bornstein (13,17), who studied over 160 TS patients on several tasks of gross motor and fine motor skills. A subset of these patients was also selected based upon the presence of ADHD. Their findings suggest that tasks of simple motor speed without visual–perceptual demands are unimpaired in TS patients. In contrast, performance on tasks of fine motor skill highly dependent on visual–perceptual skills (e.g., placing pegs into grooves of differing angles) appears consistently impaired in TS patient samples and is present regardless of the presence of comorbid ADHD. These authors concluded that the motor skill deficits observed in TS appear to occur at a higher cortical level involving more complex visuomotor coordination of movement in space. No motor tics were observed during completion of the motor tasks in the studies by Yeates and Bornstein (12) and Schultz et al. (21), suggesting that the lowered scores may represent a true impairment of motor skill and are not due to the presence of motor tics. This finding is consistent with the reported observation of greater handwriting difficulties in TS children who typically do not have motor tics of the hands or fingers (27,30).

Spatial/Perceptual Ability

The literature on spatial/perceptual deficits in TS is less extensive and has yielded inconsistent results. The methodological limitations noted previously are perhaps even more compelling, notably due to the varied and numerous tests available for testing spatial and perceptual function. The utility of comparing verbal vs. performance IQ test scores to specifically identify spatial/perceptual deficits in TS is not clinically useful as previously discussed and awaits confirmation by more rigorously controlled studies.

Brookshire et al. (46) and Schultz et al. (21) tested a component process model of visuomotor integration deficits in TS children, which included measures of visuomotor integration ability, motor skill, and spatial/perceptual ability. Both studies reported significant correlations among tasks of spatial/perceptual ability, fine motor skill, and response inhibition (presumed to be a domain of EF), suggestive of weaknesses in all of these areas in TS children, irrespective of their ADHD status. However, none of the measures employed to assess these three component processes could fully account for the deficits in visuomotor integration, suggesting a primary difficulty with the integration of both visuoperceptual and motor functions but not pure spatial/perceptual ability in TS (21). A recent study by Sheppard et al. (47) utilized a computerized line bisection task in which subjects were required to bisect horizontal lines with or without a moving background array. The sample consisted of nine TS patients and nine control subjects matched for age, sex, education, and IQ. The TS subjects were shown to be right-biased in judging the midpoint of horizontal lines, similar to that reported in unmedicated ADHD patients (48). Functional asymmetries in tasks such as line bisection are generally indicative of a functional asymmetry in the regions of the brain that are important in attentional orienting. Thus, unilateral right hemisphere dysfunction would result in a consistent rightward bias in the line bisection task. These authors suggest a lateralized (right hemisphere) fronto-striatal deficit of visuospatial attention in children with TS consistent with recent neuroimaging studies in TS.

Executive Function

Executive function covers a broad domain of cognitive and behavioral functions, including mental tracking, sustained attention, working memory, planning and organization, goal-directed behavior, cognitive flexibility (e.g., problem solving, set maintenance), and impulse control and self-regulation. EF has been linked to the frontal cortex and its extensive connections to basal ganglia structures, which suggests that EF has a shared pathophysiology with TS (42). Frontal systems have long been viewed as exerting largely an inhibitory influence. Thus, impairment of frontal cortex creates a loss of inhibitory control of motor action, cognitive processing, and behavioral control, similar to the motor deficit reported in TS. The motor deficit in TS is defined by an irritability to inhibit the urge to move and vocalize, thereby resulting in the classic motion and vocal tics. Therefore, it is reasonable to hypothesize that TS patients would have significant impairment on tasks of EF. Unfortunately, EF deficits are also commonly observed in several other neurological conditions, including ADHD (49), OCD (50,51), and most basal ganglia disorders such as Parkinson's disease and Huntington's disease. Thus, EF impairment does not appear unique to TS and may be present in a variety of neurological disorders in which impairment of fronto-striatal circuitry is involved.

Compared to visuomotor integration ability and motor skill, the literature on EF impairment in TS remains equivocal. Although studies have reported EF deficits on selected cognitive tasks, no consistent measure of EF has emerged as consistently impaired in TS patient populations. This is not surprising given the broad domain of cognitive and behavioral functions believed to be associated with EF. A number of studies of adult and child TS samples incorporating EF measures have emerged within the past decade. The results vary by type of study and measure employed. Many studies have used tests of mental flexibility such as the Wisconsin Card Sorting Test, which require subjects to sort cards according to certain rules (e.g., color, shape, and number); tests of mental tracking and sequencing such as the Trailmaking

Test, which require numeric and then alternating alphanumeric sequencing; tasks of verbal and nonverbal fluency; and a variety of tasks that assess cognitive flexibility, set-shifting, reaction time, and response inhibition. Some EF tasks such as the Trailmaking Test and various computerized reaction time tasks are also dependent upon visuomotor integration ability, which may more accurately account for the EF deficits reported to occur in TS patients.

Of the more commonly employed measures of EF, a consistent finding has emerged on measures of response time, which arguably may rely more heavily on motor skill than purely measuring EF (5). Nonetheless, three studies have investigated response time parameters using a computerized continuous performance task (CPT) in which subjects must respond based upon a predetermined response set that can be simple (e.g., pressing a key for any letter except a designated letter) or complex (e.g., pressing one of four keys based upon where a target appears in a visual field). Both children and adults with TS respond more slowly than expected on the CPT, suggesting difficulties with sustained attention (43,52,53). The study by Harris et al. (43) found that TS subjects, regardless of comorbid ADHD status, showed significantly increased response time variability compared to test-normative data, suggesting that this type of EF deficit is independent of the presence of ADHD and possibly more characteristic of TS. However, Veal et al. (54) did not control for the presence of OCD—a condition whose time and mental speed during EF tasks are also impaired.

More recently, Mahone et al. (55) examined EF in fluency and recall measures among children with TS or ADHD and normal controls. This study assessed two relevant aspects of EF. Clustering of responses on measures of verbal fluency, figural fluency, and verbal learning was examined to assess strategic response organization, and rule breaks, intrusions, and repetition errors were recorded to assess inhibition errors. Interestingly, no significant differences were found among the three groups on tasks of response organization. However, there was a significant group difference on one of the disinhibition variables, with both TS and ADHD groups showing significantly more intrusions on verbal list learning trials. Overall, both the ADHD and TS groups were largely free of EF impairment. Thus, children with uncomplicated TS (e.g., no evidence of behavioral comorbidity) may not have significant EF deficits. These results were essentially replicated in a small study by Brand et al. (56), which employed three common measures of EF (Trailmaking Test, Stroop Interference Test, and a measure of verbal fluency) in children with TS alone and TS plus ADHD. Similar to the results of Shucard et al. (53), no significant differences were found between the TS and TS plus ADHD groups on the neuropsychological tasks of EF, with the exception of verbal fluency in which the TS plus ADHD group performed significantly worse. These authors further conducted stepwise regression analyses to determine the predictors of psychosocial dysfunction and found that tic symptom severity and the presence of ADHD, but not EF impairment, were predictive of worse psychosocial functioning.

SUMMARY

The accumulated body of scientific evidence regarding intellectual ability, presence of learning disorders, and specific neuropsychological deficits in TS suggests that difficulties in these areas are present in a significant percentage of patients. Despite the numerous methodological shortcomings of past neuropsychological studies of TS, relatively robust and consistent finding have emerged. The literature to date has suggested that intellectual ability is normally distributed in TS. Whether or not individuals with TS have significant discrepancies between their verbal and nonverbal abilities remains unclear, although there does appear to be some consensus that individuals with TS may indeed have relatively lower performance IQ scores, suggesting the possibility of greater nondominant hemispheric dysfunction. The prevalence of learning disabilities in TS appears to be quite similar to the base rates reported for the general population. There is evidence to suggest that the prevalence of LDs in TS may actually be lower than the general population when strict diagnostic criteria are applied. When learning disabilities are present in TS patients, they tend to be specific for difficulties in math and written language. Specific neuropsychological deficits in TS have been consistently reported to include visuomotor integration problems, impaired fine motor skill, and executive dysfunction, although recent studies have suggested that the presence of ADHD may more accurately explain EF in TS.

The presence of comorbid behavioral conditions, notably ADHD and OCD, appears to significantly increase the likelihood that an individual with TS will also have intellectual deficits, a learning disability, or some demonstrable cognitive impairment.

When present, either a learning disability and/or a specific neuropsychological deficit may pose a greater obstacle for individuals with TS than the tic disorder itself. This is particularly salient for children with TS who maybe at a higher risk for poor school performance and academic failure. The psychosocial impact of these problems is also far-reaching. Given the recent emphasis on the early detection of academic and learning problems, it would seem prudent that children with TS suspected of having intellectual, academic, or neuropsychological difficulties be evaluated as soon as possible. There are numerous educational interventions and accommodations available to children with learning disabilities and/or specific academic weaknesses that work equally well for children with TS with similar types of problems. Many children with TS require either informal educational accommodations or meet formal requirements to receive special education placement and individualized educational plans.

The available body of scientific evidence that persons with TS have normally distributed intellectual ability would suggest a diminished role for routine IQ testing, unless there is compelling clinical evidence to suggest that the individual may have a learning disability or specific academic weakness. Given that children with TS may be particularly at risk for learning disabilities or academic deficiencies in math and written language, a complete psychoeducational work-up should be conducted for any TS child suspected of having such difficulties. This evaluation should be conducted as early as possible so that educational interventions can be implemented. Traditionally, the psychoeducational evaluation is performed by the school psychologist and should include standardized IQ assessment and academic achievement testing, which can objectively identify and quantify the nature and severity of the learning problem and recommend appropriate educational and remedial interventions.

Neuropsychological testing is indicated to identify specific cognitive deficits that might be present in TS, notably problems with visuomotor integration, motor skill, and executive function. The evaluation performed by the school psychologist typically does not assess these cognitive functions. Therefore, referral for neuropsychological testing is indicated if there is a strong clinical suspicion of cognitive deficits. However, the accumulated neuropsychological literature in TS suggests that a broad-based, comprehensive, and lengthy neuropsychological examination is not necessary. At a minimum, the neuropsychological test battery should include assessment of visuomotor integration ability, motor skills, spatial/perceptual abilities, and executive function. This type of assessment would take less time to complete, is less costly, and likely has greater sensitivity and specificity for identifying neurocognitive deficits associated with TS.

Neuropsychological functioning continues to be an important component in understanding the full neurobehavioral spectrum of TS. At present, there is great opportunity to explore neuropsychological functioning in TS with newly emerging technology such as functional magnetic resonance imaging (fMRI), positron emission tomography (PET), and related techniques, which assess cortical metabolic activity, as well as newer electrophysiological techniques. This technology, notably fMRI, allows investigation of neuropsychological functioning in vivo and may shed important clues about the neuroanatomical substrates of neuropsychological impairment and learning disabilities in TS.

REFERENCES

1. Como PG. Neuropsychological function in Tourette's syndrome. In: Cohen DJ, Jankovic J, Goetz C, eds. Advances in Neurology Tourette's Syndrome. Vol. 85. New York: Lippincott, Williams and Wilkens, 2001:103–111.
2. Robertson MM, Yakely JW. Obsessive–compulsive disorder and self-injurious behavior. In: Kurlan R, ed. Handbook of Tourette's Syndrome and Related Tic and Behavioral Disorders. New York: Marcel Dekker, 1993:45–87.
3. Towbin KE, Riddle MA. Attention deficit hyperactivity disorder. In: Kurlan R, ed. Handbook of Tourette's Syndrome and Related Tic and Behavioral Disorders. New York: Marcel Dekker, 1993:89–110.
4. Walkup JT, Khan S, Schuerholz L, Young-Suk P, Leckman JT, Schultz RT. Phenomenology and natural history of tic-related ADHD and learning disabilities. In: Leckman JF, Cohen DJ, eds. Tourette's Syndrome—Tics, Obsessions, Compulsion: Developmental Psychopathology and Clinical Care. New York: John Wiley and Sons, 1999:63–79.
5. Schultz RT, Carter AS, Scahill L, Leckman JF. Neuropsychological findings. In: Leckman JF, Cohen DJ, eds. Tourette's Syndrome—Tics, Obsessions, Compulsion: Developmental Psychopathology and Clinical Care. New York: John Wiley and Sons, 1999:80–103.
6. Shapiro AK, Shapiro E, Bruun R, Sweet RD. Gilles de la Tourette's Syndrome. New York: Raven Press, 1978.
7. Shapiro AK, Shapiro E, Young JG, Feinberg TE. Gilles de la Tourette's Syndrome. 2d ed. New York: Raven Press, 1978.
8. Apter A, Pauls DL, Bleich A, Zohar AH, Kron S, Ratzoni G, Dycian A, et al. An epidemiological study of Gilles de la Tourette's syndrome in Israel. Arch Gen Psychiatry 1993; 50:734–738.
9. Parraga HC, McDonald HG. Etiology of Tourette's disorder. J Am Acad Child Adolesc Psychiatry 1996; 35:2–3.
10. Sutherland RJ, Kolb B, Schoel WM, Whishaw IQ, Davies D. Neuropsychological assessment of children and adults with Tourette syndrome: a comparison with learning disabilities and schizophrenia. In: Friedhoff AJ, Chase TN, eds. Gilles de la Tourette Syndrome. Advances in Neurology. Vol. 35. New York: Raven Press, 1982:311–321.
11. Dykens E, Leckman J, Riddle M, et al. Intellectual, academic, and adaptive functioning of Tourette syndrome children with and without attention deficit disorder. J Abnorm Child Psychol 1990; 18:607–615.
12. Yeates KO, Bornstein RA. Attention deficit disorder and neuropsychological functioning in children with Tourette's syndrome. Neuropsychology 1994; 8:65–74.
13. Bornstein RA. Neuropsychological correlates of obsessive characteristics in Tourette syndrome. J Neuropsychiatr Clin Neurosci 1991; 3:157–162.

14. Wechsler D. Wechsler Intelligence Scale for Children. 3rd ed. San Antonio: The Psychological Corporation, 1991.
15. Lezak MD. Neuropsychological assessment. 3rd ed. New York: Oxford University Press, 1995.
16. Incagnoli T, Kane R. Neuropsychological functioning in Gilles de la Tourette's syndrome. J Clin Neuropsychol 1981; 3:165–171.
17. Bornstein RA. Neuropsychological performance in children with Tourette syndrome. Psychiatry Res 1990; 33:73–81.
18. Pennington BF. Diagnosing Learning Disorders. New York: Guildford Press, 1991.
19. Comings DE, Himes JA, Comings BG. An epidemiological study of Tourette's syndrome in a single school district. J Clin Psychiatry 1990; 51:463–469.
20. Kurlan R, McDermott MP, Deeley C, Como PG, Brower C, Eapen S, Andresen EM, Miller B. Prevalence of tics in schoolchildren and association with placement in special education. Neurology 2000; 57:1383–1388.
21. Schultz RT, Carter AS, Gladstone M, Scahill L, Leckman JF, Peterson BS, Zhang H, et al. Visual–motor integration functioning in children with Tourette syndrome. Neuropsychology 1998; 12:134–145.
22. Singer HS, Rosenberg LA. Development of behavioral and emotional problems in Tourette's syndrome. Pediatr Neurol 1989; 5:41–44.
23. Walkup JT, Rosenberg LA, Brown J, Singer HS. The validity of instruments measuring tic severity in Tourette's syndrome. J Am Acad Child Adolesc Psychiatry 1992; 31:472–477.
24. Walkup JT, Scahill L, Riddle MA. Disruptive behavior, hyperactivity, and learning disabilities in children with Tourette's syndrome. Adv Neurol 1995; 65:259–272.
25. Erenberg G, Cruse RP, Rothner AD. Tourette's syndrome. Clevel Clin Q 1986; 53:127–131.
26. Abwender DA, Como PG, Kurlan R, Parry K, Fett K, Cui AL, Plumb S, et al. School problems in Tourette's syndrome. Arch Neurol 1996; 53:509–511.
27. Hagin RA, Beecher R, Pagano G, Kreeger H. Effects of Tourette syndrome on learning. In: Friedhoff AJ, Chase TN, eds. Gilles de la Tourette Syndrome. Advances in Neurology. Vol. 35. New York: Raven Press, 1982:323–328.
28. Incagnoli T, Kane R. Developmental perspective of the Gilles de la Tourette's syndrome. Percept Mot Skills 1983; 57:1271–1281.
29. Matthews WS. Attention deficits and learning disabilities in children with Tourette's syndrome. Psychiatr Ann 1988; 18:414–416.
30. Silver AA, Hagin RA. Gilles de la Tourette syndrome. Learning Disorders in Childhood. New York: John Wiley and Sons, 1990:470–492.
31. Bornstein RA, Carroll A, King G. Relationship of age to neuropsychology deficit in Tourette syndrome. J Dev Behav Pediatr 1985; 6:284–286.
32. Golden GS. Psychologic and neuropsychologic aspects of Tourette's syndrome. Neurol Clin 1984; 2:91–102.
33. Burd L, Kauffman DW, Kerbeshian J. Tourette syndrome and learning disabilities. J Learn Disabil 1992; 25:598–604.

34. Schuerholz LJ, Baumgardner TL, Singer HS, Reiss AL, Denckla MB. Neuropsychological status of children with Tourette's syndrome with and without attention deficit hyperactivity disorder. Neurology 1996; 46:958–965.
35. Berger M, Yule W, Rutter M. Attainment and adjustment in two geographical areas: I. The prevalence of specific learning disabilities. Br J Psychiatry 1975; 126:510–526.
36. Satterfield JH, Dawson ME. Electrodermal correlates of hyperactive children. Psychophysiology 1971; 8:191–197.
37. Zametkin AJ, Rapoport JL. Neurobiology of attention deficit disorder and hyperactivity: where have we come in 50 years? J Am Acad Child Adolesc Psychiatry 1987; 26:676–686.
38. Zametkin AJ, Nordahi TE, Gross M, King C, Semple WE, Rumsey J, Hamburger S, Cohen RM. Cerebral glucose metabolism in adults with hyperactivity of childhood onset. N Engl J Med 1990; 232:1361–1366.
39. Ernst M, Liebenauer L, King A, Fitzgerald G, Cohen R, Zametkin AJ. Reduced brain metabolism in hyperactive girls. J Am Acad Child Adolesc Psychiatry 1994; 33:858–868.
40. Lombroso P, Leckman J. The neurobiology of Tourette's syndrome and tic-related disorders in children. In: Charney DS, Nestler EJ, Bunney BS, eds. Neurobiology of Mental Illness. New York: Oxford University Press, 1999:779–787.
41. McDougle CJ. The neurobiology and treatment of obsessive–compulsive disorder. In: Charney DS, Nestler EJ, Bunney BS, eds. Neurobiology of Mental Illness. New York: Oxford University Press, 1999:518–533.
42. Denckla MB, Reader MJ. Education and psychosocial interventions: executive dysfunction and its consequences. In: Kurlan R, ed. Handbook of Tourette's Syndrome and Related Tic and Behavioral Disorders. New York: Marcel Dekker, 1993:431–451.
43. Harris EL, Schuerholz LJ, Singer HS, Reader MJ, Brown JE, Cox C, Mohr J, et al. Executive function in children with Tourette syndrome and/or attention deficit hyperactivity disorder. J Int Neuropsychol Soc 1995; 1:511–516.
44. Campbell SB, Werry JS. Attention deficit disorder (hyperactivity). In: Quay HC, Werry JS, eds. Psychopathological Disorders of Childhood. 3rd ed. New York: Wiley, 1986:111–155.
45. Frost LA, Moffit TE, McGee R. Neuropsychological correlates of psychopathology in an unselected cohort of young adolescents. J Abnorm Psychol 1989; 98:307–313.
46. Brookshire BL, Butler IJ, Ewing-Cobbs L, Fletcher JM. Neuropsychological characteristics of children with Tourette Syndrome: evidence for a nonverbal learning disability. J Clin Exp Neuropsychol 1994; 16:289–302.
47. Sheppard DM, Bradshaw JL, Mattingly JB. Abnormal line bisection judgements in children with Tourette's syndrome. Neuropsychologia 2002; 40:253–259.
48. Sheppard DM, Bradshaw JL, Mattingly JB, Lee P. Effects of stimulant medication on the lateralization of line bisection judgements of ADHD children. J Neurol Neurosurg Psychiatry 1999; 66:57–63.

49. Barkley RA, Grodzinsky G, DuPaul GJ. Frontal lobe functions in attention deficit disorder with and without hyperactivity: a review and research report. J Abnorm Child Psychol 1992; 20:163–188.
50. Hollander E, Wong CM. The relationship between executive impairment and serotonergic sensitivity in obsessive compulsive disorder. Neuropsychiatry Neuropsychol Behav Neurol 1996; 9:230–233.
51. Rosenberg DR, Dick EL, Ohearn KM, Sweeney JA. Response inhibition deficits in obsessive compulsive disorder—an indicator of dysfunction of frontostriatal circuits. J Psychiatr Neurosci 1997; 22:29–38.
52. Silverstein SM, Como PG, Palumbo DR, West LL, Osborn LM. Multiple sources of attentional dysfunction in adults with Tourette's syndrome: comparison with attention deficit-hyperactivity disorder. Neuropsychology 1995; 9:157–164.
53. Shucard DW, Benedict RH, Tekok-Kilic A, Lichter DG. Slowed reaction time during a continuous performance test in children with Tourette's syndrome. Neuropsychology 1997; 11:147–155.
54. Veal DM, Sahakian BJ, Owen AM, Marks IM. Specific cognitive deficits in tests sensitive to frontal lobe dysfunction in obsessive compulsive disorder. Psychol Med 1996; 26:1261–1269.
55. Mahone EM, Koth CW, Cutting L, Singer HS, Denckla MB. Executive function in fluency and recall measures among children with Tourette's syndrome or ADHD. J Int Neuropsychol Soc 2001; 7:102–111.
56. Brand N, Geenee R, Oudenhoven M, Lindenborn B, van der Ree A, Cohen-Kettenis P, Buitelar JK. Brief report: cognitive functioning in children with Tourette's syndrome with and without comorbid ADHD. J Pediatr Psychol 2002; 27:203–208.

13

Basal Ganglia Circuits and Thalamocortical Outputs

Jonathan W. Mink
University of Rochester School of Medicine and Dentistry
Rochester, New York, U.S.A.

The basal ganglia have all the aspects of a "clearing house" that accumulates samples of ongoing projected activity and, on a competitive basis, can facilitate any one and suppress all others.

—Denny-Brown and Yanagisawa (1976) (1)

We propose that this circuit is organized anatomically and neurochemically so that the striatum can select and maintain motor behaviors .... Furthermore, the basal ganglia function to suppress other conflicting activities while reinforcing ongoing behaviors.

—Penney and Young (1983) (2)

INTRODUCTION

The basal ganglia are large subcortical structures comprising several interconnected nuclei in the forebrain, diencephalon, and midbrain. Historically, the basal ganglia have been viewed as a component of the motor system. However, there is now substantial evidence that the basal ganglia interact with all of the frontal cortex and with the limbic system. Thus, the basal ganglia have a role in cognitive and emotional function in addition to their role in motor control. Indeed, diseases of the basal ganglia often cause a combination of movement, affective, and cognitive disorders. The same may be said of Tourette's syndrome (TS), in which there is often a combination of motor, affective, and cognitive dysfunction. The fundamental pathophysiology of TS is not known, but there is now general agreement that it probably involved dysfunction of basal ganglia and frontal cortical circuits (3,4).

A popular model of basal ganglia functional anatomy in movement disorders suggests that involuntary movements, including tics, are associated with decreased inhibitory output from the basal ganglia with resulting excessive activity in frontal cortical areas (5,6). This model has also been invoked to provide a theoretical anatomic framework for understanding obsessive–compulsive disorder, depression, and other psychiatric disorders. The model has been modified more recently in light of additional anatomical and physiological data to provide a more general model of basal ganglia function and dysfunction (7–9). According to this model, the basal ganglia act to facilitate desired behaviors and inhibit potentially competing or unwanted behaviors to prevent them from interfering with the desired behavior. The anatomy and physiology underlying this model are described in this chapter. Recent advances have made it possible to suggest how specific neural mechanisms may relate to specific clinical manifestations of TS. The three major groups of symptoms associated with TS (tics, obsessive–compulsive behaviors, and attention-deficit/hyperactivity disorder) have impaired inhibition of unwanted behaviors as a common feature. The chapter concludes with a discussion of possible specific pathophysiologic mechanisms underlying these behaviors.

BASAL GANGLIA CIRCUITRY

The basal ganglia include the striatum (caudate, putamen, nucleus accumbens), the subthalamic nucleus (STN), the globus pallidus (internal segment [GPi], external segment [GPe], ventral pallidum [VP]), and the substantia nigra (pars compacta [SNpc] and pars reticulata [SNpr]) (Fig. 1). The striatum and subthalamic nucleus receive the majority of inputs from outside of the basal ganglia. Most of those inputs come from the cerebral cortex, but thalamic nuclei also provide strong inputs to the striatum. The bulk of the outputs from the basal ganglia arise from the globus pallidus internal segment, ventral pallidum, and substantia nigra pars reticulata. These outputs are inhibitory to thalamic nuclei that in turn project to the frontal lobe.

The striatum receives the bulk of extrinsic input to the basal ganglia. The striatum receives excitatory input from virtually all of the cerebral cortex

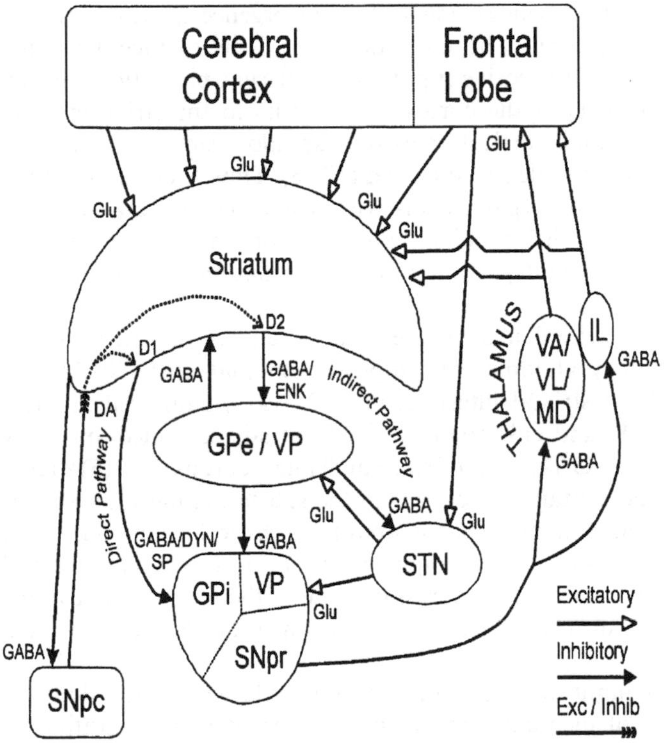

Figure 1 Simplified schematic diagram of basal ganglia–thalamocortical circuitry. Excitatory connections are indicated by open arrows, inhibitory connections by filled arrows. The modulatory dopamine projection is indicated by a three-headed arrow. Brainstem projections are not shown. dyn = dynorphin; enk = enkephalin; GABA = gamma-aminobutyric acid; glu = glutamate; GPe = globus pallidus pars externa; GPi = globus pallidus pars interna; IL = intralaminar thalamic nuclei; MD = mediodorsal nucleus; SNpc = substantia nigra pars compacta; SNpr = substantia nigra pars reticulata; SP = substance P; STN = subthalamic nucleus; VA = ventral anterior nucleus; VL = ventral lateral nucleus; VP = ventral pallidum.

(10). In addition, the ventral striatum (nucleus accumbens and rostroventral extensions of caudate and putamen) receive inputs from the hippocampus and amygdala (11,12). The cortical input uses glutamate as its neurotransmitter and terminates largely on the heads of the dendritic spines of medium spiny neurons (13,14). The projection from the cerebral cortex to striatum has a roughly topographic organization. It has been suggested that this topography provides the basis for a segregation of functionally different circuits in the basal ganglia (15). Although the topography implies a certain degree of parallel organization, there is also evidence for convergence and divergence in the corticostriatal projection. The large dendritic fields of medium spiny neurons (16) allow them to receive input from adjacent projections, which arise from different areas of the cortex (17). Inputs to the striatum from several functionally related cortical areas overlap and a single cortical area projects divergently to multiple striatal zones (17,18). Thus, there is a multiply convergent and divergent organization within a broader framework of functionally different parallel circuits. This organization provides an anatomical framework for the integration and transformation of cortical information in the striatum (19).

Medium spiny striatal neurons receive a number of other inputs, including (1) excitatory glutamatergic inputs from thalamus (20–22); (2) cholinergic input from striatal interneurons (23); (3) γ-aminobutyric acid (GABA), substance P, and enkephalin input from adjacent medium spiny striatal neurons (24); (4) GABA input from small interneurons (25); (5) a large input from dopamine-containing neurons in the substantia nigra pars compacta (SNpc) (26); and (6) a more sparse input from the serotonin-containing neurons in the dorsal and median raphe nuclei (27). The dopamine and serotonin inputs are of particular interest because of the role of medications that influence these neurotransmitters in the treatment of TS and associated symptoms.

The dopamine input to the striatum terminates largely on the shafts of the dendritic spines of medium spiny neurons where it is in a position to modulate transmission from the cerebral cortex to the striatum (14). The action of dopamine on striatal neurons depends on the type of dopamine receptor involved. Five types of G-protein-coupled dopamine receptors have been described (D1–D5) (28). These have been grouped into two families based on their linkage to adenylcyclase activity and response to agonists. The D1 family includes D1 and D5 receptors and the D2 family includes D2, D3, and D4 receptors. D1 receptors are thought to stimulate adenyl cyclase activity and may potentiate the effect of cortical input to striatal neurons, while D2 receptors are thought to inhibit adenyl cyclase activity and may decrease the effect of cortical input to striatal neurons (29). More recent data indicate that the effect of dopamine on striatal medium spiny neurons is dependent on the membrane potential of the target neurons (30). The role of dopamine in learning and reward will be discussed in further detail below.

Medium spiny striatal neurons contain the inhibitory neurotransmitter GABA (31) and are inhibitory to their targets. In addition, they have peptide neurotransmitters that are colocalized with GABA (24,32). Based on the type of neurotransmitters and the predominant type of dopamine receptor they contain, the medium spiny neurons can be divided into two populations. One population contains GABA, dynorphin, and substance P and primarily expresses D1 dopamine receptors. These neurons project to the basal ganglia output nuclei, GPi, VP, and SNpr (5,33,34). The second population contains GABA and enkephalin and primarily expresses D2 dopamine receptors. These neurons project to the external segment of the globus pallidus (GPe) (5,33,34).

Although there are no apparent regional differences in the striatum based on cell type, an intricate internal organization has been revealed with special stains. When the striatum is stained for acetylcholinesterase (AChE), there is a patchy distribution of lightly staining regions within more heavily stained regions (35). The AChE-poor patches have been called striosomes and the AChE-rich areas have been called the extrastriosomal matrix. The matrix forms the bulk of the striatal volume and receives input from most areas of the cerebral cortex. Within the matrix are clusters of neurons with similar inputs that have been termed matrisomes (19). The bulk of the output from cells in the matrix is to both segments of the GP, VP, and to the SNpr. The striosomes receive input from the prefrontal cortex and send output to the SNpc (36). Immunohistochemical techniques have demonstrated that many substances such as substance P, dynorphin, and enkephalin have a patchy distribution that may be partly or wholly in register with the striosomes (37). The striosome–matrix organization suggests a level of functional segregation within the striatum that may be important in understanding the variety of symptoms in TS. However, it is not known specifically how the striosome–matrix anatomic organization translates to functional segregation.

The subthalamic nucleus receives an excitatory, glutamatergic input from many areas of the frontal lobes with especially large inputs from motor areas of cortex (38–40). The STN also receives an inhibitory GABA input from GPe (41). The output from the STN is glutamatergic and excitatory to the basal ganglia output nuclei, GPi, VP, and SNpr (42,43). STN also sends an excitatory projection back to GPe (44). There is a somatopic organization in the STN (45,46) and a relative topographic separation of "motor" and "cognitive" inputs to the STN (47).

The primary basal ganglia output arises from the GPi, a GPi-like component of VP, and the SNpr. As described above, the GPi and SNpr receive excitatory input from the STN and inhibitory input from the striatum. They also receive an inhibitory input from the GPe. The dendritic fields of GPi, VP, and SNpr neurons span up to 1-mm diameter and thus have the potential to integrate a large number of converging inputs (48,49). The output from the GPi, VP, and SNpr is inhibitory and uses GABA as its neurotransmitter (50). The primary output is directed to thalamic nuclei that project to the frontal lobes: the ventrolateral, ventroanterior, and mediodorsal nuclei. The thalamic targets of the GPi, VP, and SNpr project, in turn, to the frontal lobe, with the strongest output going to motor areas. Collaterals of the axons projecting to the thalamus project to an area at the junction of the midbrain and pons near the pedunculopontine nucleus (51). Other output neurons (20%) project to intralaminar nuclei of the thalamus, to the lateral habenula, or to the superior colliculus (52,53).

The basal ganglia motor output has a somatotopic organization such that the body below the neck is largely represented in the GPi and the head and eyes are largely represented in the SNpr (15,46,54). The separate representation of different body parts is maintained throughout the basal ganglia. Within the representation of an individual body part, it also appears that there is segregation of outputs to different motor areas of cortex and that an individual GPi neuron sends output via the thalamus to just one area of the cortex (55,56). Thus, GPi neurons that project via the thalamus to the motor cortex are adjacent to, but separate from, those that project to the premotor cortex or supplementary motor area. GPi neurons that project via the thalamus to the prefrontal cortex are also separate from those projecting to motor areas and from VP neurons projecting via the thalamus to the orbitofrontal cortex. The anatomic segregation of basal ganglia–thalamocortical outputs suggests functional segregation, too (15,56). Functional segregation of basal ganglia–thalamocortical circuits has important implications for understanding the anatomical basis for different aspects of TS.

The GPe and the GPe-like part of VP may be viewed as intrinsic nuclei of the basal ganglia. Like the GPi and SNpr, the GPe receives an inhibitory projection from the striatum and an excitatory one from the STN. Unlike the GPi, the striatal projection to the GPe contains GABA and enkephalin but not substance P (5,34). The output of the GPe is quite different from the output of the GPi. The output is GABAergic and inhibitory and the majority of the output projects to the STN. The connections from striatum to GPe, from GPe to STN, and from STN to GPi form the "indirect" striatopallidal pathway to GPi (57) (Fig. 1). In addition, there is a monosynaptic GABAergic inhibitory output from the GPe directly to the GPi and to the SNpr (58) and a GABAergic projection back to the striatum (59). Thus, GPe neurons are in a position to provide feedback inhibition to neurons in the striatum and STN and feedforward inhibition to neurons in the GPi and SNpr. This circuitry suggests that the GPe may act to oppose, limit, or focus the effect of the striatal and STN projections to the GPi and SNpr as well as focus activity in these output nuclei.

Dopamine input to the striatum arises from the SNpc and the ventral tegmental area (VTA). The SNpc projects to most of the striatum; the VTA projects to the ventral striatum. The SNpc and VTA are made up of large dopamine-containing cells. The SNpc receives input from the striatum, specifically from the striosomes (32). This input is GABAergic and inhibitory. The SNpc and VTA dopamine neurons project to all of the caudate and putamen in a topographic manner (60,61). However, the nigral dopamine neurons receive inputs from one striatal circuit and project back to the same and to adjacent circuits (61). Thus, they appear to be in a position to modulate activity across functionally different circuits.

Although the basal ganglia intrinsic circuitry is complex, the overall picture is of two primary pathways through the basal ganglia from the cerebral cortex with the output directed via the thalamus at the frontal lobes. These pathways consist of two disynaptic pathways from the cortex to the basal ganglia output (Fig. 1). In addition, there are several multisynaptic pathways involving GPe. The two disynaptic pathways are from the cortex through (1) the striatum and 2) STN to the basal ganglia outputs (Fig. 1). These pathways have important anatomical and functional differences. First, the cortical input to STN comes only from the frontal lobe, whereas the input to the striatum arises from virtually all areas of the cerebral cortex. Second, the output from the STN is excitatory, whereas the output from the striatum is inhibitory. Third, the excitatory route through the STN is faster than the inhibitory route through the striatum (62–64). Finally, the STN projection to GPi is divergent and the striatal projection is more focused (65). Thus, the two disynaptic pathways from the cerebral cortex to the basal ganglia output nuclei, GPi and SNpr, provide fast, widespread, divergent excitation through the STN and slower, focused, inhibition through the striatum. This organization provides an anatomical basis for focused inhibition and surround excitation of neurons in the GPi and SNpr (Fig. 2). Because the output of the GPi and SNpr is inhibitory, this would result in focused facilitation and surround inhibition of basal ganglia–thalamocortical targets.

We have developed a scheme of normal basal ganglia motor function based on the results of anatomical, physiological, and lesion studies (7,66,67). This scheme is relevant to understanding the neurobiology and pathophysiology of TS (4). In this scheme, the tonically active inhibitory output of the basal ganglia acts as a "brake" on motor pattern generators (MPGs) in the cerebral cortex. When a movement is initiated by a particular MPG, basal ganglia output neurons projecting to competing MPGs increase their firing rate, thereby increasing inhibition and applying a "brake" on those generators. Other basal ganglia output neurons projecting to the generators involved in the desired movement decrease their discharge, thereby removing tonic inhibition and releasing the "brake" from the desired motor patterns. Thus, the intended movement is enabled and competing movements are prevented from interfering with the desired one.

The anatomical arrangement of the STN and striatal inputs to the GPi and SNpr form the basis for a functional center-surround organization as shown in Fig. 3. When a voluntary movement is initiated by cortical mechanisms, a separate signal is sent to the STN, exciting it. The STN projects in a

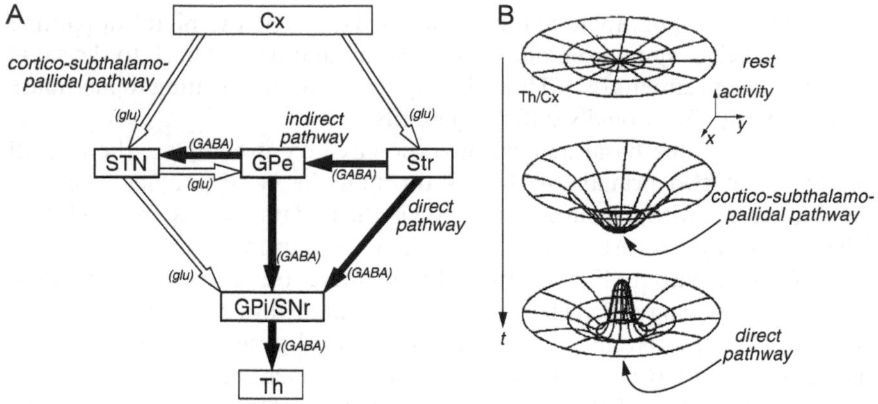

Figure 2 (A) A schematic diagram of the cortico–subthalamo–pallidal, direct cortico–striato–pallidal, and indirect cortico–striato–GPe–subthalamo–GPi pathways. White and black arrows represent excitatory glutamatergic (glu) and inhibitory GABAergic (GABA) projections, respectively. Cx = cerebral cortex; GPe = external segment of the globus pallidus; GPi = internal segment of the globus pallidus; SNr = substantia nigra pars reticulata; STN = subthalamic nucleus; Str = striatum; Th = thalamus. (B) A schematic diagram explaining the activity change in the thalamus and/or cortex (Th/Cx) following the sequential inputs through the cortico–subthalamo–pallidal (middle) and direct cortico–striato–pallidal (bottom) pathways. (From Ref. 64.)

widespread pattern and excites the GPi. The increased GPi activity causes inhibition of thalamocortical motor mechanisms. In parallel to the pathway through the STN, signals are sent from all areas of the cerebral cortex to the striatum. The cortical inputs are transformed by the striatal integrative circuitry to a focused, context-dependent output that inhibits specific neurons in the GPi. The inhibitory striatal input to the GPi is slower, but more powerful, than the excitatory STN input. The resulting focally decreased activity in the GPi selectively disinhibits the desired thalamocortical MPGs. Indirect pathways from striatum to GPi (striatum 6 GPe 6 GPi and striatum 6 GPe 6 STN6 GPi) (Fig. 1) result in further focusing of the output. The net result of basal ganglia activity during a voluntary movement is the inhibition ("braking") of competing motor patterns and focused facilitation (releasing the "brake") from the selected voluntary movement pattern generators.

This scheme provides a framework for understanding the pathophysiology of involuntary movements generally (7). Different involuntary movements such as chorea, dystonia, or tics result from different abnormalities in the basal ganglia circuits. Broad lesions of the GPi or SNpr disinhibit both desired and unwanted motor patterns leading to inappropriate activation of

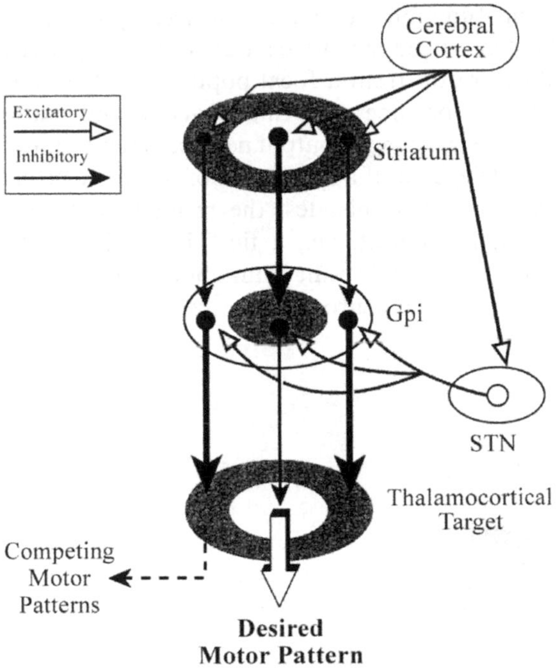

Figure 3 Schematic of normal functional organization of the basal ganglia output. Excitatory projections are indicated by open arrows; inhibitory projections are indicated by filled arrows. Relative magnitude of activity is represented by line thickness. (From Ref. 4.)

competing motor patterns, but normal generation of the wanted movement. Thus, lesions of the GPi cause cocontraction of multiple muscle groups and difficulty turning off unwanted motor patterns, but do not affect movement initiation (68). Lesions of the SNpr cause unwanted saccadic eye movements that interfere with the ability to maintain visual fixation, but do not impair the initiation of voluntary saccades (69). Lesions of VP impair the inhibition of previously learned behavioral responses, leading to perseveration (70). Lesions of putamen may cause dystonia due to the loss of focused inhibition in the GPi (71). Lesions of the STN produce continuous involuntary movements of the contralateral limbs (hemiballism or hemichorea) (72). Despite the involuntary movements, voluntary movements can still be performed. Although structural lesions of the putamen, GPi, VP, SNpr, or STN produce certain types of unwanted movements or behaviors, they do not produce tics. Tics are more likely to arise from abnormal activity patterns. Most likely, these abnormal patterns arise from the striatum.

If a scheme of basal ganglia function is to explain the pathophysiology of tics, it must account for the stereotyped repetitive nature of tics. A pattern of stereotyped motor output can result from a focal population of striatal neurons becoming active. If they become abnormally active and cause unwanted inhibition of a group of basal ganglia output neurons, an unwanted competing motor pattern can be triggered. If a specific set of striatal neurons becomes overactive in discrete repeated episodes, the result would be a repeated, stereotyped, unwanted movement, i.e., a tic. This is illustrated schematically in Fig. 4. Multiple tics would result from abnormal excessive activity of multiple discrete sets of striatal neurons. It has been hypothesized

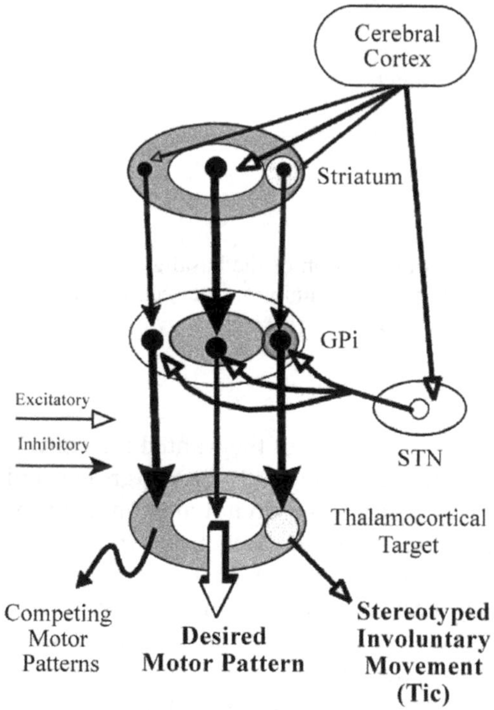

Figure 4 Schematic of hypothetical reorganization of basal ganglia output in tic disorders. Conventions are the same as in Figure 3. When a discrete set of striatal neurons becomes active inappropriately (right of figure) this leads to aberrant inhibition of a discrete set of GPi neurons. The abnormally inhibited GPi neurons disinhibit thalamocortical mechanisms involved in a specific unwanted, competing motor pattern resulting in a stereotyped involuntary movement (tic). (From Ref. 4.)

that each tic would correspond to activity of a discrete set of striatal neurons (4).

The discrete sets of striatal neurons in which overactivity can cause tics may correspond to the striatal matrisomes (19). Matrisomes are thought to be zones of functional homogeneity in an otherwise heterogeneous striatum. If these clusters of neurons become active at inappropriate times, unwanted stereotyped movements would be produced. Microstimulation in the putamen of awake monkeys elicits stereotyped movements of individual body parts (73). At some sites, movement of multiple adjacent body parts is elicited. Increasing the stimulation current can increase the number of contracting muscles, but in a stereotyped pattern for each site. These data indicate that repeated activation of discrete sets of striatal neurons can produce repeated stereotyped movements. The motor output resulting from such activation is stereotyped for each zone (matrisome) and thus could be the substrate for the stereotyped repetitive movements that tics represent. While no data exist as to what determines the temporal pattern of spontaneous activity in matrisomal neurons, it is tempting to speculate that the intrinsic membrane properties or afferent activity patterns lead to the temporal pattern of tics that is seen clinically (74).

It is widely believed that abnormalities of dopamine neurotransmission have a primary role in the pathophysiology of TS. The "dopamine hypothesis" arises in part from the clinical observation that blockade of dopamine receptors decreases tics and potentiation of dopamine transmission with stimulant medications may elicit tics or increase their severity (75). However, measures of dopamine receptors, presynaptic content, or function in pathological or functional imaging studies have produced conflicting results (see Chapters 14 and 16). Despite the conflicting data and limitations of the studies summarized above, the dopamine hypothesis of TS remains important. There may be significant abnormalities of dopamine-mediated function even in the absence of primary abnormalities of dopamine neurons or postsynaptic receptor binding.

The dopamine input of the basal ganglia largely arises from the SNpc (Fig. 1). As noted above, the action of dopamine on striatal neurons depends on the type of dopamine receptor involved. It is generally agreed that D1 receptors stimulate and D2 receptors inhibit adenyl cyclase activity. There is also evidence that dopamine transmission influences the conductance of sodium, potassium, and calcium ions (29), but it appears that these effects are primarily local and have little influence on the membrane potential of the entire cell. Both D1 and D2 receptors are located on medium spiny striatal cells. Some evidence suggests that D1 receptors are preferentially located on cells that project to the GPi or SNpr and that D2 receptors are located on cells that project to the GPe (33). However, there is evidence that some medium spiny cells contain both D1 and D2 receptors (29). In addition to the postsynaptic localization, D2 receptors are also present presynaptically on corticostriatal terminals and on other dopaminergic terminals (autoreceptors) (76).

The conventional view has been that dopamine acts at D1 receptors to facilitate the activity of postsynaptic neurons and at D2 receptors to inhibit postsynaptic neurons (5,6,33). Indeed, this is a fundamental concept for currently popular models of basal ganglia pathophysiology (5,6). However, it has been shown recently that the effect of dopamine on medium spiny striatal neurons may depend critically on the membrane potential of the medium spiny cell at the time of dopamine release (30,77). The effect of a D1 agonist on the firing rate of medium spiny neurons was studied at both depolarized and hyperpolarized membrane potentials. Normally, the membrane potential of medium spiny neurons fluctuates between two stable resting states: relatively hyperpolarized (approximately −80 mV) and relatively depolarized (approximately −55 mV) (78). In the experiments of Hernandez-Lopez et al. (30) evoked discharge was inhibited by D1 agonists at hyperpolarized membrane potentials, but was facilitated by D1 agonists at more depolarized resting potentials. This effect appears to be mediated by L-type Ca^{2+} conductance. Thus, D1 dopamine receptor activation can either inhibit or enhance evoked activity, depending on the level of membrane depolarization.

In addition to short-term facilitation or inhibition of striatal activity, there is evidence that dopamine can modulate corticostriatal transmission by mechanisms of long-term depression (LTD) and long-term potentiation (LTP) (79–81). The mechanisms of LTD and LTP are thought to rely on time-dependent changes in intracellular calcium and second messenger systems. Through these mechanisms, dopamine strengthens or weakens the efficacy of corticostriatal synapses and can thus mediate reinforcement of specific discharge patterns. LTP and LTD are thought to be fundamental to many neural mechanisms of learning and may underlie the hypothesized role of the basal ganglia in habit learning (82,83).

There is increasing evidence for a role of the basal ganglia in procedural learning. Much of the research has focused on the learning of tasks or of sequential behavior. There is increasing evidence for a role of the basal ganglia in procedural learning that leads to the formation of habits and the performance of behavioral routines once they are learned (82). Tonically active striatal neurons (TANs) and SNpc dopamine neurons fire in relation to behaviorally significant events (84,85). The activity patterns of these neurons change as the task becomes learned and when novel stimuli or events are introduced. Other striatal neurons also change activity in relation to learning. In rats performing a T-maze task, striatal neurons changed activity patterns as the task become learned and more automatic (82). In monkeys performing a discrimination learning task, striatal neurons changed activity as the animal learned new associations between stimuli and reward (86). Functional imaging studies have also shown basal ganglia activity correlated with the learning of new tasks. Striatal lesions or focal striatal dopamine depletion impairs the learning of new movement sequences (87). These findings together support a role for the basal ganglia in certain types of procedural learning.

The state-dependent effect of dopamine and the role of dopamine in LTP and LTD have potential importance to the pathophysiology of TS. Abnormalities in these mechanisms could result in aberrant action of dopamine that might be corrected by dopamine antagonists (or agonists (88)) despite normal dopamine content and transmitter–receptor interaction. Two aspects of dopamine neurotransmission discussed above are appealing candidates in the pathophysiology of tics. If a set of striatal neurons spent excessive periods of time in the depolarized resting state, the effect of dopamine via D1 receptors would be facilitatory and thus would make these cells more likely to fire in response to weak cortical inputs. This aberrant firing would elicit a tic in the manner proposed above (Fig. 4). Thus, abnormalities in the regulation of the resting potential states of striatal neurons may cause abnormal response to dopamine without a fundamental abnormality of dopamine transmission, per se. Changes in the probability of the membrane potential being in the depolarized state over time could underlie the clinical observed temporal fluctuations in tics. Alternatively, abnormally weak LTD or strong LTP of discrete sets of striatal neurons could cause excessive activity resulting in abnormal stereotyped movements as described above. Since LTP and LTD are thought to be mediated by dopamine in the striatum, this is another means by which apparently abnormal responses to dopamine may be seen without a fundamental abnormality of dopamine neurotransmission. Despite the emphasis on dopamine, it is also possible that other mechanisms including glutamate-mediated transmission and intracellular signal transduction could lead to abnormal LTP or LTD.

The scheme of basal ganglia function described above was developed specifically for the motor circuits of the basal ganglia–thalamocortical system (7). However, it is likely that the fundamental principles of function in the somatomotor, oculomotor, limbic, and cognitive basal ganglia circuits are similar. If the basic scheme of facilitation and inhibition of competing movements is extended to encompass more complex behaviors and thoughts, many features of TS can be explained as a failure to inhibit unwanted behaviors and thoughts due to abnormal basal ganglia output patterns.

The segregation of basal ganglia outputs to the frontal lobes via thalamus described above may provide the anatomical substrate for production of simple tics, complex tics, and compulsions. Abnormal activation of motor cortex via basal ganglia–thalamocortical circuits would be expected to cause relatively simple motor patterns like those seen in simple tics. Abnormal activation of premotor, supplementary motor, and cingulate motor areas would be expected to cause more elaborate motor patterns like those seen in complex tics. Abnormal activation of orbitofrontal cortex would be expected to cause even more elaborate motor patterns seen as compulsions. The premonitory symptoms would likewise be associated with abnormal activity of these areas. Thus, abnormal activation of motor areas may be associated with specific or nonspecific sensations and activation of orbitofrontal areas may be associated with obsessions. Finally, abnormal disinhibition of dorsolateral prefrontal mechanisms may be associated with attention deficits. The proposed relationship between different basal ganglia circuits and the different symptoms associated with TS is hypothetical. However, with advances in functional imaging methodology there is an opportunity to test it directly in individual with different manifestations of TS.

In summary, the scheme of basal ganglia function presented here, in conjunction with known features of anatomical organization and dopamine neurotransmission provides a hypothesis for the pathophysiology of tics. According to the hypothesis, clusters of striatal neurons (matrisomes) become abnormally active in inappropriate contexts leading to inhibition of GPi or SNpr neurons that would normally be active to suppress unwanted movements. The inhibition of these GPi or SNpr neurons would then disinhibit thalamocortical circuits, leading to the production of tics. Activity-dependent dopamine effects would inappropriately reinforce these activity patterns leading to stereotyped repetition. Over time, exactly which striatal neuronal clusters are overactive may change under various influences so that the produced movements will also change over time. This hypothesis is testable directly, but requires a better animal model of tics than what is currently available. Continued progress on basal ganglia physiology and pathophysiology, functional imaging studies, and study of dopamine modulation of striatal circuits will be important to further our understanding of brain mechanisms relevant to TS.

ACKNOWLEDGMENTS

Supported by NIH R01NS39821, R21NS40086, and the Tourette Syndrome Association.

REFERENCES

1. Denny-Brown D, Yanagisawa N. The role of the basal ganglia in the initiation of movement. In: Yahr MD, ed. The Basal Ganglia. New York: Raven Press, 1976:115–149.

2. Penney JB, Young AB. Speculations on the functional anatomy of basal ganglia disorders. Annu Rev Neurosci 1983; 6:73–94.
3. Leckman J, Cohen D. Tourette's Syndrome—Tics, Obsessions, Compulsions: Developmental Psychopathology and Clinical Care. New York: John Wiley & Sons, 1999:584.
4. Mink JW. Basal ganglia dysfunction in Tourette's syndrome: a new hypothesis. Pediatr Neurol 2001; 25:190–198.
5. Albin RL, Young AB, Penney JB. The functional anatomy of basal ganglia disorders. Trends Neurosci 1989; 12:366–375.
6. DeLong MR. Primate models of movement disorders of basal ganglia origin. Trends Neurosci 1990; 13:281–285.
7. Mink JW. The basal ganglia: focused selection and inhibition of competing motor programs. Prog Neurobiol 1996; 50:381–425.
8. Redgrave P, Prescott T, Gurney K. The basal ganglia: a vertebrate solution to the selection problem? Neuroscience 1999; 89:1009–1023.
9. Mink J. The basal ganglia and involuntary movements: impaired inhibition of competing motor patterns. Arch Neurol 2003; 60:1365–1368.
10. Kemp JM, Powell TPS. The corticostriate projection in the monkey. Brain 1970; 93:525–546.
11. Russchen F, Bakst I, Amaral D, Price J. The amygdalostriatal projections in the monkey. An anterograde tracing study. Brain Res 1985; 329:241–257.
12. Fudge J, Kunishio K, Walsh C, Richard D, Haber S. Amygdaloid projections to ventromedial striatal subterritories in the primate. Neuroscience 2002; 110: 257–275.
13. Cherubini E, Herrling PL, Lanfumey L, Stanzione P. Excitatory amino acids in synaptic excitation of rat striatal neurones in vitro. J Physiol 1988; 400:677–690.
14. Bouyer JJ, Park DH, Joh TH, Pickel VM. Chemical and structural analysis of the relation between cortical inputs and tyrosine hydroxylase-containing terminals in rat neostriatum. Brain Res 1984; 302:267–275.
15. Alexander GE, DeLong MR, Strick PL. Parallel organization of functionally segregated circuits linking basal ganglia and cortex. Annu Rev Neurosci 1986; 9:357–381.
16. Wilson CJ, Groves PM. Fine structure and synaptic connections of the common spiny neuron of the rat neostriatum: a study employing intracellular injection of horseradish peroxidase. J Comp Neurol 1980; 194:599–614.
17. Selemon LD, Goldman-Rakic PS. Longitudinal topography and interdigitation of corticostriatal projections in the rhesus monkey. J Neurosci 1985; 5:776–794.
18. Flaherty AW, Graybiel AM. Corticostriatal transformations in the primate somatosensory system. Projections from physiologically mapped body-part representations. J Neurophysiol 1991; 66:1249–1263.
19. Graybiel AM, Aosaki T, Flaherty AW, Kimura M. The basal ganglia and adaptive motor control. Science 1994; 265:1826–1831.
20. Lapper SR, Bolam JP. Input from the frontal cortex and the parafascicular nucleus to cholinergic interneurons in the dorsal striatum of the rat. Neuroscience 1992; 51:533–545.
21. Sadikot AF, Parent A, Francois C. Efferent connections of the centromedian

and parafascicular thalamic nuclei in the squirrel monkey: a PHA-L study of subcortical projections. J Comp Neurol 1992; 315:137–159.
22. McFarland NR, Haber SN. Organization of thalamostriatal terminals from the ventral motor nuclei in the macaque. J Comp Neurol 2001; 429:321–336.
23. Izzo PN, Bolam JP. Cholinergic synaptic input to different parts of spiny striatonigral neurons in the rat. J Comp Neurol 1988; 269:219–234.
24. Penny GR, Afsharpour S, Kitai ST. The glutamate decarboxylase-, leucine enkephalin-, methionine enkephalin- and substance P-immunoreactive neurons in the neostriatum of the rat and cat: evidence for partial population overlap. Neuroscience 1986; 17:1011–1045.
25. Bolam JP, Hanley JJ, Booth PA, Bevan MD. Synaptic organisation of the basal ganglia. J Anat 2000; 196:527–542.
26. Carpenter MB. Anatomy of the corpus striatum and brain stem integrating systems. In: Brooks VB, ed. Handbook of Physiology: The Nervous System. Bethesda, MD: American Physiological Society, 1981:947–995.
27. Lavoie B, Parent A. Immunohistochemical study of the serotoninergic innervation of the basal ganglia in the squirrel monkey. J Comp Neurol 1990; 299: 1–16.
28. Sibley DR, Monsma FJ. Molecular biology of dopamine receptors. Trends Pharmacol Sci 1992; 13:61–69.
29. Surmeier DJ, Reiner A, Levine MS, Ariano MA. Are neostriatal dopamine receptors co-localized? Trends Neurosci 1993; 16:299–305.
30. Hernandez-Lopez S, Bargas J, Surmeier DJ, Reyes A, Galarraga E. D1 receptor activation enhances evoked discharge in neostriatal medium spiny neurons by modulating an L-type Ca^{2+} conductance. J Neurosci 1997; 17:3334–3342.
31. Ribak CE, Vaughn JE, Roberts E. The GABA neurons and their axon terminals in rat corpus striatum as demonstrated by GAD immunocytochemistry. J Comp Neurol 1979; 187:261–283.
32. Graybiel AM. Neurotransmitters and neuromodulators in the basal ganglia. Trends Neurosci 1990; 13:244–254.
33. Gerfen CR, Engber TM, Mahan LC, Susel Z, Chase TN, Monsma FJ, Sibley DR. D_1 and D_2 dopamine receptor-regulated gene expression of striatonigral and striatopallidal neurons. Science 1990; 250:1429–1432.
34. Gerfen CR, Young WS III. Distribution of striatonigral and striatopallidal peptidergic neurons in both patch and matrix compartments: an in situ hybridization histochemistry and fluorescent retrograde tracing study. Brain Res 1988; 460:161–167.
35. Graybiel AM, Ragsdale CW. Histochemically distinct compartments in the striatum of human, monkey and cat demonstrated by acetylcholinesterase staining. Proc Natl Acad Sci USA 1978; 75:5723–5726.
36. Gerfen CR. The neostriatal mosaic: multiple levels of compartmental organization in the basal ganglia. Annu Rev Neurosci 1992; 15:285–320.
37. Graybiel AM, Ragsdale CW, Yoneika ES, Elde RP. An immunohistochemical study of enkephalins and other neuropeptides in the striatum of the cat with evidence that the opiate peptides are arranged to form mosaic patterns in

register with striosomal compartments visible with acetylcholinesterase staining. Neuroscience 1981; 6:377–397.
38. Rouzaire-Dubois B, Scarnati E. Pharmacological study of the cortical-induced excitation of subthalamic nucleus neurons in the rat: evidence for amino acids as putative neurotransmitters. Neuroscience 1987; 21:429–440.
39. Fujimoto K, Kita H. Response characteristics of subthalamic neurons to the stimulation of the sensorimotor cortex in the rat. Brain Res 1993; 609:185–192.
40. Hartmann-von Monakow K, Akert K, Kunzle H. Projections of the precentral motor cortex and other cortical areas of the frontal lobe to the subthalamic nucleus in the monkey. Exp Brain Res 1978; 33:395–403.
41. Kita H, Chang HT, Kitai ST. Pallidal inputs to subthalamus: intracellular analysis. Brain Res 1983; 264:255–265.
42. Rinvik E, Ottersen OP. Terminals of subthalamonigral fibres are enriched with glutamate-like immunoreactivity: an electron microscopic, immunogold analysis in the cat. J Chem Neuroanat 1993; 6:19–30.
43. Brotchie JM, Crossman AR. D-[^{3}H]Aspartate and [^{14}C]GABA uptake in the basal ganglia of rats following lesions in the subthalamic region suggest a role for excitatory amino acid but not GABA-mediated transmission in subthalamic nucleus efferents. Exp Neurol 1991; 113:171–181.
44. Parent A, Smith Y, Filion M, Dumas J. Distinct afferents to internal and external pallidal segments in the squirrel monkey. Neurosci Lett 1989; 96:140–144.
45. Nambu A, Takada M, Inase M, Tokuno H. Dual somatotopical representations in the primate subthalamic nucleus: evidence for ordered but reversed body-map transformations from the primary motor cortex and the supplementary motor area. J Neurosci 1996; 16:2671–2683.
46. DeLong MR, Crutcher MD, Georgopoulos AP. Primate globus pallidus and subthalamic nucleus: functional organization. J Neurophysiol 1985; 53:530–543.
47. Maurice N, Deniau J, Glowinski J, Thierry A. Relationships between the prefrontal cortex and the basal ganglia in the rat: physiology of the cortico-subthalamic circuits. J Neurosci 1998; 18:9539–9546.
48. Percheron G, Yelnik J, Francois C. A Golgi analysis of the primate globus pallidus. III. Spatial organization of the striato–pallidal complex. J Comp Neurol 1984; 227:214–227.
49. Francois C, Yelnik J, Percheron G. Golgi study of the primate substantia nigra. II. Spatial organization of dendritic arborizations in relation to the cytoarchitectonic boundaries and to the striatonigral bundle. J Comp Neurol 1987; 265: 473–493.
50. Penney JB, Young AB. GABA as the pallidothalamic neurotransmitter: implications for basal ganglia function. Brain Res 1981; 207:195–199.
51. Rye DB, Lee HJ, Saper CB, Wainer BH. Medullary and spinal efferents of the pedunculopontine tegmental nucleus and adjacent mesopontine tegmentum in the rat. J Comp Neurol 1988; 269:315–341.
52. Parent A, De Bellefeuille L. Organization of efferent projections from the

internal segment of globus pallidus in primate as revealed by fluorescence retrograde labelling method. Brain Res 1982; 245:201–213.
53. Francois C, Percheron G, Yelnik J, Tande D. A topographic study of the course of nigral axons and of the distribution of pallidal axonal endings in the centre median–parafascicular complex of macaques. Brain Res 1988; 473:181–186.
54. Georgopoulos AP, DeLong MR, Crutcher MD. Relation between parameters of step-tracking movements and single cell discharge in the globus pallidus and subthalamic nucleus of the behaving monkey. J Neurosci 1983; 3:1586–1598.
55. Middleton FA, Strick PL. Anatomical evidence for cerebellar and basal ganglia involvement in higher cognitive function. Science 1994; 266:458–461.
56. Hoover JE, Strick PL. Multiple output channels in the basal ganglia. Science 1993; 259:819–821.
57. Alexander GE, Crutcher MD. Functional architecture of basal ganglia circuits: neural substrates of parallel processing. Trends Neurosci 1990; 13:266–271.
58. Bolam JP, Smith Y. The striatum and the globus pallidus send convergent synaptic inputs onto single cells in the entopeduncular nucleus of the rat: a double anterograde labelling study combined with postembedding immunocytochemistry for GABA. J Comp Neurol 1992; 321:456–476.
59. Bevan MD, Booth PA, Eaton SA, Bolam JP. Selective innervation of neostriatal interneurons by a subclass of neuron in the globus pallidus of the rat. J Neurosci 1998; 18:9438–9452.
60. Hedreen JC, DeLong MR. Organization of striatopallidal, striatonigral, nigrostriatal projections in the macaque. J Comp Neurol 1991; 304:569–595.
61. Haber SN, Fudge JL, McFarland NR. Striatonigrostriatal pathways in primates form an ascending spiral from the shell to the dorsolateral striatum. J Neurosci 2000; 20:2369–2382.
62. Kita H. Responses of globus pallidus neurons to cortical stimulation: intracellular study in the rat. Brain Res 1992; 589:84–90.
63. Maurice N, Deniau J, Glowinski J, Thierry A. Relationships between the prefrontal cortex and the basal ganglia in the rat: physiology of the cortico-nigral circuits. J Neurosci 1999; 19:4674–4681.
64. Nambu A, Tokuno H, Hamada I, Kita H, Imanishi M, Akazawa T, Ikeuchi Y, Hasegawa N. Excitatory cortical inputs to pallidal neurons via the subthalamic nucleus in the monkey. J Neurophysiol 2000; 84:289–300.
65. Parent A, Hazrati L-N. Anatomical aspects of information processing in primate basal ganglia. Trends Neurosci 1993; 16:111–116.
66. Mink JW, Thach WT. Basal ganglia intrinsic circuits and their role in behavior. Curr Opin Neurobiol 1993; 3:950–957.
67. Thach WT, Mink JW, Goodkin HP, Keating JG. Combining versus gating motor programs: differential roles for cerebellum and basal ganglia. In: Mano N, Hamada I, DeLong MR, eds. Role of the Cerebellum and Basal Ganglia in Voluntary Movement. Amsterdam: Elsevier Science Publishers, 1993:235–245.
68. Mink JW, Thach WT. Basal ganglia motor control. III. Pallidal ablation: normal reaction time, muscle cocontraction, slow movement. J Neurophysiol 1991; 65:330–351.

69. Hikosaka O, Wurtz RH. Modification of saccadic eye movements by GABA-related substances. II. Effects of muscimol in monkey substantia nigra pars reticulata. J Neurophysiol 1985; 53:292–308.
70. Ferry A, Lu X-C, Price JL. Effects of excitotoxic lesions in the ventral striato-pallidal–thalamocortical pathway on odor reversal learning: inability to extinguish an incorrect response. Exp Brain Res 2000; 131:320–335.
71. Perlmutter JS, Tempel LW, Black KJ, Parkinson D, Todd RD. MPTP induces dystonia and parkinsonism. Clues to the pathophysiology of dystonia. Neurology 1997; 49:1432–1438.
72. Carpenter MB, Carpenter CS. Analysis of somatotopic relations of the corpus Luysi in man and monkey. J Comp Neurol 1951; 95:349–370.
73. Alexander GE, DeLong MR. Microstimulation of the primate striatum. II. Somatotopic organization of striatal microexcitable zones and their relation to neuronal response properties. J Neurophysiol 1985; 53:1417–1430.
74. Peterson B, Leckman J. The temporal dynamics of tics in Gilles de la Tourette syndrome. Biol Psychiatry 1998; 44:1337–1348.
75. Singer HS. Neurobiological issues in Tourette syndrome. Brain Dev 1994; 16:353–364.
76. Kalsner S, Westfall TC. Presynaptic receptors and the question of autoregulation of neurotransmitter release. Ann NY Acad Sci 1990; 604:652–655.
77. Nicola S, Surmeier J, Malenka R. Dopaminergic modulation of neuronal excitability in the striatum and nucleus accumbens. Annu Rev Neurosci 2000; 23:185–215.
78. Wilson CJ, Kawaguchi Y. The origins of two-state spontaneous membrane potential fluctuations of neostriatal spiny neurons. J Neurosci 1996; 16:2397–2410.
79. Groves PM, Garcia-Munoz M, Linder JC, Manley MS, Martine ME, Young SJ. Elements of the intrinsic organization and information processing in the neostriatum. In: Houk JC, Davis JL, Beiser DG, eds. Models of Information Processing in the Basal Ganglia. Cambridge, MA: MIT Press, 1995:51–96.
80. Wickens J, Kotter R. Cellular models of reinforcement. In: Houk JC, Davis JL, Beiser DG, eds. Models of Information Processing in the Basal Ganglia. Cambridge, MA: MIT Press, 1995:187–214.
81. Centonze D, Gubellini P, Picconi B, Calabresi P, Giacomini P, Bernardi G. Unilateral dopamine denervation blocks corticostriatal LTP. J Neurophysiol 1999; 82:3575–3579.
82. Jog M, Kubota Y, Connolly C, Hillegaart V, Graybiel A. Building neural representations of habits. Science 1999; 286:1745–1749.
83. Knowlton B, Mangels J, Squire L. A neostriatal habit learning system in humans. Science 1996; 273:1399–1402.
84. Aosaki T, Kimura M, Graybiel AM. Temporal and spatial characteristics of tonically active neurons of the primate's striatum. J Neurophysiol 1995; 73:1234–1252.
85. Schultz W, Romo R, Ljungberg T, Mirenowicz J, Hollerman JR, Dickinson A. Reward-related signals carried by dopamine neurons. In: Houk JC, Davis JL,

Beiser DG, eds. Models of Information Processing in the Basal Ganglia. Cambridge, MA: MIT Press, 1995:233–249.
86. Tremblay L, Hollerman J, Schultz W. Modifications of reward expectation-related neuronal activity during learning in primate striatum. J Neurophysiol 1998; 80:964–977.
87. Matsumoto N, Hanakawa T, Maki S, Graybiel AM, Kimura M. Role of nigrostriatal dopamine system in learning to perform sequential motor tasks in a predictive manner. J Neurophysiol 1999; 82:978–998.
88. Gilbert D, Sethuraman G, Sine L, Peters S, Sallee F. Tourette's syndrome improvement with pergolide in a randomized, double-blind, crossover trial. Neurology 2000; 54:1310–1315.

14

Neurobiological Issues in Tourette's Syndrome

Harvey S. Singer and Karen Minzer
Johns Hopkins University School of Medicine
Baltimore, Maryland, U.S.A.

INTRODUCTION

Tourette's syndrome (TS) is characterized by the presence of chronic motor and vocal tics and is commonly associated with a variety of behavioral and emotional problems. In his manuscript published in 1885, Gilles de la Tourette (1) noted no anatomical or pathological cause in the syndrome that bears his name and referred scientists interested in pursuing pathophysiological mechanisms to the field of psychology. Although much information has been acquired pertaining to the underlying anatomy and physiology of tic disorders, many perplexing questions remain. The fact that tics resolve or diminish in many individuals suggests the possibility of a developmental alteration rather than a fixed or progressive disorder. There is convincing evidence that cortico-striatal-thalamo-cortical (aka frontal-subcortical) pathways are involved in the expression of TS and its accompanying neuropsychiatric problems, but the precise location(s) remains speculative. A two-pathway model of circuits (direct and indirect) through the basal ganglia is often cited in discussions of hyperkinetic and hypokinetic movement disorders, but this concept represents an oversimplification of complex interactions and newer models have been proposed. Intrinsic neurotransmitters utilized within cortico-striatal-thalamo-cortical pathways are well established, but each has its own complex system of message transduction as well as interaction with other transmitter agents. Although TS is generally accepted as a genetic disorder, environmental factors, such as streptococci infection, have been proposed as contributing factors.

This chapter focuses on three neurobiological issues relating to TS. 1) What is the neuroanatomical localization for tics and comorbid neurobehavioral problems? 2) What is happening at the cellular level, i.e., what is the role of abnormalities of synaptic neurotransmission? 3) Is there a neuroimmunological basis for tic disorders? We begin by defining the cortico-striatal-thalamo-cortical circuits from anatomical and neurochemical perspectives. We then present evidence, both direct and indirect, supporting the involvement of these pathways. We review proposed pathophysiological hypotheses as defined at several levels of specificity, i.e., neuroanatomical localization, physiological abnormality, and neurochemical basis. Lastly, we review clinical characteristics of three movement disorders: Sydenham's chorea (SC), Tourette's syndrome, and pediatric autoimmune neuropsychiatric disorders associated with streptococcal infection (PANDAS) that have been hypothesized to be autoimmune-initiated and discuss the laboratory evidence pertaining to these discussions.

NEUROANATOMICAL LOCALIZATION OF TOURETTE'S SYNDROME

Before defining a neuroanatomical localization, it is essential to clarify the specific components or symptoms of the syndrome that one wishes to localize. In this instance, tics, the essential components of TS, comprise an enormous range of sudden, rapid, repetitive, nonrhythmic movements or vocalizations. They are paroxysmal and abrupt in character, typically wax and wane, often occur in bursts, evolve over time, are exacerbated by anxiety or fatigue, frequently resolve in adulthood, and differ widely in individual patients and families (2). In addition, patients with tic disorders often have a variety of comorbid findings, including attention-deficit/hyperactivity disorder (ADHD), obsessive-compulsive disorder (OCD), mood disorders, executive function deficits, and other problems.

Neuroanatomical Pathways

Cortico-Striatal-Thalamo-Cortical Circuits

Cortical to striatal pathways: In this section, an overview of circuitry and its associated neurochemistry is presented in order to provide a framework for understanding proposed pathophysiological mechanisms. Despite historical emphasis on the striatum (caudate and putamen), it has become evident that newer proposals require knowledge of the entire circuit.

Five distinct parallel circuits have been described in primates with each subserving a different function (3,4). Although presented as distinct pathways, there is evidence to suggest, however, that these circuits may be more integrated than was previously thought (5). This multiple convergent and divergent organization provides the capacity for integration and transformation of cortical information (6). The *motor* circuit, a potential site for generation of tics, originates primarily from the supplementary motor cortex and projects to the putamen in a somatotopic distribution. The *oculomotor* circuit, a potential site of origin for ocular tics, begins principally in the frontal eye fields and connects to the central region of the caudate. The *dorsolateral prefrontal* (*cognitive*) circuit links Brodmann areas 9 and 10 with the dorsolateral head of the caudate and appears to be involved with executive function and motor planning. Dysfunction of this pathway could lead to attentional difficulties and poor results on Letter Word Fluency Testing (7). The *lateral orbitofrontal* (*personality*) circuit originates in the inferolateral prefrontal cortex and projects to the ventromedial caudate. Orbitofrontal injury is associated with OCD, personality changes, disinhibition, irritability, and mania. Lastly, the *anterior cingulate* (*limbic*) circuit arises in the anterior cingulate gyrus and projects to the ventral striatum (olfactory tubercle, nucleus accumbens, and ventral medial aspect of the caudate and putamen) which receives additional input from the amygdala, hippocampus, and entorhinal and perirhinal cortex. Mutism, apathy, and OCD are associated with this circuit.

Striatal to thalamic pathways: The commonly diagramed striatothalamic circuit is subdivided into two pathways ("direct" and "indirect") from the striatum to globus pallidus interna (GPi) and substantia nigra pars reticulata (SNpr) and one extending from these neurons to the thalamus (Fig. 1). The direct pathway transmits striatal information monosynaptically to the GPi and SNpr, whereas the indirect system conveys information to these same regions via a disynaptic relay from globus pallidus externa (GPe) to the subthalamic nucleus (STN). These parallel pathways have opposing effects on GABAergic GPi/SNpr output neurons (i.e., the direct pathway inhibits and the indirect pathway stimulates) and, in turn, produce a reverse effect on thalamocortical (VA-VL) neurons. Striatal output innervates both the GPi and SNpr in a somatotopic organization; head and eyes represented in SNpr and the rest of the body in the GPi (8,9). Although the aforementioned two-pathway circuit appears relatively straightforward and easy for most to comprehend, available anatomical data suggest the presence of a more complex basal ganglia circuit with output to a variety of functional systems (10–13). For example, outputs from GPi/SNpr project to medial dorsal thalamic nuclei, centromedian-parafascicular thalamic complex,

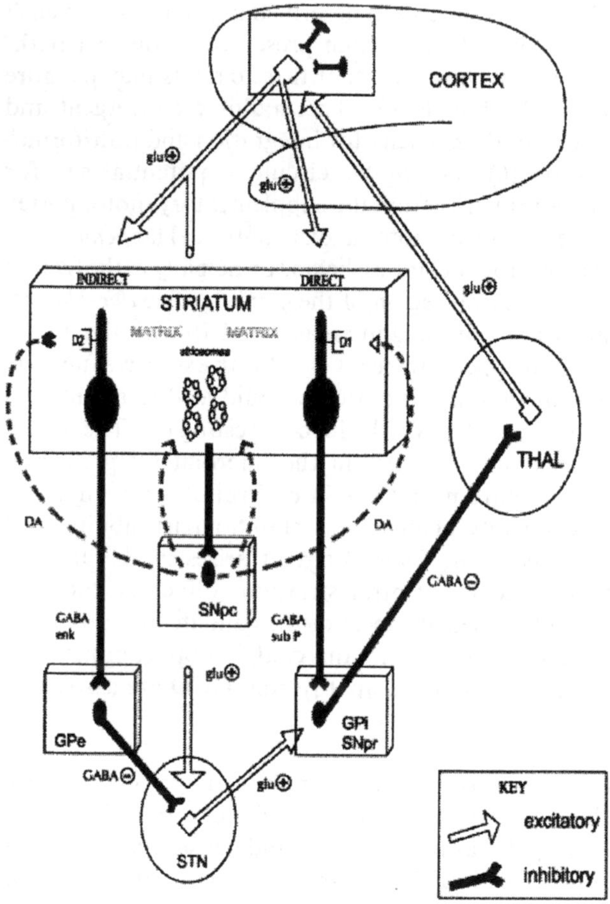

Figure 1 Striatal pathways: direct, indirect, and striosomal. The inhibitory direct pathway transmits information monosynaptically to the GPi. The excitatory *indirect* pathway connects disynaptically to the GPi via the GPe and STN. The *striosomal* pathway transmits information to the SNpc, which in turn exerts dopaminergic influence back to the striatum. SNpc = substantia nigra pars compacta; GPe = globus pallidus externa; GPi = globus pallidus interna; STN = subthalamic nucleus; THAL = thalamus.

pedunculopontine tegmental nucleus, and habenula. The SNpr projects to the superior colliculus.

In addition to the aforementioned two-pathway system, a striosomal pathway has been described (14). In brief, on the basis of its intrinsic anatomical organization, the striatum is composed of two neurochemically defined compartments (15,16). These compartments have been variably designated striosomes and extrastriosomal matrix, patches and matrix, or island and matrix. This neostriatal organization was initially defined and established in the rodent, cat, and human through the use of catecholamine fluorescence (17), opiate receptor autoradiography (18), and acetylcholinesterase (AChE) histochemistry (19,20). For example, AChE staining shows patchy areas of lightly stained regions called striosomes amidst the bulk of a more heavily stained striatal area (called matrix). Cells within the matrix (matrisomes) receive innervation from sensorimotor and association areas of the neocortex and represent the site of origin of both direct and indirect pathways. Smaller striosomal areas receive input from the orbitofrontal, anterior cingulate, and posterior medial prefrontal cortex and project to the substantia nigra pars compacta (SNpc) and its immediate area (21). The SNpc, in turn, gives rise to the dopaminergic nigrostriatal tract.

Thalamocortical pathway: The thalamic targets of GPi/SNpr innervation, in turn, project to the frontal lobe, with the VA-VL thalamic complex providing excitatory innervation to motor-related cortical areas. Topographical representation noted in the striatum and globus pallidus is maintained within the thalamus and subsequent projections to the premotor and motor cortex.

Distribution of Classical Neurotransmitters Within Cortico-Striatal-Thalamo-Cortical Pathways

The distribution of classical neurotransmitters within the basal ganglia and cortico-striatal-thalamo-cortical circuits makes it possible for a variety of transmitters to be involved in the pathobiology of TS (6,22). In the striatum, projecting medium-sized spiny neurons (MSSN) comprise more than 90% of striatal neurons, plus there are three subpopulations of interneurons: large aspiny cholinergic neurons; medium-sized aspiny neurons expressing somatostatin, neuropeptide Y, and nitric oxide synthase; and medium-sized aspiny GABAergic neurons expressing parvalbumin, a calcium-binding protein.

Modulating Influences on Projecting Medium-Sized Spiny Neurons

Medium-sized spiny neurons receive massive input from the cerebral cortex (glutamate), intralaminar nuclei of the thalamus (glutamate), mesencephalon (dopamine), from the SNpc and ventral tegmental area (VTA), subpopulations of striatal interneurons (acetylcholine or peptides), and from other MSSN (GABA, substance P, and enkephalin) (Fig. 2). Corticostriatal inputs release glutamate, which via α-amino-3-hydroxy-5-methyl-4-isoxazole-4-propionate (AMPA) receptors elicit an excitatory synaptic potential (EPSP). *N*-methyl-D-aspartate (NMDA) receptors, acting via voltage-gated ion chan-

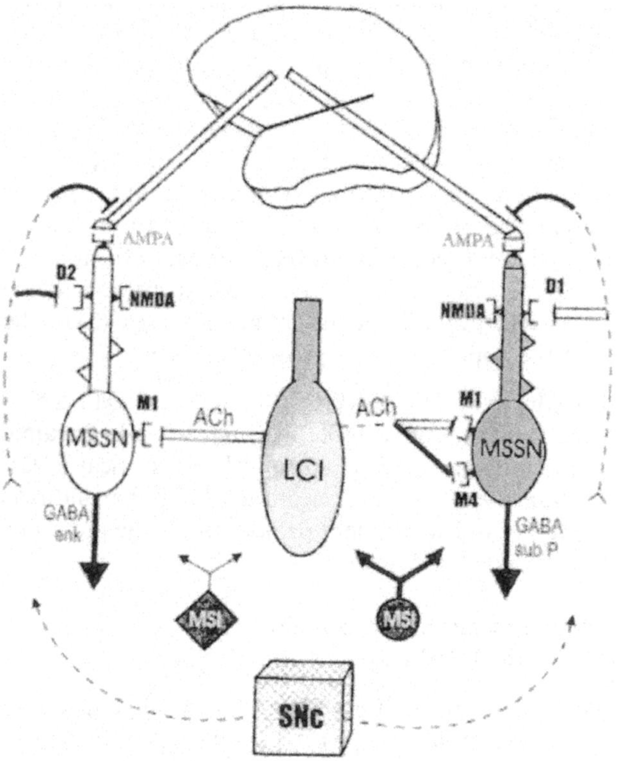

Figure 2 Several modulatory influences on striatal MSSN (medium-sized spiny neurons). Modulatory afferent projections shown in this figure arise from the cortex (glutamate), SNpc (dopamine), LCI (acetylcholine), and MSI (GABA and neuropeptides). Dopaminergic influences arise from SNpc and influence presynaptic cortical receptors and D_1 (excitatory) and D_2 (inhibitory) receptors on the MSSN. LCI act on muscarinic M1 (excitatory) and M4 (inhibitory) receptors. Additionally, voltage-gated NMDA receptors are hypothesized to influence striatal activity. (MSSN = medium-sized spiny neurons, LCI = large aspiny, cholinergic neurons, MSI = medium-sized aspiny interneurons, NMDA = *N*-methyl-D-aspartate receptors, SNpc = substantia nigra pars compacta). Other inputs not shown include serotonergic inputs from the median raphe, glutamatergic inputs from the thalamus, and dopaminergic inputs from the ventral tegmental area. (From Ref. 105.)

nels, have also been hypothesized to modulate striatal activity (23). Dopaminergic input from the SNpc can have either an excitatory or inhibitory effect depending on the receptor subtype; D_1 receptors stimulate adenylate cyclase and enhance activity, whereas D_2 receptors inhibit adenylate cyclase and decrease activity. Dopamine has been hypothesized to influence cortical input via either dopamine receptors on presynaptic glutamatergic corticostriatal terminals (24) or postsynaptic D_1 and D_2 receptors. In the former, the activation of presynaptic D_2 receptors would reduce the release of excitatory transmitters. D_2 receptors are also present on MSSN contributing to the indirect pathway (striato-GPe), whereas D_1 receptors are primarily located on the direct pathway (striato-GPi/SNpr) neurons as well as on cholinergic interneurons. Large aspiny acetylcholine (ACh) interneurons (LCI) send outputs to medium-sized aspiny interneurons (MSI) and to MSSN. Direct-pathway projecting MSSN have both muscarinic M1 and M4 receptors, whereas indirect pathway MSSN have primarily M1 receptors. Hence the effects of ACh and dopamine on MSSN are influenced by the presence of specific receptor subtypes that are segregated, in part, to specific neurons.

Projections from Striatal Neurons

Medium-sized spiny neurons in the matrix region of the striatum provide GABAergic projections to the globus pallidus and SNpr. "Indirect" MSSN are GABAergic and express enkephalins, whereas "direct" MSSN are GABAergic but contain tachykinins such as substance P. Striosomes project to the SNpc.

CONFIRMATION OF A CORTICO-STRIATAL-THALAMO-CORTICAL CIRCUIT ABNORMALITY

A variety of circumstantial and direct evidence supports a dysfunction within cortico-striatal-thalamo-cortical circuits. Inferred evidence includes: the association of basal ganglia dysfunction with other movement disorders; the induction or ablation of stereotypic behaviors after microinjection of dopaminergic agents into rodent striatum (14,25); pathological studies in individuals with tics secondary to encephalitis (26,27); and tic suppression following neurosurgical treatments that disrupt cortico-striatal-thalamo-cortical circuitry, e.g., leukotomies and thalamotomies (28). Direct evidence for pathophysiological involvement of cortico-striatal-thalamo-cortical circuits in TS is provided by neurophysiological evaluation, volumetric MRI studies, area measurements of the corpus callosum, functional imaging of glucose metabolism and blood flow, and examination of ocular movements. In this section, we review the contribution of a variety of approaches to our understanding of TS.

Standard Approaches Used to Evaluate the Neuroanatomical Localization in Tourette's Syndrome

Physical Examination

In contrast to other established movement disorders, such as Huntington's and Parkinson's disease, the physical examination in TS fails to provide direct clues as to neuroanatomical localization of the dysfunction. In children with TS without ADHD, the physical and neurological examination of subtle signs (PANESS) has shown no difficulties in performance of simple and complex motor tasks (7). Voluntary movements in TS have been studied with several paradigms, including assessment of serial choice reaction time by use of a button pushing procedure (29) and unimanual/bimanual rhythmical tasks with handheld objects (30). In the former, increased movement sequencing deficits, without progressive slowing as the level of advanced information was reduced, were thought to be suggestive of frontal striatal dysfunction involving the motor or dorsolateral prefrontal cortex (29). In the second study, manipulative tasks showed inaccuracies in precision grip, which were associated with reduced activation of secondary motor areas on fMRI, indicative of movement organization difficulties (30). Lastly, a lateralized frontostriatal deficit affecting visuospatial attention has been hypothesized on the basis of results showing an abnormally right-biased line bisection task (31).

The presence of comorbid features such as ADHD and OCD and results of formal neuropsychological evaluations have provided further evidence to support a disorder of cortico-striatal-thalamo-cortical abnormalities in TS. Neuroimaging studies in children with ADHD and adolescents and adults with OCD have shown abnormalities within the basal ganglia or its circuits (32–35). Comprehensive psychological evaluations in children with TS, with or without ADHD, have repeatedly identified the presence of executive dysfunction (36–39). Executive function is a term used to refer to self-regulating behaviors necessary to select and sustain actions and guide behavior within the context of goals or rules. Essential components of executive function—initiation, planning, shifting of thought or attention, organization, inhibition of inappropriate thought or behavior, and sustained and sequenced behavior—are thought to involve the prefrontal cortex (4,40,41).

Neuroradiology

Routine noninvasive neuroradiographic studies (CT and MRI) have identified only isolated defects that are considered to be incidental nonspecific findings, unrelated to the basic pathology (42–44). In two publications, localized lesions have been associated with clinical symptoms. One report described a 17-year-old male with TS and comorbid OCD, ADHD, stuttering, and gait disturbance who had bilateral symmetrical globus pallidus lesions on MRI (45), and the other report described an 11-year-old male with TS who had multicystic changes predominantly in the gyrus rectus of the left frontal lobe on MRI (Fig. 3) (46).

Neurophysiology

A variety of electrophysiological studies have been performed, including electroencephalography (EEG), evoked potentials, polysomnography, and event-related potentials. EEG, computed EEG topography (brain mapping), and evoked responses have generally been normal (47–49). The absence of Bereitschaft potentials (negative electrical potentials that normally precede the performance of routine volitional motor activities) before involuntary spontaneous simple tics previously suggested that these movements were not generated from typical pathways (50). Other studies, however, demonstrate that not all voluntary movements are preceded by these potentials, making the interpretation of results in TS more difficult (51). Polysomnographical studies in patients with TS have shown markedly altered sleep quality and difficulties with initiating and maintaining sleep (52–55). Based on a positive correlation between variables of sleep disturbance and the severity of TS, some investigators have suggested a disorder of hyperarousal (52). Prepulse inhibition of the startle reflex, a measure of inhibitory sensorimotor gating, is deficient in TS (56). Impairment of various attention-related behaviors has also been used to support alterations within cortico-striatal-thalamo-cortical circuits, e.g., studies of visual attention on tactile performance (57), a vibrotactile choice reaction time task (58), and visual modalities (59).

Event-related brain potentials (ERPs) are small voltage fluctuations recorded from the scalp that vary as a function of stimulus perception or in conjunction with cognitive processes (60). ERPs have been measured in TS subjects during different paradigms and results have been used to support hypotheses of either altered inhibitory processes or sustaining difficulties (59–63). Using two responsive-locked ERPs, Bereitschaft and motor potentials, investigators have suggested an abnormal modulation of circuits involving motor excitation or inhibition (64).

Neuropathology

Routine postmortem studies have failed to identify a specific focus of abnormality. Although the authors are aware of several unpublished evaluations in which brains were normal, there have been two single case reports that contain detailed neuropathological examinations (65). In the first case, the patient had the onset of symptoms at age 18 and his neurological illness was progressive (66). A detailed histological evaluation, which included motor areas, cerebellar system, red nucleus, basal ganglia, olivary nucleus, and the

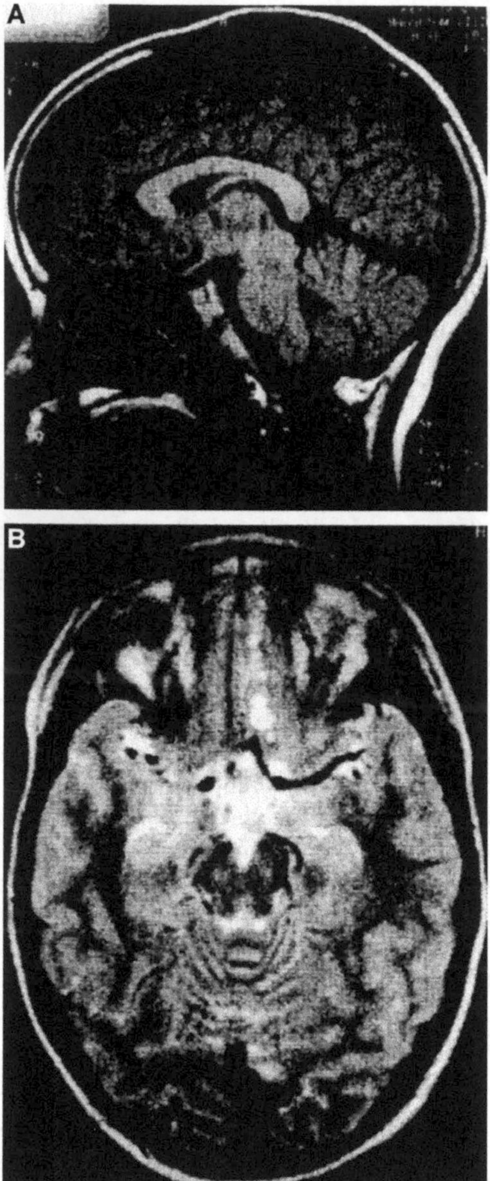

Figure 3 Localized lesions in a TS patient. Sagittal T_1-weighted and axial T_2-weighted MRI of an 11-year-old boy with TS demonstrate multicystic changes in the left gyrus rectus and superior frontal gyrus. (From Ref. 46.)

anterior horns of the cervical spinal cord, showed no evidence for a disease process. In a second case, findings in a 42-year-old suggested "arrested development" of the striatum (67). More specifically, examination showed an increased packing density of neurons in the caudate nucleus and putamen, closely resembling that seen in a 1-year-old child. Additionally, the number of small neurons was increased compared to those in normal controls and in non-TS pathological controls.

Neuropathological and radiographic investigations in individuals with secondary tics ("acquired Tourette's") also confirm associations with structural abnormalities. For example, in a postmortem study of encephalitis lethargica, individuals with acquired tics differed from those without tics by the presence of an array of small focal lesions in the central gray matter that extended into the midbrain tegmentum (26,27). Tourette-like symptoms have appeared in association with a variety of acute and chronic neurological disorders, such as after encephalitis (68), head injury (69), peripheral (non-CNS) injury (70), stroke (71), cardiovascular surgery (72), and the use of drugs (73,74). Sporadic tics, either motor or vocal, also occur in some patients with torsion dystonia, Huntington's disease, and neuroacanthocytosis. A lesion in the midbrain tegmentum has been suggested on the basis of resolution of tics following an abnormality to this area, caused by thiamine deficiency (75).

Glucose Metabolism and Blood Flow Studies in Cortex and Striatum

Corticostriatal glucose metabolism and blood flow studies have identified abnormalities within the basal ganglia and cortical areas in patients with TS. Examination by positron emission tomography (PET) following injection of [^{18}F]2-fluoro-2-deoxyglucose showed bilateral symmetrical increases or decreases of glucose utilization within the basal ganglia and decreased activity in frontal, cingulate, and insular cortices (76–78). In a study assessing functional coupling of regional cerebral metabolic rates for glucose, connectivity of the ventral striatum differentiated TS from control groups (79). TS subjects also had positive coupling between motor and orbitofrontal circuits.

Studies of cerebral blood flow by single photon emission computed tomography (SPECT) have identified hypoperfusion of the basal ganglia (80) and, in one report, a decreased blood flow to the left lenticular region (81). Comparison of perfusion imaging between children with chronic motor tics and TS showed decreased perfusion primarily affecting the left hemisphere in the TS group (82). Perfusion differences, however, were thought to be related to comorbid symptoms rather than tics. With use of a new cerebral blood flow imaging agent, Tc-99m-ECD, regional blood flows were found to be significantly lower, in the left caudate, cingulum, right cerebellum, and right and left dorsolateral prefrontal regions in 38 children with TS as compared to 18 controls (83). No correlation was detected between the severity of motor tics and blood flow, but there was a positive correlation between the severity of vocal tics and several regions. Functional neuroimaging of tics has been evaluated using event-related [^{15}O]H_2O PET combined with time-synchronized videotaping (84). Brain regions that significantly correlated with tic occurrence included medial and lateral premotor cortices, anterior cingulate cortex, dorsolateral-rostral prefrontal cortex, inferior parietal cortex, putamen, caudate, primary motor cortex, the Broca's area, superior temporal gyrus, insula, and claustrum. Which of these regions accounts for the initiation, rather than execution, of diverse motor and vocal behaviors remains unknown.

Volumetric Magnetic Resonance Imaging Studies

Direct evidence for pathophysiological involvement of cortico-striatal-thalamo-cortical circuits in TS is provided from volumetric MRI studies. Several structural studies have been reported that show that either the caudate or the lenticular nuclei are abnormal in volume or asymmetry compared to control subject (85–88). For example, one study showed significant differences in the symmetry of the putamen; that is, TS patients have a right-sided predominance, whereas a left-sided predominance was observed in controls (87). MRI studies have shown that the corpus callosum was abnormal in individuals with TS, predominantly males (Fig. 4) (88–90). In a study of children with TS and ADHD, symptom-dependent changes were present in the rostral area of the corpus callosum; the diagnosis of TS was associated with significant increases in size and ADHD with significant decreases in size (89). Since the rostral callosum carries interhemispheric connections, a larger or smaller region suggests disruption of communication between frontal lobes with a likely alteration in hemispheral function. Of interest is the subsequent finding

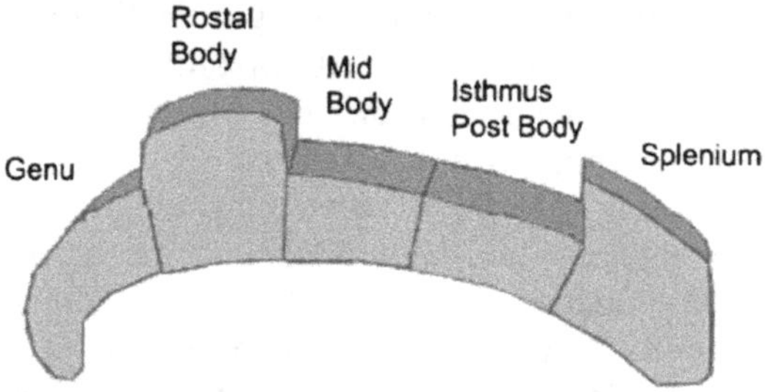

Figure 4 Diagrammatic representation corpus callosum area measurement. MRI study of corpus callosum in a primarily male population found increased size in rostral body and spelium in TS patients as compared to control subjects. (From Ref. 89.)

that differences in basal ganglia asymmetry or volume as well as changes in the corpus callosum do not distinguish girls with TS from matched controls (91,92). Several recent studies have further assessed the importance of cortical inputs to basal ganglia structures by comparing the volumes of various cortical brain regions in TS to those in controls. One investigation showed the dorsal prefrontal and parieto-occipital regions to be larger in TS (93), whereas others identified differences in cortical white matter; for example, the right frontal lobe has a larger percentage of white matter (94) or volumetric decreases are present in the deep left frontal white matter (95). Changes in white matter, especially deep white matter, suggest that abnormalities are present in long association and projection fiber bundles.

Functional Magnetic Resonance Imaging

Preliminary functional MRI studies have suggested that the pathogenesis of tics involves neuronal activity within subcortical neuronal circuits. Investigators have compared images acquired during periods of voluntary tic suppression with those acquired when subjects were allowed spontaneous expression of their tics (96). Results showed significant changes in signal intensity between paradigms in the basal ganglia and thalamus as well as in connected cortical regions. The magnitude of regional signal change in the basal ganglia and thalamus correlated inversely with tic severity. On the basis of these studies, it has been suggested that voluntary tic suppression involves activation of the prefrontal cortex and caudate and bilateral deactivation of the putamen and globus pallidus (96). Other investigators have studied activation of the sensorimotor cortex during a standard motor task paradigm to determine whether an abnormal organization of motor functions could be detected in TS patients (97). Functional MRI imaging of five patients with TS during repetitive finger tapping showed an increased area of cerebral activation in both sensorimotor cortex and supplementary motor area as compared to healthy subjects. These data support the suggestion that cortico-striatal-thalamo-cortical pathways contribute to the pathogenesis of TS. Functional imaging during the performance of manipulative tasks in TS patients showed greatly reduced activation of secondary motor areas as compared with those at baseline (98). Equal metabolic activity in these areas during rest and task performance suggests that these areas are continuously involved in movement preparation.

Oculomotor Paradigms

Oculomotor testing has been used to investigate the mechanism by which the brain controls movement in TS (Fig. 5) (99–102). Neurophysiologically, the control of various types of saccades has been attributed to different cerebral areas; the frontal eye field and posterior parietal cortex are associated with

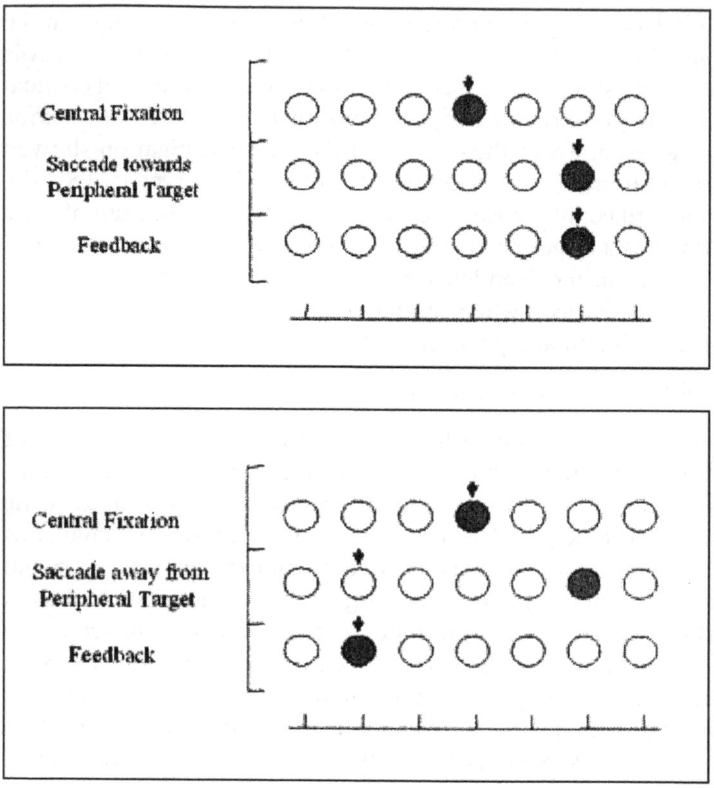

Figure 5 Diagrammatic representation of eye movement protocol. Subjects sit in front of a tangent screen, on which an array of light-emitting diodes appeared at 10°, 20°, and 30° to the right and left of center. Top: prosaccade paradigm. Subjects were instructed to change their gaze to the peripheral target light as soon as it appeared. The paradigm tested the subject's ability to initiate saccades to a suddenly appearing, unpredictable visual stimulus as measured by latency. Bottom: antisaccade paradigm. This paradigm was used to test for the ability to inhibit a prosaccade. The subject was instructed to look in the direction *opposite* to the target, at its mirror location in the opposite visual field. The number of errors and latency of movement was measured. Oculomotor findings suggest that TS is associated with delay in initiation of motor response as evidenced by prolonged latency on prosaccade testing. (From Ref. 101.)

initiating saccades; the dorsolateral prefrontal cortex, supplementary eye field, and cingulate cortex are involved with more volitional and cognitive aspects of saccade control; and all of the aforementioned areas interact with the basal ganglia. Thus findings of delays in initiating a motor response to a visual stimulus in TS, as evidenced by prolonged latency on prosaccades, are believed to be secondary to abnormalities in circuits involving motor/premotor cortices (including frontal eye field). In contrast, the presence of comorbid ADHD appears to be associated with deficits in inhibiting looking toward the stimulus during an antisaccade task and excessive variability in motor response to a visual stimulus (101). Anatomically, these excessive directional antisaccade errors are most likely related to dysfunction of the dorsolateral prefrontal cortex or caudate (103,104).

SPECIFIC PATHWAY HYPOTHESES IN TOURETTE'S SYNDROME

In general, current pathophysiological hypotheses for TS are defined at several levels of specificity, i.e., neuroanatomical localization, physiological abnormality, and neurochemical basis. For example, neuroanatomical proposals include abnormalities within specific portions of the cortico-striatal-thalamo-cortical pathway or specific regions within the striatum, e.g., striosomes. At the physiological level, the two most common hypotheses are disinhibited afferent thalamocortical signals or impaired inhibition at the cortical level. The final pathophysiological level attempts to define hypotheses on the presence of specific abnormalities at the cellular level, i.e., a neurochemical basis.

Neuroanatomical Basis

Cortico-Striatal-Thalamo-Cortical Pathway Abnormality

Over the years, investigators have suggested that TS may be produced by alterations within the basal ganglia, by abnormalities of its major fiber pathways, and by lesions in other brain regions that have prominent interconnections with the basal ganglia, i.e., cortico-striatal-thalamo-cortical circuits (2,105). An important aspect of a circuit hypothesis is that lesions in one part (e.g., globus pallidus) of a circuit could produce signs and symptoms similar to those caused by a lesion in another region of the circuit (e.g., prefrontal cortex). Hence analogous to the situation at a racetrack, a poor showing (or abnormal behavior) could result from an abnormal circuit, with the problem arising anywhere within the oval (frontal lobe, basal ganglia, or thalamus).

The major focus in this pathway, however, has been on the striatothalamic circuit, i.e., direct and indirect pathways from the striatum to GPi neurons, which act similar to a brake or an accelerator. As previously discussed, these parallel pathways have opposing effects on GABAergic GPi output neurons (i.e., the direct pathway inhibits and the indirect pathway stimulates) and, in turn, a reverse effect on thalamocortical (VA-VL) neurons. In sum, it is hypothesized that disinhibition of excitatory neurons in the thalamus results in hyperexcitability of cortical motor areas and the release of tics.

Striatal Compartment (Striosomes/Matrix) Abnormality

Both striatal compartments (striosomes and matrix): 1) receive specific cortical afferents (striosomes receive convergent limbic and prelimbic inputs, and the matrix receives converging inputs from ipsilateral motor and sensorimotor cortices and contralateral primary motor cortex); 2) are innervated by distinct subcortical afferents (cholinergic and aspiny GABA interneurons play intermediary roles); and 3) have a preferential distribution of axons (striosomes to SNpc and matrix to the globus pallidus) (Fig. 6). Recognizing that TS is considered by many to be a developmental disorder, it is of interest to note that there are changes in the density of neurotransmitter uptake sites and receptors in certain compartments during the development of the striatum (106). The striosome–matrix organization implies a level of functional segregation that could be important to the understanding of TS. What remains unknown, however, is how this organization translates to specific symptoms.

Suggestions that a compartment abnormality may be involved in TS have been based on studies assessing the pathobiology of motor stereotypies (involuntary, patterned, coordinated, repetitive, seemingly purposeful, rhythmic, and suppressible movements). Pathophysiologically, the nigrostriatal system has a major role in the production of stereotypies; that is, movements can be induced in response to directly acting dopamine agonists (apomorphine) or to indirectly acting dopamine receptor agonists (amphetamine, cocaine) (107,108). Combined activation of both D_1 and D_2 receptors is required to induce stereotypies (109,110), and the behavioral effect can be blocked by dopamine receptor antagonists (108). In response to dopamine agonists, investigators have identified a variety of changes affecting components of dopamine neurotransmission, second messengers, neuropeptides, and the expression of genes encoding specific transcription factors (14,15,111,112). Further monitoring of the inducibility of immediate-early genes for the Fos/Fra family of transcription factors subsequently led to the discovery of variations within the striosomal and matrix portion of the striatum (14,15). More specifically, the relative enhancement of striosome over matrix, especially in the anterior and lateral (sensorimotor) part of the striatum, was an excellent predictor of the amount of stereotypy. Extending

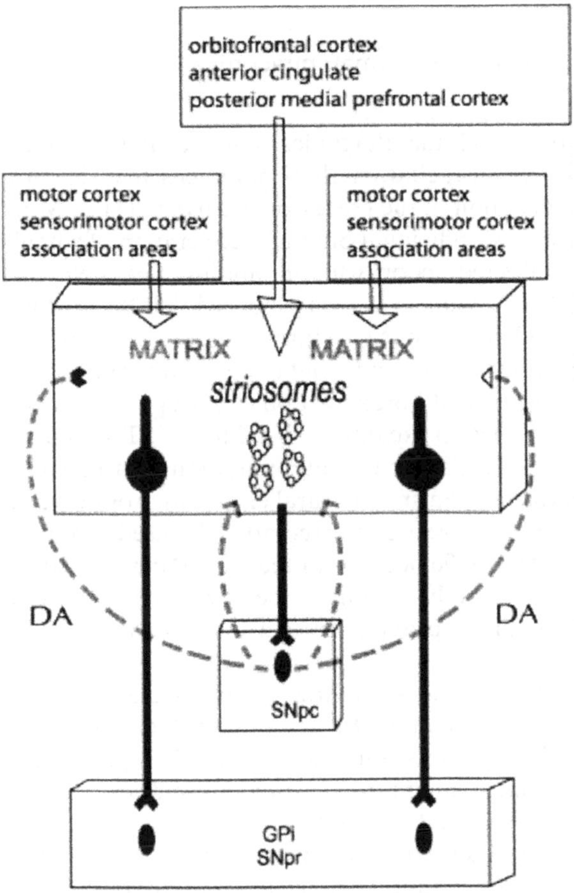

Figure 6 Striatal compartment abnormality hypothesis. The striatum can be divided into two components: striosomes and matrix. Striosomes innervate the SNpc, which in turn gives rise to the dopaminergic nigrostriatal tract. Abnormal striosomal activity has been found in the production of stereotypies and may have implications for tics. SNpc = substantia nigra pars compacta; DA = dopamine; D_1 = dopamine 1 receptor; D_2 = dopamine 2 receptor; SNpc = substantia nigra pars compacta; GPi = globus pallidus interna; SNpr = substantia nigra pars reticulata.

the striosome/matrix hypothesis to tics, Mink (113) has hypothesized that overactivity in the matrisome can cause tics. More specifically, their abnormal activity could result in unwanted inhibitions of GPi or SNpr neurons that are normally active in suppressing unwanted movements. Hence inhibition of these motor activities in a discrete repetitive fashion could trigger an unwanted competing motor pattern, e.g., tic.

Physiological Abnormalities

Excess Thalamic Excitation or Abnormal Intracortical Inhibition

The basic tenet to most hypotheses is that the tonically active inhibitory GPi/SNpr output acts like a brake on excitatory thalamic nuclei that, in turn, influences motor pattern generation in the cortex or brainstem (113). More specifically, it is proposed that the individual braking/acceleration of specific motor patterns enables the desired action while inhibiting any competing actions. In an elegant hypothesis, Mink (113) has proposed that the anatomical arrangement of the subthalamic nucleus (an excitatory nucleus that receives cortical input from frontal areas) and striatal inputs to the GPi/SNpr form the basis for a "center-surround" organization. As proposed, cortical initiation of a movement generates an excitatory signal to the STN, and the STN then diffusely excites the GPi/SNpr causing inhibition of a thalamocortical and brainstem motor mechanism. In parallel, inputs from cortical areas projecting to the striatum are transferred to a focused, context-dependent output that inhibits specific neurons in the GPi/SNpr. The latter, slower but stronger pathway selectively disinhibits the desired motor pattern (Fig. 7). Lastly, the indirect pathway provides further focuses on the output signal.

Intracortical inhibitory pathways provide a second major site of proposed pathophysiological abnormality. In order to further investigate this possibility, transcranial magnetic stimulation (TMS) has provided a valuable approach. The two most common measures utilized are *prepulse inhibition* (PPI), aka intracortical inhibition (ratio of amplitude of motor action potential generated by a superthreshold stimulus to that after a conditioning paradigm that uses a subthreshold stimulus followed by a standard suprathreshold stimulus), and *cortical silent period* (period of electrical silence after the TMS-evoked motor-evoked potential (MEP) in a voluntarily contracted muscle). Although TMS results are somewhat variable among TS studies, all showed either a reduced PPI and/or shortened cortical silent period (114–116). These findings suggest that tics originate from either a primarily subcortical disorder affecting the motor cortex through disinhibited afferent signals, from impaired inhibition directly at the level of the motor cortex, or both.

Neurochemical Basis

Specific Neurotransmitter Abnormality

Neurochemical hypotheses tend to be based on extrapolations from clinical trials evaluating the response to specific medications, from CSF, blood, and

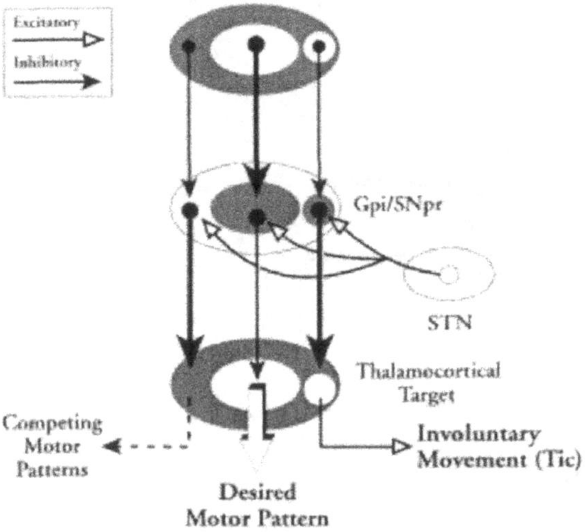

Figure 7 Excess thalamic excitation hypothesis. Mink has proposed that the anatomic arrangement of the subthalamic nucleus and striatal inputs to the GPi/SNpr form the basis for a "center-surround" organization. See text for further discussion. GPi = globus pallidus pars interna; SNpr = substantia nigra pars reticulata; STN = subthalamic nucleus. (From Ref. 113.)

urine studies in relatively small numbers of patients, from neurochemical assays on a few postmortem brain tissues, and from PET/SPECT studies. Most neurotransmitters involved in cortico-striatal-thalamo-cortical circuitry, including the dopaminergic (DA), glutamatergic, GABAergic, serotonergic, cholinergic, noradrenergic, and opioid systems, have all been implicated (105,117). Which, if any, of these proposals represents the primary pathological factor remains to be definitively determined. Although the authors' bias is that the DA system has a significant role, because many transmitter systems are interrelated in the production of complex actions, it is indeed possible, if not probable, that imbalances exist within several transmitter systems.

Dopamine: The possibility of a dopaminergic abnormality in TS continues to receive strong consideration because of the therapeutic response to neuroleptics, preliminary data from postmortem studies, and a variety of nuclear imaging protocols (105,118,119). If TS is associated with excess nigrostriatal dopaminergic activity, whether via supersensitive dopamine receptors, dopamine hyperinnervation, or abnormal presynaptic terminal function, a significant hyperkinetic effect is expected (Fig. 8). As

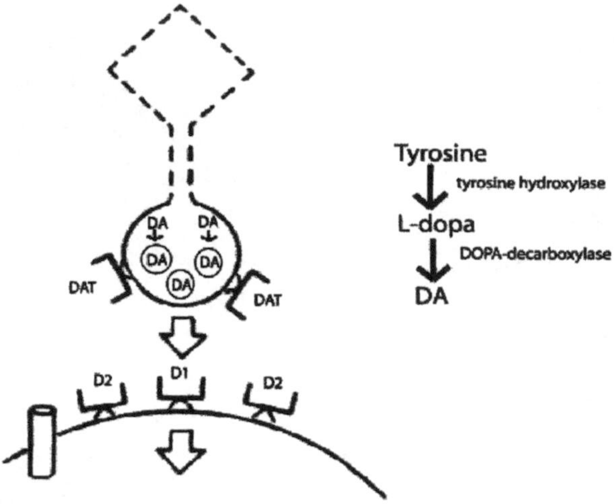

Figure 8 Dopaminergic synapse: possible abnormality in TS. Hypothesized dopaminergic abnormalities include 1) receptor abnormality; 2) dopamine hyper-innervation; and 3) abnormal presynaptic terminal function. DA = dopamine; DAT = dopamine transporter; DRD1 = dopamine receptor D_1; DRD2 = dopamine receptor D_2.

noted previously, excitatory D_1 dopamine receptors are expressed mainly on striatal MSSN of the direct pathway and inhibitory D_2 receptors on MSSN of the indirect pathway. Activation of D_1 receptors is excitatory to the movement-releasing direct pathway, whereas activation of D_2 receptors inhibits the indirect pathway that, in turn, inhibits movement. Hence the result of either action is the disinhibition of excitatory neurons in the thalamus that, in turn, could cause hyperexcitability or disinhibition of cortical motor areas and the release of tics. In addition to short-term effects, DA can modulate corticostriatal transmission by the mechanism of long-term depression or potentiation (120–122). This modulation either strengthens or weakens the efficacy of corticostriatal synapses and can, in turn, mediate reinforcement of specific discharge patterns (113). DA-induced fluctuating abnormalities in the resting potential of striatal neurons have been hypothesized to influence tic waxing and waning and also explain the lack of identifiable abnormality in DA transmission (113). Lastly, besides the important role of dopamine in the "two-pathway system," it also has an essential role in the learning process suggested in the striosome circuit (15,123).

Supersensitive postsynaptic dopamine receptors. The possibility of abnormal postsynaptic receptors was initially suggested by findings of reduced basal and turnover levels of a dopamine metabolite, homovanillic acid, in cerebrospinal fluid that were restored to normal after the administration of haloperidol (124–126). Limited studies of D_1 and D_2 receptor binding in postmortem striatal tissue have shown trends, but no significant differences between TS and control subjects (119). Investigations of D_2 dopamine receptors by PET and SPECT have produced inconsistent findings in studies comparing TS patients and controls (127–130). Two studies support the hypothesis that the dopamine receptor is involved in the neurobiology of TS. In a study of five sets of identical twins, increased binding of [^{123}I]iodobenzamide ([^{123}I]-IBZM) was observed in the head of the caudate nucleus in association with increased tic severity (129). In our PET study with a spiperone derivative, 3-N [^{11}C]methylspiperone, Bmax levels above the 95th percentile prediction limit (normal regressed against age) were observed in 4 of 20 adult subjects, and multiple linear regression analyses revealed a trend between the severity of vocal tics and Bmax values (130). In contrast to these studies reporting changes of D_2 receptors, others using [^{123}I]IBZM or [^{11}C]raclopride did not show differences (127,128).

Dopamine hyperinnervation. Attempts to provide support for postulated dopamine hyperinnervation (increased number of dopamine terminals) by PET or SPECT binding have resulted in conflicting reports. For example, a study of five adults with TS that used [^{123}I]β-CIT SPECT found that striatal dopamine transporter (DAT) binding was higher than in controls (131). In a second study, with a similar technique, the mean striatal activity ratio was significantly higher in TS patients and 5/12 TS subjects showed striatum/occipital cortex ratios more than 2 standard deviations above the normal mean (132). In contrast, other investigators using SPECT or PET techniques in adult patients with TS showed no difference in DAT binding as compared to controls (133–135). Evaluation of dorsal striatal dopaminergic innervation by use of in vivo measures of vesicular monoamine transporter type 2 (VMAT2) binding with the ligand (+)-alpha-[^{11}C]dihydrotetrabenazine showed no differences between TS subjects and age-compatible normal controls (136). These results suggest that there is no increased striatal innervation, but do not exclude an abnormality in the regulation of dopamine release or reuptake.

Presynaptic dopaminergic abnormality. A presynaptic dopamine abnormality involving dopa decarboxylase activity has been proposed. In a PET study, 11 adolescents with TS accumulated [^{18}F]fluorodopa at a level 25% higher in the left caudate nucleus and 53% higher in the right midbrain compared with levels in control subjects (137). The authors suggest that upregulation of dopa decarboxylase activity could explain these alterations and that the process reflects deficits in a variety of functional elements of the dopamine system.

Elevated intrasynaptic dopamine release. In order to evaluate dopamine release in TS, we pretreated seven adults with TS and five age-matched comparison subjects with intravenously administered amphetamine, a central stimulant that enhances dopamine release and blocks its reuptake, and with saline (138). Each subject underwent two [^{11}C]raclopride PET scans: one after intravenous pretreatment with saline and the second after intravenously administered amphetamine to induce dopamine release (Fig. 9). In the putamen, after amphetamine challenge, the mean value of intrasynaptic dopamine determined by the TREMBLE method for TS subjects was increased by 21% and for controls was reduced by 0.02% ($p = 0.04$). Dopamine release was not significantly different in the caudate region. Explanations for the higher intrasynaptic dopamine levels in the putamen of TS subjects after amphetamine stimulation are speculative. Among several possibilities are an increased release of dopamine from the presynaptic terminal secondary to a localized defect in the release mechanism, a lack of presynaptic inhibition, an increased firing of presynaptic neurons, or a functional defect in dopamine

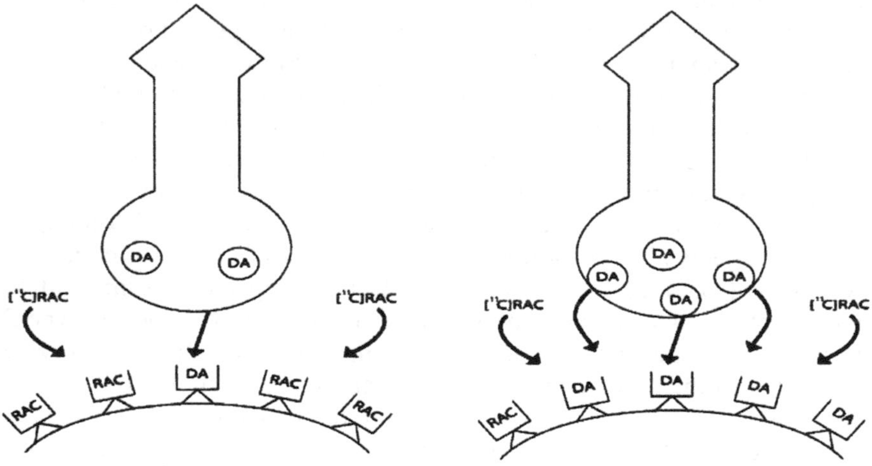

Figure 9 Elevated intrasynaptic dopamine release hypothesis PET study. Each subject underwent two [^{11}C]raclopride PET scans. (Left) saline + [^{11}C]raclopride; RAC competes with endogenous synaptic DA. (Right) amphetamine + [^{11}C]raclopride challenge; increased levels of DA induced by the stimulant compete with RAC. Larger percentage reductions in RAC binding between postsaline and postamphetamine scans were found in the putamen of TS subjects when compared with controls, indicating greater dopamine release. (From Ref. 138.)

reuptake from the synaptic cleft. An alternative unifying hypothesis, which we favor, involves the tonic-phasic model of dopamine release (139). Tonic dopamine, which exists extracellularly in low concentration, determines the long-term or homeostatic mechanism. This "basal" level of dopamine is defined primarily as an extrasynaptic measure and is calculated by use of microdialysis and electrophysiological measurements. Dopamine autoreceptors (D_2 and D_3 subtypes) are proposed as regulators of tonic dopamine control (140). Phasic dopamine is the spike-dependent dopamine released primarily into the synapse. It can escape the synaptic cleft with sufficient stimulation or when an uptake blocker is given in high concentrations. Intrasynaptic dopamine release induced by the use of stimulant challenges, such as with amphetamine, has been proposed as a surrogate measurement for phasic dopamine.

Clinical and imaging studies, including our dopamine release data, are consistent with the possibility that the underlying pathobiology in TS is an abnormal regulation of the phasic dopamine response resulting in a hyperresponsive spike-dependent dopaminergic system. The basic mechanism proposed for alteration of the phasic dopamine is a decrease in tonic dopamine levels. Although there are other potential explanations (e.g., decreased phasic overflow from the synaptic cleft to the extracellular space or diminished cortical afferent input), we believe that decreased tonic dopamine levels are secondary to increased activity of the dopamine transporter since the reuptake transporter determines the concentration of extrasynaptic dopamine. Hence we have proposed that the essential underlying mechanism in TS could be an overactive dopamine transporter system (138). This situation would create reduced levels of extracellular dopamine, higher concentrations of dopamine in the axon terminal, increased stimulus-dependent dopamine release, autoreceptor supersensitivity at the presynaptic site, and increased sensitivity to low-dose neuroleptics. Several clinical findings in TS patients support the overactive dopamine transporter hypothesis. For example, the exacerbation of tics by stimulant medications (141,142) could be secondary to greater dopamine release from the axon terminal. Environmental stimuli, such as stress, anxiety, and medications, well known to exacerbate tics, have been shown to increase phasic bursts of dopamine. Lastly, tic suppression with very low doses of neuroleptics (143) may occur because a reduced amount of tonic dopamine is available for the neuroleptic to block.

Glutamate: Glutamate is the excitatory neurotransmitter of corticostriatal neurons, output neurons from the subthalamic nucleus, and thalamostriatal and thalamocortical projections. Very limited data are available to assess adequately the potential role of glutamate in TS. Reduced levels of this amino acid were detected in four postmortem TS samples in GPi,

GPe, and SNpr (144). Since, in the same study, levels of glutamate and aspartate were normal in a variety of cortical regions, further studies are necessary to clarify the meaning of glutamate changes. Based on the reduction of glutamate in pallidal areas and MRI volumetric studies showing reduction in the size of the left globus pallidus, a role for reduced subthalamic nucleus glutamate output (either excessive inhibition from GPe projections or a primary developmental abnormality of the STN) has been proposed (144,145). In the latter hypothesis, reduced STN glutamate would result in diminished excitation of the inhibitory GPi/SNpr and ultimately increased thalamocortical excitation.

Gamma-aminobutyric acid: GABAergic MSSN are the primary projection neurons from the striatum for both striato-GPi (direct) and striato-GPe (indirect) pathways. It has been hypothesized that in TS, a decrease in striatal GABAergic projections involving both the direct and indirect pathway would, in turn, cause insufficient inhibition of excitatory thalamocortical neurons, with the ultimate result being increased glutamatergic cortical excitation, and tic behavior. A second proposed GABAergic mechanism for tic production is an impairment of cortical inhibition of thalamocortical afferent signals. This deficiency has been hypothesized to be secondary to reduced activity of GABAergic interneurons. Despite the described specificity of the aforementioned hypotheses, there are a few data to support an abnormality of GABA in TS. Benzodiazepines, which enhance the inhibitory effect of GABA, have some efficacy in tic suppression (146). Nevertheless, the activity of glutamate decarboxylase, the highly specific presynaptic marker for GABAergic interneurons in the cerebral cortex, is normal in postmortem cortex (147), as are levels of GABA in various brain regions, whole blood, and CSF (144,145,148). From a developmental perspective, both GABAergic MSSN and many cortical GABAergic interneurons migrate from similar embryonic regions in the ganglionic eminence (149). It has therefore been postulated in TS that a single adverse event during development could affect both striatal and cortical inhibitory function (150).

Serotonin: Serotonergic fibers project from the medial raphe to the striatum, substantia nigra, and cortex. In OCD, pharmacological studies strongly support a role for serotonin in causing these symptoms. Hence since OCD is common in TS, there has been a concerted effort to assess this neurotransmitter in this population. In CSF studies, 5-hydroxyindole acetic acid (5-HIAA), the principal metabolite of serotonin, is reduced in some, but not all, patients with TS (124–126,151). Levels of this metabolite in the cerebral cortex are normal (147), whereas tryptophan and 5-HIAA may be globally decreased in basal ganglia regions (144,145). Plasma tryptophan, whole-blood serotonin, and 24-hr excretion of serotonin have also been reported to be reduced in TS subjects (151,152). A β-CIT SPECT binding study has reported a negative correlation between overall tic severity and binding in the midbrain (serotonergic receptors) and thalamus (serotonin or noradrenergic receptors) (133). There was no overall reduction in density of serotonin transporters in TS patients. The authors suggest that serotonergic transmission is a modifying, but not causal, factor in the pathogenesis of tics.

Second Messenger System Abnormality

Identification of a postreceptor defect involving a second messenger system could potentially explain the presence of reported abnormalities within a variety of neurotransmitter systems in TS. For example, for multiple neurotransmitters, an interaction exists with adenosine 3′,5′-monophosphate (cAMP): D_1 and α-adrenergic receptors activate adenylate cyclase activity, whereas opiate (μ and δ), α-2-adrenergic, D_2, serotonergic (5-HT_{1A}), and muscarinic (M4) receptors inhibit cyclase activity (Fig. 10). Hence an abnormality involving a second messenger could unify findings of alterations within multiple transmitter systems. In a small number of postmortem brain samples from individuals with TS, amounts of cAMP were 34–56% of normal in frontal, temporal, and occipital cortices and 23% of normal in the putamen (119,147). In a follow-up study evaluating specific steps involved in the

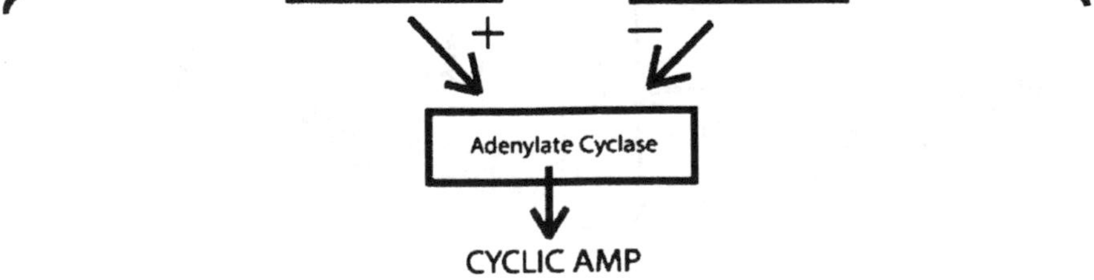

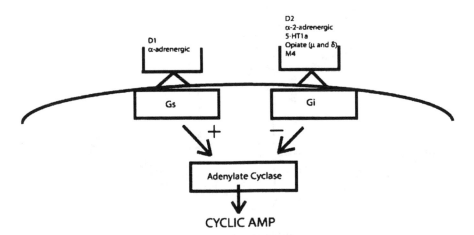

Figure 10 Second messenger system abnormality hypothesis. Multiple neurotransmitters interact with the second messenger system utilizing adenosine 3′,5′-monophosphate (cyclic AMP). Postmortem studies have shown some increase of control cAMP but follow-up studies have not supported an important role for second messenger systems (205). D_1 = dopamine 1 receptor; D_2 = dopamine 2 receptor; 5-HT_{1A} = serotonergic receptor; M4 = muscarinic 4 receptor; Gs = stimulatory G protein; Gi = inhibitory G protein.

production and catabolism of cAMP as well as binding of [^{3}H]inositol 1,4,5-triphosphate (IP_3) to IP_3 receptors and [^{3}H]phorbol ester to protein kinase C, phosphatidylinositol second messenger generating systems were not thought to be major contributing factors in the development of TS (153).

Vesicular Docking Protein Abnormality

Because PET studies suggested a possible abnormality in neurotransmitter release, the relative binding of vesicle-docking proteins has been investigated. This first step in vesicle release involves synaptic vesicle-docking proteins, known as the SNARE (soluble *N*-ethylmaleimide-sensitive factor attachment protein receptors) proteins (Fig. 11). The vesicle-SNARE (v-SNARE) VAMP-2 (also called synaptobrevin), found on the vesicle membrane, forms a complex with the presynaptic target membrane SNAREs (t-SNAREs) SNAP-25 and syntaxin. Fusion of the three SNARE proteins, along with synaptotagmin, which is thought to act as a calcium sensor, into a vesicle-docking complex mediates vesicle fusion and release. Western blotting assays

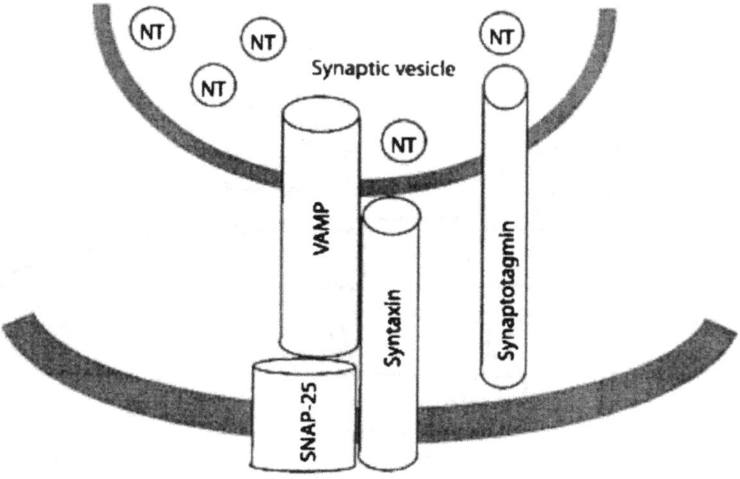

Figure 11 Vesicular docking complex and associated proteins. SNARE (soluble *N*-ethylmaleimide-sensitive factor attachment protein receptors) proteins VAMP-2, SNAP-25, and syntaxin form the vesicle-docking complex along with synaptotagmin. Using a semiquantitative analysis, Western blotting assays run on postmortem TS and control brain tissue have shown some alterations in these proteins. (From Ref. 154.)

run on postmortem TS ($n = 3$) and control ($n = 3$) brain tissue have not shown consistent changes in vesicle-docking protein expression (154).

IS THERE A NEUROIMMUNOLOGICAL BASIS FOR TIC DISORDERS?

Since most experts concur that TS is an inherited disorder, why do we even consider the possibility of an environmentally related tic disorder? For example, strong support for a genetic etiology of chronic tic disorders is derived from an 86% concordance rate in monozygotic twins compared with a rate of only 20% in dizygotic twins (155,156). One answer to the aforementioned question is that further evaluation of these same monozygotic twins identified that genotype does not predict phenotype; for example, twins show great variability in the frequency and severity of tic symptoms. Further evidence that epigenetic factors and gene–environment interactions play an important role in determining tic severity in TS has been provided by multiple investigators (157–160).

A hypothesized role for environmental factors, especially infections, in the presentation or exacerbation of neuropsychiatric diseases, such as tics and OCD, is not a new phenomenon (161–164). Proposals of relationships between tics and infectious agents are not limited to Group A β-hemolytic streptococcal infection (GABHS), but have also been reported in isolated cases following acute infections with *Streptococcus pyogenes*, Lyme borreliosis, and *Mycoplasma pneumoniae* (165–167). More specific hypotheses suggesting that tic disorders represent immune phenomena are derived primarily based from the model proposed for Sydenham's chorea (SC). In this latter condition, antibodies produced against GABHS are believed to cross-react with neuronal tissue through the process of molecular mimicry (Fig. 12). But are SC, TS (chronic tic disorder), and pediatric autoimmune neuropsychiatric disorder associated with streptococcal infection (acronym PANDAS) the same and is there sufficient confirmatory evidence for an autoimmune mechanism in any of these disorders?

Defining Separate Disorders

The importance of correctly defining the clinical disorder is based on the fact that some investigators have attempted to use studies in one disorder to support findings in a different entity. For example, studies of antistreptococcal or antibasal ganglia antibodies in classical TS patients have been proposed as evidence supporting the existence of PANDAS. Hence a critical starting point for the assessment of existing data is a brief review of the disorders under consideration.

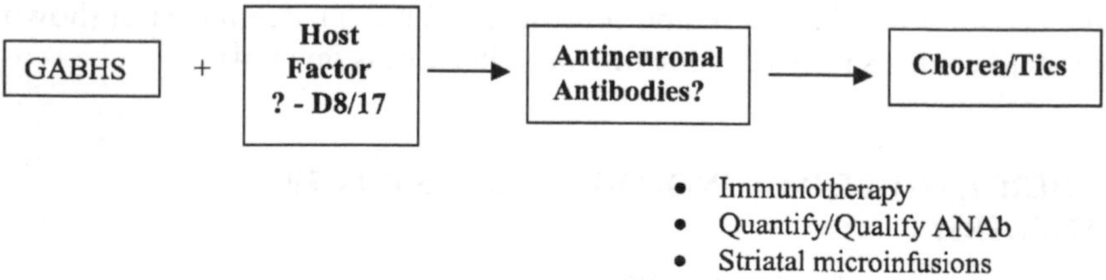

Figure 12 Proposed mechanism for autoimmune neurologic disorders. Antibodies against Group A β-hemolytic streptococci (GABHS), in the presence of a host-derived factor, cross-react with striatal neurons, resulting in clinical symptoms (tics, chorea). Attempts to confirm an autoimmune mechanism have included results from immunotherapy, quantification of antineuronal antibodies, and striatal micro-infusions.

1. Sydenham's chorea is considered the prototype for an infectious agent triggering an autoimmune disorder that, in turn, causes a variety of neuropsychiatric symptoms. SC has a clearly defined association with rheumatic fever (168) and connection with a preceding GABHS infection (169). It typically occurs between the ages of 5 and 15 years, and a female predominance has been observed in large studies. The distinguishing clinical feature of this disorder is the presence of chorea that ranges in severity, is usually generalized, and typically involves the face and extremities. Most patients have concomitant psychological dysfunction presenting as personality changes, obsessive-compulsive symptoms, emotional irritability, distractibility, and age-regressed behaviors (170,171). Motor or vocal tics and oculogyric crises have also been reported in patients with SC (172,173). The outcome in SC is quite favorable; most cases resolve in 1–6 months, although mild to moderate chorea may persist (174).

2. Tourette's syndrome characteristics have been extensively discussed in this text and are typified by a childhood onset, waxing and waning course, evolving involuntary motor and vocal tics, and a time course of greater than 1 year. Tics are exacerbated by stress, anxiety, and fatigue and may improve during activities that require concentration.

3. PANDAS (i.e., pediatric autoimmune neuropsychiatric disorders associated with streptococcal infection) was initially proposed to represent a subset of tic disorder (or OCD) patients (175). Its criteria include the presence of OCD and/or tic disorder, prepubertal age at onset, sudden, "explosive" onset of symptoms and/or a course of sudden exacerbations and remissions, a temporal relationship between symptoms and GABHS, and the presence of neurological abnormalities including hyperactivity and choreiform move-

ments. The existence of PANDAS has been supported by clinical, neuroradiographic, and laboratory studies. More specifically, additional cohorts have been described (176), familial studies showed that first-degree relatives of children with PANDAS have higher rates of tic disorders and OCD than those in the general population (177), volumetric analyses in children with PANDAS identified that the average size of the caudate, putamen, and globus pallidus was significantly larger in PANDAS than in healthy children (178), and a trait marker for susceptibility in rheumatic fever (the monoclonal antibody D8/17) has been found to have an expanded expression in individuals with PANDAS (179). Nevertheless, despite these findings, concerns have been raised about the existing clinical criteria used to define this disorder (180,181). A variety of diagnostic shortcomings for PANDAS have been identified, with the most important deficiency being the absence of a prospective epidemiological study confirming that an antecedent GABHS infection is associated with either the onset or exacerbation of tic disorders (or OCD). A review of other diagnostic concerns is discussed in detail in a recent publication (181).

Existing Evidence for or Against an Autoimmune Mechanism

Sydenham's chorea. The autoimmune hypothesis in SC is supported by the proposed success of immunomodulatory therapies (182,183) and the measurement of serum antineuronal antibodies. For the latter, investigators have quantified antineuronal antibodies using a variety of methodologies: immunofluorescent antibody staining in human caudate and subthalamic nuclei (171,184,185); direct immunofluorescence on unfixed frozen sections from rat striatum (186); and enzyme-linked immunosorbent assays (ELISA) on human postmortem basal ganglia tissue (187,188). In a study by Church et al. (187), positive antibasal ganglia antibodies (ABGA) were found in 95% of acute and 56% of persistent SC patients. Furthermore, in the same population, Western blotting identified IgG reactivity against basal ganglia proteins in all acute SC subjects (20/20) compared to an absence of binding in healthy controls (187). In a separate study, elevated ABGA were confirmed in SC patients and analysis of immunoblots showed significant differences in the mean binding patterns of SC and controls (Fig. 13) (188). In conclusion, although current data suggest an autoimmune process in SC, a specific disease-related brain autoantigen, with a monoclonal antibody that also cross-reacts with streptococcal proteins, has yet to be identified.

Tourette syndrome. In the TS population, antineuronal antibodies have been quantified by ELISA (against human basal ganglia and human neuroblastoma cells) and immunofluorescent (against human basal ganglia and rat striatum) methods (186,189–191). One ELISA study showed that, compared

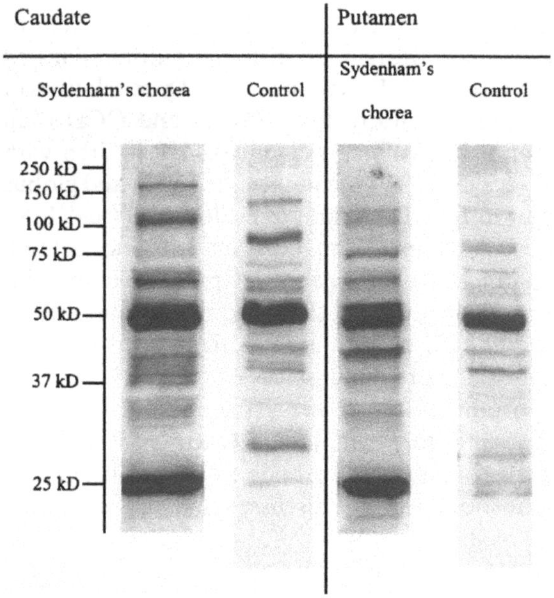

Figure 13 Western blotting of SC serum to human caudate and putamen. Antibasal ganglia antibody binding patterns are shown for SC patients and control subjects. Discriminant analysis of multiple bands showed significant differences in the mean binding patterns of SC and controls. (From Ref. 188).

with control subjects ($n=39$), children with TS ($n=41$) had a significant increase in the mean and median optical density (OD) levels of serum antibodies against the putamen, but not the caudate or globus pallidus (189). The authors, however, found no simple association between putamen ELISA OD levels and indicators of streptococcal infection. In addition, a risk ratio calculation for abnormal antistreptococcal titers in children with TS was similar to that in controls. Total antineural antibodies, measured by immunofluorescence on frozen sections of rat striatum, were higher in 81 subjects with TS (age 8–51 years) compared to controls. The difference in antibody titers, however, was not significant when children and adolescents with TS ($n=54$) were compared to normal controls (186).

Several studies using single-point-in-time measurements have shown higher mean antistreptolysin O (ASO) titers in patients with TS compared with controls (171,180,192). In one, ASO titers correlated with tic severity (192). In contrast, other investigators have shown no association between antistreptococcal antibodies and TS (193–195), but in one report, a correlation was identified with the diagnosis of ADHD (196). The necessity of longitudinal rather than single-point-in-time measurements to compare laboratory and clinical associations cannot be overemphasized.

Difficulties in interpreting measurements of total antineuronal antibody levels have prompted investigators to perform *Western blot analyses* in order to identify disease-specific changes in regional brain epitopes. Using a direct visual analysis, Singer et al. (189) showed that antibodies to caudate/putamen occurred more frequently in TS subjects at 83, 67, and 60 kDa. Using a similar approach, Trifiletti and Packard (197) confirmed the presence of a specific brain protein at an apparent molecular weight of 83 kDa that was recognized by antibodies in the serum of 80–90% of patients with TS or OCD. Recent methodological advances (e.g., multivariate analysis of discriminance) have enhanced the ability to detect and quantify minor changes in the antigenic composition of autoantibody repertoires. For example, a comparison between visual and discriminant techniques showed that numerous, rather than only three, molecular weight values contributed to the overall difference between TS and control antibody repertoires against striatal epitopes (198). Results from this study suggest that the 60-kDa region is representative of TS antibody repertoires, whereas antibodies against 83- and 67-kDa antigens did not differentiate as strongly between groups. Sequence analysis of the 60-kDa protein has identified it as a human heat shock protein, an antigenic structure that is not exclusive to neuronal tissue (Hoekstra et al., personal communication).

Since the presence of autoantibodies in the serum of TS patients does not imply causation (autoantibodies are also found in controls), *animal models* have been developed to study whether serum (IgG) can induce stereotypies that may be analogous to human tics in rodents. Cannulas are placed in regions of the neostriatum known to induce stereotypies, either serum or IgG is microinfused, and animals are observed for development of movements or utterances. Results from three studies have been intriguing but, unfortunately, inconsistent. Hallett et al. (199) infused dilute serum from five TS patients, with high antibody titers against human neuroblastoma, bilaterally into the lateral striatal region of the rat and showed a significant increase in stereotypic behaviors (e.g., licks and forepaw shakes) and episodic utterances in the TS group. Taylor et al. (200) infused serum from 12 TS patients, with high antibody titers against rat striatum, bilaterally into the ventrolateral striatal region of rats and showed a significant increase of oral stereotypies. Loiselle et al. (201) microinfused serum from five TS children, with high antibody titers against human postmortem putamen, bilaterally into the rodent ventral striatum and ventrolateral striatum. In this study, despite infusion of patient sera at the same coordinates used in the Hallett et al. and Taylor et al. protocols, no rat developed any audible abnormality and there was no significant increase in stereotypic behaviors. Further studies using TS sera are in progress. In summary, despite some data suggesting the possibility of an autoimmune mechanism in some cases with TS, strong consistent, confirmatory evidence is lacking as are data supporting involvement of streptococcal infection.

PANDAS. Despite the proposal that PANDAS is modeled after SC (e.g., an infectious agent, GABHS, triggering an autoimmune disorder) and there is an expanding list of proposed poststreptococcal autoimmune disorders [e.g., paroxysmal dyskinesias (193), acute disseminated encephalomyelitis (194), dystonia (195), myoclonus (202), and anorexia nervosa] (203), limited evidence exists confirming an autoimmune disorder. Support for this hypothesis is derived from a single study that examined the response of patients with PANDAS to two forms of immunomodulatory therapy, intravenous immunoglobulin (IVIG) and plasmapheresis (PEX) (204). Twenty-nine children with PANDAS, obtained from a nationwide search, were randomized in a partially double-blind fashion (no sham apheresis) to an IVIG, IVIG placebo (saline), and PEX group. One month after treatment, the severity of obsessive-compulsive symptoms (OCS) were improved by 58% and 45% in the PEX and IVIG groups, respectively, compared to only 3% in the IVIG control. In contrast, tic scores were only improved after PEX treatment, i.e., reductions of 49% (PEX), 19% (IVIG), and 12% (IVIG placebo). Improvements in both tics and OCS were sustained for 1 year.

Antibasal ganglia antibodies have been measured in 15 children with the diagnosis of PANDAS and compared to 15 controls (Singer et al., abstract). ELISA and Western immunoblotting methods were used to detect ABGA against supernatant, pellet, and synaptosomal preparations from adult postmortem caudate, putamen, and globus pallidus. ELISA optical density values did not differ between PANDAS patients and controls across all preparations. Immunoblotting identified multiple bands in all subjects with no significant differences in the number of bands or their total density. Discriminant analysis, used to assess mean immunoblotting binding patterns, showed that PANDAS patients differed from controls only for the caudate supernatant fraction, with PANDAS-primarily tic subjects providing the greatest discrimination. Among the epitopes contributing to differences between PANDAS and control in the caudate supernatant fraction, the epitope at 183 kDa was the most different between groups. In conclusion, ELISA measurements do not significantly differentiate between PANDAS and controls. Discriminant analysis of immunoblot curves assayed using a caudate supernatant fraction raises the possibility of different antibody repertoires in PANDAS subjects, especially in those who primarily have tics.

In preliminary rodent microinfusion studies, bilateral infusions of serum from children with classical PANDAS failed to induce dysfunction after injections into either lateral or ventrolateral rodent striatal sites (201).

SUMMARY

This chapter has presented neuroanatomical and physiological background for understanding current and future hypotheses pertaining to the neurobiology of TS. A variety of research approaches have been used to explore the underlying mechanisms of tic disorders. In summary, a growing body of evidence indicates that an abnormality in cortico-striatal-thalamo-cortical circuits and its neurotransmitter systems is likely to be associated with the clinical and comorbid characteristics in TS. Physiologically, theories include excess cortical excitement, deficient intracortical inhibition, or disruption of a center-surround organization. Neurochemically, evidence continues to support involvement of the dopamine system, but other transmitters within abnormal circuits may also be involved. Autoimmune-mediated mechanisms, based on results of immunomodulatory therapy and measurement of antineuronal antibodies, have been reported as possible candidates for a variety of movement disorders. Limited data from distinctly different disorders should not be merged, but rather considered as individual pieces of a large puzzle. To date, the strongest evidence for an immune disorder is available for SC. In TS, elevated antineuronal antibodies have been identified, but the precise correlation with symptomatology is lacking. Although PANDAS is an intriguing hypothesis, convincing evidence supporting an immune-mediated process is not yet available. Lastly, for TS, SC, and PANDAS, no specific disease-related brain autoantigen with a monoclonal antibody that also cross-reacts with streptococcal proteins has been identified. In conclusion, the precise neurobiological abnormality in TS remains undefined and an ongoing challenge.

ACKNOWLEDGMENTS

This is supported in part by a grant from the Tourette Syndrome Association. We thank Dr. Pamala Talalay for her review of the manuscript.

REFERENCES

1. dela Tourette G. Étude sur une affection nerveuse caractérisée par l'incoordination motrice accompagnée d'écholalie et de copralalie. Arch Neurol 1885; 9:19–42, 158–200.
2. Singer HS, Walkup JT. Tourette syndrome and other tic disorders: diagnosis, pathophysiology, and treatment. Medicine (Baltimore) 1991; 70:15–32.
3. Alexander GE, DeLong MR, Strick PL. Parallel organization of functionally segregated circuits linking basal ganglia and cortex. Annu Rev Neurosci 1986; 9:357–381.
4. Cummings JL. Frontal-subcortical circuits and human behavior. Arch Neurol 1993; 50:873–880.

5. Gerfen CR, Wilson CJ. The Basal Ganglia: Handbook of Chemical Neuroanatomy. Amsterdam: Elsevier, 1996.
6. Graybiel AM, Aosaki T, Flaherty AW, Kimura M. The basal ganglia and adaptive motor control. Science 1994; 265:1826–1831.
7. Schuerholz LJ, Singer HS, Denckla MB. Gender study of neuropsychological and neuromotor function in children with Tourette syndrome with and without attention-deficit hyperactivity disorder. J Child Neurol 1998; 13:277–282.
8. Georgopoulos AP, DeLong MR, Crutcher MD. Relations between parameters of step-tracking movements and single cell discharge in the globus pallidus and subthalamic nucleus of the behaving monkey. J Neurosci 1983; 3:1586–1598.
9. DeLong MR, Crutcher MD, Georgopoulos AP. Primate globus pallidus and subthalamic nucleus: functional organization. J Neurophysiol 1985; 53:530–543.
10. Smith Y, Bevan MD, Shink E, Bolam JP. Microcircuitry of the direct and indirect pathways of the basal ganglia. Neuroscience 1998; 86:353–387.
11. Filion M. Physiologic basis of dyskinesia. Ann Neurol 2000; 47:S35–S40. Discussion S40–1.
12. Parent A, Hazrati LN. Functional anatomy of the basal ganglia. I. The cortico-basal ganglia-thalamo-cortical loop. Brain Res Brain Res Rev 1995; 20:91–127.
13. Parent A, Hazrati LN. Functional anatomy of the basal ganglia. II. The place of subthalamic nucleus and external pallidum in basal ganglia circuitry. Brain Res Brain Res Rev 1995; 20:128–154.
14. Graybiel AM, Canales JJ, Capper-Loup C. Levodopa-induced dyskinesias and dopamine-dependent stereotypies: a new hypothesis. Trends Neurosci 2000; 23:S71–S77.
15. Canales JJ, Graybiel AM. A measure of striatal function predicts motor stereotypy. Nat Neurosci 2000; 3:377–383.
16. Brown LL, Feldman SM, Smith DM, Cavanaugh JR, Ackermann RF, Graybiel AM. Differential metabolic activity in the striosome and matrix compartments of the rat striatum during natural behaviors. J Neurosci 2002; 22:305–314.
17. Olson L, Seiger A, Fuxe K. Heterogeneity of striatal and limbic dopamine innervation: highly fluorescent islands in developing and adult rats. Brain Res 1972; 44:283–288.
18. Pert CB, Kuhar MJ, Snyder SH. Opiate receptor: autoradiographic localization in rat brain. Proc Natl Acad Sci USA 1976; 73:3729–3733.
19. Graybiel AM, Ragsdale CW Jr. Histochemically distinct compartments in the striatum of human, monkeys, and cat demonstrated by acetylthiocholinesterase staining. Proc Natl Acad Sci USA 1978; 75:5723–5726.
20. Graybiel AM, Ragsdale CW Jr. Clumping of acetylcholinesterase activity in the developing striatum of the human fetus and young infant. Proc Natl Acad Sci USA 1980; 77:1214–1218.
21. Gerfen CR. The neostriatal mosaic: multiple levels of compartmental organization in the basal ganglia. Annu Rev Neurosci 1992; 15:285–320.
22. Graybiel AM. Neurotransmitters and neuromodulators in the basal ganglia. Trends Neurosci 1990; 13:244–254.

23. Di Chiara G, Morelli M, Consolo S. Modulatory functions of neurotransmitters in the striatum: ACh/dopamine/NMDA interactions. Trends Neurosci 1994; 17:228–233.
24. Calabresi P, Pisani A, Mercuri NB, Bernardi G. The corticostriatal projection: from synaptic plasticity to dysfunctions of the basal ganglia. Trends Neurosci 1996; 19:19–24.
25. Delfs JM, Schreiber L, Kelley AE. Microinjection of cocaine into the nucleus accumbens elicits locomotor activation in the rat. J Neurosci 1990; 10:303–310.
26. Sacks OW. Acquired Tourettism in adult life. Adv Neurol 1982; 35:89–92.
27. Wohlfart GID, Hellberg AM. Compulsory shouting (Benedek's klazomania) associated with oculogyric spasms in chronic epidemic encephalitis. Acta Psychiatr Scand 1961; 36:369–377.
28. Rauch SL, Baer L, Cosgrove GR, Jenike MA. Neurosurgical treatment of Tourette's syndrome: a critical review. Compr Psychiatry 1995; 36:141–156.
29. Sheppard DM, Bradshaw JL, Georgiou N, Bradshaw JA, Lee P. Movement sequencing in children with Tourette's syndrome and attention deficit hyperactivity disorder. Mov Disord 2000; 15:1184–1193.
30. Serrien DJ, Nirkko AC, Loher TJ, Lovblad KO, Burgunder JM, Wiesendanger M. Movement control of manipulative tasks in patients with Gilles de la Tourette syndrome. Brain 2002; 125:290–300.
31. Sheppard DM, Bradshaw JL, Mattingley JB. Abnormal line bisection judgements in children with Tourette's syndrome. Neuropsychologia 2002; 40:253–259.
32. Lou HC, Henriksen L, Bruhn P, Borner H, Nielsen JB. Striatal dysfunction in attention deficit and hyperkinetic disorder. Arch Neurol 1989; 46:48–52.
33. Zametkin AJ, Nordahl TE, Gross M, et al. Cerebral glucose metabolism in adults with hyperactivity of childhood onset. N Engl J Med 1990; 323:1361–1366.
34. Castellanos FX, Giedd JN, Eckburg P, et al. Quantitative morphology of the caudate nucleus in attention deficit hyperactivity disorder. Am J Psychiatry 1994; 151:1791–1796.
35. Hynd GW, Hern KL, Novey ES, et al. Attention deficit-hyperactivity disorder and asymmetry of the caudate nucleus. J Child Neurol 1993; 8:339–347.
36. Harris EL, Schuerholz LJ, Singer HS, et al. Executive function in children with Tourette syndrome and/or attention deficit hyperactivity disorder. J Int Neuropsychol Soc 1995; 1:511–516.
37. Schuerholz LJ, Baumgardner TL, Singer HS, Reiss AL, Denckla MB. Neuropsychological status of children with Tourette's syndrome with and without attention deficit hyperactivity disorder. Neurology 1996; 46:958–965.
38. Mahone EM, Koth CW, Cutting L, Singer HS, Denckla MB. Executive function in fluency and recall measures among children with Tourette syndrome or ADHD. J Int Neuropsychol Soc 2001; 7:102–111.
39. Muller SV, Johannes S, Wieringa B, et al. Disturbed monitoring and response inhibition in patients with Gilles de la Tourette syndrome and co-morbid obsessive compulsive disorder. Behav Neurol 2003; 14:29–37.

40. Denckla MB, Reiss AL. Prefrontal-subcortical circuits in developmental disorders. In: Krasnegot NA, Lyon GR, Goldman-Rakic PS, eds. Development of the Prefrontal Cortex: Evolution, Neurobiology, and Behavior. Baltimore: Brookes Publishing, 1997:283–293.
41. Levin HSCK, Hartmann J, Evankovich K, Mattson AJ, Harward H, Ringholz G, Ewing-Cobbs L, Fletcher JM. Developmental changes in performance on tests of purported frontal lobe functioning. Dev Neuropsychol 1991; 7:377–395.
42. Chase TN, Geoffrey V, Gillespie M, Burrows GH. Structural and functional studies of Gilles de la Tourette syndrome. Rev Neurol 1986; 142:851–855.
43. Harcherik DF, Cohen DJ, Ort S, et al. Computed tomographic brain scanning in four neuropsychiatric disorders of childhood. Am J Psychiatry 1985; 142:731–734.
44. Robertson MM, Trimble MR, Lees AJ. The psychopathology of the Gilles de la Tourette syndrome. A phenomenological analysis. Br J Psychiatry 1988; 152: 383–390.
45. Demirkol A, Erdem H, Inan L, Yigit A, Guney M. Bilateral globus pallidus lesions in a patient with Tourette syndrome and related disorders. Biol Psychiatry 1999; 46:863–867.
46. McAbee GN, Wark JE, Manning A. Tourette syndrome associated with unilateral cystic changes in the gyrus rectus. Pediatr Neurol 1999; 20:322–324.
47. Krumholz A, Singer HS, Niedermeyer E, Burnite R, Harris K. Electrophysiological studies in Tourette's syndrome. Ann Neurol 1983; 14:638–641.
48. Drake ME Jr, Hietter SA, Padamadan H, Bogner JE. Computerized EEG frequency analysis in Gilles de la Tourette syndrome. Clin Electroencephalogr 1991; 22:250–253.
49. Drake ME Jr, Hietter SA, Padamadan H, Bogner JE, Andrews JM, Weate S. Auditory evoked potentials in Gilles de la Tourette syndrome. Clin Electroencephalogr 1992; 23:19–23.
50. Obeso JA, Rothwell JC, Marsden CD. Simple tics in Gilles de la Tourette's syndrome are not prefaced by a normal premovement EEG potential. J Neurol Neurosurg Psychiatry 1981; 44:735–738.
51. Papa SM, Artieda J, Obeso JA. Cortical activity preceding self-initiated and externally triggered voluntary movement. Mov Disord 1991; 6:217–224.
52. Cohrs S, Rasch T, Altmeyer S, et al. Decreased sleep quality and increased sleep related movements in patients with Tourette's syndrome. J Neurol Neurosurg Psychiatry 2001; 70:192–197.
53. Glaze DG, Frost JD Jr, Jankovic J. Sleep in Gilles de la Tourette's syndrome: disorder of arousal. Neurology 1983; 33:586–592.
54. Drake ME Jr, Hietter SA, Bogner JE, Andrews JM. Cassette EEG sleep recordings in Gilles de la Tourette syndrome. Clin Electroencephalogr 1992; 23:142–146.
55. Silvestri R, De Domenico P, Di Rosa AE, Bramanti P, Serra S, Di Perri R. The effect of nocturnal physiological sleep on various movement disorders. Mov Disord 1990; 5:8–14.
56. Swerdlow NR, Karban B, Ploum Y, Sharp R, Geyer MA, Eastvold A. Tactile

prepuff inhibition of startle in children with Tourette's syndrome: In search of an "fMRI-friendly" startle paradigm. Biol Psychiatry 2001; 50:578–585.
57. Georgiou N, Bradshaw JL, Phillips JG. Directed attention in Gilles de la Tourette syndrome. Behav Neurol 1998; 11:85–91.
58. Howells D, Georgiou-Karistianis N, Bradshaw J. The ability to orient attention in Gilles de la Tourette syndrome. Behav Neurol 1998; 11:205–209.
59. Johannes S, Kube C, Wieringa BM, Matzke M, Munte TF. Brain potentials and time estimation in humans. Neurosci Lett 1997; 231:63–66.
60. Johannes S, Wieringa BM, Nager W, Muller-Vahl KR, Dengler R, Munte TF. Electrophysiological measures and dual-task performance in Tourette syndrome indicate deficient divided attention mechanisms. Eur J Neurol 2001; 8:253–260.
61. Johannes S, Wieringa BM, Nager W, Muller-Vahl KR, Dengler R, Munte TF. Excessive action monitoring in Tourette syndrome. J Neurol 2002; 249:961–966.
62. Oades RD, Dittmann-Balcar A, Schepker R, Eggers C, Zerbin D. Auditory event-related potentials (ERPs) and mismatch negativity (MMN) in healthy children and those with attention-deficit or Tourette/tic symptoms. Biol Psychol 1996; 43:163–185.
63. van Woerkom TC, Roos RA, van Dijk JG. Altered attentional processing of background stimuli in Gilles de la Tourette syndrome: a study in auditory event-related potentials evoked in an oddball paradigm. Acta Neurol Scand 1994; 90:116–123.
64. O'Connor K, Lavoie ME, Robert M. Preparation and motor potentials in chronic tic and Tourette syndromes. Brain Cogn 2001; 46:224–226.
65. Richardson EP Jr. Neuropathological studies of Tourette syndrome. Adv Neurol 1982; 35:83–87.
66. Dewult A, van Bogaret L. Études anatomocliniques de syndrôme hypercinétiques complexes. Monatsschr Psychiatr Neurol 1941; 104:53–61.
67. Balthasar K. Über das anatomische Substrat der generalisierten Tic-Krankheit: Entwicklungshemmung des corpus striatum. Arch Psychiatr Berlin 1957; 195:531–549.
68. Northam RS, Singer HS. Postencephalitic acquired Tourette-like syndrome in a child. Neurology 1991; 41:592–593.
69. Majumdar A, Appleton RE. Delayed and severe but transient Tourette syndrome after head injury. Pediatr Neurol 2002; 27:314–317.
70. Factor SA, Molho ES. Adult-onset tics associated with peripheral injury. Mov Disord 1997; 12:1052–1055.
71. Kwak CH, Jankovic J. Tourettism and dystonia after subcortical stroke. Mov Disord 2002; 17:821–825.
72. Singer HS, Dela Cruz PS, Abrams MT, Bean SC, Reiss AL. A Tourette-like syndrome following cardiopulmonary bypass and hypothermia: MRI volumetric measurements. Mov Disord 1997; 12:588–592.
73. Klawans HL, Falk DK, Nausieda PA, Weiner WJ. Gilles de la Tourette syndrome after long-term chlorpromazine therapy. Neurology 1978; 28:1064–1066.

74. Singer WD. Transient Gilles de la Tourette syndrome after chronic neuroleptic withdrawal. Dev Med Child Neurol 1981; 23:518–521.
75. Pantoni L, Poggesi L, Repice A, Inzitari D. Disappearance of motor tics after Wernicke's encephalopathy in a patient with Tourette's syndrome. Neurology 1997; 48:381–383.
76. Baxter LR. Brain imaging as a tool in establishing a theory of brain pathology in obsessive compulsive disorder. J Clin Psychiatry 1990; 51(suppl):22–25. Discussion 26.
77. Baxter LR Jr, Schwartz JM, Guze BH, Bergman K, Szuba MP. PET imaging in obsessive compulsive disorder with and without depression. J Clin Psychiatry 1990; 51(suppl):61–69. Discussion 70.
78. Stoetter B, Braun AR, Randolph C, et al. Functional neuroanatomy of Tourette syndrome. Limbic-motor interactions studied with FDG PET. Adv Neurol 1992; 58:213–226.
79. Jeffries KJ, Schooler C, Schoenbach C, Herscovitch P, Chase TN, Braun AR. The functional neuroanatomy of Tourette's syndrome: an FDG PET study III: functional coupling of regional cerebral metabolic rates. Neuropsychopharmacology 2002; 27:92–104.
80. Hall CDM, Shields J, et al. Brain perfusion patterns with $^{99}Tc^{m}$-HMPAO/SPECT in patients with Gilles de la Tourette syndrome—Short report. Nuclear Medicine: The State of the Art of Nuclear Medicine in Europe. Stuttgart: Schattauer, 1991:243–245.
81. Riddle MA, Rasmusson AM, Woods SW, Hoffer PB. SPECT imaging of cerebral blood flow in Tourette syndrome. Adv Neurol 1992; 58:207–211.
82. Chiu NT, Chang YC, Lee BF, Huang CC, Wang ST. Differences in 99mTc-HMPAO brain SPET perfusion imaging between Tourette's syndrome and chronic tic disorder in children. Eur J Nucl Med 2001; 28:183–190.
83. Diler RS, Reyhanli M, Toros F, Kibar M, Avci A. Tc-99m-ECD SPECT brain imaging in children with Tourette's syndrome. Yonsei Med J 2002; 43:403–410.
84. Stern E, Silbersweig DA, Chee KY, et al. A functional neuroanatomy of tics in Tourette syndrome. Arch Gen Psychiatry 2000; 57:741–748.
85. Peterson B, Riddle MA, Cohen DJ, et al. Reduced basal ganglia volumes in Tourette's syndrome using three-dimensional reconstruction techniques from magnetic resonance images. Neurology 1993; 43:941–949.
86. Hyde TM, Stacey ME, Coppola R, Handel SF, Rickler KC, Weinberger DR. Cerebral morphometric abnormalities in Tourette's syndrome: a quantitative MRI study of monozygotic twins. Neurology 1995; 45:1176–1182.
87. Singer HS, Reiss AL, Brown JE, et al. Volumetric MRI changes in basal ganglia of children with Tourette's syndrome. Neurology 1993; 43:950–956.
88. Moriarty J, Varma AR, Stevens J, Fish M, Trimble MR, Robertson MM. A volumetric MRI study of Gilles de la Tourette's syndrome. Neurology 1997; 49:410–415.
89. Baumgardner TL, Singer HS, Denckla MB, et al. Corpus callosum morphology in children with Tourette syndrome and attention deficit hyperactivity disorder. Neurology 1996; 47:477–482.

90. Peterson BS, Leckman JF, Duncan JS, et al. Corpus callosum morphology from magnetic resonance images in Tourette's syndrome. Psychiatry Res 1994; 55: 85–99.
91. Mostofsky SH, Wendlandt J, Cutting L, Denckla MB, Singer HS. Corpus callosum measurements in girls with Tourette syndrome. Neurology 1999; 53:1345–1347.
92. Zimmerman AM, Abrams MT, Giuliano JD, Denckla MB, Singer HS. Subcortical volumes in girls with Tourette syndrome: support for a gender effect. Neurology 2000; 54:2224–2229.
93. Peterson BS, Staib L, Scahill L, et al. Regional brain and ventricular volumes in Tourette syndrome. Arch Gen Psychiatry 2001; 58:427–440.
94. Fredericksen KA, Cutting LE, Kates WR, et al. Disproportionate increases of white matter in right frontal lobe in Tourette syndrome. Neurology 2002; 58: 85–89.
95. Kates WR, Frederikse M, Mostofsky SH, et al. MRI parcellation of the frontal lobe in boys with attention deficit hyperactivity disorder or Tourette syndrome. Psychiatry Res 2002; 116:63–81.
96. Peterson BS, Skudlarski P, Anderson AW, et al. A functional magnetic resonance imaging study of tic suppression in Tourette syndrome. Arch Gen Psychiatry 1998; 55:326–333.
97. Biswal BB, Ulmer JL. Blind source separation of multiple signal sources of fMRI data sets using independent component analysis. J Comput Assist Tomogr 1999; 23:265–271.
98. Serrien DJ, Burgunder JM, Wiesendanger M. Control of manipulative forces during unimanual and bimanual tasks in patients with Huntington's disease. Exp Brain Res 2002; 143:328–334.
99. Farber RH, Swerdlow NR, Clementz BA. Saccadic performance characteristics and the behavioural neurology of Tourette's syndrome. J Neurol Neurosurg Psychiatry 1999; 66:305–312.
100. Narita AS, Shawkat FS, Lask B, Taylor DS, Harris CM. Eye movement abnormalities in a case of Tourette syndrome. Dev Med Child Neurol 1997; 39:270–273.
101. Mostofsky SH, Lasker AG, Singer HS, Denckla MB, Zee DS. Oculomotor abnormalities in boys with Tourette syndrome with and without ADHD. J Am Acad Child Adolesc Psych 2001; 40:1464–1472.
102. Dursun SM, Burke JG, Reveley MA. Antisaccade eye movement abnormalities in Tourette syndrome: evidence for cortico-striatal network dysfunction? J Psychopharmacol 2000; 14:37–39.
103. Lasker AG, Zee DS. Ocular motor abnormalities in Huntington's disease. Vis Res 1997; 37:3639–3645.
104. Guitton D, Buchtel HA, Douglas RM. Frontal lobe lesions in man cause difficulties in suppressing reflexive glances and in generating goal-directed saccades. Exp Brain Res 1985; 58:455–472.
105. Singer HS. Neurobiology of Tourette syndrome. Neurol Clin 1997; 15:357–379.
106. Lowenstein PR, Slesinger PA, Singer HS, et al. Compartment-specific changes

in the density of choline and dopamine uptake sites and muscarinic and dopaminergic receptors during the development of the baboon striatum: a quantitative receptor autoradiographic study. J Comp Neurol 1989; 288:428–446.
107. Fog R, Pakkenberg H. Behavioral effects of dopamine and *p*-hydroxyamphetamine injected into corpus striatum of rats. Exp Neurol 1971; 31:75–86.
108. Ridley RM. The psychology of perserverative and stereotyped behaviour. Prog Neurobiol 1994; 44:221–231.
109. Clark D, White FJ. D1 dopamine receptor–the search for a function: a critical evaluation of the D1/D2 dopamine receptor classification and its functional implications. Synapse 1987; 1:347–388.
110. Delfs JM, Kelley AE. The role of D1 and D2 dopamine receptors in oral stereotypy induced by dopaminergic stimulation of the ventrolateral striatum. Neuroscience 1990; 39:59–67.
111. Robinson TE, Becker JB. Enduring changes in brain and behavior produced by chronic amphetamine administration: a review and evaluation of animal models of amphetamine psychosis. Brain Res 1986; 396:157–198.
112. Dumartin B, Caille I, Gonon F, Bloch B. Internalization of D1 dopamine receptor in striatal neurons in vivo as evidence of activation by dopamine agonists. J Neurosci 1998; 18:1650–1661.
113. Mink JW. Basal ganglia dysfunction in Tourette's syndrome: a new hypothesis. Pediatr Neurol 2001; 25:190–198.
114. Ziemann U, Paulus W, Rothenberger A. Decreased motor inhibition in Tourette's disorder: evidence from transcranial magnetic stimulation. Am J Psychiatry 1997; 154:1277–1284.
115. Moll GH, Wischer S, Heinrich H, Tergau F, Paulus W, Rothenberger A. Deficient motor control in children with tic disorder: evidence from transcranial magnetic stimulation. Neurosci Lett 1999; 272:37–40.
116. Moll GH, Heinrich H, Trott GE, Wirth S, Bock N, Rothenberger A. Children with comorbid attention-deficit-hyperactivity disorder and tic disorder: evidence for additive inhibitory deficits within the motor system. Ann Neurol 2001; 49:393–396.
117. Leckman PDJF, Cohen DJ. Tic disorders. In: Bloom FEKD, ed. Psychopharmacology: Fourth Generation of Progress. New York: Raven Press, 1995:1665–1674.
118. Singer HS, Butler IJ, Tune LE, Seifert WE Jr, Coyle JT. Dopaminergic dysfunction in Tourette syndrome. Ann Neurol 1982; 12:361–366.
119. Singer HS, Hahn IH, Moran TH. Abnormal dopamine uptake sites in postmortem striatum from patients with Tourette's syndrome. Ann Neurol 1991; 30:558–562.
120. Centonze D, Gubellini P, Picconi B, Calabresi P, Giacomini P, Bernardi G. Unilateral dopamine denervation blocks corticostriatal LTP. J Neurophysiol 1999; 82:3575–3579.
121. Groves P, Garcia-Munoz M, Linder J, Manley M, Martine M, Young S. Elements of the intrinsic organization and information processing in the neostriatum. In: Houk J, Davis J, Beiser D, eds. Models of Information Processing in the Basal Ganglia. Cambridge, MA: MIT Press, 1995:51–96.

122. Wickens JR, Kotter R, Alexander ME. Effects of local connectivity on striatal function: stimulation and analysis of a model. Synapse 1995; 20:281–298.
123. Aosaki T, Tsubokawa H, Ishida A, Watanabe K, Graybiel AM, Kimura M. Responses of tonically active neurons in the primate's striatum undergo systematic changes during behavioral sensorimotor conditioning. J Neurosci 1994; 14:3969–3984.
124. Singer HS, Tune LE, Butler IJ, Zaczek R, Coyle JT. Clinical symptomatology, CSF neurotransmitter metabolites, and serum haloperidol levels in Tourette syndrome. Adv Neurol 1982; 35:177–183.
125. Butler IJ, Koslow SH, Seifert WE Jr, Caprioli RM, Singer HS. Biogenic amine metabolism in Tourette syndrome. Ann Neurol 1979; 6:37–39.
126. Cohen DJ, Shaywitz BA, Caparulo B, Young JG, Bowers MB Jr, Chronic, multiple tics of Gilles de la Tourette's disease. CSF acid monoamine metabolites after probenecid administration. Arch Gen Psychiatry 1978; 35:245–250.
127. George MS, Robertson MM, Costa DC, et al. Dopamine receptor availability in Tourette's syndrome. Psychiatry Res 1994; 55:193–203.
128. Turjanski N, Sawle GV, Playford ED, et al. PET studies of the presynaptic and postsynaptic dopaminergic system in Tourette's syndrome. J Neurol Neurosurg Psychiatry 1994; 57:688–692.
129. Wolf SS, Jones DW, Knable MB, et al. Tourette syndrome: prediction of phenotypic variation in monozygotic twins by caudate nucleus D2 receptor binding. Science 1996; 273:1225–1227.
130. Wong DF, Singer HS, Brandt J, et al. D2-like dopamine receptor density in Tourette syndrome measured by PET. J Nucl Med 1997; 38:1243–1247.
131. Malison RT, McDougle CJ, van Dyck CH, et al. [^{123}I]beta-CIT SPECT imaging of striatal dopamine transporter binding in Tourette's disorder. Am J Psychiatry 1995; 152:1359–1361.
132. Muller-Vahl KR, Berding G, Brucke T, et al. Dopamine transporter binding in Gilles de la Tourette syndrome. J Neurol 2000; 247:514–520.
133. Heinz A, Knable MB, Wolf SS, et al. Tourette's syndrome: [^{123}I]beta-CIT SPECT correlates of vocal tic severity. Neurology 1998; 51:1069–1074.
134. Wong DF, Ricaurte G, Grunder G, et al. Dopamine transporter changes in neuropsychiatric disorders. Adv Pharmacol 1998; 42:219–223.
135. Stamenkovic M, Schindler SD, Asenbaum S, et al. No change in striatal dopamine re-uptake site density in psychotropic drug naive and in currently treated Tourette's disorder patients: a [^{123}I]beta-CIT SPECt-study. Eur Neuropsychopharmacol 2001; 11:69–74.
136. Meyer P, Bohnen NI, Minoshima S, et al. Striatal presynaptic monoaminergic vesicles are not increased in Tourette's syndrome. Neurology 1999; 53:371–374.
137. Ernst M, Zametkin AJ, Jons PH, Matochik JA, Pascualvaca D, Cohen RM. High presynaptic dopaminergic activity in children with Tourette's disorder. J Am Acad Child Adolesc Psych 1999; 38:86–94.
138. Singer HS, Szymanski S, Giuliano J, et al. Elevated intrasynaptic dopamine release in Tourette's syndrome measured by PET. Am J Psychiatry 2002; 159:1329–1336.

139. Grace AA. Cortical regulation of subcortical dopamine systems and its possible relevance to schizophrenia. J Neural Transm Gen Sect 1993; 91:111–134.
140. Gobert A, Rivet JM, Audinot V, et al. Functional correlates of dopamine D3 receptor activation in the rat in vivo and their modulation by the selective antagonist, (+)-S 14297: II Both D2 and "silent" D3 autoreceptors control synthesis and release in mesolimbic, mesocortical and nigrostriatal pathways. J Pharmacol Exp Ther 1995; 275:899–913.
141. Erenberg G, Cruse RP, Rothner AD. Gilles de la Tourette's syndrome: effects of stimulant drugs. Neurology 1985; 35:1346–1348.
142. Price RA, Leckman JF, Pauls DL, Cohen DJ, Kidd KK. Gilles de la Tourette's syndrome: tics and central nervous system stimulants in twins and nontwins. Neurology 1986; 36:232–237.
143. Singer HS, Rabins P, Tune LE, Coyle JT. Serum haloperidol levels in Gilles de la Tourette syndrome. Biol Psychiatry 1981; 16:79–84.
144. Anderson GM, Pollak ES, Chatterjee D, Leckman JF, Riddle MA, Cohen DJ. Postmortem analysis of subcortical monoamines and amino acids in Tourette syndrome. Adv Neurol 1992; 58:123–133.
145. Anderson GM, Pollak ES, Chatterjee D, Leckman JF, Riddle MA, Cohen DJ. Brain monoamines and amino acids in Gilles de la Tourette's syndrome: a preliminary study of subcortical regions. Arch Gen Psychiatry 1992; 49:584–586.
146. Gonce M, Barbeau A. Seven cases of Gilles de la Tourette's syndrome: partial relief with clonazepam: a pilot study. Can J Neurol Sci 1977; 4:279–283.
147. Singer HS, Hahn IH, Krowiak E, Nelson E, Moran T. Tourette's syndrome: a neurochemical analysis of postmortem cortical brain tissue. Ann Neurol 1990; 27:443–446.
148. Van Woerkom T, Rosenbaum D, Enna S. Overview of pharmacological approaches to therapy for Tourette syndrome. In: Friedhoff A, Chase T, eds. Advances in Neurology. Vol 35. New York: Raven Press, 1982:369–375.
149. Anderson SA, Eisenstat DD, Shi L, Rubenstein JL. Interneuron migration from basal forebrain to neocortex: dependence on Dlx genes. Science 1997; 278:474–476.
150. Leckman JF. Tourette's syndrome. Lancet 2002; 360:1577–1586.
151. Leckman JF, Goodman WK, Anderson GM, et al. Cerebrospinal fluid biogenic amines in obsessive compulsive disorder. Tourette's syndrome, and healthy controls. Neuropsychopharmacology 1995; 12:73–86.
152. Comings DE. Blood serotonin and tryptophan in Tourette syndrome. Am J Med Genet 1990; 36:418–430.
153. Singer HS, Dickson J, Martinie D, Levine M. Second messenger systems in Tourette's syndrome. J Neurol Sci 1995; 128:78–83.
154. Lee O, Loiselle CR, Becker KG, Kwak NG, Comi AM, Singer HS. Neurochemical markers and microarrays in postmortem Tourette syndrome putamen and brain area 9. Ann Neurol 2002; 52(suppl 1), S101.
155. Hyde TM, Aaronson BA, Randolph C, Rickler KC, Weinberger DR. Relationship of birth weight to the phenotypic expression of Gilles de la Tourette's syndrome in monozygotic twins. Neurology 1992; 42:652–658.

156. Price RA, Kidd KK, Cohen DJ, Pauls DL, Leckman JF. A twin study of Tourette syndrome. Arch Gen Psychiatry 1985; 42:815–820.
157. Whitaker AH, Van Rossem R, Feldman JF, et al. Psychiatric outcomes in low-birth-weight children at age 6 years: relation to neonatal cranial ultrasound abnormalities. Arch Gen Psychiatry 1997; 54:847–856.
158. Burd L, Severud R, Kerbeshian J, Klug MG. Prenatal and perinatal risk factors for autism. J Perinat Med 1999; 27:441–450.
159. Lichter DG, Dmochowski J, Jackson LA, Trinidad KS. Influence of family history on clinical expression of Tourette's syndrome. Neurology 1999; 52:308–316.
160. Hanna PA, Janjua FN, Contant CF, Jankovic J. Bilineal transmission in Tourette syndrome. Neurology 1999; 53:813–818.
161. Selling L. The role of infection in the etiology of tics. Arch Neurol Psychiatry 1929; 22:1163–1171.
162. Brown EE. Tics (habit spasms) secondary to sinusitis. Arch Pediatr 1957; 74: 39–46.
163. Kondo K, Kabasawa T, Greenberg BD, et al. Improvement in Gilles de la Tourette syndrome after corticosteroid therapy: symptom exacerbation of vocal tics and other symptoms associated with streptococcal pharyngitis in a patient with obsessive-compulsive disorder and tics Lyme disease presenting as Tourette's syndrome and *Mycoplasma pneumoniae* infection. Ann Neurol 1978; 4:387.
164. Kiessling LS. Tic disorders associated with evidence of invasive group A beta hemolytic streptococcal disease, abstracted. Dev Med Child Neurol 1989; 31:48.
165. Greenberg BD, Murphy DL, Swedo SE. Symptom exacerbation of vocal tics and other symptoms associated with streptococcal pharyngitis in a patient with obsessive-compulsive disorder and tics. Am J Psychiatry 1998; 155:1459–1460.
166. Riedel M, Straube A, Schwarz MJ, Wilske B, Muller N. Lyme disease presenting as Tourette's syndrome. Lancet 1998; 351:418–419.
167. Muller N, Riedel M, Forderreuther S, Blendinger C, Abele-Horn M. Tourette's syndrome and *Mycoplasma pneumoniae* infection. Am J Psychiatry 2000; 157:481–482.
168. Bright R. Cases of spasmodic disease accompanying affections of the pericardium. Med-Chir Trans 1838; 22:1–19.
169. Schwartzman JD, McDonald DH. Sydenham's chorea: Report of 140 cases and review of the recent literature. Arch Pediatr 1948; 65:6–24.
170. Freeman JM, Aron AM, Collard JE, Mackay MC. The emotional correlates of Sydenham's chorea. Pediatrics 1965; 35:42–49.
171. Swedo SE, Leonard HL, Schapiro MB, et al. Sydenham's chorea: physical and psychological symptoms of St Vitus dance. Pediatrics 1993; 91:706–713.
172. Cardoso F, Eduardo C, Silva AP, Mota CC. Chorea in fifty consecutive patients with rheumatic fever. Mov Disord 1997; 12:701–703.
173. Mercadante MT, Campos MC, Marques-Dias MJ, Miguel EC, Leckman J. Vocal tics in Sydenham's chorea. J Am Acad Child Adolesc Psych 1997; 36:305–306.

174. Cardoso F, Vargas AP, Oliveira LD, Guerra AA, Amaral SV. Persistent Sydenham's chorea. Mov Disord 1999; 14:805–807.
175. Swedo SE, Leonard HL, Garvey M, et al. Pediatric autoimmune neuropsychiatric disorders associated with streptococcal infections: clinical description of the first 50 cases. Am J Psychiatry 1998; 155:264–271.
176. Murphy ML, Pichichero ME. Prospective identification and treatment of children with pediatric autoimmune neuropsychiatric disorder associated with group A streptococcal infection (PANDAS). Arch Pediatr Adolesc Med 2002; 156:356–561.
177. Lougee L, Perlmutter SJ, Nicolson R, Garvey MA, Swedo SE. Psychiatric disorders in first-degree relatives of children with pediatric autoimmune neuropsychiatric disorders associated with streptococcal infections (PANDAS). J Am Acad Child Adolesc Psych 2000; 39:1120–1126.
178. Giedd JN, Rapoport JL, Garvey MA, Perlmutter S, Swedo SE. MRI assessment of children with obsessive-compulsive disorder or tics associated with streptococcal infection. Am J Psychiatry 2000; 157:281–283.
179. Swedo SE, Leonard HL, Mittleman BB, et al. Identification of children with pediatric autoimmune neuropsychiatric disorders associated with streptococcal infections by a marker associated with rheumatic fever. Am J Psychiatry 1997; 154:110–112.
180. Kurlan R. Tourette's syndrome and 'PANDAS': will the relation bear out? Pediatric autoimmune neuropsychiatric disorders associated with streptococcal infection. Neurology 1998; 50:1530–1534.
181. Singer H, Loiselle C. PANDAS: a commentary. J Psychosom Res 2003; 55:31–39.
182. Green LN. Corticosteroids in the treatment of Sydenham's chorea. Arch Neurol 1978; 35:53–54.
183. Garvey MA, Swedo SE. Sydenham's chorea. Clinical and therapeutic update. Adv Exp Med Biol 1997; 418:115–120.
184. Husby G, van de Rijn I, Zabriskie JB, Abdin ZH, Williams RC Jr, Antibodies reacting with cytoplasm of subthalamic and caudate nuclei neurons in chorea and acute rheumatic fever. J Exp Med 1976; 144:1094–1110.
185. Kotby AA, El Badawy N, El Sokkary S, Moawad H, El Shawarby M. Antineuronal antibodies in rheumatic chorea. Clin Diagn Lab Immunol 1998; 5:836–839.
186. Morshed SA, Parveen S, Leckman JF, et al. Antibodies against neural, nuclear, cytoskeletal, and streptococcal epitopes in children and adults with Tourette's syndrome. Sydenham's chorea, and autoimmune disorders. Biol Psychiatry 2001; 50:566–577.
187. Church AJ, Cardoso F, Dale RC, Lees AJ, Thompson EJ, Giovannoni G. Anti-basal ganglia antibodies in acute and persistent Sydenham's chorea. Neurology 2002; 59:227–231.
188. Singer HS, Loiselle CR, Lee O, Garvey MA, Grus FH. Anti-basal ganglia antibody abnormalities in Sydenham chorea. J Neuroimmunol 2003; 136:154–161.
189. Singer HS, Giuliano JD, Hansen BH, et al. Antibodies against human putamen in children with Tourette syndrome. Neurology 1998; 50:1618–1624.

190. Singer HS, Giuliano JD, Hansen BH, et al. Antibodies against a neuron-like (HTB-10 neuroblastoma) cell in children with Tourette syndrome. Biol Psychiatry 1999; 46:775–780.
191. Kiessling LS, Marcotte AC, Culpepper L. Antineuronal antibodies in movement disorders. Pediatrics 1993; 92:39–43.
192. Singer HS, Loiselle CR, Wendlandt JT, Swedo SE, Grus FH. Antineuronal antibodies in Sydenham's chorea and PANDAS: an ELISA and Western blot analysis. Neurology 2002; 58:A372.
193. Dale RC, Church AJ, Surtees RA, Thompson EJ, Giovannoni G, Neville BG. Post-streptococcal autoimmune neuropsychiatric disease presenting as paroxysmal dystonic choreoathetosis. Mov Disord 2002; 17:817–820.
194. Dale RC, Church AJ, Cardoso F, et al. Poststreptococcal acute disseminated encephalomyelitis with basal ganglia involvement and auto-reactive antibasal ganglia antibodies. Ann Neurol 2001; 50:588–595.
195. Dale RC, Church AJ, Benton S, et al. Post-streptococcal autoimmune dystonia with isolated bilateral striatal necrosis. Dev Med Child Neurol 2002; 44:485–489.
196. Peterson BS, Leckman JF, Tucker D, et al. Preliminary findings of antistreptococcal antibody titers and basal ganglia volumes in tic, obsessive-compulsive, and attention deficit/hyperactivity disorders. Arch Gen Psychiatry 2000; 57:364–372.
197. Trifiletti RR, Packard AM. Immune mechanisms in pediatric neuropsychiatric disorders. Tourette's syndrome, OCD, and PANDAS. Child Adolesc Psychiatr Clin N Am 1999; 8:767–775.
198. Wendlandt JT, Grus FH, Hansen BH, Singer HS. Striatal antibodies in children with Tourette's syndrome: multivariate discriminant analysis of IgG repertoires. J Neuroimmunol 2001; 119:106–113.
199. Hallett JJ, Harling-Berg CJ, Knopf PM, Stopa EG, Kiessling LS. Anti-striatal antibodies in Tourette syndrome cause neuronal dysfunction. J Neuroimmunol 2000; 111:195–202.
200. Taylor JR, Morshed SA, Parveen S, et al. An animal model of Tourette's syndrome. Am J Psychiatry 2002; 159:657–660.
201. Loiselle CR, Lee O, Moran TH, Singer HS. Striatal microinfusion of Tourette syndrome and PANDAS sera: failure to induce behavioral changes. Mov Disord 2003. In press.
202. DiFazio MP, Morales J, Davis R. Acute myoclonus secondary to group A beta-hemolytic streptococcus infection: a PANDAS variant. J Child Neurol 1998; 13:516–518.
203. Sokol MS. Infection-triggered anorexia nervosa in children: clinical description of four cases. J Child Adolesc Psychopharmacol 2000; 10:133–145.
204. Perlmutter SJ, Leitman SF, Garvey MA, et al. Therapeutic plasma exchange and intravenous immunoglobulin for obsessive-compulsive disorder and tic disorders in childhood. Lancet 1999; 354:1153–1158.
205. Singer HS. Neurochemical analysis of postmortem cortical and striatal brain tissue in patients with Tourette syndrome. Adv Neurol 1992; 58:135–144.

15

Infection and Autoimmune Factors in Tourette's and Related Disorders

William M. McMahon and Michael Johnson
University of Utah
Salt Lake City, Utah, U.S.A.

INTRODUCTION

This chapter summarizes the evidence regarding the following question: Do infections or autoimmune processes contribute to onset or exacerbation of Tourette's syndrome (TS), obsessive–compulsive disorder (OCD), and associated disorders? This question is a controversial one, with important implications for treatment and prevention. It is also a very difficult one to answer. This chapter first summarizes the emergence of hypotheses linking Tourette's syndrome to infection or immune processes. Next, the psychiatric symptoms and neuroimmune mechanism of Sydenham's chorea (SC) are examined. Subsequently, the evidence for pediatric autoimmune neuropsychiatric disorders associated with streptococcus (PANDAS) is evaluated.

INFECTION AND TICS

TS was originally described as hereditary by Gilles de la Tourette in 1885 (1). Modern twin, adoption, and segregation analysis studies have supported a genetic etiology, although nongenetic mechanisms such as head injury, infection, and autoimmunity may also contribute to etiology (2–5) (see below).

Recent concerns about infection as a potential etiologic factor for Tourette's and related disorders have focused on group A β-hemolytic streptococci (GAβHS). In so far as SC is considered a useful model for understanding movement disorders triggered by infection, it is noteworthy that over a dozen bacterial, viral, and fungal pathogens have been implicated in causing chorea and dystonia (6).

Anecdotal case reports suggest possible etiologic associations between tics and nonstreptococcal infections although systematic and controlled studies examining tics or OCD symptoms are lacking. In a recent review, Garvey et al. (7) note reports of tics following acute sinusitis published in 1929 and 1957. More recently, *Mycoplasma pneumoniae* infection was reported in two children: a 7-year-old boy and a 13-year-old girl both with prior histories of tics in early childhood and exacerbation of tics with the onset of infection. In these two cases, antibiotic treatment was followed by partial or complete tic remission and decreased *M. pneumoniae* titer (8). Lyme disease has been implicated in the report of a 9-year-old boy with a prior transient blinking tic at age 4. Subsequent onset of vocal and multiple oral–facial tics at age 9 years was associated with a peak immunoglobulin G (IgG) titer to *Borrelia burgodorferi* of 100 U/mL. These tics remitted following intravenous ceftriaxone treatment. Follow-up 1 year later disclosed no recurrence of tics, and low *B. burgodorferi* titers (11 U/mL) (9). A 40-year-old male with advanced HIV disease and *Mycobacterium avium* infections suffered an onset of "sudden, involuntary, recurrent, stereotyped" vocalizations and movements involving the upper extremities. There was no past history of tics in the patient or other family members (10).

Three publications document co-occurrence of tics and herpes infection (11–13). The first case report described a 19-year-old woman with the onset of vocal tics involving words or barks and complex motor tics (13). A 6-year-old girl with presumed herpes encephalitis developed a hemorrhagic lesion of the right mesial temporal region, along with edema of the right temporal lobe, basal ganglia, and thalamus. She was treated with a 10-day course of acyclovir and 2 weeks following discharge she was noted to have frequent eye-blinking tics that rapidly progressed to multiple motor tics and vocalizations, including complex tics, with some tics occurring every 5–10 sec. The authors concluded that the lack of any family history for tics combined with the patient's acute presentation argued against encephalopathy as a nonspecific factor that merely uncovered a preexisting TS genetic predisposition (12). An 11-year-old girl with a past history of tics starting at age 5 was reported to have significant worsening of tics several weeks after suffering an outbreak of Herpes simplex type I lesions. After she was started on acyclovir, her tic symptoms were noted to decrease within 48 hr. A second exacerbation in tics several months later was also noted to respond to acyclovir (11).

From the cases summarized above, it seems possible that several infectious agents may precipitate tics or Tourette's disorder. Possible mechanisms include direct infection, specific autoimmune reactions, or nonspecific effects of a heightened inflammatory response. Any of these mechanisms could interfere with the function of the cortico–thalamo–striatal–cortical loop and result in tics. Curiously, four of the seven published cases document a prior history of tics. Increased body temperature may exacerbate tics in some individuals (14,15). Because infection may be associated with fever, a possible mechanism relating tics and infection may involve a temperature-sensitive mechanism. Other neurogenetic disorders have been associated with temperature sensitivity. "Generalized febrile seizures plus" is an epilepsy disorder associated with a mutation in the sodium channel α_2 subunit (16). Finally, autoimmune antibodies against basal ganglia could be initiated or exacerbated by infectious agents other than strep. Indeed, the first publication that proposed a neuroimmune model for tics and OCD [pediatric, infection-triggered, autoimmune neuropsychiatric disorders associated with Streptococcus (PITANDS)] included viral infections as well as strep (17). Autoimmune disorders may be initiated or exacerbated by specific bacterial or viral agents presenting antigens that mimic components of human tissue. The resulting immune antibodies then bind both the infectious agent and cross-reacting components of human tissue. Such a mechanism of molecular mimicry has been proposed for GAβHS in rheumatic fever (RF; reviewed in Cunningham 2002). SC, the brain manifestation of RF, has been proposed as a model for GAβHS-triggered tics and OCD. But before examining RF and SC, an introduction to PANDAS is in order.

THE BIRTH OF PANDAS

The hypothesis that TD and OCD may be triggered by streptococcal infection had roots in OCD studies of the 1980s. At the National Institute of Mental Health (NIMH), studies of childhood OCD led Judith Rapoport to develop a theory of etiology involving the basal ganglia (18,19). Susan Swedo, a pediatrician and member of the NIMH team, examined children with SC, a known disorder of the basal ganglia. SC is one of the major manifestations of acute rheumatic fever (RF). Swedo et al. (20) reported that 82% of patients with SC had concomitant onset of obsessions and compulsions, and one-third met requirements for OCD. Louise Kiessling and colleagues (21) at Brown University noted an increase in tic disorders in children following a community outbreak of strep-throat in Providence, Rhode Island. Not only did the tics begin abruptly following the infection, but also antineuronal antibodies directed against human caudate were found in 45% of tic cases ($n=30$), compared to a rate of 20% in controls without tics. The authors pointed out that a previous study of antibodies against caudate in SC patients found a similar positive rate of 46% (22). They speculated that some cases of TD result from an attack of basal ganglia by antibodies that cross-react with streptococcal antigens, in a process similar to SC. In 1995, the NIMH group reported four cases that suggested a new, infection-triggered, autoimmune subtype of pediatric OCD and TD (17). All cases were males aged 10 to 14 years with abrupt, severe onset, or worsening of OCD or tics. One had Tourette's syndrome, one had OCD, and two had both. Two of the cases had evidence of recent GAβHS, and the two others had histories of recent viral illnesses. These cases were proposed to represent a subgroup of pediatric OCD patients with sudden, distinct onset of clinically significant symptoms, followed by waning of symptoms, a pattern very similar to the pattern of SC. Subsequent reports by the NIMH group and other investigators have focused on GAβHS as the putative infectious trigger and Swedo coined the term Pediatric Autoimmune Neuropsychiatric Disorders Associated with Streptococcus (PANDAS). Because SC has been proposed as a model for the study of PANDAS (23), a review of SC is first in order before examining PANDAS in more detail.

SYDENHAM'S CHOREA

In 1668, Thomas Sydenham described the childhood syndrome that bears his name. SC is a disorder most commonly occurring in childhood that varies in intensity from severe incapacity caused by marked weakness, incoordination, and exaggerated movements of the limbs and trunk to subtle tic-like movements of facial or finger muscles. Dr. Sydenham also recognized behavioral and emotional changes (24). SC is one of the major manifestations of RF and usually occurs about 6 weeks after pharyngitis caused by GAβHS. At the turn of the century, RF was a dread disease, frequently causing severe morbidity and mortality in the United States, but it began to abate even before the development of antibiotics (25). Public and professional concern about RF was reawakened in the late 1980s when several epidemics of RF with attendant heart disease and SC reemerged (25–27). SC, like the other major manifestations of RF (carditis, polyarthritis, erythema marginatum, and subcutaneous nodules), results from an autoimmune attack on the affected organs. The course of SC is variable. Movements may remit in weeks to months, or they may persist beyond 2 years. Sydenham patients also have tic-like movements in addition to the chorea, and true tics have been reported in 2 cases of SC (28). Brazilian investigators found that persistence of chorea may be increased in females and in SC with RF carditis (29). A relationship to female gender is also evident in the increased ratio of females to males and the association of chorea during early pregnancy, apparently in women with prior history of RF (30). While a great deal is known about SC, much is still unknown. In a recent review, Dale (24, p. 184) states that "despite being recognized over 300 years ago, the disease remains enigmatic and poorly understood."

Psychiatric Symptoms of SC

Psychiatric symptoms have long been associated with SC (24). Studies by the NIMH group suggested that OCD was associated with SC, but not RF without SC. Using a 20-item adaptation of the Leyton Obsessional Inventory and telephone interviews, 3/20 SC cases, but 0/14 RF without SC cases were diagnosed with OCD (31). Subsequently, direct examination of SC children has disclosed high rates of obsessive–compulsive symptoms (9/11 or 82%) and of full syndrome OCD (4/11 or 36%) in children with acute SC (20). Furthermore, the course of OC symptoms waxed and waned with SC symptoms. Curiously, onset of OC and other psychiatric symptoms could begin days to weeks before the onset of SC. Using a prospective study design of new onset cases, Brazilian investigators similarly found abrupt onset OCD and OC symptoms to be increased in 30 SC cases compared to 20 non-SC RF cases (32). Follow-up occurred every 2 months for 6 months and revealed the course of OC symptoms. OC symptom severity peaked during the first 2 months of SC in 17% of cases with OCD and 70% of cases with OC symptoms, with symptom severity subsiding within 4 months of SC onset in most children. The same investigators from the University of Sao Paulo subsequently reported an increased risk of OCD and OC symptoms associated with SC when SC recurred (33).

Another Brazilian study systematically assessed all children with acute RF, ages 5 through 16 (34). Rates of psychopathology were compared between three groups: RF with SC ($n=22$), RF without SC ($n=20$), and age- and gender-matched controls with other diseases ($n=20$). Thirteen percent of the SC group were found to meet DSM-IV criteria for OCD, whereas 10% of the RF without SC group and none of the controls met the same criteria. Furthermore, the SC group had significantly higher rates of the combined type of attention-deficit/hyperactivity disorder (ADHD, 45.5%), TD (9.1%), any type of tic disorder (72%), and major depression (40.9%). Onset of major depression occurred at the same time or following onset of RF in 8 of 9 SC cases with depression. However, onset of psychiatric symptoms predated onset of RF in 78% with obsessive–compulsive symptoms and for 45% of tic disorders. Remarkably, ADHD onset preceded RF onset by an average of 4 years and was predictive of RF associated with SC. The authors suggested "that in some cases, ADHD, tic disorders and obsessive–compulsive symptoms may reflect a vulnerability to developing" (34, p. 2037) RF and SC. The high rate of OCD in RF without SC varied from earlier studies but is consistent with findings from Utah. A mail survey of 65 Utah SC cases and 35 non-SC RF cases found evidence for OCD in 25% of SC compared to 9% of non-SC RF (35). Thus, it appears that OCD, tics, ADHD, depression, and other psychiatric symptoms occur at increased rates in children with SC, and perhaps in children with RF without SC as well. A consistent finding has been that OC symptoms associated with SC begin abruptly days to weeks before, at the same time, or soon after the onset of chorea. The suggestion by Mercadante et al. (34) that pre-existing ADHD is associated with vulnerability to SC and RF deserves further investigation. Likewise, further investigation is needed to test the hypothesis that shared genetic vulnerability increases risk for both psychiatric disorders (e.g., tics, OCD, ADHD) and for RF with and without SC.

GAβHS STRAIN SPECIFICITY

Some strains of GAβHS have been associated more frequently with outbreaks of RF than other strains. Strains of GAβHS can be distinguished in a number of ways, most commonly using M-typing and T-typing (36). Virulence for RF corresponds to the type of M protein on the bacterial cell surface that confers resistance to phagocytosis by human polymorphonuclear leukocytes. Antigenic differences in M protein allow the recognition of 80 or more different group A streptococcal strains, of which eight (M types 1, 3, 5, 6, 14,18,19, and 24) are associated with epidemic RF (37–39). A provocative, but unreplicated study by Bronze and Dale (40) reported that an epitope of certain M proteins evoke antibodies that cross-react with the human brain. Antibodies against digests of M6 protein were bound to human basal ganglia and other brain regions. Anti-M6 antibody binding was partially inhibited by M5 and M19, but not M25 proteins. The brain-reactive epitope was an amino acid sequence, Ala–Lys–Glu, localized to a decapeptide in the B repeat region of the M6 protein. The authors hypothesized that this amino acid sequence initiates the production of antibodies that cross-react with both GAβHS and brain tissue, an autoimmune mechanism known as *molecular mimicry* (41). More recent genetic studies of GAβHS have extended knowledge gained from previous serological M protein typing with molecular knowledge of the *emm* gene. The *emm* gene encodes the M protein and allows comparison of DNA sequences between specific isolates of the same strain. For example, increased occurrence of serotype M18 has been associated with increased incidence of RF in Utah (42). Molecular analysis of isolates from those Utah throat cultures disclosed very restricted genetic variation for M18 GAβHS. Future studies of

RF outbreaks may be able to identify a specific strep DNA sequence involved in the pathogenesis of RF in specific cases.

Superantigens

GAβHS, like some other bacteria and viruses, are capable of producing superantigens (43). Streptococcal superantigens appear to play a role in toxic shock syndrome and severe invasive disease. Superantigens provoke inflammatory cytokine and T-cell responses that may contribute to autoimmune processes (36). Guttate psoriasis is an autoimmune disorder associated with the streptococcal pyrogenic exotoxin C. Whether superantigens play a role in RF or PANDAS is not clear.

Human Susceptibility

Not all children appear equally vulnerable to RF. Even during an epidemic of GAβHS, only an estimated 3–6% of children with untreated rheumatogenic GAβHS pharyngitis develop RF (44). Susceptibility to RF appears familial, but the mode of inheritance is uncertain. Massell has reviewed studies using clinical history of the familiality of RF published before 1956: 4 studies that used blood group serologic markers published between 1956 and 1964, 13 studies that used human leukocyte antigen (HLA) markers published between 1973 and 1993, and 4 studies using D8/17 published between 1985 and 1991 (44). Although methods vary across studies, evidence for a major gene that confers susceptibility is relatively consistent. Perhaps the most impressive early family study was published by Wilson and Schweitzer (45) in 1954: 646 children from 291 families were observed for the development of RF for 10 years. In the 52 families at genetic risk for RF, 33% of children (40/121) developed RF, compared to 0.6% (3/525) of children in non-RF families, which was interpreted by the authors as support for a recessive model. Twin studies by Taranta and colleagues (46) found 3 of 16 monozygotic twin pairs to be concordant for the same exact manifestation of RF. Only 2 of 23 same-sex dizygotic pairs were concordant for any manifestation of RF, only 1 of these was concordant for the exact type of RF manifestation (46). Taranta subsequently added 17 additional dizygotic pairs and found that the RF rate for monozygotic pairs was seven times greater than for dizygotic twin pairs (47). Brazilian investigators studied HLA markers for cosegregation with RF status in 55 RF cases and 61 controls in 22 families. Using all members of these families, a trend for segregation of HLA type and susceptibility for RF was found, and subsequent analysis of affected sib pairs supported an autosomal dominant model with penetrance between 0.5 and 0.9 and a gene frequency of at least 1% (48).

HLA Association Studies

Association studies of HLA Class II markers in RF support a hypothesis that the HLA region contains an RF susceptibility gene. A variety of HLA Class I antigens have been studied in diverse ethnic samples, with inconsistent results. The Class II antigens, HLA antigens that occur only on B lymphocytes and macrophages, show more consistent RF associations, particularly with HLA-DR4. Three laboratories have reported positive associations between DR4 and RF: Ayoub et al. (49,50) found DR4 in 62.5% with RF and 31% in non-RF controls; Annastasiou-Nana et al. (51) found DR4 in 52% of RF subjects compared to 32% of controls, and an additional negative association with DR6, which occurred in only 6% of RF cases but 26% of controls; and Rajapakse et al. (52) found DR4 in 72% of cases with rheumatic heart disease vs. 12% of controls. The first three studies used samples of U.S. Caucasians, while the last study analyzed a sample from Saudi Arabia. RF in a number of other racial/ethnic groups has been associated with other HLA markers: DR3 and Dqw2 in natives of New Delhi, India; DR6 in blacks in South Africa; Drw53 and DR7 in Sao Paolo, Brazil; and B16 in Turkey. Thus evidence for HLA association with RF varies among different ethnic groups.

D8/17

In 1989, Khanna et al. (53) found a B-cell antigen that was present in cases of rheumatic fever. The development of the assay for this antigen, known as D8/17, built on previous attempts to define an RF-specific antigen test. D8/17 antibody was derived from a fusion hybridoma obtained following injection of B cells from a patient who had well documented RF 20 years earlier. Initial studies used immunofluorescence microscopy to detect D8/17 positive B cells. RF populations from the United States, Mexico, Chile, and the former Soviet Union showed high D8/17 expression (54). Binding studies suggested that the D8/17 antibody binds contractile proteins present in heart, skeletal and smooth muscle, and that it may also share epitopes with some components of group A streptococci (55).

More recently, flow cytometry detection has been used in an attempt to increase assay objectivity and efficiency (56). Sensitivity of D8/17 may be decreased in some ethnic groups, at least in India (57). In Israel, blood from 22 RF children from three ethnic groups was found to have significantly higher ($p < 0.001$) mean D8/17 expression (11.5%) than 13 control children (4.2%) (58). Hill (59) and Murphy and Goodman (60) have described difficulties with establishing the flow cytometry method, including need for positive and negative controls for calibration, matched isotype control, standardization of instrument settings, antibody dilutions, and reagents.

Genetics of D8/17

Although formal segregation analysis was not performed, Khanna et al. (53) concluded that their D8/17 study suggests an autosomal recessive mode of inheritance based on the segregation pattern of the phenotypes defined by the D8/17 positive cells within HLA-typed RF families. In 1992, Herdy and colleagues (61) found the percentage of D8/17 positive B cell to average 38.5% in 10 patients, siblings, fathers, and mothers, 4.5% in normal controls, and 27.5% in the other 2 controls with a family history of RF. The increased percentage of D8/17 cells in family members of RF probands has been interpreted as a marker of genetic risk. One case report supports this view: a family member of an RF proband who was found to have a positive D8/17 assay (30%), but who had no other evidence of RF, developed RF 6 months later (62). D8/17 has subsequently been studied in children with tics and OCD (reviewed below).

Environmental Factors

The limited data from twin studies suggests that environmental factors contribute to risk for RF (46). In the 14 pairs of monozygotic twins reported by Taranta and colleagues (46), only 3 were concordant for RF manifestation. Besides the genetic variability of the strep organism, other environmental risks may contribute. Crowding and winter weather increase risk, probably by promoting proximity of strep-carrying individuals and increasing transmission of the strep organism through a community. Furthermore, repeated exposures to GAβHS may be needed activate immune response resulting in RF in susceptible individuals (37).

IMMUNE RESPONSES IN THE HUMAN HOST

Immunoglobulin G (IgG) antibodies in serum from children with SC bind brain tissue from the caudate, putamen, and subthalamic nuclei, regions thought to be involved in the pathogenesis of SC (20,22,40,63–67). Early studies using an indirect immunofluorescent (IF) method depended on subjective judgments of antibody binding to brain tissue. Church et al. (63) in London have compared IF and newer methods of detection of antibasal ganglia antibodies, ELISA, and Western blotting (WB), using serum from Brazilian SC cases. SC serum was tested against brain protein from homogenized caudate, putamen, and globus pallidus from a patient with no evidence of neurologic disease. Using ELISA, they found that 95% of 20 acute SC cases (symptomatic less than 2 years) had antibasal ganglia antibodies in serum, compared to 56% in 16 persistent SC cases, 13% of 16 acute RF without SC, and 0% of 10 normal pediatric controls. Using Western blotting, even higher rates of specific antibodies were found: 100% for acute SC, 69% for persistent SC, and 13% for acute RF; whereas no antibody binding to basal ganglia was found in normal controls. The results using IF were nearly identical to ELISA and WB methods. The authors concluded that antibasal ganglia antibodies (ABGA) "are universal in acute SC" and are "central to the pathology of SC, possibly by alteration of corticostriatal circuits" (63, p. 231). The same group replicated and extended this finding by testing both serum and cerebrospinal fluid (CSF) in a new Brazilian sample of 14 acute SC, 4 persistent SC, and 10 control children and adolescents (64). On WB, serum IgG ABGA was found in 93% of acute SC, 50% of persistent SC, and none of the controls. Antibodies binding to three antigens were common to the SC samples, at 40, 45, and 60 kDa. CSF ABGA were positive in 3 of 4 acute SC and both of the persistent SC samples available for testing, and the basal ganglia antigens appeared the same as in the serum samples. Abnormal oligoclonal antibody patterns were found in paired serum–CSF samples in only the acute SC samples.

Singer et al. (67) tested sera from 9 NIH-ascertained children with acute SC and 9 age- and sex-matched controls. ELISA and WB methods were used to test SC serum in supernatant, pellet, and synaptosomal fractions of human adult caudate, putamen, and basal ganglia. ELISA detected elevated antibodies in all SC samples, but differences from controls were not significant. Comparison of adult vs. pediatric basal ganglia tissues resulted in similar ABGA results. The authors concluded that ABGA studies need not use pediatric brain samples. WB results showed multiple bands binding to adult basal ganglia in both subjects and controls. Discriminant analysis of WB showed SC to be significantly different from controls, with caudate supernatant the most discriminant. Caudate supernatant bands at 126 and 113 kDa were the two bands with the highest discriminant power. The findings of Singer et al. vary from the two reports from the London group in several ways, including a lower rate of ABGA positivity and the size of the antigen binding to antibody. These differences may reflect small SC sample size, variance in sample handling, method of processing brain tissue (pooled basal ganglia homogenate vs. separate samples for caudate, putamen, and globus pallidus), and variance associated with ABGA in controls. Nevertheless, both of these studies support the hypothesis that ABGA can be found in SC subjects.

In summary, published studies support the presence of antibasal ganglia antibodies in serum from SC subjects. One small study of CSF found ABGA to be the same as those in serum. The paucity of material from SC cases, along with the complexity of sampling and assay methodology contribute to the challenging nature of this research. Progress in characterizing both the relevant antibodies and the related basal ganglia antigens is ongoing. Such research will require the cooperation of patients, clinicians, and laboratory scientists.

Antibodies, Cervical Lymph Nodes, and the Blood–Brain Barrier

Even if antibasal ganglia antibodies circulate are found in the serum of SC patients, it is not clear how such antibodies develop in the brain. The process of developing autoantibodies within the brain is not well characterized. Based on survival of tissue allografts, the brain has been considered a site of limited immune reactivity, a concept known as immune privilege (68). However, Knopf et al. (69) have used a rat model to demonstrate specific antibody synthesis within the brain against a peripherally introduced antigen, despite an intact blood–brain barrier. This model provides direct evidence that specific B cells migrate from periphery to brain where antibody is produced. Furthermore, Knopf et al. showed that immunizing the rat model with the antigen prior to introducing the antigen to brain accelerates the subsequent production of antibody within the brain. The cervical lymph system appears to play an important role. Could this mechanism explain how GAβHS pharyngitis with a particular epitope mimicking basal ganglia triggers the production of ABGA peripherally and within brain? The experiments have yet to be carried out.

Cytokines

Mittleman (70) reported that TH 1 type cytokines are elevated in CSF and in supernatants of peripheral blood mononuclear cell cultures from subjects with SC (and also PANDAS, see below). Elevation of TH 1 type cytokines was interpreted as supporting the active involvement of cell-mediated rather than humoral immunity. Church et al. (64) found increased levels of TH 2 type interleukin-4 (IL-4) in both CSF and serum of acute and persistent SC subjects. Interleukin-10 (IL-10) levels were elevated in acute, but not persistent, sera and CSF samples. The authors interpreted their results as supporting B-cell activation and a humoral mechanism, but noted that T-cell activation and cellular involvement could not be ruled out. The increases in cytokine levels were small, a finding consistent with focal CNS disease restricted to basal ganglia. The authors also noted that elevated CSF IL-4 may indicate intrathecal TH 2 type humoral activity, although the source of IL-4 (intrathecal or from outside the brain) could not be determined.

Is SC an Autoimmune Disorder?

Five criteria for establishing that a disorder is an autoimmune disorder have been stated (71):

1. Auto-antibodies in serum or CSF increased compared to controls
2. Auto-antibodies in brain
3. Induction of disease in animal model by passive transfer of antibody
4. Induction of disease by autoantigen immunization

5. Improvement of clinical symptoms after removal of antibodies with plasma exchange

SC appears to meet Criterion 1, although published results vary regarding the rates of antibasal ganglia antibodies in SC cases and controls. In addition, the molecular mass of the antigens to which antibodies from SC serum bind has been inconsistent between reports. Pathology studies of brain are limited, and so far none tests basal ganglia for autoantibodies. Because SC is transient and not a fatal disease, brain samples from SC patients are unlikely to be directly examined, except in rare cases. As direct examination of human brain tissue is not readily possible, neuroimaging studies may be an acceptable approximation. Giedd et al. (72) have reported increased size of caudate, putamen, and globus pallidus in 24 SC cases as compared to 48 controls. Total cerebral, thalamic, prefrontal, and midfrontal volumes did not differ. These findings support the involvement of basal ganglia, but do not address the issue of antibodies. Traill et al. (73) reported a serial MRI neuroimaging study of an SC subject, who manifested abnormally increased bilateral signal involving the putamen, globus pallidus, and head of the caudate nucleus during the acute phase of SC, with subsequent resolution of the movement disorder. This limited literature suggests a need for longitudinal studies of MRI volume. Clinical symptoms and levels of serum and/or CSF antibasal ganglia antibodies could indirectly address Criterion 2. Criterion 3 has yet to be achieved, as no animal model has yet been established. A preliminary report by Hallett and Kiessling (74) suggests that a rat model demonstrates abnormal movements after passive transfer of antibodies in serum from a patient with SC was infused into the subthalamic nucleus. If replicated, this animal model could allow for demonstration of autoantibodies that target specific brain regions, and give valuable information about cellular targets. Criterion 4, active immunization of an animal model, has also not been achieved. Criterion 5, clinical response to immune modulating treatments has been reported anecdotally (23,75), but no controlled trial has been published.

Recent reviews have come to similar conclusions regarding the need for more evidence of an autoimmune etiology in SC. Loiselle and Singer (76, p. 1236) emphasize the need for caution by concluding that "the current wide acceptance of SC as an "established" model for CNS autoimmunity highlights the need for further studies of this hypothesis." Dale (24) concludes that published studies support antineuronal antibodies as mediators of SC, but raises questions about alternative immune mechanisms. These include possible cytotoxic T-lymphocyte attack, cytokine-mediated neuronal dysfunctions and even superantigen-mediated immunity. Thus, significant evidence supports the hypothesis that SC is an autoimmune disorder triggered by GAβHS, but this evidence does not reach the standard of mechanistic proof reached by a number of other neuroimmune disorders (71).

PANDAS

The hypothesis that GAβHS triggers tics and OCD by an autoimmune mechanism has been critiqued by several authors, including the NIMH group themselves (7,77–79). Kurlan (77,80) has pointed out several challenges for the PANDAS hypothesis. The exacerbating effect of nonspecific stress on TD severity is well known and could contribute to episodes of exacerbation. Antineuronal antibodies are found in only some cases of PANDAS, and they are also found in control subjects without PANDAS. If PANDAS were similar to RF, heart or other manifestations would be expected in PANDAS children, and increased RF would be found in relatives of PANDAS cases. Hoekstra et al. (81, p. 443) concluded that the PANDAS concept "is ill defined, is not supported by unique" immune findings in unselected patients and is "phenomenologically unsound." Despite these issues, determining the pathogenesis of this autoimmune form of TD/OCD is of critical importance, as new opportunities for treatment and prevention would follow (80). Furthermore, recognition of a PANDAS phenotype would accelerate research by highlighting brain mechanisms and by enabling genetics research to discriminate between etiologic subtypes of TD in linkage studies. If proven, the PANDAS hypothesis could also partially answer one of the most puzzling questions about TD: Why does it wax and wane?

Working Criteria for Diagnosing PANDAS

In 1998, Swedo et al. (82) published a summary of 50 PANDAS cases along with the "working diagnostic criteria" used to define them. The working criteria proposed by the NIMH PANDAS group are:

1. Onset after the age of 3 and before puberty
2. Presence of OCD or tic disorder
3. Course characterized by abrupt onset and/or dramatic exacerbations
4. Temporal association with GAβHS infection
5. Temporal association with neurologic abnormalities including motor hyperactivity and adventitious movements (including tics and choreiform movements but not chorea).

These criteria provide a useful focus for research on strep-triggered tics and OCD. However, a comparison of the criteria to what is known about TD raises a question about limitations in the definition of PANDAS.

Age

Criterion 1 requires PANDAS children to be between age 3 years and puberty. This is not significantly different from TD. Mean age at onset for the 50 PANDAS cases was 6.3 years for tics and 7.4 years for OCD. For TD, the mean age at onset was 6.7 + 3 years in 221 TD Yale cases (83). Furthermore, abrupt onset of OCD following severe pharyngitis has been reported in a 25-year-old male (84). If PANDAS shares mechanistic features with SC, it is likely that age at onset could extend into young adulthood.

Nature of Psychiatric Symptoms

Criterion 2 requires presence of tics or OCD. Among the 50 NIMH PANDAS cases, 48% had a primary diagnosis of OCD. Motor tics were present in 80% and primary diagnosis of a tic disorder was assigned in 52%. In the majority of these cases, tics and OCD were comorbid. Similarly, TD co-occurs with OCD or OC symptoms in up to 85% of cases reported in 16 published reports (83). Likewise, ADHD co-occurs in 50% or more in both PANDAS (82) and of idiopathic TD (85). Furthermore, case reports suggest that PANDAS may include anorexia nervosa (86), body dysmorphic disorder (87), and myoclonic movements (88,89). Finally, emotional lability, oppositional defiant disorder, major depression, separation anxiety, and regressive behaviors were described as common in the original NIMH 50 (82). Thus, comorbidity beyond tics and OCD appears common and diverse in what is largely a literature of anecdotal and retrospective reports. If PANDAS results from an autoimmune attack of only basal ganglia, diverse comorbidity could be expected. If the autoimmune mechanism were not confined to basal ganglia, comorbidity would be likely. Perhaps the most distinctive feature to be emphasized in future research should be the nature and timing of onset of ADHD. Onset of ADHD after the age of 7 years would be unusual and could be a distinctive feature.

Episodic Course

PANDAS is defined as having an episodic course with abrupt onset and exacerbations (Criterion 3). Idiopathic TD is usually episodic, and abrupt onset or exacerbation is common. Singer et al. (79) have reported that 42 (52%) of 80 consecutive TS clinic cases described a sudden, explosive onset or worsening. Only 15 of these gave a history of infection within 6 weeks of the explosive episode. History compatible with GAβHS was found in only 9 cases, or 11% of the total sample. Records of throat culture or serology were not sought in this study. The authors concluded that abrupt onset or exacerbation commonly occurs in TS. Historical report of GAβHS was evident in only a minority of cases with abrupt episodes. The course of childhood OCD is less well-documented, but 18% of 83 consecutive cases evaluated for a treatment trial of childhood OCD were judged to have sudden onset (90). For both tics and OCD, defining the term "abrupt" appears to be critical. Swedo et al. have used the term "explosive" to describe the rapid spikes of increased severity followed by gradual improvement (82). Garvey et al. (7, p. 414) have indicated that "Onset of a specific symptom exacerbation can often be assigned to a particular day or week, at which time symptoms seemed to 'explode' in severity." These descriptors appear useful to define the type of onset in new cases, but may need to be better operationalized for assessing exacerbations in children with ongoing symptoms. Lin et al. (91) have applied bootstrap methods to quantify exacerbation thresholds based on symptom ratings in the previous month. Further development of these analytic methods will be helpful. However, the greatest limitation of the present literature derives from the selected and retrospective nature of reports of abrupt onset or exacerbation associated with GAβHS. Prospective studies in unselected samples of TD and OCD are needed to provide objective and concurrent evidence of the course of psychiatric symptoms (and GAβHS infection as described below).

Temporal Association with GAβHS

Criterion 4 requires tic and OCD symptom onset or exacerbation to be associated with GAβHS infection. This means that psychiatric symptoms should rise after infection, and then remit in the absence of reinfection. The temporal association with GAβHS is the most distinctive feature (92), but it appears to be the most problematic. Among the original NIMH 50 cases, 42% had a documented infection prior to tic or OC symptom onset, 2% had a known GAβHS exposure, and 28% recalled an undiagnosed sore throat with no serologic evidence of infection. These numbers account for 72% of cases. Each of the 50 cases also had at least one exacerbation of symptoms occurring within 6 weeks of documented GAβHS. So the lifetime pattern is the deciding factor, with at least two documented rises in symptoms following GAβHS necessary to meet the NIMH PANDAS criterion for temporal association (82).

Because PANDAS has been modeled after RF, it is useful to recall the Jones Criteria, the standard for establishing the diagnosis of RF (93). The 1992 update of the Jones Criteria requires findings on physical exam and the demonstration of an antecedent streptococcal infection. Evidence of antecedent infection can be positive throat culture, rapid strep test or antistreptococcal antibodies (ASO and/or antiDNase-B). However, GAβHS HS isolates can frequently be cultured from young children, and a positive culture may represent carrier status or active pharyngitis (94). Clinically, the degree of illness in a child with an episode of GAβHS pharyngitis triggering

RF can be so mild as to escape notice by the child and parents. For example, only 28% of RF cases could recall a sore throat and only 18% had sought medical care during the recent outbreak of RF in Utah (26). As a result, GAβHS can be isolated from throat cultures of only 25% of untreated patients with RF, resulting in a false negative result (95). Serum ASO and/or antiDNase-B antibody titers are more reliable evidence of antecedent strep infection but false positive and false negative results are not uncommon (96). For SC, both ASO and antiDNase-B titers may return to normal before onset of SC, which may not occur for up to 9 months after GAβHS pharyngitis (7). In one early SC study, antibody titers were found to have declined to normal levels in 40–50% of cases (97). Furthermore, false positive results for ASO serology can occur as a result of the presence of streptococcal strains other than pyogenes and in the presence of high lipoprotein concentrations (96,98).

A strategic test of Criterion 4 has been reported by Murphy and Pichichero (99). They prospectively identified 12 children with PANDAS presenting to a primary care suburban pediatric clinic over a 3-year period. New-onset OCD was associated with positive throat culture or rapid antigen-detection assay in 6 cases at presentation of OCD symptoms and within the previous month in 4 other cases. Of the remaining two cases, one presented with antiDNase-B titer > 1360 and the other manifest GAβHS pharyngitis during a recurrence of PANDAS symptoms. Curiously, antibiotic treatment of pharyngitis resulted in resolution of OC symptoms within a mean of 14 days, with two children showing symptom resolution within 6 days. The authors noted that this rapid response seems inconsistent with a mechanism involving neuronal antibodies. They suggested a possible role for super-antigens. Conclusions from this study were limited by the sample selection and size, as well as the possibility of placebo response. Furthermore, no estimates could be made for population prevalence of PANDAS. Likewise, they could not address the possibility that association of neuropsychiatric symptoms with GAβHS occur spuriously or as the result of nonspecific stress. Better understanding of these issues will require larger and more comprehensive study designs. Future research progress would also be made if GAβHS throat culture isolates could be prospectively stored for later biochemical and genetic analysis (42) before onset of PANDAS. In the case of SC, there may be a period of several months to a year before symptom onset after a streptococcal infection is noted. Thus, these tests may give false negative results if the triggering infection occurred months earlier.

In studying TD cases, Peterson et al. (100) found elevated ASO in 19% and antiDNase-B in 24% of 37 normal controls. Furthermore, Church and Dale (101) tested ASO in 50 adult controls and concluded that the usual upper limit for ASO in children (200 IU/mL) is too low for adults. They recommended that the upper limit for adults be 270 IU/mL. Thus, the interpretation of high serology titers is a complex topic. Ayoub and Harden (96) have recommended that proper interpretation of assays performed in any lab require norms established for normal populations for each age group in each geographic region.

Criterion 5: Neurological Abnormalities

Finally, formal testing for choreiform movements and/or motor hyperactivity was positive in 25/26 of the 50 NIMH PANDAS children (82). Garvey et al. have indicated that the term "choreiform" should not be confused with overt chorea, but that this historical term should be used until the electrophysiologic mechanism is discovered. The question arises, how many garden-variety TD cases (or controls) would also manifest these subtle choreiform movements that were previously described in children with diverse neurodevelopmental disorders? (102). On the other hand, Garvey et al. (7) also reports deterioration of handwriting as a feature observed in some cases of PANDAS. Even if an uncommon indicator, handwriting samples could provide further objectivity as a measure of transient neurologic abnormality.

Evidence for PANDAS as an Autoimmune Disorder

Some published evidence exists for PANDAS relevant to three of the five criteria of Archelos and Hartung (71) for neuroimmune disorders. Specifically, investigators have reported neuronal antibodies in serum, passive transfer of antibodies to an animal model and improvement in symptoms after plasma exchange. There is no report of autoantibodies in human brain. Like SC, brain tissue of children with PANDAS is not likely to be available for study except in rare cases. Neuroimaging studies of treatment cases and one systematic study of 34 PANDAS children disclose acute enlargement of basal ganglia (103). No study has yet attempted active immunization to produce the disease in an animal model.

Antibodies

Kiessling et al. (21) first reported an increased rate of antibasal ganglia antibodies in two successive cohorts referred for clinic evaluation of ADHD, behavior disorders, and learning disabilities. Serum ABGA were tested by using indirect immunofluorescence against caudate and other cerebral tissues from brains from two adult victims of sudden death. When cases were divided into subsets with and without movement disorders, antibodies against caudate were more frequent in movement disorder cases (44%) than in those without movement disorders (21%). These investigators replicated and extended their findings in a new sample of 19 children with ADHD combined with tics or OCD cases, compared to 19 children with ADHD but without tics or OCD (104). This study used indirect immunofluorescence with tissue from caudate, putamen, and other cortical regions obtained from an adult victim of a sudden death. ABGA were found in 63% of tic/OCD cases and in 37% of non-tic/OCD cases (odds ratio 2.9, 95% CI 1.5–5.7). Antibodies against putamen were slightly more frequent than those against caudate in both subject groups. Curiously, over 40% of both groups had some serologic evidence of recent strep infection (ASO or anti-DNase B), but only the ADHD with tics/OCD group were positive on both tests. Singer et al. found antineuronal antibodies against putamen to be increased using ELISA on serum for 41 children with TD compared to 39 controls (105). Human brain tissue from a 78-year-old man was used as the target tissue. These investigators used ELISA optical density results to stratify TD and controls into the highest and lowest 10 cases for characterizing antibodies by WB. Antibody bands were found for 83 kDa in 13 cases and 5 controls, at 67 kDa for 11 cases and 8 controls, and at 60 kDa in 9 cases and 3 controls. Using sucrose gradient separation, the brain antigens were shown to reside in the synaptosomal fraction. Curiously, the only clinical variable that correlated with elevated ELISA optical density was a positive family history of tics ($p=0.04$). Serologic titers of ASO above 166 and anti-DNase B above 170 were also significantly associated with elevated ELISA. The authors point out that 33% of controls had ELISA evidence for antineuronal antibodies and that finding an association does not prove causation. Trifeletti et al. (106,107) have reported finding a protein in the blood of 25 of 29 TD/OCD adults tested and in 11 out of 11 TD/OCD children. This 83-kDa protein, called ts83, is found in normal brain, but not in blood. Furthermore, 1 of 8 SC subjects tested also had ts83. Interestingly, anti-ts83 antibodies were found to be high in three patients when their TD/OCD symptoms were severe, and these antibody levels dropped with successful treatment. In two cases, the treatment was immunological (IVIg in one, corticosteroids in another) (106). It is not clear whether this antibody, ts83, is the same as the 83-kDa antibody reported by Singer et al. (105).

Morshed et al. (66) tested serum from an array of children and adults for antibodies against rat striatum, and for antibodies against nuclear, cytoskeletal, and streptococcal epitopes. Subjects included patients with TD (81), SC (27), autoimmune disorders (52), and controls (67) who were matched for age and geography (postal zip code) to the TD sample. Total and IgG antibodies against rat brain striatum were visualized by indirect IF, using subject serum that was diluted 1:10. Positive sera were then quantified by serial twofold dilution. Results were then rank-ordered, and means for dilution rank orders were compared across subject categories. The subjects with autoimmune disorders ranked significantly highest on antineural antibodies, with SC second, TD third, and normal controls lowest. Mean rank of antineural antibodies for TD subjects were significantly higher than controls, and significantly lower than SC and autoimmune subjects. However, when subjects were stratified into child and adult samples, TD adult subjects were significantly different than controls ($p = 0.045$), while the difference between child samples was nearly significant ($p = 0.051$). Surprisingly, the TD subjects also ranked significantly higher than normal controls and SC subjects on antinuclear antibodies. Autoimmune subjects ranked higher than TD subjects on antinuclear antibodies. IF staining of striatal cells for the highest-ranking TD cases most commonly showed an "antinuclear" binding pattern. This antinuclear pattern was not found with SC serum, where the staining of neurons was diverse, including cytoplasmic, blood vessel, antinuclear, and matrix. No significant differences were found for TD or for IgG class totals, cytoskeletal antibodies, ASO, or antiDNase-B. No distinctive banding pattern was found for any subject group on WB. No phenotypic features were found to be correlated with antibody findings. The authors conclude that their findings support an autoimmune process in TD, but that it appears to involve antibodies more directed against neuronal nuclei, unlike SC. The authors also acknowledge that their findings are limited by the use of rat striatum instead of human tissue, that indirect IF may be less robust than ELISA and that their TD phenotype measures did not include type of onset or course of illness.

Peterson et al. (100) reported ASO and antiDNase-B to be elevated in ADHD cases compared to chronic tic disorder, OCD, or control individuals. In ADHD and OCD subjects, higher antibody titers correlated with larger volumes of putamen and globus pallidus.

In summary, evidence for antibasal ganglia antibodies in TD/OCD serum comes from several laboratories using a variety of techniques. However, published studies vary greatly in sample characteristics (age, type of onset, course), dilution of serum, source of target brain tissue (rat or human, homogenized or separated striatal cell components), and method of detection (indirect IF, ELISA, WB). It is not surprising that the nature of reported antibodies also varies greatly.

D8/17 and PANDAS

The D8/17 assay developed for RF has been studied in children with tics and OCD [reviewed by Murphy and Goodman (60)]. In Swedo's (108) study, 23 of 27 (85%) PANDAS patients, 8 of 9 (89%) SC patients, and 4 of 24 (17%) healthy children were D8/17 positive. Individuals were defined as positive if greater than 12% of B cells were D8/17 positive. The results of the Swedo study appear to be consistent with a study by Murphy et al. (109), in which 31 patients with childhood-onset OCD and/or TD or chronic tic disorder had an average of 22% D8/17-positive B cells with a standard deviation of 5% and 21 comparison subjects had an average of 9% D8/17-positive B cells with a standard deviation of 2%. Using 11.8% as a cutoff for positive, all patients with OCD/TD were positive and only one of the comparison subjects was positive. Subsequent studies have reported D8/17 to be elevated in eating disorders and in autism, but not in OCD in adults (110–112). Thus, the specificity of D8/17 for neuropsychiatric disorders is not clear. More recent studies have attempted to use flow cytometry instead of fluorescent microscopy (113). Hoekstra et al. (114) used flow cytometry and found elevated D8/17 expression levels in 33 TD cases, compared to levels in 20 controls. Murphy and Goodman (60) have reported challenges in adopting the methodology and advise caution in using D8/17 for diagnosis or treatment. While differences between cases and controls have been found, the distribution of D8/17 expression appears continuous and does not define separate subpopulations (60,114).

Animal Models

Two independent laboratories have described an animal model consistent with the PANDAS hypothesis. Hallett and colleagues at Brown first provided evidence for the role of antibodies in producing tic-like repetitive movements and sounds in rats (115–117). They microinfused three substances: serum from 5 TD cases; control serum and IgG derived from TD serum. Five male Fisher 344 rats were tested with each substance via an osmotic pump in a cannula placed at the medial edge of the lateral striatum. Cannula placement was confirmed by histological examination. Oral stereotypies and noises resulted in control rats. The noises were of sufficient loudness to be heard by the observer "standing five feet from the cage." Immunohistochemistry confirmed selective binding of IgG antibody to striatum from TD patients but not with controls.

This model was partially replicated and extended by Taylor et al. (118) at Yale. Sera from TD and controls were first screened for antineural or antinuclear antibodies. Cannulae were implanted in the ventrolateral striatum, a subregion previously demonstrated to produce oral stereotypies when infused with amphetamine. Serum from TD cases with high antibodies produced significantly more oral stereotypies than serum from TD with low levels of antibodies and from controls. Genital grooming was also found to increase in rats receiving the high antibody serum compared to the low antibody and normal control sera. The striking phonic stereotypies reported by Hallett et al. (117) were not reported by Taylor et al., perhaps due to the slightly more ventral and lateral locations for infusion. This positional difference is likely to result in very different stereotypic movement profiles (119). Another methodological difference between the two studies was in the ascertainment scheme. Hallett et al. began with PANDAS cases. Taylor et al. began with unselected TD before dichotomizing by antibody level. Taylor et al. attempted to diagnose PANDAS via pediatric records and parent interview. Documentation was available to address the PANDAS criteria in only 6 of the 12 high antibody TD cases, and none of them met the NIH criteria. Further work is needed to identify the nature and selectivity of the serum antibodies from TD serum. It is also not clear whether antibodies in serum have a relationship to GAβHS infection, and whether M-type or other GAβHS strain differences contribute to a mechanism. Relevant to this point, Muller et al. (120) have reported increased ELISA titers of antibodies against M12 and M19 proteins in serum from 25 TD adults as compared to 25 normal adult controls.

Treatment Studies

Besides the temporal association with GAβHS, the concept of PANDAS is supported by reports of clinical improvement following immunological or antibiotic treatment. Two of the patients in the first NIMH PANDAS cases described by Allen et al. (17) were treated with plasmapheresis, one with intravenous immunoglobulin, and one with immunosuppressive doses of prednisone. All had clinically significant response immediately after treatment. Giedd et al. reported serial MRI changes in a 12-year-old boy experimentally treated for PANDAS, using plasma exchange (121). Treatment was associated with dramatic clinical improvement and with changes in basal ganglia volume. Caudate decreased by 24%, putamen, by 12% and globus pallidus by 24%. From Topeka, Kansas, Sokol and Gray (122) have reported three cases of apparent postinfectious eating disorders, one in a 12-year-old boy with strep-throat and compulsive exercising and a prior history of tics. Penicillin treatment was associated with remarkable improvement, with subsequent deterioration when penicillin was discontinued and improvement again when it was reinstituted. Tucker et al. (123) at Yale have also reported improvement with both penicillin and with plasmapheresis in a 12-year-old girl with TD/OCD associated with strep-throat. Antibodies against rat striatal homogenates and antibodies reactive against the strep M6 protein were found in the girl's blood. Serial volumetric brain MRIs taken early in the course of illness, just before plasmapheresis and 2 weeks after plasmapheresis showed globus pallidus enlargement relative to baseline that decreased after the procedure and correlated with clinical improvement.

Perlmutter et al. (124) reported the first controlled trial of immune modulating therapy for children with PANDAS. Outcome at 1 month and 1 year were compared for three treatment groups: plasma exchange (5 single-volume treatments over 2 weeks for 10 children); intravenous immunoglobulin given (IVIg given at a dose of 1 g/kg per day for 2 consecutive days, $n=9$); and sham IVIg (saline given in the same manner as the active IVIg, $n=10$). At 1 month, both active treatments produced improvement in OCD, anxiety and overall function. Tic symptoms improved with plasma exchange. Remarkably, treatment gains were also found at 1-year follow-up.

A pilot study testing penicillin prophylaxis for tics and OCD used a double-blind, balanced cross-over design in 37 children with PANDAS (125). Each child received twice-daily oral 250 mg penicillin V and placebo, each for 4 months. No differences in tic or OCD symptoms were found, nor were there differences in the rate of GAβHS infection. The authors concluded that prophylaxis was not adequate to eliminate infections, and that future studies should be carried out using a more effective method of prophylaxis.

In summary, there is one controlled trial in a small sample of PANDAS cases and several individual case reports that support immune modulating treatments. Treatment with antibiotics has been reported as unsuccessful in a prophylactic trial and as efficacious in the open treatment trial of acute GAβHS pharyngitis associated with onset of PANDAS. This preliminary evidence points out the need for further study, but does not justify clinical use of these treatments outside of approved research trials.

Genetics of PANDAS

A family study of PANDAS suggests that tics and OCD occur at rates higher than those in the general population and similar to rates in families ascertained for tics and OCD (126). Lougee et al. found that 21% of 54 PANDAS subjects had at least one first-degree relative with a history of tics and that 26% had OCD. Furthermore, there may be overlapping susceptibility between PANDAS and RF. Swedo (92) has reported that rates of RF in parents and grandparents of children with SC probands are similar to rates of RF in PANDAS families, 4% for SC and 6.7% for PANDAS, as compared to 1.4% for control children.

CONCLUSIONS

Proving that a subset of TD cases result from a GAβHS-triggered autoimmune process will be very difficult. PANDAS does not currently meet criteria as an established neuroimmune disorder. The implications for new treatment and prevention methods heighten the need to validate and refine the PANDAS hypothesis. Sydenham's chorea (SC) serves to illustrate that GAβHS can trigger neuropsychiatric disorders. The boundaries between SC and PANDAS, once thought to be clear, now appear genetically more fuzzy, with a possible common susceptibility. In community samples, the high background rate of GAβHS infection and carrier status means that false positive associations pose a great challenge to study design. Treatment and prophylaxis trials have produced mixed results on a small number of subjects. Defining specific antibasal ganglia antibodies and their pathogenic mechanism appear feasible using a combination of human clinical studies and animal models. Larger treatment trials, which incorporate antibody assays and neuroimaging, may be necessary to establish the PANDAS concept. An animal model appears promising, especially for testing mechanisms of diseases and treatment.

ACKNOWLEDGMENTS

We thank Jenise Jensen, M.S., L. George Veasy, M.D., and Harry Hill, M.D. for thoughtful review of this manuscript. This work was supported in part by MH58868 and by NS40034.

REFERENCES

1. Goetz CG, Klawans HL. Gilles de la Tourette on Tourette syndrome. Adv Neurol 1982; 35:1–16.
2. Beskind DL, Keim SM. Choreoathetotic movement disorder in a boy with *Mycoplasma pneumoniae* encephalitis. Ann Emerg Med 1994; 23:1375–1378.
3. Comings D. Tourette Syndrome and Human Behavior. Duarte, CA: Hope Press, 1990.
4. Pauls DL, Leckman JF. The inheritance of Gilles de la Tourette's syndrome and associated behaviors. Evidence for autosomal dominant transmission. N Engl J Med 1986; 315:993–997.
5. Shapiro A, Shapiro E, Young J, Feinberg T. Signs, symptoms, and clinical course. In: Shapiro A, Shapiro E, Young J, Feinberg T, eds. Gilles de la Tourette Syndrome. New York: Raven Press, 1988:127–193.
6. Janavs JL, Aminoff MJ. Dystonia and chorea in acquired systemic disorders. J Neurol Neurosurg Psychiatry 1998; 65:436–445.
7. Garvey MA, Giedd J, Swedo SE. PANDAS: the search for environmental triggers of pediatric neuropsychiatric disorders. Lessons from rheumatic fever. J Child Neurol 1998; 13:413–423.
8. Muller N, Riedel M, Forderreuther S, Blendinger C, Abele-Horn M. Tourette's syndrome and *Mycoplasma pneumoniae* infection. Am J Psychiatry 2000; 157:481–482.
9. Riedel M, Straube A, Schwarz MJ, Wilske B, Muller N. Lyme disease presenting as Tourette's syndrome. Lancet 1998; 351:418–419.
10. McDaniel JS, Summerville MB. Tic disorder associated with encephalopathy in advanced HIV disease. Gen Hosp Psychiatry 1994; 16:298–300.
11. Budman CL, Kerjakovic M, Bruun RD. Viral infection and tic exacerbation. J Am Acad Child Adolesc Psychiatry 1997; 36:162.

12. Northam RS, Singer HS. Postencephalitic acquired Tourette-like syndrome in a child. Neurology 1991; 41:592–593.
13. Turley JM. Tourette-like disorder after herpes encephalitis. Am J Psychiatry 1988; 145:1604–1605.
14. Lombroso PJ, Mack G, Scahill L, King RA, Leckman JF. Exacerbation of Gilles de la Tourette's syndrome associated with thermal stress: a family study. Neurology 1991; 41:1984–1987.
15. Scahill L, Lombroso PJ, Mack G, Van Wattum PJ, Zhang H, Vitale A, Leckman JF. Thermal sensitivity in Tourette syndrome: preliminary report. Percept Mot Skills 2001; 92:419–432.
16. Mulley JC, Scheffer IE, Petrou S, Berkovic SF. Channelopathies as a genetic cause of epilepsy. Curr Opin Neurol 2003; 16:171–176.
17. Allen AJ, Leonard HL, Swedo SE. Case study: a new infection-triggered, autoimmune subtype of pediatric OCD and Tourette's syndrome. J Am Acad Child Adolesc Psychiatry 1995; 34:307–311.
18. Swedo SE. Rituals and releasers: an ethological model of obsessive–compulsive disorder. In: Rapoport JL, ed. Obsessive–Compulsive Disorder in Children and Adolescents. Washington, DC: American Psychiatric Press, 1989:269–288.
19. Wise SP, Rapoport JL. Obsessive–compulsive disorders: is it basal ganglia dysfunction? In: Rapoport JL, ed. Obsessive–Compulsive Disorder in Children and Adolescents. Washington, DC: American Psychiatric Press, 1989:327–346.
20. Swedo SE, Leonard HL, Schapiro MB, Casey BJ, Mannheim GB, Lenane MC, Rettew DC. Sydenham's chorea: physical and psychological symptoms of St. Vitus dance. Pediatrics 1993; 91:706–713.
21. Kiessling LS, Marcotte AC, Culpepper L. Antineuronal antibodies in movement disorders. Pediatrics 1993; 92:39–43.
22. Husby G, van de Rijn I, Zabriskie JB, Abdin ZH, Williams RC Jr, Antibodies reacting with cytoplasm of subthalamic and caudate nuclei neurons in chorea and acute rheumatic fever. J Exp Med 1976; 144:1094–1110.
23. Swedo SE. Sydenham's chorea. A model for childhood autoimmune neuropsychiatric disorders. J Am Med Assoc 1994; 272:1788–1791.
24. Dale RC. Autoimmunity and the basal ganglia: new insights into old diseases. Q J Med 2003; 96:183–191.
25. Bronze MS, Dale JB. The reemergence of serious group A streptococcal infections and acute rheumatic fever. Am J Med Sci 1996; 311:41–54.
26. Veasy LG. Five "lessons" derived from the ten year experience with the resurgence of rheumatic fever in the intermountain area of the United States. XIIIth Lancefield International Symposium on Streptococci and Streptococcal Diseases, Paris, France, September 16–20, 1996.
27. Veasy LG, Wiedmeier SE, Orsmond GS, Ruttenberg HD, Boucek MM, Roth SJ, Tait VF, Thompson JA, Daly JA, Kaplan EL, et al. Resurgence of acute rheumatic fever in the intermountain area of the United States. N Engl J Med 1987; 316:421–427.
28. Mercadante MT, Campos MC, Marques-Dias MJ, Miguel EC, Leckman J.

Vocal tics in Sydenham's chorea. J Am Acad Child Adolesc Psychiatry 1997; 36:305–306.
29. Cardoso F, Vargas AP, Oliveira LD, Guerra AA, Amaral SV. Persistent Sydenham's chorea. Mov Disord 1999; 14:805–807.
30. Cardoso F. Chorea gravidarum. Arch Neurol 2002; 59:868–870.
31. Swedo SE, Rapoport JL, Cheslow DL, Leonard HL, Ayoub EM, Hosier DM, Wald ER. High prevalence of obsessive–compulsive symptoms in patients with Sydenham's chorea. Am J Psychiatry 1989; 146:246–249.
32. Asbahr FR, Negrao AB, Gentil V, Zanetta DM, da Paz JA, Marques-Dias MJ, Kiss MH. Obsessive–compulsive and related symptoms in children and adolescents with rheumatic fever with and without chorea: a prospective 6-month study. Am J Psychiatry 1998; 155:1122–1124.
33. Asbahr FR, Ramos RT, Negrao AB, Gentil V. Case series: increased vulnerability to obsessive–compulsive symptoms with repeated episodes of Sydenham chorea. J Am Acad Child Adolesc Psychiatry 1999; 38:1522–1525.
34. Mercadante MT, Busatto GF, Lombroso PJ, Prado L, Rosario-Campos MC, do Valle R, Marques-Dias MJ, Kiss MH, Leckman JF, Miguel EC. The psychiatric symptoms of rheumatic fever. Am J Psychiatry 2000; 157:2036–2038.
35. McMahon WM, Filloux FM, Ashworth JC, Jensen J. Movement disorders in children and adolescents. Neurol Clin 2002; 20:1101–1124.
36. Cunningham MW. Pathogenesis of group A streptococcal infections. Clin Microbiol Rev 2000; 13:470–511.
37. Bisno AL. Group A streptococcal infections and acute rheumatic fever. N Engl J Med 1991; 325:783–793.
38. Facklam R, Beall B, Efstratiou A, Fischetti V, Johnson D, Kaplan E, Kriz P, Lovgren M, Martin D, Schwartz B, Totolian A, Bessen D, Hollingshead S, Rubin F, Scott J, Tyrrell G. *emm* typing and validation of provisional M types for group A streptococci. Emerg Infect Dis 1999; 5:247–253.
39. Fischetti VA. Streptococcal M protein: molecular design and biological behavior. Clin Microbiol Rev 1989; 2:285–314.
40. Bronze MS, Dale JB. Epitopes of streptococcal M proteins that evoke antibodies that cross-react with human brain. J Immunol 1993; 151:2820–2828.
41. Fujinami RS, Oldstone MB. Molecular mimicry as a mechanism for virus-induced autoimmunity. Immunol Res 1989; 8:3–15.
42. Smoot JC, Korgenski EK, Daly JA, Veasy LG, Musser JM. Molecular analysis of group A Streptococcus type emm18 isolates temporally associated with acute rheumatic fever outbreaks in Salt Lake City, Utah. J Clin Microbiol 2002; 40:1805–1810.
43. Bessen DE, Lombroso PJ. Group A streptococcal infections and their potential role in neuropsychiatric disease. Adv Neurol 2001; 85:295–305.
44. Massell B. Rheumatic Fever and Streptococcal Infection. Boston: The Francis A. Countway Library of Medicine, 1997.
45. Wilson M, Schweitzer M. Pattern of hereditary susceptibility in rheumatic fever. Circulation 1954; 10:699–704.

46. Taranta A, Torosdag S, Metrakos JD, Jegier W, Uchida I. Rheumatic fever in monozygotic and dizygotic twins. Circulation 1959; 20:778.
47. Taranta A, Markowitz M. Rheumatic Fever. Boston: Kluwer Academic Publishers, 1989.
48. Gerbase-DeLima M, Scala LC, Temin J, Santos DV, Otto PA. Rheumatic fever and the HLA complex. A cosegregation study. Circulation 1994; 89:138–141.
49. Ayoub EM. The search for host determinants of susceptibility to rheumatic fever: the missing link. T. Duckett Jones Memorial Lecture. Circulation 1984; 69:197–201.
50. Ayoub EM, Barrett DJ, Maclaren NK, Krischer JP. Association of class II human histocompatibility leukocyte antigens with rheumatic fever. J Clin Invest 1986; 77:2019–2026.
51. Anastasiou-Nana MI, Anderson JL, Carlquist JF, Nanas JN. HLA-DR typing and lymphocyte subset evaluation in rheumatic heart disease: a search for immune response factors. Am Heart J 1986; 112:992–997.
52. Rajapakse C, Halim K, Al-Orainey M, Al-Nozha M, Al-Aska A. A genetic marker for rheumatic heart disease. Br Heart J 1987; 58:659–662.
53. Khanna AK, Buskirk DR, Williams RC Jr, Gibofsky A, Crow MK, Menon A, Fotino M, Reid HM, Poon-King T, Rubinstein P, et al. Presence of a non-HLA B cell antigen in rheumatic fever patients and their families as defined by a monoclonal antibody. J Clin Invest 1989; 83:1710–1716.
54. Gibofsky A, Khanna A, Suh E, Zabriskie JB. The genetics of rheumatic fever: relationship to streptococcal infection and autoimmune disease. J Rheumatol Suppl 1991; 30:1–5.
55. Kemeny E, Husby G, Williams RC Jr, Zabriskie JB. Tissue distribution of antigen(s) defined by monoclonal antibody D8/17 reacting with B lymphocytes of patients with rheumatic heart disease. Clin Immunol Immunopathol 1994; 72:35–43.
56. Chapman F, Visvanathan K, Carreno-Manjarrez R, Zabriskie JB. A flow cytometric assay for D8/17 B cell marker in patients with Tourette's syndrome and obsessive compulsive disorder. J Immunol Methods 1998; 219:181–186.
57. Ganguly NK, Anand IS, Koicha M, Jindal S, Wahi PL. Frequency of D8/17 B lymphocyte alloantigen in north Indian patients with rheumatic heart disease. Immunol Cell Biol 1992; 70(Pt 1):9–14.
58. Harel L, Zeharia A, Kodman Y, Straussberg R, Zabriskie JB, Amir J. Presence of the d8/17 B-cell marker in children with rheumatic fever in Israel. Clin Genet 2002; 61:293–298.
59. Hill HR. Group A streptococcal infections and the pathogenesis of acute rheumatic fever. Scientific proceedings of the 49th annual meeting of the American Academy of Child and Adolescent Psychiatry, San Francisco, October, 2002.
60. Murphy T, Goodman W. Genetics of childhood disorders: XXXIV. Autoimmune disorders, part 7: D8/17 reactivity as an immunological marker of susceptibility to neuropsychiatric disorders. J Am Acad Child Adolesc Psychiatry 2002; 41:98–100.

61. Herdy GV, Zabriskie JB, Chapman F, Khanna A, Swedo S. A rapid test for the detection of a B-cell marker (D8/17) in rheumatic fever patients. Braz J Med Biol Res 1992; 25:789–794.
62. Regelmann WE, Talbot R, Cairns L, Martin D, Miller LC, Zabriskie JB, Braun D, Gray ED. Distribution of cells bearing "rheumatic" antigens in peripheral blood of patients with rheumatic fever/rheumatic heart disease. J Rheumatol 1989; 16:931–935.
63. Church AJ, Cardoso F, Dale RC, Lees AJ, Thompson EJ, Giovannoni G. Anti-basal ganglia antibodies in acute and persistent Sydenham's chorea. Neurology 2002; 59:227–231.
64. Church AJ, Dale RC, Cardoso F, Candler PM, Chapman MD, Allen ML, Klein NJ, Lees AJ, Giovannoni G. CSF and serum immune parameters in Sydenham's chorea: evidence of an autoimmune syndrome? J Neuroimmunol 2003; 136: 149–153.
65. Kotby AA, El Badawy N, El Sokkary S, Moawad H, El Shawarby M. Antineuronal antibodies in rheumatic chorea. Clin Diagn Lab Immunol 1998; 5:836–839.
66. Morshed SA, Parveen S, Leckman JF, Mercadante MT, Bittencourt Kiss MH, Miguel EC, Arman A, Yazgan Y, Fujii T, Paul S, Peterson BS, Zhang H, King RA, Scahill L, Lombroso PJ. Antibodies against neural, nuclear, cytoskeletal, and streptococcal epitopes in children and adults with Tourette's syndrome. Sydenham's chorea, and autoimmune disorders. Biol Psychiatry 2001; 50:566–577.
67. Singer HS, Loiselle CR, Lee O, Garvey MA, Grus FH. Anti-basal ganglia antibody abnormalities in Sydenham chorea. J Neuroimmunol 2003; 136:154–161.
68. Cserr HF, Knopf PM. Cervical lymphatics, the blood–brain barrier, and the immunoreactivity of the brain. In: Keane RW, Hickey WF, eds. Immunology of the Nervous System. Oxford: Oxford University Press, 1997:134–150.
69. Knopf PM, Harling-Berg CJ, Cserr HF, Basu D, Sirulnick EJ, Nolan SC, Park JT, Keir G, Thompson EJ, Hickey WF. Antigen-dependent intrathecal antibody synthesis in the normal rat brain: tissue entry and local retention of antigen-specific B cells. J Immunol 1998; 161:692–701.
70. Mittleman BB. Cytokine networks in Sydenham's chorea and PANDAS. In: Horaud T, Bouvet A, Leclercq R, Montclos HD, Sicard M, eds. Streptococci and the Host. New York: Plenum Press, 1997:933–935.
71. Archelos JJ, Hartung HP. Pathogenetic role of autoantibodies in neurological diseases. Trends Neurosci 2000; 23:317–327.
72. Giedd JN, Rapoport JL, Kruesi MJ, Parker C, Schapiro MB, Allen AJ, Leonard HL, Kaysen D, Dickstein DP, Marsh WL. Sydenham's chorea: magnetic resonance imaging of the basal ganglia. Neurology 1995; 45:2199–2202.
73. Traill Z, Pike M, Byrne J. Sydenham's chorea: a case showing reversible striatal abnormalities on CT and MRI. Dev Med Child Neurol 1995; 37:270–273.
74. Hallett J, Kiessling L. Genetics of childhood disorders: XXXV. Autoimmune disorders, part 8: animal models for noninflammatory autoimmune disorders of the brain. J Am Acad Child Adolesc Psychiatry 2002; 41:223–225.

75. Garvey MA, Swedo SE. Sydenham's chorea: Clinical and therapeutic update. In: Horaud T, Bouvet A, Leclercq R, Montclos HD, Sicard M, eds. Streptococci and the Host. New York: Plenum Press, 1997:115–120.
76. Loiselle CR, Singer HS. Genetics of childhood disorders: XXXI. Autoimmune disorders, part 4: is Sydenham chorea an autoimmune disorder? J Am Acad Child Adolesc Psychiatry 2001; 40:1234–1236.
77. Kurlan R. Tourette's syndrome and 'PANDAS': will the relation bear out? Pediatric autoimmune neuropsychiatric disorders associated with streptococcal infection. Neurology 1998; 50:1530–1534.
78. Murphy TK, Goodman WK, Ayoub EM, Voeller KK. On defining Sydenham's chorea: where do we draw the line? Biol Psychiatry 2000; 47:851–857.
79. Singer HS, Giuliano JD, Zimmerman AM, Walkup JT. Infection: a stimulus for tic disorders. Pediatr Neurol 2000; 22:380–383.
80. Kurlan R. Investigating Tourette syndrome as a neurologic sequela of rheumatic fever. CNS Spectr 1999; 4:62–67.
81. Hoekstra PJ, Kallenberg CG, Korf J, Minderaa RB. Is Tourette's syndrome an autoimmune disease? Mol Psychiatry 2002; 7:437–445.
82. Swedo SE, Leonard HL, Garvey M, Mittleman B, Allen AJ, Perlmutter S, Lougee L, Dow S, Zamkoff J, Dubbert BK. Pediatric autoimmune neuropsychiatric disorders associated with streptococcal infections: clinical description of the first 50 cases. Am J Psychiatry 1998; 155:264–271.
83. Leckman JL, King RA, Cohen DJ. Tics and tic disorders. In: Leckman JL, Cohen DJ, eds. Tourette's Syndrome—Tics, Obsessions, Compulsions: Developmental Psychopathology and Clinical Care. New York: Wiley & Sons, 1999.
84. Bodner SM, Morshed SA, Peterson BS. The question of PANDAS in adults. Biol Psychiatry 2001; 49:807–810.
85. Spencer T, Biederman J, Coffey BJ, Geller D, Faraone S, Wilens T. Tourette disorder and ADHD. In: Cohen D, Jankovic J, Goetz CG, eds. Advances in Neurology: Tourette Syndrome. Vol. 85. Philadelphia, PA: Lippincott, Williams & Williams, 2001:57–78.
86. Sokol MS. Infection-triggered anorexia nervosa in children: clinical description of four cases. J Child Adolesc Psychopharmacol 2000; 10:133–145.
87. Mathew SJ. PANDAS variant and body dysmorphic disorder. Am J Psychiatry 2001; 158:963.
88. DiFazio MP, Morales J, Davis R. Acute myoclonus secondary to group A beta-hemolytic streptococcus infection: a PANDAS variant. J Child Neurol 1998; 13:516–518.
89. Martinelli P, Ambrosetto G, Minguzzi E, Battaglia S, Rizzo G, Scaglione C. Late-onset PANDAS syndrome with abdominal muscle involvement. Eur Neurol 2002; 48:49–51.
90. Giulino L, Gammon P, Sullivan K, Franklin M, Foa E, Maid R, March JS. Is parental report of upper respiratory infection at the onset of obsessive–compulsive disorder suggestive of pediatric autoimmune neuropsychiatric disorder associated with streptococcal infection? J Child Adolesc Psychopharmacol 2002; 12:157–164.

91. Lin H, Yeh CB, Peterson BS, Scahill L, Grantz H, Findley DB, Katsovich L, Otka J, Lombroso PJ, King RA, Leckman JF. Assessment of symptom exacerbations in a longitudinal study of children with Tourette's syndrome or obsessive–compulsive disorder. J Am Acad Child Adolesc Psychiatry 2002; 41:1070–1077.
92. Swedo SE. Pediatric autoimmune neuropsychiatric disorders associated with streptococcal infections (PANDAS). Mol Psychiatry 2002; 7(suppl 2) S24–25.
93. Special Writing Group of the Committee on Rheumatic Fever, Endocarditis, and Kawasaki Disease, Council on Cardiovascular Disease in the Young, American Heart AssociationGuidelines for the diagnosis of initial attack of rheumatic fever. J Am Med Assoc 1992; 268, 2069.
94. Kaplan EL. Recent epidemiology of group A streptococcal infections in North America and abroad: an overview. Pediatrics 1996; 97:945–948.
95. Kavinsky CJ, Parrillo JE. Rheumatic fever and other cardiovascular disease. In: Austen KF, Frank MM, Atkinson JP, Cantor H, eds. Samter's Immunologic Diseases. 6th ed. Vol. II. Philadelphia, PA: Lippincott, Williams & Williams, 2001:546–560.
96. Ayoub EM, Harden E. Immune response to streptococcal antigens: diagnostic methods. In: Rose NR, Hamilton RG, Detrick B, eds. Manual of Clinical Laboratory Immunology. Washington, DC: ASM Press, 2002:409–416.
97. Ayoub EA, Wannamaker LW. Streptococcal antibody titers in Sydenham's chorea. Pediatrics 1966; 38:946–956.
98. Gray GC, Struewing JP, Hyams KC, Escamilla J, Tupponce AK, Kaplan EL. Interpreting a single antistreptolysin O test: a comparison of the "upper limit of normal" and likelihood ratio methods. J Clin Epidemiol 1993; 46:1181–1185.
99. Murphy ML, Pichichero ME. Prospective identification and treatment of children with pediatric autoimmune neuropsychiatric disorder associated with group A streptococcal infection (PANDAS). Arch Pediatr Adolesc Med 2002; 156:356–361.
100. Peterson BS, Leckman JF, Tucker D, Scahill L, Staib L, Zhang H, King R, Cohen DJ, Gore JC, Lombroso P. Preliminary findings of antistreptococcal antibody titers and basal ganglia volumes in tic, obsessive–compulsive, and attention deficit/hyperactivity disorders. Arch Gen Psychiatry 2000; 57:364–372.
101. Church AJ, Dale RC. Antistreptolysin-O titers: implications for adult PANDAS. Pediatric autoimmune neuropsychiatric disorders associated with streptococcal infections. Am J Psychiatry 2002; 159:320.
102. Touwen BC, Sporrel T. Soft signs and MBD. Dev Med Child Neurol 1979; 21:528–530.
103. Giedd JN, Rapoport JL, Garvey MA, Perlmutter S, Swedo SE. MRI assessment of children with obsessive–compulsive disorder or tics associated with streptococcal infection. Am J Psychiatry 2000; 157:281–283.
104. Kiessling LS, Marcotte AC, Culpepper L. Antineuronal antibodies: tics and obsessive–compulsive symptoms. J Dev Behav Pediatr 1994; 15:421–425.
105. Singer HS, Giuliano JD, Hansen BH, Hallett JJ, Laurino JP, Benson M,

Kiessling LS. Antibodies against human putamen in children with Tourette syndrome. Neurology 1998; 50:1618–1624.
106. Trifiletti RR, Altemus M, Packard AM, Bandele AN, Zabriskie JB. Changes in antineuronal antibodies following conventional and immunosuppressive therapy for Tourette's syndrome and obsessive–compulsive disorder. Ann Neurol 1998; 44:561.
107. Trifiletti RR, Altemus M, Solomon GE, Packard AM, Bandele AN, Zabriskie JB. TS83: candidate target brain autoantigen in Tourette's syndrome and obsessive–compulsive disorder. Ann Neurol 1998; 44:561.
108. Swedo SE. Repetitive behaviors and D8/17 positivity-letter. Am J Psychiatry 1997; 154:1630–1631.
109. Murphy TK, Goodman WK, Fudge MW, Williams RC Jr, Ayoub EM, Dalal M, Lewis MH, Zabriskie JB. B lymphocyte antigen D8/17: a peripheral marker for childhood-onset obsessive–compulsive disorder and Tourette's syndrome? Am J Psychiatry 1997; 154:402–407.
110. Eisen JL, Leonard HL, Swedo SE, Price LH, Zabriskie JB, Chiang SY, Karitani M, Rasmussen SA. The use of antibody D8/17 to identify B cells in adults with obsessive– compulsive disorder. Psychiatry Res 2001; 104:221–225.
111. Hollander E, DelGiudice-Asch G, Simon L, Schmeidler J, Cartwright C, DeCaria CM, Kwon J, Cunningham-Rundles C, Chapman F, Zabriskie JB. B lymphocyte antigen D8/17 and repetitive behaviors in autism. Am J Psychiatry 1999; 156:317–320.
112. Sokol MS, Ward PE, Tamiya H, Kondo DG, Houston D, Zabriskie JB. D8/17 expression on B lymphocytes in anorexia nervosa. Am J Psychiatry 2002; 159:1430–1432.
113. Murphy TK, Benson N, Zaytoun A, Yang M, Braylan R, Ayoub E, Goodman WK. Progress toward analysis of D8/17 binding to B cells in children with obsessive compulsive disorder and/or chronic tic disorder. J Neuroimmunol 2001; 120:146–151.
114. Hoekstra PJ, Bijzet J, Limburg PC, Steenhuis MP, Troost PW, Oosterhoff MD, Korf J, Kallenberg CG, Minderaa RB. Elevated D8/17 expression on B lymphocytes, a marker of rheumatic fever, measured with flow cytometry in tic disorder patients. Am J Psychiatry 2001; 158:605–610.
115. Hallett JJ, Harling-Berg CZ, Agrawal JR, Kiessling LS. Tic-like phonation and dyskinesia after intracaudate microinfusion of sera from children with Tourette syndrome. FASEB J 1996; 10:A1357.
116. Hallett JJ, Stopa EG, Harling-Berg CZ, Agrawal JR, Kiessling LS. Neuroanatomical correlates of Tourette syndrome IgG induced dyskinesias in rats. Soc Neuroschi Abstr 1997.
117. Hallett JJ, Harling-Berg CJ, Knopf PM, Stopa EG, Kiessling LS. Anti-striatal antibodies in Tourette syndrome cause neuronal dysfunction. J Neuroimmunol 2000; 111:195–202.
118. Taylor JR, Morshed SA, Parveen S, Mercadante MT, Scahill L, Peterson BS, King RA, Leckman JF, Lombroso PJ. An animal model of Tourette's syndrome. Am J Psychiatry 2002; 159:657–660.

119. Dickson PR, Lang CG, Hinton SC, Kelley AE. Oral stereotypy induced by amphetamine microinjection into striatum: an anatomical mapping study. Neuroscience 1994; 61:81–91.
120. Muller N, Kroll B, Schwarz MJ, Riedel M, Straube A, Lutticken R, Reinert RR, Reineke T, Kuhnemund O. Increased titers of antibodies against streptococcal M12 and M19 proteins in patients with Tourette's syndrome. Psychiatry Res 2001; 101:187–193.
121. Giedd JN, Rapoport JL, Leonard HL, Richter D, Swedo SE. Case study: acute basal ganglia enlargement and obsessive–compulsive symptoms in an adolescent boy. J Am Acad Child Adol Psychiatry 1996; 35:913–915.
122. Sokol MS, Gray NS. Case study: an infection-triggered, autoimmune subtype of anorexia nervosa. J Am Acad Child Adolesc Psychiatry 1997; 36:1128–1133.
123. Tucker DM, Leckman JF, Scahill L, Wilf GE, LaCamera R, Cardona L, Cohen P, Heidmann S, Goldstein J, Judge J, Snyder E, Bult A, Peterson BS, King R, Lombroso P. A putative poststreptococcal case of OCD with chronic tic disorder, not otherwise specified. J Am Acad Child Adolesc Psychiatry 1996; 35:1684–1691.
124. Perlmutter SJ, Leitman SF, Garvey MA, Hamburger S, Feldman E, Leonard HL, Swedo SE. Therapeutic plasma exchange and intravenous immunoglobulin for obsessive–compulsive disorder and tic disorders in childhood. Lancet 1999; 354:1153–1158.
125. Garvey MA, Perlmutter SJ, Allen AJ, Hamburger S, Lougee L, Leonard HL, Witowski ME, Dubbert B, Swedo SE. A pilot study of penicillin prophylaxis for neuropsychiatric exacerbations triggered by streptococcal infections. Biol Psychiatry 1999; 45:1564–1571.
126. Lougee L, Perlmutter SJ, Nicolson R, Garvey MA, Swedo SE. Psychiatric disorders in first-degree relatives of children with pediatric autoimmune neuropsychiatric disorders associated with streptococcal infections (PANDAS). J Am Acad Child Adolesc Psychiatry 2000; 39:1120–1126.

16

Imaging in Tourette's Syndrome

Andrew Feigin and David Eidelberg
North Shore-Long Island Jewish Research Institute
North Shore University Hospital
Manhasset
and New York University School of Medicine
New York, New York, U.S.A.

INTRODUCTION

Tourette's syndrome (TS) is characterized by multiple clinical phenomena including tics as well as behavioral disorders. The clinical characteristics of TS vary between individuals with regard to severity and physical and temporal distribution. Because functional and even structural imaging may reflect both clinical symptomatology as well as actual disease pathology, imaging in TS presents significant challenges. Nonetheless, strides have been made in the neuroimaging of TS, contributing to the understanding of the pathophysiology of the disease and potentially leading to new therapies. This chapter will review the current status of imaging with magnetic resonance imaging (MRI), positron emission tomography (PET), and single photon emission computed tomography (SPECT) in TS, and the potential application of these methodologies to clinical trials and genetic studies.

Neuroimaging studies have either focused on changes associated with TS in general, or have attempted to tease apart the different neuroanatomical and functional manifestations of varying clinical syndromes associated with TS. Given that the most commonly associated behavioral disorders in TS are attention-deficit/hyperactivity disorder (ADHD) and obsessive–compulsive disorder (OCD), this chapter will address imaging findings in TS in general, and in these associated disorders as well.

TOURETTE'S SYNDROME

MRI

MRI abnormalities have been identified in TS patients in several brain regions, including the basal ganglia, corpus callosum, limbic areas, and frontal white matter. Basal ganglia structures that have been found to have reduced volume in TS include the lentiform nuclei (1,2) and the caudate (3,4). Although several studies have found significant asymmetries of volume loss in these structures, it is not clear if these asymmetries are true features of TS, or simply variations due to relatively small sample sizes (5) and perhaps differences in handedness. In addition, basal ganglia volumetric differences between TS and controls have not been consistently identified (6). For example, in a study of girls with TS, no intracerebral morphometric differences were found between the TS subjects and matched controls, except for reduced lateral ventrical size in the TS subjects (7). When potentially confounding variables such as intersubject differences in sex, age, symptoms of ADHD and OCD, and antistreptococcal antibody titers are accounted for, volume reductions appear to be most prominent in bilateral putamen (8). Even so, the volume reductions are of a relatively small magnitude, in the range of 5% less than matched subjects. Nonetheless, taken together, these observations suggest that the movement disorder of TS may, in part, arise from a structural abnormality in the lentiform nuclei, and perhaps more specifically in the putamen.

Several studies have examined corpus callosum volumes in TS. As with the basal ganglia, these studies have produced conflicting results, with some studies demonstrating reduced (9)—and others increased—corpus callosum volumes (10,11). The differences between these studies might be due to differences in the clinical characteristics of the study subjects, as the latter studies found reduced corpus callosum volumes in those subjects with ADHD.

Changes in corpus callosum volume might reflect differences in frontal lobe volume as opposed to representing primary TS pathology (12,13). One study has demonstrated increased right frontal white matter volume in TS (12), and another found increased dorsal prefrontal volumes (14). Again, the effect of associated behavioral abnormalities and small sample sizes on these studies remains to be fully elucidated.

PET and SPECT

Early PET studies of regional brain metabolism in TS found relative hypometabolism in the ventral striatum, midbrain, and paralimbic and ventral prefrontal cortex, and increased metabolic rates in primary motor and motor association cortices (15,16). Hexamethylpropyleneamine oxime (HMPAO)/SPECT studies (measuring cerebral blood flow) have generally confirmed these observations (17–19). In a more recent PET blood flow study, the on-line measurement of tic severity and frequency was associated with brain activation in premotor and motor cortices, anterior cingulate, dorsolateral prefrontal cortex, inferior parietal cortex, and striatum (20). These studies suggest that the signs of TS may be generated by abnormal modulation of the limbic and motor basal ganglia thalamocortical pathways.

Studies utilizing a method of assessing regional covariation in metabolic rates, thereby describing potential functional interactions between brain regions (networks), have confirmed and extended these observations. We have successfully used a comprehensive brain network modeling approach for the detection and quantification of regional metabolic interactions in several neurological disorders (21) including TS (22). In TS, two patterns of brain metabolism were identified—one was characterized by metabolic increases in lateral premotor and supplementary motor association cortices and in the midbrain, and the other was characterized by covariate decreases in caudate and thalamic metabolism associated with smaller reductions in lentiform and hippocampal metabolism. We have recently confirmed these findings in a new cohort of 12 unmedicated adult TS patients (23). In this study, a voxel-based comparison between the TS subjects and 14 age-matched controls using statistical parametric mapping (SPM99) demonstrated decreased metabolism in bilateral lentiform nuclei, and increased metabolism in bilateral sensorimotor cortex (Fig. 1). Network analysis revealed a pattern characterized by striatal and thalamic hypometabolism covarying with hypermetabolism in calcarine cortex and pons; individual subject expression of this pattern

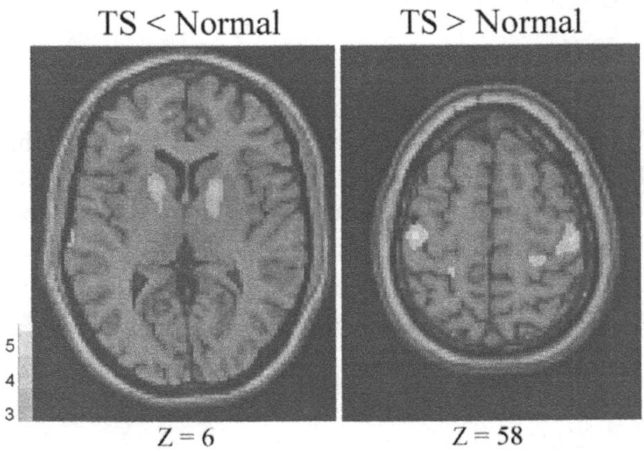

Figure 1 SPM analysis of FDG/PET images, comparing 12 unmedicated adult TS patients to 14 age-matched and sex-matched controls. TS is characterized by hypometabolism in bilateral lentiform nuclei and hypermetabolism in bilateral sensorimotor cortex.

separated the TS subjects from controls at a high degree of statistical significance ($p < 0.0001$), and correlated with an independent clinical measure of functional disability (the Global Impairment Index of the Yale Global Tic Severity Score).

Several imaging studies have evaluated the possible involvement of dopaminergic systems in TS. Early PET studies assessing presynaptic dopaminergic terminals and postsynaptic dopamine D_2 receptors with fluorodopa and raclopride, respectively, failed to identify differences between TS and controls (24,25). Some subsequent studies have identified changes in dopamine D_2 receptor binding in TS (26), but others have not (27). One study described increased fluorodopa (FDOPA) uptake in the left caudate and right midbrain in TS subjects (28), but this has not been confirmed. Assessments of dopamine transporter (DAT) integrity with $[^{123}I]\beta$-CIT and SPECT have produced conflicting results, with some studies demonstrating increased striatal DAT binding in TS (29) and others suggesting that decreased DAT binding correlates with more severe tics (30). Given the conflicting results of imaging studies of the dopaminergic system, it is not possible to draw conclusions about whether this neurotransmitter is primarily involved in the pathogenesis of TS (5). Nonetheless, even if there is relative structural integrity of the dopaminergic system, there could be changes in the function of dopaminergic neurons. In fact, a recent study utilizing PET to measure raclopride displacement after treatment with amphetamine has found that TS is characterized by increases in putamenal dopamine release compared to controls (31). As with other imaging studies, however, it is impossible to know whether these findings are due to the presence or increase in tics in the TS subjects, or actually reflective of the underlying pathophysiology of the disorder.

ADHD

Approximately 50% of children with TS also have ADHD. Whether the pathophysiology of ADHD in TS is the same as when it occurs independently from TS remains unknown. Because very few neuroimaging studies have attempted to identify abnormalities due specifically to ADHD in children with TS, this section will review neuroimaging studies of ADHD in general. Overall, imaging findings in ADHD have focused on regions that have also been identified as important in the pathophysiology of TS.

MRI

As mentioned above, changes in corpus callosum have been identified in TS patients with ADHD. Specifically, smaller anterior regions of the corpus callosum have been reported (10,32,33). These observations were not found in another study (34), but subsequently were confirmed when intersubject differences in brain volume were accounted for (35).

Several studies have found that children with ADHD have reduced total cerebral volumes (36,37). As in TS in general, most studies have further demonstrated frontal lobe abnormalities in ADHD. Frontal lobe regions reported to have reduced volumes in ADHD include the orbitofrontal cortex (38), deep frontal white matter (39), and both premotor and prefrontal cortices (37).

The caudate nucleus has also been implicated in the pathophysiology of ADHD. Reductions in caudate nucleus volume (34,36) as well as changes in caudate asymmetry (40,41) have been described. Supporting the clinical significance of these changes is the added observation that frontal gray matter and caudate volumes correlate with parent-rates and clinician-rated ADHD severity measures (36)

Cerebellar vermis volume appears to be reduced in children with ADHD. Two studies have found reduced volumes in the posterior inferior lobe of the cerebellar vermis in boys with ADHD (42,43), suggesting that an abnormality in cerebello-thalamo-prefrontal circuits may be involved in the pathophysiology of ADHD.

Several studies have applied functional MRI (fMRI) techniques to the study of ADHD. One study found that boys with ADHD, as compared to matched controls, demonstrate increased striatal activation during an attentional task when treated with methylphenidate (44). Another study examining the effects of methylphenidate found an increase in cerebellar vermis T2 relaxation times with methylphenidate in children with ADHD, and the effect was greatest in those children with the most hyperactivity (45). Another study found reduced frontal activation during task performance in untreated children with ADHD (46). These studies generally confirm prior observations using structural resting state imaging methods. Future imaging studies in ADHD will likely focus on activation paradigms, as resting state brain abnormalities may not be as prominent as functional changes that occur during task performance.

PET and SPECT

PET and SPECT imaging have been utilized to assess cerebral metabolism and blood flow in ADHD as well as the dopaminergic system. In general, because of ethical considerations, these studies have been limited to adults with ADHD or a history of ADHD, as the use of child controls for studies involving exposure to radiation has been felt to be inappropriate.

Overall, PET and SPECT studies have been in accord with MRI studies. Decreased frontal lobe metabolism has been observed in ADHD (47) and left anterior frontal lobe metabolism has been found to inversely correlate with ADHD severity (48). Similarly, cerebral blood flow studies utilizing various SPECT and PET ligands have found decreased resting state perfusion in the frontal cortex (49–52), striatum (49), and cerebellum (52).

Neuroimaging studies have implicated the dopaminergic system in the pathogenesis of ADHD, although the exact nature of the defect has remained elusive. Prefrontal reductions in FDOPA uptake have been observed (53), although this was not confirmed in another study that suggested elevated midbrain FDOPA uptake in ADHD (54). Several studies utilizing SPECT imaging of DAT have found elevations in striatal DAT binding in adults (55 56 57) and children (58) with ADHD, but another recent study has failed to confirm this (59). The reasons for the many conflicting results of imaging studies in ADHD remain uncertain but likely relate to small numbers of subjects, differences in imaging methodologies, and perhaps heterogeneity of the disease processes underlying ADHD. Finally, one SPECT study in untreated children with ADHD found increased striatal D_2 receptor binding compared to historical controls; the extent of the increase correlated with measures of hyperactivity (but not measures of inattention) and predicted responses to methylphenidate (60). These observations suggest that different aspects ADHD may be mediated by abnormalities in different brain regions, and perhaps even different neurotransmitter systems.

OCD

OCD affects approximately 50% of TS patients, and genetic studies suggest an etiological link between OCD and TS. The clinical similarity between some compulsive behaviors such as repetitive checking, counting, or touching and complex motor tics underscores the potential relationship between these phenomena. It remains unknown whether OCD occurring in TS is fundamentally different from sporadic OCD, and several clinical studies have suggested differences in the phenomenology of OCD between these groups (61,62).

MRI

As in TS and ADHD, volumetric MRI studies of OCD have produced somewhat inconsistent results. Some studies have demonstrated reduced frontal and striatal volumes (63,64), whereas others found no change (65), and still others found increases in striatal volumes (66). More recent studies have reported increased gray matter in the orbitofrontal cortex and thalamus in patients with OCD (67), and decreased volume of corpus callosum (68). Despite the inconsistent volumetric MRI results, the brain regions that appear to be involved in OCD are largely the same as those identified in neuroimaging studies of TS.

PET and SPECT

PET and SPECT studies also suggest a pathophysiological relationship between TS and OCD. [^{18}F]fluorodeoxyglucose/PET studies in subjects with OCD have demonstrated metabolic increases in the orbitofrontal cortex and striatum (69–71). Similarly, studies in TS patients have found that the presence of behavioral abnormalities, specifically OCD, is also associated with metabolic increases in the orbitofrontal cortex (72,73). SPECT blood flow studies have confirmed these observations (74).

Imaging studies of therapies for OCD have extended many of these observations as well. For example, metabolic increases in the cingulate cortex, thalamus, and lentiform nuclei in OCD are normalized after successful medical treatment for OCD (75). Similarly, HMPAO/SPECT demonstrates increased blood flow in the medial frontal cortex, cingulate, and striatum in OCD patients, and normalization of these values following successful neurosurgical treatment with limbic leucotomy (76). Reductions in caudate metabolism as measured by FDG/PET have been found to correlate with clinical improvement after treatment with paroxetine (77). Taken together, these studies support the idea that the behavioral manifestations of TS may result from alterations in the modulation of specific limbic basal ganglia thalamocortical pathways.

OVERALL MODEL

The symptoms of TS appear to arise from abnormalities in several overlapping but distinct cortico-striato-thalamo-cortical (CSTC) circuits (6). Although the underlying primary pathology of TS remains unknown, neuroimaging studies have provided clues as to how individual differences in the manifestations of TS are generated in the brain. The hyperkinetic movement disorder of TS appears to be generated by an abnormality in the motor CSTC loop, perhaps primarily originating from a defect in the lentiform nuclei, and perhaps more specifically in the putamen. Increased activity in sensorimotor cortices results from these changes, producing tics. In contrast, the behavioral manifestations of TS appear to arise from abnormalities in separate limbic CSTC circuits involving the ventral striatum and its connections with the frontal lobe. The factors that determine the extent to which these different networks are abnormal in individual TS patients and the exact relationships, if any, between the expression of one network and another remain unknown.

CONCLUSION

Applications of modern neuroimaging technologies to the study of TS have led to an improved knowledge of the underlying pathophysiology of the disorder. Nonetheless, many questions remain. A basic issue that has yet to be resolved is whether the changes seen with neuroimaging simply reflect the presence of abnormal signs and symptoms of TS, or are they more basic to the pathophysiology of TS? In the future, neuroimaging methods could be used for assessing therapies for the different aspects of TS, and for studying the genetics of TS. With regard to the latter, the wide spectrum of the clinical manifestations of TS combined with the apparent incomplete penetrance of the disorder may cause difficulty in identifying individuals within a family that carry a gene (or genes) predisposing to TS. The development of a reliable imaging marker that could be used for identifying individuals that might be gene carriers even in the absence of tics could provide a powerful tool in isolating the gene or genes responsible for causing TS.

REFERENCES

1. Peterson B, Riddle MA, Cohen DJ, Katz LD, Smith JC, Hardin MT, Leckman JF. Reduced basal ganglia volumes in Tourette's syndrome using three-dimensional reconstruction techniques from magnetic resonance images. Neurology 1993; 43(5):941–949.
2. Singer SH, Reiss AL, Brown JE, Aylward EH, Shih B, Chee E, Harris EL, Reader MJ, Chase GA, Bryan RN, et al. Volumetric MRI changes in basal ganglia of children with Tourette's syndrome. Neurology 1993; 43(5):950–956.
3. Castellanos FX, Giedd JN, Eckburg P, Marsh WL, Vaituzis AC, Kaysen D, Hamburger SD, Rapoport JL. Quantitative morphology of the caudate nucleus in attention deficit hyperactivity disorder. Am J Psychiatry 1994; 151(12):1791–1796.
4. Hyde TM, Stacey ME, Coppola R, Handel SF, Rickler KC, Weinberger DR. Cerebral morphometric abnormalities in Tourette's syndrome: a quantitative MRI study of monozygotic twins. Neurology 1995; 45(6):1176–1182.
5. Peterson BS. Neuroimaging studies of Tourette syndrome: a decade of progress. Adv Neurol 2001; 85:179–196.
6. Swerdlow NR, Young AB. Neuropathology in Tourette syndrome: an update. Adv Neurol 2001; 85:151–161.
7. Zimmerman AM, Abrams MT, Giuliano JD, Denckla MB, Singer HS. Subcortical volumes in girls with Tourette syndrome: support for a gender effect. Neurology 2000; 54(12):2224–2229.
8. Peterson BS, Leckman JF, Tucker D, Scahill L, Staib L, Zhang H, King R, Cohen DJ, Gore JC, Lombroso P. Preliminary findings of antistreptococcal antibody titers and basal ganglia volumes in tic, obsessive–compulsive, and attention deficit/hyperactivity disorders. Arch Gen Psychiatry 2000; 57(4):364–372.
9. Peterson BS, Leckman JF, Duncan JS, Wetzles R, Riddle MA, Hardin MT,

Cohen DJ. Corpus callosum morphology from magnetic resonance images in Tourette's syndrome. Psychiatry Res 1994; 55(2):85–99.
10. Baumgardner TL, Singer HS, Denckla MB, Rubin MA, Abrams MT, Colli MJ, Reiss AL. Corpus callosum morphology in children with Tourette syndrome and attention deficit hyperactivity disorder. Neurology 1996; 47(2):477–482.
11. Mostofsky SH, Wendlandt J, Cutting L, Denckla MB, Singer HS. Corpus callosum measurements in girls with Tourette syndrome. Neurology 1999; 53(6):1345–1347.
12. Fredericksen KA, Cutting LE, Kates WR, Mostofsky SH, Singer HS, Cooper KL, Lanham DC, Denckla MB, Kaufmann WE. Disproportionate increases of white matter in right frontal lobe in Tourette syndrome. Neurology 2002; 58(1):85–89.
13. Moriarty J, Varma AR, Stevens J, Fish M, Trimble MR, Robertson MM. A volumetric MRI study of Gilles de la Tourette's syndrome. Neurology 1997; 49(2):410–415.
14. Peterson BS, Staib L, Scahill L, Zhang H, Anderson C, Leckman JF, Cohen DJ, Gore JC, Albert J, Webster R. Regional brain and ventricular volumes in Tourette syndrome. Arch Gen Psychiatry 2001; 58(5):427–440.
15. Chase TN, Geoffrey V, Gillespie M, Burrows GH. Structural and functional studies of Gilles de la Tourette syndrome. Rev Neurol 1986; 142(11):851–855.
16. Braun AR, Stoetter B, Randolph C, Hsiao JK, Vladar K, Gernert J, Carson RE, Herscovitch P, Chase TN. The functional neuroanatomy of Tourette's syndrome: an FDG–PET study: I. Regional changes in cerebral glucose metabolism differentiating patients and controls. Neuropsychopharmacology 1993; 9(4):277–291.
17. George MS, Trimble MR, Costa DC, Robertson MM, Ring HA, Ell J. Elevated frontal cerebral blood flow in Gilles de la Tourette syndrome: a 99Tcm-HMPAO SPECT study. Psychiatry Res 1992; 45(3):143–151.
18. Moriarty J, Costa DC, Schmitz B, Trimble MR, Ell J, Robertson MM. Brain perfusion abnormalities in Gilles de la Tourette's syndrome. Br J Psychiatry 1995; 167(2):249–254.
19. Riddle MA, Rasmusson AM, Woods SW, Hoffer B. SPECT imaging of cerebral blood flow in Tourette syndrome. Adv Neurol 1992; 58:207–211.
20. Stern E, Silbersweig DA, Chee KY, Holmes A, Robertson MM, Trimble M, Frith CD, Frackowiak RS, Dolan RJ. A functional neuroanatomy of tics in Tourette syndrome. Arch Gen Psychiatry 2000; 57(8):741–748.
21. Eidelberg D. Functional brain networks in movement disorders. Curr Opin Neurol 1998; 11(4):319–326.
22. Eidelberg D, Moeller JR, Antonini A, Kazumata K, Dhawan V, Budman C, Feigin A. The metabolic anatomy of Tourette's syndrome. Neurology 1997; 48(4):927–934.
23. Feigin A, Budman C, Zgaljardic D, Dhawan V, Eidelberg D. Metabolic brain networks in Tourette syndrome. Mov Disord 2002; 17(suppl 5):S339.
24. Singer HS, Wong DF, Brown JE, Brandt J, Krafft L, Shaya E, Dannals RF, Wagner HN Jr, Positron emission tomography evaluation of dopamine D-2 receptors in adults with Tourette syndrome. Adv Neurol 1992; 58:233–239.

25. Turjanski N, Sawle GV, Playford ED, Weeks R, Lammerstma AA, Lees AJ, Brooks DJ. PET studies of the presynaptic and postsynaptic dopaminergic system in Tourette's syndrome. J Neurol Neurosurg Psychiatry 1994; 57(6):688–692.
26. Wolf SS, Jones DW, Knable MB, Gorey JG, Lee KS, Hyde TM, Coppola R, Weinberger DR. Tourette syndrome: prediction of phenotypic variation in monozygotic twins by caudate nucleus D2 receptor binding. Science 1996; 273(5279):1225–1227.
27. Wong DF, Singer HS, Brandt J, Shaya E, Chen C, Brown J, Kimball AW, Gjedde A, Dannals RF, Ravert HT, Wilson D, Wagner HN Jr. D2-like dopamine receptor density in Tourette syndrome measured by PET. J Nucl Med 1997; 38(8):1243–1247.
28. Ernst M, Zametkin AJ, Jons H, Matochik JA, Pascualvaca D, Cohen RM. High presynaptic dopaminergic activity in children with Tourette's disorder. J Am Acad Child Adolesc Psychiatry 1999; 38(1):86–94.
29. Malison RT, McDougle CJ, van Dyck CH, Scahill L, Baldwin RM, Seibyl JP, Price LH, Leckman JF, Innis RB. (^{123}I)beta-CIT SPECT imaging of striatal dopamine transporter binding in Tourette's disorder. Am J Psychiatry 1995; 152(9):1359–1361.
30. Heinz A, Knable MB, Wolf SS, Jones DW, Gorey JG, Hyde TM, Weinberger DR. Tourette's syndrome: (^{123}I)beta-CIT SPECT correlates of vocal tic severity. Neurology 1998; 51(4):1069–1074.
31. Singer HS, Szymanski S, Giuliano J, Yokoi F, Dogan AS, Brasic JR, Zhou Y, Grace AA, Wong DF. Elevated intrasynaptic dopamine release in Tourette's syndrome measured by PET. Am J Psychiatry 2002; 159(8):1329–1336.
32. Hynd GW, Semrud-Clikeman M, Lorys AR, Novey ES, Eliopulos D, Lyytinen H. Corpus callosum morphology in attention deficit–hyperactivity disorder: morphometric analysis of MRI. J Learn Disabil 1991; 24(3):141–146.
33. Giedd JN, Castellanos FX, Casey BJ, Kozuch P, King AC, Hamburger SD, Rapoport JL. Quantitative morphology of the corpus callosum in attention deficit hyperactivity disorder. Am J Psychiatry 1994; 151(5):665–669.
34. Castellanos FX, Giedd JN, Hamburger SD, Marsh WL, Rapoport JL. Brain morphometry in Tourette's syndrome: the influence of comorbid attention-deficit/hyperactivity disorder. Neurology 1996; 47(6):1581–1583.
35. Castellanos FX. Neural substrates of attention-deficit hyperactivity disorder. Adv Neurol 2001; 85:197–206.
36. Castellanos FX, Lee P, Sharp W, Jeffries NO, Greenstein DK, Clasen LS, Blumenthal JD, James RS, Ebens CL, Walter JM, Zijdenbos A, Evans AC, Giedd JN, Rapoport JL. Developmental trajectories of brain volume abnormalities in children and adolescents with attention-deficit/hyperactivity disorder. JAMA 2002; 288(14):1740–1748.
37. Mostofsky SH, Cooper KL, Kates WR, Denckla MB, Kaufmann WE. Smaller prefrontal and premotor volumes in boys with attention-deficit/hyperactivity disorder. Biol Psychiatry 2002; 52(8):785–794.
38. Hesslinger B, Tebartz van Elst L, Thiel T, Haegele K, Hennig J, Ebert D.

Frontoorbital volume reductions in adult patients with attention deficit hyperactivity disorder. Neurosci Lett 2002; 328(3):319–321.
39. Kates WR, Frederikse M, Mostofsky SH, Folley BS, Cooper K, Mazur-Hopkins P, Kofman O, Singer HS, Denckla MB, Pearlson GD, Kaufmann WE. MRI parcellation of the frontal lobe in boys with attention deficit hyperactivity disorder or Tourette syndrome. Psychiatry Res 2002; 116(1–2):63–81.
40. Hynd GW, Hern KL, Novey ES, Eliopulos D, Marshall R, Gonzalez JJ, Voeller KK. Attention deficit-hyperactivity disorder and asymmetry of the caudate nucleus. J Child Neurol 1993; 8(4):339–347.
41. Mataro M, Garcia-Sanchez C, Junque C, Estevez-Gonzalez A, Pujol J. Magnetic resonance imaging measurement of the caudate nucleus in adolescents with attention-deficit hyperactivity disorder and its relationship with neuropsychological and behavioral measures. Arch Neurol 1997; 54(8):963–968.
42. Berquin C, Giedd JN, Jacobsen LK, Hamburger SD, Krain AL, Rapoport JL, Castellanos FX. Cerebellum in attention-deficit hyperactivity disorder: a morphometric MRI study. Neurology 1998; 50(4):1087–1093.
43. Mostofsky SH, Reiss AL, Lockhart P, Denckla MB. Evaluation of cerebellar size in attention-deficit hyperactivity disorder. J Child Neurol 1998; 13(9):434–439.
44. Vaidya CJ, Austin G, Kirkorian G, Ridlehuber HW, Desmond JE, Glover GH, Gabrieli JD. Selective effects of methylphenidate in attention deficit hyperactivity disorder: a functional magnetic resonance study. Proc Natl Acad Sci U S A 1998; 95(24):14494–14499.
45. Anderson CM, Polcari A, Lowen SB, Renshaw F, Teicher MH. Effects of methylphenidate on functional magnetic resonance relaxometry of the cerebellar vermis in boys with ADHD. Am J Psychiatry 2002; 159(8):1322–1328.
46. Rubia K, Overmeyer S, Taylor E, Brammer M, Williams SC, Simmons A, Bullmore ET. Hypofrontality in attention deficit hyperactivity disorder during higher-order motor control: a study with functional MRI. Am J Psychiatry 1999; 156(6):891–896.
47. Zametkin AJ, Nordahl TE, Gross M, King AC, Semple WE, Rumsey J, Hamburger S, Cohen RM. Cerebral glucose metabolism in adults with hyperactivity of childhood onset. N Engl J Med 1990; 323(20):1361–1366.
48. Zametkin AJ, Liebenauer LL, Fitzgerald GA, King AC, Minkunas DV, Herscovitch P, Yamada EM, Cohen RM. Brain metabolism in teenagers with attention-deficit hyperactivity disorder. Arch Gen Psychiatry 1993; 50(5):333–340.
49. Amen DG, Carmichael BD. High-resolution brain SPECT imaging in ADHD. Ann Clin Psychiatry 1997; 9(2):81–86.
50. Gustafsson P, Thernlund G, Ryding E, Rosen I, Cederblad M. Associations between cerebral blood-flow measured by single photon emission computed tomography (SPECT), electro-encephalogram (EEG), behaviour symptoms, cognition and neurological soft signs in children with attention-deficit hyperactivity disorder (ADHD). Acta Paediatr 2000; 89(7):830–835.
51. Lou HC, Henriksen L, Bruhn P. Focal cerebral hypoperfusion in children with dysphasia and/or attention deficit disorder. Arch Neurol 1984; 41(8):825–829.

52. Kim BN, Lee JS, Shin MS, Cho SC, Lee DS. Regional cerebral perfusion abnormalities in attention deficit/hyperactivity disorder. Statistical parametric mapping analysis. Eur Arch Psychiatry Clin Neurosci 2002; 252(5):219–225.
53. Ernst M, Zametkin AJ, Matochik JA, Jons H, Cohen RM. DOPA decarboxylase activity in attention deficit hyperactivity disorder adults. A (fluorine-18)fluorodopa positron emission tomographic study. J Neurosci 1998; 18(15):5901–5907.
54. Ernst M, Zametkin AJ, Matochik JA, Pascualvaca D, Jons H, Cohen RM. High midbrain (^{18}F)DOPA accumulation in children with attention deficit hyperactivity disorder. Am J Psychiatry 1999; 156(8):1209–1215.
55. Dresel S, Krause J, Krause KH, LaFougere C, Brinkbaumer K, Kung HF, Hahn K, Tatsch K. Attention deficit hyperactivity disorder: binding of (99mTc)TRODAT-1 to the dopamine transporter before and after methylphenidate treatment. Eur J Nucl Med 2000; 27(10):1518–1524.
56. Dougherty DD, Bonab AA, Spencer TJ, Rauch SL, Madras BK, Fischman AJ. Dopamine transporter density in patients with attention deficit hyperactivity disorder. Lancet 1999; 354(9196):2132–2133.
57. Krause KH, Dresel SH, Krause J, Kung HF, Tatsch K. Increased striatal dopamine transporter in adult patients with attention deficit hyperactivity disorder: effects of methylphenidate as measured by single photon emission computed tomography. Neurosci Lett 2000; 285(2):107–110.
58. Cheon KA, Ryu YH, Kim YK, Namkoong K, Kim CH, Lee JD. Dopamine transporter density in the basal ganglia assessed with ((123)I)IPT SPET in children with attention deficit hyperactivity disorder. Eur J Nucl Med Mol Imaging 2003; 30(2):306–311.
59. van Dyck CH, Quinlan DM, Cretella LM, Staley JK, Malison RT, Baldwin RM, Seibyl JP, Innis RB. Unaltered dopamine transporter availability in adult attention deficit hyperactivity disorder. Am J Psychiatry 2002; 159(2):309–312.
60. Ilgin N, Senol S, Gucuyener K, Gokcora N, Sener S. Is increased D2 receptor availability associated with response to stimulant medication in ADHD? Dev Med Child Neurol 2001; 43(11):755–760.
61. Holzer JC, Goodman WK, McDougle CJ, Baer L, Boyarsky BK, Leckman JF, Price LH. Obsessive–compulsive disorder with and without a chronic tic disorder. A comparison of symptoms in 70 patients. Br J Psychiatry 1994; 164(4):469–473.
62. Eapen V, Robertson MM, Alsobrook JP II, Pauls DL. Obsessive compulsive symptoms in Gilles de la Tourette syndrome and obsessive compulsive disorder: differences by diagnosis and family history. Am J Med Genet 1997; 74(4):432–438.
63. Jenike MA, Breiter HC, Baer L, Kennedy DN, Savage CR, Olivares MJ, O'Sullivan RL, Shera DM, Rauch SL, Keuthen N, Rosen BR, Caviness VS, Filipek A. Cerebral structural abnormalities in obsessive–compulsive disorder. A quantitative morphometric magnetic resonance imaging study. Arch Gen Psychiatry 1996; 53(7):625–632.
64. Rosenberg DR, Keshavan MS, O'Hearn KM, Dick EL, Bagwell WW, Seymour AB, Montrose DM, Pierri JN, Birmaher B. Frontostriatal measurement in treatment-naive children with obsessive–compulsive disorder. Arch Gen Psychiatry 1997; 54(9):824–830.

65. Aylward EH, Harris GJ, Hoehn-Saric R, Barta E, Machlin SR, Pearlson GD. Normal caudate nucleus in obsessive–compulsive disorder assessed by quantitative neuroimaging. Arch Gen Psychiatry 1996; 53(7):577–584.
66. Scarone S, Colombo C, Livian S, Abbruzzese M, Ronchi P, Locatelli M, Scotti G, Smeraldi E. Increased right caudate nucleus size in obsessive–compulsive disorder: detection with magnetic resonance imaging. Psychiatry Res 1992; 45(2): 115–121.
67. Kim JJ, Lee MC, Kim J, Kim IY, Kim SI, Han MH, Chang KH, Kwon JS. Grey matter abnormalities in obsessive–compulsive disorder: statistical parametric mapping of segmented magnetic resonance images. Br J Psychiatry 2001; 179, 330–334.
68. Farchione TR, Lorch E, Rosenberg DR. Hypoplasia of the corpus callosum and obsessive–compulsive symptoms. J Child Neurol 2002; 17(7):535–537.
69. Baxter LR Jr, Phelps ME, Mazziotta JC, Guze BH, Schwartz JM, Selin CE. Local cerebral glucose metabolic rates in obsessive–compulsive disorder. A comparison with rates in unipolar depression and in normal controls. Arch Gen Psychiatry 1987; 44(3):211–218.
70. Saxena S, Brody AL, Ho ML, Alborzian S, Ho MK, Maidment KM, Huang SC, Wu HM, Au SC, Baxter LR Jr, Cerebral metabolism in major depression and obsessive–compulsive disorder occurring separately and concurrently. Biol Psychiatry 2001; 50(3):159–170.
71. Swedo SE, Schapiro MB, Grady CL, Cheslow DL, Leonard HL, Kumar A, Friedland R, Rapoport SI, Rapoport JL. Cerebral glucose metabolism in childhood-onset obsessive–compulsive disorder. Arch Gen Psychiatry 1989; 46(6): 518–523.
72. Braun AR, Randolph C, Stoetter B, Mohr E, Cox C, Vladar K, Sexton R, Carson RE, Herscovitch P, Chase TN. The functional neuroanatomy of Tourette's syndrome: an FDG–PET Study: II. Relationships between regional cerebral metabolism and associated behavioral and cognitive features of the illness. Neuropsychopharmacology 1995; 13(2):151–168.
73. Baxter LR, Guze BH. Neuroimaging. In: Kurlan R, ed. Handbook of Tourette's Syndrome and Related Tic and Behavioral Disorders. New York: Marcel Dekker, 1993:289–304.
74. Alptekin K, Degirmenci B, Kivircik B, Durak H, Yemez B, Derebek E, Tunca Z. Tc-99m HMPAO brain perfusion SPECT in drug-free obsessive–compulsive patients without depression. Psychiatry Res 2001; 107(1):51–56.
75. Perani D, Colombo C, Bressi S, Bonfanti A, Grassi F, Scarone S, Bellodi L, Smeraldi E, Fazio F. (^{18}F)FDG PET study in obsessive–compulsive disorder. A clinical/metabolic correlation study after treatment. Br J Psychiatry 1995; 166(2): 244–250.
76. Kim MC, Lee TK, Son BC, Choi CR, Lee C. Regional cerebral blood flow changes in patients with intractable obsessive compulsive disorders treated by limbic leukotomy. Stereotact Funct Neurosurg 2001; 76(3–4):249–255.
77. Hansen ES, Hasselbalch S, Law I, Bolwig TG. The caudate nucleus in obsessive–compulsive disorder. Reduced metabolism following treatment with paroxetine: a PET study. Int J Neuropsychopharmacol 2002; 5(1):1–10.

17

The Inheritance Pattern

Maria C. Rosario-Campos
Yale University School of Medicine
New Haven, Connecticut, U.S.A.

David L. Pauls
Massachusetts General Hospital
and Harvard University School of Medicine
Boston, Massachusetts, U.S.A.

INTRODUCTION

Although the familial nature of Tourette's syndrome (TS) has been observed since 1885 by Gilles de la Tourette himself, it was not until the late 1970s that studies (1,2) demonstrated an increased frequency of a positive family history of tics in families of TS patients. These early studies did not estimate rates of illness among relatives. The first study to do so was reported by Kidd et al. (3). This study combined TS and chronic tics (CT) into a single category and showed that the risk to relatives was significantly elevated over what would be expected by chance.

In fact, all the early studies combined TS and CT into a single category. This was based on the assumption that CT represented a milder variant manifestation of TS. In 1981, Pauls et al. (4) reanalyzed the data collected by Kidd et al. (3) as well as family history data collected from a sample of consecutive TS clinic patients to examine empirically this hypothesis of a relationship between TS and CT. The results of those analyses demonstrated that: (1) CT appeared to represent a variant expression of TS; (2) the increased risk for TS and CT was consistent across the two samples; and (3) the patterns of occurrence within families of TS probands were consistent with hypotheses of vertical transmission.

As indicated, all these studies relied on family history data. That is, not all the relatives were personally assessed and the diagnoses of the relatives were based on information obtained from one—or at most two—informants. However, it has been demonstrated that family history data underestimate the "true" rates of TS and CT obtained with direct interviews (5).

FAMILY STUDIES

To address the potential problem of reporting biases in family history studies, the Yale Family Study of Tourette's Syndrome was undertaken in 1981. In this study, all available first-degree relatives were personally assessed using a structured psychiatric interview. These interview data were then used to assign a range of diagnoses, including TS, CT, and obsessive–compulsive disorder (OCD). Two raters who were blind to the diagnosis of the proband made all diagnoses independently. The results from that study reinforce the idea that TS is familial and that CT and some forms of OCD are variant expressions of TS (6).

The hypothesis that OCD is a variant manifestation of the syndrome grew out of a number of studies that documented the increased frequency of obsessive–compulsive (OC) symptomatology in TS patients (7–16) and was reinforced by the Yale Family Study data suggesting that OCD could represent a variant expression of TS (17). Several subsequent clinical (18–22) as well as family genetic studies have supported these findings (6,23–26). These studies report that the rate of OCD is significantly higher in families of TS probands regardless of whether the proband has a concomitant diagnosis of OCD. That is, the rate of OCD is equally high in families of probands with both TS and OCD, and in families of probands with TS only. It is important to note that a recent TS family study conducted in Japan reported lower rates of TS, CT, OCD, and subclinical OCD, when compared to the rates reported in Western family studies (24). Interestingly, OCD by itself appears to occur more frequently in female relatives of TS probands (6), suggesting some sex-related expression of the syndrome, with males being more likely to express TS and tics and females being more likely to express OCD in the absence of any tics.

Similarly, OCD genetic family studies have also provided evidence that at least some TS and OCD patients share the same genetic vulnerability (27,28). These studies present higher rates of tics and/or TS in first-degree relatives of OCD patients, when compared to control relatives. Even when a comorbid diagnosis of TS in the OCD probands was an exclusion criterion for the study, their relatives presented significantly higher rates of tics than control relatives (28).

Additional support for a genetic component in the etiology of TS came from twin studies (29,30), which show concordance rates for TS in monozygotic (MZ) twins to range between 60% and 80%, compared to less than 20% from dizygotic (DZ) twins (29,30). When the phenotype assessed is expanded to include all kinds of chronic tics, the concordance rates increase to almost 100% in MZ twins (23).

In summary, twin and family genetic studies have provided strong evidence that genetic factors are involved in the vertical transmission within families of a vulnerability to TS and related disorders (31). Once a genetic basis of a disorder is established, a logical next step is to examine whether specific genetic models can explain patterns of transmission within families. Segregation analyses allow an examination of specific genetic and nongenetic models by testing the goodness-of-fit of the pattern of inheritance specified by a hypothesized genetic model to that of the observed patterns of transmission.

ANALYSES OF GENETIC DATA

In the 1980s, five separate studies (32–36) used family history data to test specific genetic hypotheses regarding the inheritance of TS and CT. All studies reported that the pattern of inheritance within families was consistent with a genetic hypothesis that postulated the existence of a single gene of major effect that conferred susceptibility to TS and/or CT. Although the single-locus hypothesis provided the best fit to the data, the hypothesis of multifactorial–polygenic transmission could not be rejected (33). This hypothesis posits that there are many genes, each with equal and additive effect, contributing to the expression of the disorder. Similarly, Comings et al. (34) also could not reject the multifactorial–polygenic hypothesis unless extended relatives were included and the population prevalence for TS and CT was restricted to less than 0.0075.

Nevertheless, the conclusion in all these studies was that a two-allele single major locus genetic model best explained the observed data. A single locus with two alleles results in three possible genotypes. Let TS represent the susceptibility allele for the TS spectrum of behaviors and let "TSTS, TSts, and tsts" represent the three possible genotypes. The probability that a specific genotype will result in a particular phenotype (e.g., TS or CT) is defined as the penetrance. By convention, f_2 is the penetrance for the genotype with two susceptibility alleles (in the above example, f_2 is the penetrance for the TSTS genotype), f_1 is the penetrance for the heterozygous genotype (TSts), and f_0 is the penetrance for the genotype with no susceptibility alleles (tsts). For classic autosomal dominant Mendelian inheritance, $f_2 = f_1 = 1.0$ and $f_0 = 0.0$. For recessive inheritance, $f_2 = 1.0$ and $f_1 = f_0 = 0.0$. When f_2 is less than 1.0, the disorder is said to be incompletely penetrant, and is referred to as a complex disorder because the pattern of inheritance is not strictly Mendelian. If $f_2 > f_1 > f_0$, then the disorder does not follow either a dominant or a recessive pattern and each genotype has a unique probability of expressing the phenotype. It is important to mention that the estimates of penetrance (f_2, f_1, f_0) varied considerably from study to study. Thus, although the results from all studies were consistent with a single-locus hypothesis, not all studies supported an identical model of inheritance. Although some concluded that the most likely mode of inheritance for TS and CT was an autosomal dominant transmission with sex-specific penetrances (32,34,36), others reported unequal f_2 and f_1 values that were not consistent with dominant inheritance (33,35). Nevertheless, all models predicted that males were more likely to develop TS and/or CT if they inherited the susceptibility allele.

Another study suggested that the mode of inheritance for TS was not strictly dominant or recessive, and that the inheritance of TS may be best described as "semidominant, semirecessive" (37). This hypothesis was based on the assumption that wide ranges of other behaviors are also manifestations of the TS susceptibility genes. However, this study used family history data and no formal segregation analyses were presented to support their hypothesis.

Results from analyses presented by Pauls et al. (5) suggested that there was a consistent underestimation of rates in the parents of TS probands in the family history studies of Kidd et al. (3,4) and Kidd and Pauls (33). This same bias could have occurred in the study by Devor (35) because he analyzed families previously reported in the literature. Therefore, the genetic model parameters resulting from these genetic analyses are most likely inaccurate. Specifically, the penetrances for the heterozygotes would be expected to be underestimated because, in any single-locus model, at least one of the parents would be heterozygous for the susceptibility allele. If parents were systematically being incorrectly identified as unaffected, the penetrance estimates for the heterozygotes would be too low.

Another shortcoming of family history studies might be the high number of phenocopies reported. For example, Baron et al. (32) predicted that approximately 70% of the males and 50% of the females would be phenocopies (individuals with the disorder but without the gene for the condition). It is possible that consistent underreporting of the condition for parents and/or females could have been responsible for the high phenocopy estimate. Because fewer parents and female relatives would have been included as affected, there would have been more families in which the proband was an isolated case. This would yield a higher estimate of the rate of phenocopies.

As mentioned above, family study data result in higher estimates of the rates of TS and CT in the first-degree relatives of TS probands, when compared to the rates obtained from family history studies (5). Pauls and Leckman (38) demonstrated that the pattern within families was consistent with autosomal dominant transmission. Segregation analyses were also undertaken with data collected for a linkage study of TS (39). The results from segregation analyses of the multigenerational family data are remarkably similar to the results from the nuclear family data reported by Pauls and Leckman (38). In both sets of analyses, an autosomal dominant hypothesis was supported when: (1) only relatives with TS were included as affected; (2) relatives with TS or CT were included as affected; and (3) relatives with TS, CT, or OCD were included as affected.

Although more recent segregation analyses generally continue to support the presence of a major locus, the reported characteristics of this predisposition gene have varied. Hasstedt et al. (40) found the pattern of inheritance to be consistent with a genetic model in which the penetrance of the heterozygote was between the penetrances of the two homozygotes. Walkup et al. (41) observed a similar solution but with a significant multifactorial background. A number of studies have emphasized that there is a frequent occurrence of bilineal transmission (from both maternal and paternal sides) in studied families (41–43). Contrary to these results, Seuchter et al. (44) reported that in their sample, the pattern of transmission of TS and other related tic disorders was not consistent with Mendelian inheritance. They evaluated 108 extended TS families, with a total of 1784 individuals assessed, and also reported lower rates of OCD and subclinical OCD in the relatives than previous studies.

One possible explanation for the differences in the reported results so far is that TS is, in fact, a heterogeneous disorder. Among the frequent comorbid diagnoses, OCD has been constantly identified as representing an alternative expression of the TS phenotype. Trying to better dissect the phenotype of these TS + OCD patients, a recent study (26) has analyzed the data from the sibpair study of the Tourette Syndrome Association International Consortium for Genetics (TSAICG). The authors completed univariate and complex segregation analyses using quantitative OC symptom dimensions scores. These dimensions had been previously identified by Leckman et al. (45) and include: aggressive, sexual, and religious obsessions and checking compulsions (FACTOR1); symmetry and ordering obsessions and compulsions (FACTOR2); contamination obsessions and cleaning/washing compulsions (FACTOR3); and hoarding obsessions and compulsions (FACTOR4). FACTORS 1 and 2 were significantly correlated in the sibpairs concordant for TS, and mother–child correlations were significant for these two factors as well. Segregation analyses were consistent with dominant major gene effects for both FACTOR1 and FACTOR2, whereas for FACTOR3 and FACTOR4, the most parsimonious solution was consistent with recessive inheritance.

Alsobrook et al. (46) analyzed lifetime tic symptom data obtained from direct structured interviews of 85 TS probands and 28 affected first-degree relatives. Without any a priori assumptions concerning the relatedness of symptoms, the 29 tic symptoms were grouped by using agglomerative hierarchical clustering in 12 symptom clusters. Scores for the probands' symptom clusters were then used as variables in a principal component factor analysis, with varimax rotation. Four factors were identified, accounting for 61% of the symptomatic variance. FACTOR1, which accounted for 20% of the variance, was characterized by aggressive behaviors that included being argumentative, having temper fits, kicking, self-injurious behavior, and coprolalia. FACTOR2, which accounted for 17% of the variance, was characterized primarily by simple tics (both motor and phonic). FACTOR3, which accounted for 14% of the variance, was characterized by compulsive behaviors such as throat clearing and repetitive actions (including touching of others or objects and repeating speech sounds). Finally, FACTOR4, which accounted for 10% of the variance, was characterized by the absence of grunting tics and the presence of tapping (which was distinguished from finger and hand tics, or touching of others or objects). This innovative study also examined the relationships of the resulting factor scores to comorbidity in probands and recurrence risks in relatives. In addition, intraclass correlations were calculated for within-family factor scores of 36 families. FACTOR3 (compulsive phenomena) was associated with an earlier age at onset of TS; high scores on FACTOR1 and FACTOR3 were associated with ADHD comorbidity in the probands; and male subjects had higher FACTOR2 scores than did female probands. Furthermore, high scores on FACTOR3 were significantly associated with both ADHD and OCD in the relatives. The authors also calculated intraclass correlation coefficients for 36 independent proband–relative pairs. The correlation between the proband and relative factor scores was significant for three of the factors (FACTOR1, FACTOR3, and FACTOR4). Even though these results need to be replicated in larger independent samples, these results indicate that these factors may represent a valid structure with clinical and genetic relevance.

In sum, despite the differences in findings, methodologies, and proposed models of inheritance, the bulk of family, twin, and segregation analyses studies supports the idea that genes play a major role in the etiology of TS and related disorders (47).

THE SEARCH FOR THE GENES

The overt nature of tics, the belief that TS was a homogeneous disorder, the hypothesis of having an autosomal dominant pattern of inheritance, and the advances in molecular biology techniques caused researchers to be enthusiastic about using linkage and association methods to find the susceptibility gene(s) causing TS. Unfortunately, to date, no genetic loci have been identified.

Genetic linkage studies provide a powerful method for confirming the conclusions of segregation analysis studies because linkage results can demonstrate the existence of a major locus and help clarify the pattern of inheritance even in the absence of a known association between a biological abnormality and TS. One reason that linkage studies have been disappointing in the localization of the TS gene(s) may be that the initial studies used parametric analyses of the data. These analyses are dependent on the accurate specification of the transmission pattern, which remains to be established.

Therefore, assuming autosomal dominant transmission and genetic homogeneity, almost 90% of the genome has been excluded by different investigators (47–51). Nevertheless, even performing a model-based linkage analysis, a recent study of a large French Canadian family identified evidence for linkage with an LOD score of 3.24 on chromosome 11 (11q23) (52). It is important to mention that this study used markers previously identified in linkage studies of population isolates in South Africa and the 11q23 locus was also found to be associated with the TS phenotype in this identity-by-descent (IBD) study (53,54).

Given current uncertainties regarding the inheritance parameters, nonparametric methods such as the sibpair approach were undertaken by the TSAICG. The sibpair method is suited for diseases with an unclear mode of inheritance, and has been successful in other complex disorders (31). This study reported two regions of the genome (on chromosomes 4q and 8p) with LOD scores higher than 2 (55).

Using the same sibpair data collected by the TSAIGC, a recent genome scan of the hoarding phenotype reported significant allele sharing for markers at 4q34–35, 5q35, and 17q25 (25). It is important to mention that the 4q site is in close proximity to the region previously linked to TS in the sibpair study (55).

Another genome scan using the affected pedigree method (APM) was completed on a series of multigenerational families and revealed eight markers with possible linkage in at least one of the families (56). Interestingly, one of the regions presented in this study (19p) also reached an LOD score higher than 1 in the TSAIGC sibpair study (55,57).

Association studies use a "case–control" design and assess the relationship between alleles and a disorder within populations. Several association studies have examined a variety of candidate genes in TS patients and controls. Some of the evaluated genes include dopamine receptors (DRD1, DRD2, DRD4, and DRD5), dopamine transporter, various noradrenergic genes (*ADRA2a*, *ADRA2C*, and *DBH*), and some serotoninergic genes (5-

HTT) (53,58–67). Nevertheless, their results must be interpreted with caution given the known potential pitfalls of this approach.

An additional approach is the search for cytogenetic abnormalities in TS patients. Some of the findings include translocation involving chromosomes 18 and 7 (68,69), breakpoints in chromosome 7 (70,71), and fragile sites on chromosome 16q22–23 (72). Unfortunately, none of the chromosomal regions in which cytogenetic abnormalities have been found to cosegregate with TS has shown any convincing evidence for linkage in the high-density families, the sibpair study, or the population isolates studies (73).

FUTURE WORK

The localization of a gene or genes responsible for the expression of TS will be a major step forward in our understanding of the genetic/biological risk factors important for the expression of this syndrome. In addition, this work will allow the potential identification of nongenetic factors associated with the manifestation or the amelioration of the symptoms of the disorders (74,75). On one hand, the identification of a linked marker will permit the design of much more incisive studies to illuminate the physiological/biochemical etiology of TS by examination of the gene product and its impact on the manifestation of the syndrome. On the other hand, by controlling for genetic factors, it will be possible to document more carefully the environmental/nongenetic factors important for the expression of the TS spectrum.

Once the location of a gene or genes has been verified, it will be possible to type the unaffected children in high-risk families to determine with a high probability who is carrying a susceptibility gene. It will then be possible to examine in more detail the interaction between genotype and environment. Linked genetic markers can serve as the basis for defining an appropriate control group for a "genetic case–control" design.

The ability to utilize genetic linkage and other aspects of genetic studies to design and carry out a study of nongenetic etiological factors of a psychiatric illness is a significant methodological advancement that has not been possible so far. Data from prospective studies of children at risk will make it possible to examine individuals with specific genotypes to determine which factors protect some from manifesting the syndrome. It is important to begin data collection now, before genes are localized. After the genes are localized, it will be ethically unacceptable to withhold the test for identification of carriers from individuals at risk, and knowledge of carrier status may change the caregiving environment.

Until this day comes, all efforts will be directed toward improving existing genetic techniques such as the identification of more specific markers, as well as developing more advanced and accurate ones. At the same time, the search for more homogeneous phenotypes and more comprehensive assessment tools needs to be emphasized.

ACKNOWLEDGMENTS

This work was supported, in part, by grants from the Tourette Syndrome Association and the Obsessive Compulsive Foundation to Dr. Rosario-Campos, and grants from the National Institutes of Health [NS16648, MH00508 (an RSA), and NS40024] to Dr. Pauls.

REFERENCES

1. Eldridge R, Sweet R, Lake CR, Ziegler M, Shapiro AK. Gilles de la Tourette's syndrome: clinical, genetic, psychological and biochemical aspects in 21 selected families. Neurology 1977; 27:115–124.
2. Shapiro AK, Shapiro ES, Bruun RD, Sweet RD. Gilles de la Tourette's Syndrome. New York: Raven Press, 1978.
3. Kidd KK, Prusoff BA, Cohen DJ. The familial pattern and transmission of Gilles de la Tourette syndrome and multiple tics. Arch Gen Psychiatry 1980; 37:1336–1339.
4. Pauls DL, Cohen DJ, Heimbuch R, Detlor J, Kidd KK. Familial pattern and transmission of Gilles de la Tourette syndrome and multiple tics. Arch Gen Psychiatry 1981; 38:1091–1093.
5. Pauls DL, Kruger SD, Leckman JF, Cohen DJ, Kidd KK. The risk of Tourette Syndrome (TS) and Chronic Multiple Tics (CMT) among relatives of TS patients: obtained by direct interview. J Am Acad Child Psychiatry 1984; 23:134–137.
6. Pauls DL, Raymond CL, Leckman JF, Stevenson JM. A family study of Tourette's syndrome. Am J Hum Genet 1991; 48:154–163.
7. Kelman DH. Gilles de la Tourette's disease in children: a review of the literature. J Child Psychol Psychiatry 1965; 6:219–226.
8. Fernando SJM. Gilles de la Tourette's syndrome. Br J Psychiatry 1967; 113:115–124.
9. Morphew JA, Sim M. Gilles de la Tourette's syndrome: a clinical and psychopathological study. Br J Med Psychol 1969; 42:293–301.
10. Nee LE, Caine ED, Polinsky RJ, Eldridge R, Ebert MH. Gilles de la Tourette syndrome: clinical and family study of 50 cases. Ann Neurol 1980; 7:41–49.
11. Yaryura-Tobias JA, Neziroglu F, Howard S, Fuller B. Clinical aspects of Gilles de la Tourette syndrome. Orthomol Psychiatry 1981; 10:263–268.
12. Jagger J, Prusoff BA, Cohen DJ, Kidd KK, Carbonari CM, John K. The epidemiology of Tourette's syndrome: a pilot study. Schizophr Bull 1982; 8:267–278.
13. Montgomery MA, Clayton PJ, Friedhoff AJ. Psychiatric illness in Tourette

syndrome patients and first-degree relatives. In: Friedhoff AJ, Chase TN, eds. Gilles de la Tourette Syndrome. New York: Raven Press, 1982:335–339.
14. Nee LE, Polinsky RJ, Ebert MH. Tourette syndrome: clinical and family studies. In: Friedhoff AJ, Chase TN, eds. Gilles de la Tourette Syndrome. New York: Raven Press, 1982:291–295.
15. Stefl ME. Mental health needs associated with Tourette syndrome. Am J Public Health 1984; 74:1310–1313.
16. Cummings JL, Frankel M. Gilles de la Tourette syndrome and neurological basis of obsessions and compulsions. Biol Psychiatry 1985; 20:1117–1126.
17. Pauls DL, Towbin KE, Leckman JF, Zahner GEP, Cohen DJ. Gilles de la Tourette syndrome and obsessive compulsive disorder: evidence supporting an etiological relationship. Arch Gen Psychiatry 1986; 43:1180–1182.
18. Robertson MM, Trimble MR, Lees AJ. The psychopathology of the Gilles de la Tourette: a phenomenological analysis. Br J Psychiatry 1988; 152:383–390.
19. Robertson MM. The Gilles de la Tourette syndrome: the current status. Br J Psychiatry 1989; 154:147–169.
20. Robertson MM. Tourette syndrome, associated conditions and the complexities of treatment. Brain 2000; 123:425–462.
21. Frankel M, Cummings JL, Robertson MM, Trimble MR, Hill MA, Benson DF. Obsessions and compulsions in the Gilles de la Tourette syndrome. Neurology 1986; 36:379–382.
22. Pitman RK, Green RC, Jenike MA, Mesulam MM. Clinical comparison of Tourette's disorder and obsessive–compulsive disorder. Am J Psychiatry 1987; 144:1166–1171.
23. Walkup JT, Leckman JF, Price RA, Harden MT, Ort S, Cohen DJ. The relationship between Tourette syndrome and obsessive compulsive disorder: a twin study. Psychopharmacol Bull 1988; 24:375–379.
24. Kano Y, Ohta M, Nagai Y, Pauls DL, Leckman JF. A family study of Tourette syndrome in Japan. Am J Med Genet (Neuropsychiatr Genet) 2001; 105:414–421.
25. Zhang H, Leckman JF, Tsai C-P, Kidd KK, Rosario Campos MC. The Tourette Syndrome Association International Consortium for Genetics. Genome wide scan of hoarding in sibling pairs both diagnosed with Gilles de la Tourette syndrome. Am J Hum Genet 2002; 70:896–904.
26. Leckman JF, Pauls DL, Zhang H, Rosario-Campos MC, Katsovich L, Kidd KK, Pakstis AJ, Alsobrook JP, Robertson MM, McMahon WM, Walkup JT, van de Wetering BJ, King RA, Cohen DJ. Obsessive–compulsive symptom dimensions in affected sibling pairs diagnosed with Gilles de la Tourette syndrome. Am J Med Genet 2003; 116B(1):60–68.
27. Pauls DL, Alsobrook JP II, Goodman W, Rasmussen S, Leckman JF. A family study of obsessive–compulsive disorder. Am J Psychiatry 1995; 152:76–84.
28. Grados MA, Riddle MA, Samuels JF, Liang K-Y, Hoehn-Saric R, Bienvenu OJ, Walkup JT, Song D, Nestadt G. The familial phenotype of obsessive–compulsive disorder in relation to tic disorders: the Hopkins OCD Family Study. Biol Psychiatry 2001; 50:559–565.

29. Price RA, Kidd KK, Cohen DJ, Pauls DL, Leckman JF. A twin study of Tourette syndrome. Arch Gen Psychiatry 1985; 42:815–820.
30. Hyde TM, Aaronson BA, Randolph C, Rickler KC, Weinberger DR. Relationship of birth weight to the phenotypic expression of Gilles de la Tourette's syndrome in monozygotic twins. Neurology 1992; 42:652–658.
31. Leckman JF. Gilles de la Tourette's Syndrome. Lancet 2002; 360:1577–1586.
32. Baron M, Shapiro E, Shapiro A, Ranier JD. Genetic analysis of Tourette syndrome suggesting a major gene. Am J Hum Genet 1981; 33:767–775.
33. Kidd KK, Pauls DL. Genetic hypotheses from Tourette syndrome. In: Friedhoff AJ, Chase TN, eds. Gilles de la Tourette Syndrome. New York: Raven Press, 1982:243–249.
34. Comings DE, Comings BG, Devor EJ, Cloninger CR. Detection of a major gene for Gilles de la Tourette syndrome. Am J Hum Genet 1984; 36:586–600.
35. Devor EJ. Complex segregation analysis of Gilles de la Tourette syndrome: further evidence for a major locus mode of transmission. Am J Hum Genet 1984; 36:704–709.
36. Price RA, Pauls DL, Kruger SD, Caine ED. Family data support a dominant major gene for Tourette syndrome. Psychiatry Res 1988; 24:251–261.
37. Comings DE, Comings BG, Knell E. Hypothesis: homozygosity in Tourette syndrome. Am J Med Genet 1989; 34:413–421.
38. Pauls DL, Leckman JF. The inheritance of Gilles de la Tourette's syndrome and associated behaviors: evidence for autosomal dominant transmission. N Engl J Med 1986; 315:993–997.
39. Pauls DL, Pakstis AJ, Kurlan R, Kidd KK, Leckman JF, Cohen DJ, Kidd JR. Segregation and linkage analyses of Gilles de la Tourette's syndrome and related disorders. J Am Acad Child Adolesc Psychiatry 1990; 29:195–203.
40. Hasstedt SJ, Leppert M, Filloux F, van de Wetering BJM, McMahon WM. Intermediate inheritance of Tourette syndrome, assuming assortive mating. Am J Hum Genet 1995; 57:682–689.
41. Walkup JT, LaBuda MC, Singer HS, Brown J, Riddle MA, Hurko O. Family study and segregation analysis of Tourette syndrome: evidence for a mixed model of inheritance. Am J Hum Genet 1996; 59:684–693.
42. Kurlan R, Eapen V, Stern J, McDermott MP, Robertson MM. Bilineal transmission in Tourette's syndrome families. Neurology 1994; 44:2336–2342.
43. McMahon WM, van de Wetering BJM, Filloux F, Betit K, Coon H, Leppert M. Bilineal transmission and phenotypic variation of Tourette's disorder in a large pedigree. J Am Acad Child Adolesc Psychiatry 1996; 35:672–680.
44. Seuchter SA, Hedebrand J, Klug B, Knapp M, Lehmkuhl G, Poustka F, Schmidt M, Remschmidt H, Baur MP. Complex segregation analysis of families ascertained through Gilles de la Tourette syndrome. Genet Epidemiol 2000; 18: 33–47.
45. Leckman JF, Grice DE, Boardman J, Zhang H, Vitale A, Bondi C, Alsobrook J, Peterson BS, Cohen DJ, Rasmussen SA, Goodman WK, McDougle CJ, Pauls DL. Symptoms of obsessive compulsive disorder. Am J Psychiatry 1997; 154: 911–917.

46. Alsobrook JP II, Leckman JF, Goodman WK, Rasmussen SA, Pauls DL. Segregation analysis of obsessive–compulsive disorder using symptom-based factor scores. Am J Med Genet (Neuropsychiatr Genet) 1999; 88:669–675.
47. State MW, Lombroso PJ, Pauls DL, Leckman JF. The genetics of childhood psychiatric disorders: a decade of progress. J Am Acad Child Adolesc Psychiatry 2000; 39(8):946–962.
48. Barr CL, Sandor P. Current status of genetic studies of Gilles de la Tourette syndrome. Can J Psychiatry 1998; 43:351–357.
49. Heutnik P, van de Wetering BJ, Breedveld GJ, Weber J, Sandkuyl LA, Devor EJ, Heiberg A, Niermeijer MF, Oostra BA. No evidence for genetic linkage of Gilles de la Tourette syndrome on chromosomes 7 and 18. J Med Genet 1990; 27:433–436.
50. Pakstis AJ, Heutnik P, Pauls DL, Kurlan R, van de Wetering BJ, Leckman JF, Sandkuyl LA, Kidd JR, Breedveld GJ, Castiglione CM, et al. Progress in the search for genetic linkage with Tourette syndrome: an exclusion map covering more than 50% of the autosomal genome. Am J Hum Genet 1991; 48:281–294.
51. Patel PI. Quest for the elusive basis of Tourette's syndrome. Am J Hum Genet 1996; 50:980–982.
52. Mérette C, Brassard A, Potvin A, Bouvier H, Rousseau F, Émond C, Bissonnette L, Roy M-A, Maziade M, Ott J, Caron C. Significant linkage for Tourette syndrome in a large French Canadian family. Am J Hum Genet 2000; 67:1008–1013.
53. Simonic I, Gericke GS, Ott J, Weber JL. Identification of genetic markers associated with Gilles de la Tourette syndrome in an Afrikaner population. Am J Hum Genet 1998; 63:839–846.
54. Simonic I, Nyholt DR, Gericke GS, Gordon D, Matsumoto N, Ledbetter DH, Ott J, Weber JL. Further evidence for linkage of Gilles de la Tourette syndrome (GTS) susceptibility loci on chromosomes 2p11, 8q22 and 11q23–24 in South African Afrikaners. Am J Med Genet 2001; 105:163–167.
55. The Tourette Syndrome Association International Consortium for Genetics. A complete genome screen in sib pairs affected by Gilles de la Tourette syndrome. Am J Hum Genet 1999; 65:1428–1436.
56. Barr CL, Wigg KG, Pakstis AJ, Kurlan R, Pauls DL, Kidd KK, Tsui L-C, et al. Genome scan for linkage to Gilles de la Tourette syndrome. Am J Med Genet 1999; 88:437–445.
57. Singer HS. Current Issues in Tourette Syndrome. Mov Disord 2000; 15:1051–1063.
58. Comings DE, Comings BG, Muhleman D, Dietz G, Shahbahrami B, Tast D, Knell E, Kocsis P, Baumgarten R, Kovacs BW, et al. The dopamine D2 receptor locus as a modifying gene in neuropsychiatric disorders. JAMA 1991; 266:1793–1800.
59. Comings DE, Muhleman D, Dietz G, Dino M, LaGro L, Gade R. Association between Tourette's syndrome and homozygosity at the dopamine D3 receptor gene. Lancet 1993; 341:906.
60. Nöthen MM, Chichon S, Hemmer S, Hebebrand J, Remschmidt H, Lehmkuhl

G, Poustka F, Schmidt M, Catalano M, Fimmers R, et al. Human dopamine D4 receptor gene: frequent occurrence of a null allele and observation of homozygosity. Hum Mol Genet 1994; 3:2207–2212.
61. Nöthen MM, Hebebrand J, Knapp H, Hebebrand K, Camps A, von Gontard A, Wettke-Schafer R, Lisch S, Cichon S, Poustka F, et al. Association analysis of the dopamine D2 receptor gene in Tourette's syndrome using the haplotype relative risk method. Am J Med Genet 1994; 54:249–252.
62. Grice DE, Leckman JF, Pauls DL, Kurlan R, Kidd KK, Pakstis AJ, Chang FM, et al. Linkage disequilibrium between an allele at the dopamine D4 receptor locus and Tourette syndrome, by the transmission-disequilibrium test. Am J Hum Genet 1996; 59:644–652.
63. Comings DE, Wu S, Chiu C, et al. Polygenic inheritance of Tourette syndrome, stuttering, attention deficit hyperactivity, conduct, and oppositional defiant disorder. Am J Med Genet (Neuropsychiatr Genet) 1996; 67:264–288.
64. Thompson M, Comings DE, Feder L, George SR, O'Dowd BF. Mutation screening of the dopamine D1 receptor gene in Tourette's syndrome and alcohol dependent patients. Am J Med Genet 1998; 81:241–244.
65. Comings DE, Gonzales N, Wu S, Gade R, Muhleman D, Saucier G, Johnson P, Verde R, Rosenthal RJ, Lesieur HR, Rugle LJ, Miller WB, MacMurray JP. Studies of the 48 bp repeat polymorphism of the *DRD4* gene in impulsive, compulsive, addictive behaviors: Tourette syndrome, ADHD, pathological gambling, and substance abuse. Am J Med Genet 1999; 4:213–215.
66. Stober G, Hedebrand J, Cichon S, Bruss M, Bonisch H, Lehmkuhl G, Poustka F, Schmidt M, Remschmidt H, Propping P, Nothen MM. Tourette syndrome and the norepinephrine transporter gene: results of a systematic mutation screening. Am J Med Genet 1999; 88:158–163.
67. Cavallini MC, Di Bella D, Catalano M, Bellodi L. An association study between 5-HTTLPR polymorphism. COMT polymorphism and Tourette's syndrome. Psychiatry Res 2000; 97:93–100.
68. Boghosian–Sell L, Comings DE, Overhauser J. Tourette syndrome in a pedigree with a 7:18 translocation: identification of a YAC spanning the translocation breakpoint at 18q22.3. Am J Hum Genet 1996; 59:999–1005.
69. Donnai D. Gene location in Tourette syndrome. Lancet 1997; 14:627–1005.
70. Kroisel PM, Petek E, Emberger W, Windpassinger C, Wladika W, Wagner K. Candidate region for Gilles de la Tourette syndrome at 7q31. Am J Med Genet 2001; 101:259–261.
71. Petek E, Windpassinger C, Vincent JB, Cheung J, Boright AP, Scherer SW, Kroisel PM, Wagner K. Disruption of a novel gene (*IMMP2L*) by a breakpoint in 7q31 associated with Tourette syndrome. Am J Hum Genet 2001; 97:93–100.
72. Kerbeshian J, Severud R, Burd L, Larson L. Peek-a-boo fragile site at 16d associated with Tourette syndrome, bipolar disorder, autistic disorder, and mental retardation. Am J Med Genet 2000; 96:69–73.
73. State MW, Greally JM, Cuker A, Bowers PN, Henegariu O, Morgan TM, Gunel M, DiLuna M, King RA, Nelson C, Donovan A, Anderson GM, Leckman JF, Hawkins T, Pauls DL, Lifton RP, Ward DC. Epigenetic abnormalities associated

with a chromosome 18(q21–q22) inversion and a Gilles de la Tourette syndrome phenotype. Proc Natl Acad Sci USA 2003; 100(8):4684–4689.

74. Pauls DL. Emerging genetic markers and their role in potential preventive intervention strategies. In: Muehrer P, ed. Conceptual Research Models for Preventing Mental Disorders. Rockville, MD: NIMH, 1990:184–195.
75. Leckman JF, Doinansky ES, Hardin M, Clubb M, Walkup JT, Stevenson J, Pauls DL. The perinatal factors in the expression of Tourette's syndrome. J Am Acad Child Adolesc Psychiatry 1990; 29:220–226.

18

Progress in Gene Localization

Cathy L. Barr
University of Toronto
The Toronto Western Hospital Research Institute
and The Hospital for Sick Children
Toronto, Ontario, Canada

OVERVIEW

Despite very strong evidence for a genetic basis for the susceptibility to develop Gilles de la Tourette syndrome (GTS), as of this date, a gene contributing to GTS has not convincingly been identified. The failure to identify genes contributing to GTS may be the result of multiple factors including a more complex mode of inheritance than previously suspected, locus heterogeneity with a number of risk genes located at different chromosomal locations, and uncertainties about how best to define the phenotype for genetic studies. Chromosomal abnormalities have been reported in isolated cases of GTS, but thus far, genes identified at breakpoints in these chromosomes do not appear to contribute to a large percentage of families with GTS. Results from several genome scans have pointed to the likely locations of GTS susceptibility genes and these regions are currently under study, with the goal of narrowing these regions for gene identification. Alternative phenotypes and statistical methods are being used in the linkage analyses to further refine the search for genes and these approaches appear promising. While it is difficult for an animal model to fully represent the complex phenotype of GTS, some progress has been made in the understanding of stereotypic movements, hyperlocomotion, and excessive grooming in experimental animal models. Such models can therefore provide important insights as to the types of genes that are likely to contribute to GTS, which will help to guide future genetic studies.

LINKAGE FINDINGS FROM GENOME SCANS

The search for genetic factors contributing to the susceptibility to GTS has been investigated by a number of groups using linkage and association studies (1,2). These studies include genome scans for GTS using multigenerational families (3,4), nuclear families with affected sibling pairs (5), and studies using pools of DNA from individuals with GTS from the South African Afrikaner population compared with those of control subjects (6). These studies are summarized in the following sections.

The genome scan of 110 affected sibling pairs from 76 families, carried out as part of an international consortium, identified several regions that provided some evidence for linkage, although the findings did not reach genome-wide significance levels (5). The most significant regions identified using single-point analysis were on 4q (D4S1625) and 8p (D8S1106). Other markers with a single-point LOD score greater than 1 were D1S1728, D4S403, D4S2623, D4S1644, D6S1053, D8S1130, D8S1145, D8S136, D10S1213, D11S912, D14S592, and D17S1298. Two regions, 4q and 8p, were found to have multipoint LOD scores greater than 2, and four additional regions on chromosomes 1, 10, 13, and 19, were found to have multipoint LOD scores greater than 1. This study is continuing and 200 additional affected sibling pairs are currently being collected to increase the power of the sample to confirm linkage and, if confirmed, to narrow the linked region for gene identification.

One of the regions identified in the genome scan of affected sibling pairs (19p13.3) overlaps with a region with some evidence for linkage identified in the author's genome scan of multigenerational families. That study of seven multigenerational families, ranging in size from 15 to 67 family members, used a panel of 386 to 109 markers across the genome and analyzed the data using both parametric (autosomal dominant with reduced penetrance) and two nonparametric methods (4). For the parametric analyses, no regions were identified that reached the accepted genome-wide significance levels; however, several regions produced suggestive evidence for linkage. The two regions with the most robust support for linkage were chromosome 19p13.3 in a large pedigree collected in Oregon (47 family members) and the centromeric region of chromosome 5 in a pedigree designated T008 (32 family members). For the nonparametric analyses, eight markers were observed with *P*-values less than 0.00005, providing significant evidence for linkage, in at least one family, that included markers in the chromosome 19 and 5 regions. The nonparametric methods used are known to have a high false positive rate; therefore additional support should be obtained before it is concluded that these regions are linked to GTS.

Capitalizing on the relative homogeneity of the South African Afrikaner population, Simonic et al. (6) compared the allele frequencies in pooled DNA from GTS individuals with that of controls using 1167 polymorphic markers distributed across the genome. Fifteen of the markers in 11 chromosomal regions showed significant differences in the distributions of alleles between the GTS and control groups. The regions that were significant and that were also supported by multiple markers were the centromeric region of chromosome 2 (D2S1790, D2S440), 8q (D8S257, D8S1132, D8S1119), 11q (D11S933, D11S1377), distal 20q (D20S1085, D20S469, D20S468), and 21q (D21S1252, GATA45C03). These five regions were further studied in 91 nuclear families (affected siblings and parents) using the transmission disequilibrium test (TDT) and haplotype relative risk (HRR) analysis (7). Single-marker TDT analysis supported the regions 2p11 (D2S139), 8q22 (GATA28F12), and 11q23–24 (D11S1377). Extended, two-locus analysis supported the regions on chromosomes 2 and 8. The chromosome 8 region was particularly interesting because this region, and specifically the marker D8S257, was previously supported by some evidence for linkage (LOD score 1.57, theta = 0.10) (8) in a large GTS pedigree collected in Utah (9). Further supporting the 8q region is the finding of a balanced translocation of chromosomes 1 and 8 in a person with GTS and in additional family members, with the chromosome 8 breakpoint being in this region. This translocation finding is further discussed in Section 5.

Linkage to the chromosome 11q23 region was reported in a single large multigenerational pedigree (127 members) from the French Canadian population (10). This study focused on the 24 markers that were previously identified by Simonic et al. (6) as being significant in the South African Afrikaner population. The most significant result in the French Canadian family was in the 11q23 region, found using multipoint analysis (LOD score of 3.24 or 3.18 after correction for multiple testing) across the markers D11S1377 and D11S933. Interestingly, one of the markers in the linked region (D11S933) is located 7 cM from the marker D11S912 that resulted in a LOD score of between 1 and 2 in the Tourette Syndrome Association genome scan. This region is therefore supported by three studies and remains very promising.

FACTORS INFLUENCING THE SUCCESS OF GENETIC LINKAGE STUDIES

Given that there is strong support for a genetic basis to GTS, it is surprising that the genome scans did not provide more significant evidence for linkage. A number of factors may have contributed to this outcome, including misspecifications of the genetic model for the parametric analyses, misdiagnosis of individuals, the choice of phenotype for genetic studies, family structure, locus heterogeneity, and phenocopies.

The original genetic studies of GTS focused on multigenerational families because GTS was assumed to be an uncommon phenotype with a relatively simple mode of inheritance. A number of segregation studies supported an autosomal dominant transmission with reduced penetrance (11–14), but some studies could not rule out multifactorial polygenic inheritance (15,16). Intermediate models (lower penetrance for heterozygotes of the disease gene than homozygotes) have also been supported (17,18). Under the assumptions of a major locus effect, large families are quite powerful for identifying linkage using parametric analyses if the mode of inheritance is specified correctly (19). However, large families are less powerful for complex modes of inheritance and are relatively weak for nonparametric analytical methods. Furthermore, if there is a high degree of locus heterogeneity, as we now suspect for GTS, then a limited number of large pedigrees will not be able to detect all of the susceptibility genes.

An unexpected complication in the study of extended pedigrees with GTS was the finding that among the large families with many affected individuals collected for linkage studies, many were bilineal; that is, the susceptibility genes were transmitted from both sides of the pedigree (20,21). Kurlan et al. (20) studied 39 high-density families defined as having 5 or more individuals with GTS and observed that 33% of these pedigrees were bilineal for GTS and 41% were bilineal for obsessive-compulsive behaviors. This was an unexpected finding at the time, given that GTS was considered, until very recently, to be a relatively uncommon disorder (22–24).

A large number of small nuclear families can be used as an alternative or a complement to linkage studies with the large families. This approach for GTS has had some success, as in the TSA genetic consortium affected sibling pair study. That is, interesting regions were identified; however, no one region reached the appropriate significance levels for the number of tests performed. The results suggest that there may be many genes contributing to the GTS phenotype located in different chromosomal locations and that no one gene contributes to a large percentage of cases. If this is indeed the case, a larger collection of families is crucial for gene identification.

A collection of small pedigrees can also be used to narrow large regions of linkage that are characteristic following a genome scan. The most power from these small pedigrees is gained from linkage disequilibrium studies that use either a dense set of markers across the region or markers in candidate genes in the region. Hence a combination approach of linkage studies using evenly spaced, highly informative markers (microsatellite markers), followed by a dense map of markers across the linked region with some markers located in candidate genes, and statistical methods that rely on linkage disequilibrium can be used to narrow the linked region and identify genes. This complementary strategy optimizes the power of the families and the chance of success.

PHENOTYPES FOR LINKAGE ANALYSIS

A number of factors characteristic of GTS present difficulties in diagnosis and are problematic for the definition of the phenotype for genetic studies. These include the change of symptoms over time (waxing and waning), variability in symptoms and severity among family members, and gender and age effects. Whereas chronic multiple tics in family members of GTS probands are a logical milder phenotype of GTS susceptibility genes (25–27), the genetic relationship of commonly occurring comorbid disorders is less clear. Obsessive-compulsive disorder (OCD), obsessive-compulsive behavior (OCB), and attention-deficit/hyperactivity disorder (ADHD) are often found in individuals with GTS and their family members. Family and twin studies support that OCD and OCB may be alternative expression of GTS susceptibility genes (27–29). The genetic relationship of GTS with ADHD and other phenotypes are currently uncertain (30–32).

The classification of affected status is more critical for extended families because the status of connecting individuals can dramatically influence the results of the linkage analysis depending on the position of the individuals in the pedigree. Thus misdiagnosis of crucial linking individuals can result in significant changes in LOD score as was seen for the linkage findings for bipolar disorder in an extended pedigree (33,34). Affected sibling pair studies are less impacted by the classification of individuals if only clearly affected individuals are selected for inclusion in the study. However, information may be lost using a restricted definition of the phenotype.

Recent studies have explored alternative phenotypes as a way to maximize the power of the sample and identify genetically meaningful phenotypes. The genotype data from the genome scan of the affected sibling pairs with GTS (5) were analyzed for the phenotype of hoarding, a component of OCD (35). This phenotype was analyzed both as a dichotomous trait and quantitative trait using standard linkage analysis (Haseman–Elston methods) and a novel analysis with recursive partitioning. Significant evidence for linkage was found for the 4q34–35 region ($P=0.0007$) previously identified in the genome scan with suggestive evidence for linkage to the GTS phenotype and also to two regions not previously identified in the genome scan, 5q35.2–35.3 ($P=0.000002$) and 17q25 ($P=0.00002$). Recursive partitioning was used to examine multiple markers simultaneously, and the results suggest joint effects of the 5q and 4q loci ($P=0.000003$). Although not significant, some evidence for linkage was previously reported for the 17q25 region (marker D17S802, LOD score 2.21, theta = 0.001) from analysis of a large kindred collected in Utah (8), further supporting this region as a susceptibility locus.

CHROMOSOMAL ABNORMALITIES REPORTED IN GTS

While the majority of individuals with GTS do not have chromosomal changes, a number of chromosomal abnormalities have been reported (36). These findings may be extremely valuable for gene identification; however, in sporadic cases, it may be impossible to determine if the chromosomal change is related to the development of GTS or a chance event that happens to co-occur in the individual. If the chromosomal change is found to be segregating with the disorder in multiple affected individuals within a family or if a number of individuals are found with the same change in the population, then this change is more likely to be related to GTS. While genes identified through chromosomal abnormalities in a single individual may be a rare cause of GTS, any gene identified could provide insight into the neurobiological basis of GTS and may lead to the identification of other genes in the pathway.

The 7q22 region has received particular interest because of two independent chromosomal events implicating this region: a balanced translocation t(7;18) that maps to the region 7q22 to 7q31 within the 14-cM interval flanked by the markers D7S515 and D7S522 (37) and an inverted duplication of chromosome 7q22.1–q31.1 (38).

The reciprocal translocation of chromosome 7 and 8, t(7;18)(q22;q22.1), was found in a patient with GTS and six relatives (37). No support for linkage was found between the breakpoint on chromosome 7q22 and the COLA1 locus at 7q21.3–q22.1 leading the authors to conclude that a GTS locus was located on the 18q region in this family (39). Furthermore, a patient with a deletion of the long arm of chromosome 18 at 18q22.1 was reported with mild hypoplastic mid-face, tic-like movements, mild OCD, panic attacks, and visual hallucinations supporting the assumption that a gene contributing to GTS was localized at 18q22.1 (40). The genome scans and a number of linkage studies that specifically investigated the 7q22 and 18q22 regions thus far have not been able to confirm linkage to either of these regions (41).

The patient with the inverted duplication of chromosome 7q22.1–q31.1 was reported to have GTS, moderate mental retardation, plus minor physical anomalies (38). A novel gene, IMP2, located between the markers D7S515 and D7S522, has been found to be disrupted by the distal breakpoint and the duplication (42). IMP2 is thought to be the human homologue of the *Saccharomyces cerevisiae* mitochondrial inner membrane peptidase subunit II gene based on 42% homology. Expression of this gene was observed in a wide range of tissues with the exception of adult liver and lung (42). While the breakpoint in IMP2 implicates this gene as an underlying factor for GTS in this patient, it is also possible that the phenotype results from the additional copy of genes in the duplicated region. Other genes located in the duplicated region are the Leu-Rch Rep gene, suggested to play a role in the development of the nervous system by protein–protein interactions, CAGH44, a polyglutamine repeat protein from brain, and neuronal cell adhesion molecule (NRCAM), a member of the cell adhesion molecules (CAMs) (42).

A balanced translocation of chromosomes 1 and 8, (t1;8)(q21.1;q22.1), was identified in a nuclear family with seven children (43). Of the six children with the translocation, one had GTS, one had modest tics and Asperger's syndrome, two had mild tics, and the two youngest were unaffected, but were still very young and not through the age of risk. The seventh child did not carry the translocation and did not exhibit any symptoms. The 8q22.1 breakpoint was supported as a susceptibility locus in the study of Simonic et al. (7) and by some evidence for linkage (marker D8S257, LOD score 1.57, theta = 0.10) in the large pedigree collected in Utah (8). The breakpoint of this translocation was cloned and no genes were identified at the breakpoint; however, the gene for core-binding factor, alpha subunit 2, translocated to 1 (CBFA2T1), a transcription factor, was identified 11 kb distal to the breakpoint at 8q22.1 (44). Positional effects of the translocation on CBFA2T1 could not be ruled out as a causative mechanism in this family; however, no GTS specific DNA changes in this gene were identified in an additional 37 unrelated GTS subjects (44).

A deletion of the very distal segment of the short arm of chromosome 9p23-pter was reported in a GTS patient also presenting with OCD, ADHD, mildly dysmorphic features with microcephaly, prominent supraorbital ridges, slight mid-facial hypoplasia, and a number of other characteristics consistent with 9p deletion syndrome (45). Another female patient with GTS has been reported with a deletion of the short arm of 9p distal to p22 and mosaicism of triple X (46). This patient also was reported to have a history of grand mal seizures, physical abnormalities, schizophrenia, mild mental retardation, and violent and aggressive behavior. No evidence for linkage of the 9pter region to GTS has been found in linkage studies thus far; however, a recent genome scan for early-onset obsessive-compulsive disorder did find evidence for linkage to the 9p24 region, 9.03 cM from 9pter (NPL score 3.19, $P = 0.0032$) (47). Interestingly, the probands in the genome scan for OCD were seven children or adolescents (age 6–17), three with a history of GTS (47).

One patient with a balanced translocation of chromosomes 3 and 8, 46XY, t(3;8) (p21.3;q24.1), has been reported (48). When this family was further studied, however, family members with GTS were identified that did not have the translocation suggesting that the translocation was not related to GTS in this family (48). However, because of the finding in the original patient, a linkage study was carried out for markers in the chromosome 3 and 8 regions that initially found a multipoint LOD score of 2.99 for markers in the chromosome 3p region (49). When more informative markers were genotyped, this result became less significant (LOD score 1.77), and multipoint analysis excluded the region of the translocation. Other linkage studies using independent families have not found support for this region (4,50).

A number of GTS patients have been reported with autism or Asperger's syndrome (51–55). The frequency of the co-occurrence of GTS in autism and Asperger's syndrome has been reported to be higher than expected by chance, leading some investigators to hypothesize a causal link (53,54,56). The exact frequency of the overlap is not known, however, and the diagnosis is complicated by the difficulty in distinguishing rituals from complex tics (56). A single patient with a de novo duplication of 16p13.1 to pter and GTS and autism has been reported (57). This patient had considerable behavior problems, was socially withdrawn and self-isolating, exhibited evident simple and complex motor and vocal tics, had poor concentration, and was easily distracted. Autistic symptoms included memory for details of street names, telephone numbers, and birth dates. Discrete dysmorphic features were also apparent. The chromosomal finding in this patient is particularly interesting given the recent reports of suggestive evidence for linkage (maximum LOD scores 2.9, 0.74, and 2.19) to the 16p13 region from genome scan studies of autism (58,59) and significant evidence for linkage of ADHD to this region (60) in a follow-up of the first genome scan for ADHD (61).

STUDIES OF CANDIDATE GENES AND REGIONS

Several positive findings with candidate genes have been reported but, as of yet, not convincingly replicated. It is important to keep in mind that for all linkage and association studies of complex traits, the results should be interpreted cautiously and the conclusions concerning the involvement of a particular gene from a single study are limited to the families studied and by the power of the sample. All studies should be extensively replicated before definitive conclusions are reached.

The focus of candidate gene studies has been on genes involved in the regulation of neurotransmitters with particular focus on the dopamine system because of the success of neuroleptics and other agents interacting with the dopaminergic system in the suppression of tics. Genes reported to be linked to GTS include the dopamine receptors D2, D3, and D4 (1). Other candidate genes have been tested for linkage, but no evidence for linkage was reported. These genes include dopamine receptors D1 and D5, tyrosine hydroxylase, dopamine beta hydroxylase, tyrosinase, dopamine transporter, serotonin transporter, tryptophan oxygenase, and the serotonin receptors 1A, 6, and 7 (1).

The serotonin receptor 1B (formerly 1Dβ) gene has been reported to be associated with obsessive-compulsive disorder (62,63). Interestingly, we have found evidence for linkage of this gene to ADHD in a sample that excludes subjects with evidence for GTS or chronic multiple tics (64). However, children with anxiety disorders were not excluded from this sample, and obsessive-compulsive behaviors were reported by parents for 10% of the children seen at the clinic from which the sample was taken (Arnold et al., unpublished). This linkage finding in the ADHD sample, which was based on the analysis of the polymorphic C to G nucleotide change at position 861, was more significant when the results were analyzed by parental transmissions—the allele transmissions from the fathers were significantly biased in transmission to the probands, but not from mothers to probands. However, in our GTS samples of nuclear families and multigenerational families, we found no significant evidence for linkage to the alleles or haplotypes of two polymorphisms, C861G (*Hin*cII) and A-129T (*Nla*III). However, similar to our finding in the ADHD sample, there was a trend for the biased transmission of the alleles when analyzed separately by parent for the C861G polymorphism (Barr et al., unpublished). This finding may prove to be a promising lead and is currently being further investigated.

The reports of sudden onset of tics and obsessive-compulsive symptoms associated with group A beta-hemolytic streptococcal infection, designated pediatric autoimmune neuropsychiatric disorders associated with streptococcal infection (PANDAS) (65,66), and the findings of high levels of autoantibodies in the sera of some individuals with GTS suggest a link between GTS and immune dysfunction, presumably autoimmunity (67–70). These findings suggest the possibility that the risk for GTS may be related to genes contributing to immune function. As with other autoimmune conditions, the genes encoding the human leukocyte antigens (HLA) are prime suspects. The two studies that have directly examined HLA class I (71,72) and class II types in GTS (72) found no association. Comings et al. specifically investigated HLA class I after noticing that the symptoms of several GTS cases seen at the clinic had an infectious disease preceding the onset of GTS symptoms by 1–4 months. Their study typed the HLA-A and -B antigens of 12 GTS subjects and found no difference in distribution compared to the North American population. The study of Caine et al. (72) used 5 small families, with 3 or 4 generations each, with a total of 37 individuals. The authors found no evidence of a shared haplotype between the five probands for the HLA-A, -B, -C, and -DR antigens and no evidence for sharing of the haplotypes between affected family members in 4 of the 5 pedigrees. Because of the small size of the samples tested, these studies may lack sufficient power to detect an association if the percentage of GTS cases resulting from autoimmunity is small. No evidence for linkage to markers in the region of the HLA has been found in genome scans or direct studies of this region (4,8), further indicating that the HLA is not a major genetic susceptibility locus or at least not in families collected for linkage studies with more than one affected individual. The possibility remains that the HLA contributes to GTS in some sporadic cases. Other immune system-related genes could be involved and this should be kept in mind while gene identification progresses in regions linked to GTS. An additional possibility is that the cases that result from streptococcal infection are phenocopies. That is, a genetic susceptibility to GTS is not inherited in these cases, and the disorder results entirely from environmental risk factors.

ANIMAL MODELS

Animal models, including transgenic and knockout mice, have been extremely useful in identifying genes or pathways involved in other genetic disorders, including some complex disorders. For example, the unexpected identification of the hypocretin receptor 2 as the susceptibility gene for narcolepsy in the canine model led to the finding that this pathway is involved in narcolepsy in humans as well (73). Prior to the cloning of the canine susceptibility gene, a very strong association of narcolepsy with the HLA class II genes had been reported and extensively replicated in studies worldwide (74–76). The identification of the hypocretin receptor 2 as the susceptibility gene in the canine model (77) led to the finding that the hypocretin peptides are completely absent in the cerebrospinal fluid of the majority of patients tested (73,78). The preliminary investigation of three genes involved in this pathway, the hypocretin preprohormone and the receptors 1 and 2, found that abnormal hypocretin levels in the cerebrospinal fluid are rarely associated with genetic changes at these three genes (79,80). These findings, in total, suggest that while the hypocretin genes are not generally altered in human narcolepsy, this pathway is undoubtedly involved, possibly via autoimmune destruction of the cells in the hypothalamus that contain hypocretin (81). Treatment with hypocretin receptor agonists may become a therapy for patients with no evidence of hypocretin in their cerebrospinal fluid (81).

Animal models for hyperlocomotion, anxiety, and obsessive-compulsive behaviors such as excessive grooming appear to have characteristics resembling human behaviors. Therefore such models may be very useful for the identification of genes involved in ADHD and OCD that may also be related to these behaviors in individuals with GTS. The recent report of excessive grooming behavior leading to hair removal in a mouse line homozygous for a loss-of-function allele of the Hoxb8 gene shows promise in the elucidation of pathways involved in grooming behavior in animals and potentially OCD in humans (82). This mouse line spent twice as much time grooming as did wild-type littermates, with some animals inducing skin lesions. Furthermore, these animals were also involved in excessive grooming of their cagemates, suggesting that this behavior is not a function of skin or sensory abnormalities.

An animal model for hyperlocomotion that appears to translate to the genetic susceptibility to ADHD in humans is the coloboma mouse, a mutant strain that is hemizygous for a 2-cM deletion of mouse chromosome 2 containing the synaptosomal-associated protein of 25 kDa (SNAP-25) gene (83). These mice are characterized by several features, most notably, marked hyperactivity that begins between postnatal days 11 and 14 (83). Other characteristics include head bobbing, prominent eye dysmorphology, and paroxysmal circling activity (83). Expression of a transgene encoding SNAP-25 rescues the hyperactivity but not the head bobbing or ophthalmic deformation (84), suggesting that the SNAP-25 gene is responsible for the observed hyperactivity but that the other characteristics of coloboma are the result of other genes in this deleted region. The coloboma strain is also delayed in some developmental milestones—the righting reflex and bar holding, a task designed to measure motor coordination. These delays are compensated over time such that the mice have comparable abilities to their normal littermates at a later age (85). Interestingly, D-amphetamine (2 or 4 mg/kg) reduced locomotor activity in coloboma mice, but increased activity in control mice, promoting comparisons to hyperactivity in children. However, methylphenidate, another stimulant commonly used in the treatment of ADHD, increased locomotor activity in both coloboma and control mice at doses of 2–32 mg/kg (84). The same dose of D-amphetamine that reduced locomotor activity in the coloboma mice, when administered to the mouse line rescued with the SNAP-25 transgene, resulted in an increase in activity that was comparable to the effect seen in wild types, indicating that hyperlocomotion and the response to D-amphetamine is attributable to the SNAP-25 gene, arguing for the role of this component of neurotransmitter release in the etiology of hyperlocomotion (84). Interestingly, a mouse line with a single copy of this gene "knocked out" created on the C57B1/6 strain background did not exhibit the hyperlocomotion phenotype (86). Thus the genetic background of the knockout line differed from the coloboma line (C3H/HeSnJ), indicating that differences in the genetic background of the mouse lines influence the phenotype. This leads the way for the identification of modifier genes influencing the hyperlocomotion phenotype. We have found significant evidence for linkage of the SNAP-25 gene to ADHD in a sample of ADHD families (87), and further support for this gene as a susceptibility factor in ADHD has been recently reported in additional samples (88–90).

Further support for the usefulness of animal models in the search for genes contributing to ADHD is provided by the hyperlocomotive phenotype of a mouse line in which the dopamine transporter gene has been knocked out (91). Evidence for linkage or association of the dopamine transporter gene in ADHD has been replicated by a number of studies (92–95).

Animal models for tics and repetitive behaviors have only recently been developed. The transgenic mouse model (D1CT-7) exhibits repetitive climbing and leaping, episodes of perseverance, or repetition of normal behaviors such as nonaggressive repeated biting and skin pulling of cagemates during grooming (96). This strain was constructed by expressing a neuropotentiating cholera toxin transgene under the control of the dopamine receptor D1 promoter, thereby expressing this gene in a subset of dopamine D1 receptor-expressing neurons. The cholera toxin enzyme chronically activates stimulatory G-protein (Gs) signal transduction, resulting in elevated cAMP levels, and constitutive activation of cAMP-dependent cellular changes. This model suggests that behaviors resembling tics and OCD in this strain result from chronic potentiation of the activity of cortical and limbic D1 receptor-expressing neurons. Pharmacological interventions in this strain further suggest that the behaviors are mediated by the induction of cortical-limbic glutamate output to the striatum (97). Based on these findings, the authors suggest that OCD behaviors and tics in humans result from excessive forebrain glutamate output to striatal motor pathways (97).

The finding of high levels of autoimmune antibodies in sera from GTS subjects, and immunohistological studies in which serum immunoglobulins from GTS patients were shown to bind to basal ganglia of human cadaver brains (69,70), led to the direct test of the involvement of these antibodies in producing tics using an animal model. Neural infusion of either whole sera or purified gamma immunoglobulins (IgG) from five children with GTS with antineuronal IgG antibodies induced increased stereotypies (e.g., licking and forepaw shaking) and vocal utterances in rats (98). The vocalizations, described as repetitive, medium-pitched sounds of short duration, were particularly interesting as these are not common in unprovoked animals and were often observed simultaneously with expression of oral, head, or forelimb stereotypies. Immunohistochemical analysis confirmed the presence of IgG selectively bound to striatal neurons in the animals that had been infused with sera from GTS subjects, providing a connection between the antibodies binding to the basal ganglia and the behaviors.

These findings were further confirmed in an additional study by the same authors (99). Stereotypic behavior was induced by injecting sera from GTS patients ($n = 12$), with high levels of antineural or antinuclear antibodies, into the ventrolateral striatum of rats, an area associated with oral stereotypy. These rats were observed to have increased oral stereotypies compared to rats that received sera injections from non-GTS controls ($n = 12$) or GTS patients ($n = 11$) with low levels of autoantibodies (99). These studies support the idea that a subset of GTS cases results from an autoimmune reaction involving IgG autoantibodies.

While animal models cannot completely duplicate the complexities of human behavior, particularly the cognitive component (e.g., obsessions, premonitory urges), these findings suggest that some less complex aspects of behavior can be modeled and hold promise for gene identification for GTS and other related human behavioral disorders.

SUMMARY

In summary, the identification of genes contributing to GTS has been surprisingly challenging given the strong heritability estimates for this disorder. The finding of a high percentage of bilineal pedigrees was particularly unexpected and may have been a factor in reducing the power of studies that used large multigenerational families. Findings suggestive of linkage have been reported for several chromosomal regions, and significant evidence has been obtained for others. These regions, however, have not always been convincingly replicated by other studies, although some recent overlap in the linkage findings is promising. Chromosomal abnormalities have been identified in several regions, but the genes identified at translocation breakpoints thus far do not seem to account for a large percentage of GTS cases. The results suggest that there may be substantial locus heterogeneity. The use of alternative phenotypes in linkage studies, as evident from the genome scan using the hoarding phenotype, appears promising. Finally, the possibility of an autoimmune etiology for GTS points to additional avenues of research for gene identification.

REFERENCES

1. Barr CL, Sandor P. Current status of genetic studies of Gilles de la Tourette syndrome. Can J Psychiatry 1998; 43(4):351–357.
2. Pauls DL. Update on the Genetics of Tourette syndrome. In: Cohen DJ, Goetz CG, Jankovic J, eds. Tourette Syndrome. Philadelphia: Lippincott Williams & Wilkins, 2001:281–293.
3. Pakstis AJ, Heutink P, Pauls DL, Kurlan R, van de Wetering BJ, Leckman JF, Sandkuyl LA, Kidd JR, Breedveld GJ, Castiglione CM, Weber J, Sparkes RS, Cohen DJ, Kidd KK, Oostra BA. Progress in the search for genetic linkage with Tourette syndrome: an exclusion map covering more than 50% of the autosomal genome. Am J Hum Genet 1991; 48(2):281–294.
4. Barr CL, Wigg KG, Pakstis AJ, Kurlan R, Pauls D, Kidd KK, Tsui LC,

Sandor P. Genome scan for linkage to Gilles de la Tourette syndrome. Am J Med Genet 1999; 88(4):437–445.
5. The Tourette Syndrome Association International Consortium for Genetics. A complete genome screen in sib pairs affected by Gilles de la Tourette syndrome. Am J Hum Genet 1999; 65(5):1428–1436.
6. Simonic I, Gericke GS, Ott J, Weber JL. Identification of genetic markers associated with Gilles de la Tourette syndrome in an Afrikaner population. Am J Hum Genet 1998; 63(3):839–846.
7. Simonic I, Nyholt DR, Gericke GS, Gordon D, Matsumoto N, Ledbetter DH, Ott J, Weber JL. Further evidence for linkage of Gilles de la Tourette syndrome (GTS) susceptibility loci on chromosomes 2p11, 8q22 and 11q23–24 in South African Afrikaners. Am J Med Genet 2001; 105(2):163–167.
8. Leppert M, Peiffer A, Snyder B, van de Wetering BJM, Filloux F, Coon H, McMahon WM. Two loci of interest in a family with Tourette syndrome. Am J Hum Genet 1996; 59:A225.
9. McMahon WM, Leppert M, Filloux F, van de Wetering BJ, Hasstedt S. Tourette symptoms in 161 related family members. Adv Neurol 1992; 58:159–165.
10. Merette C, Brassard A, Potvin A, Bouvier H, Rousseau F, Emond C, Bissonnette L, Roy MA, Maziade M, Ott J, Caron C. Significant linkage for Tourette syndrome in a large French Canadian family. Am J Hum Genet 2000; 67(4):1008–1013.
11. Devor EJ. Complex segregation analysis of Gilles de la Tourette syndrome: Further evidence for a major locus mode of transmission. Am J Hum Genet 1984; 36(3):704–709.
12. Pauls DL, Pakstis AJ, Kurlan R, Kidd KK, Leckman JF, Cohen DJ, Kidd JR, Como P, Sparkes R. Segregation and linkage analyses of Tourette's syndrome and related disorders. J Am Acad Child Adolesc Psych 1990; 29(2):195–203.
13. Curtis D, Robertson MM, Gurling HM. Autosomal dominant gene transmission in a large kindred with Gilles de la Tourette syndrome. Br J Psychiatry 1992; 160:845–849.
14. Cavallini MC, Macciardi F, Pasquale L, Bellodi L, Smeraldi E. Complex segregation analysis of obsessive compulsive and spectrum related disorders. Psychiatr Genet 1995; 5:3131.
15. Kidd KK, Pauls DL. Genetic hypothesis for Tourette syndrome. In: Friedhoff AJ, Chase TN, eds. Gilles de la Tourette Syndrome. New York: Raven Press, 1982:243–249.
16. Comings DE, Comings BG, Devor EJ, Cloninger CR. Detection of major gene for Gilles de la Tourette syndrome. Am J Hum Genet 1984; 36(3):586–600.
17. Walkup JT, LaBuda MC, Singer HS, Brown J, Riddle MA, Hurko O. Family study and segregation analysis of Tourette syndrome: Evidence for a mixed model of inheritance. Am J Hum Genet 1996; 59(3):684–693.
18. Hasstedt SJ, Leppert M, Filloux F, van de Wetering BJ, McMahon WM. Intermediate inheritance of Tourette syndrome, assuming assortative mating. Am J Hum Genet 1995; 57(3):682–689.

19. Clerget-Darpoux F, Bonaiti-Pellie C, Hochez J. Effects of misspecifying genetic parameters in lod score analysis. Biometrics 1986; 42(2):393–399.
20. Kurlan R, Eapen V, Stern J, McDermott MP, Robertson MM. Bilineal transmission in Tourette's syndrome families. Neurology 1994; 44(12):2336–2342.
21. McMahon WM, van de Wetering BJ, Filloux F, Betit K, Coon H, Leppert M. Bilineal transmission and phenotypic variation of Tourette's disorder in a large pedigree. J Am Acad Child Adolesc Psych 1996; 35(5):672–680.
22. Hornse H, Banerjee S, Zeitlin H, Robertson M. The prevalence of Tourette syndrome in 13–14-year-olds in mainstream schools. J Child Psychol Psychiatry 2001; 42(8):1035–1039.
23. Kurlan R, Whitmore D, Irvine C, McDermott MP, Como PG. Tourette's syndrome in a special education population: a pilot study involving a single school district. Neurology 1994; 44(4):699–702.
24. Comings DE, Himes JA, Comings BG. An epidemiologic study of Tourette's syndrome in a single school district. J Clin Psychiatry 1990; 51(11):463–469.
25. Kidd KK, Prusoff BA, Cohen DJ. Familial pattern of Gilles de la Tourette syndrome. Arch Gen Psychiatry 1980; 37(12):1336–1339.
26. Pauls DL, Cohen DJ, Heimbuch R, Detlor J, Kidd KK. Familial pattern and transmission of Gilles de la Tourette syndrome and multiple tics. Arch Gen Psychiatry 1981; 38(10):1091–1093.
27. Pauls DL, Raymond CL, Stevenson JM, Leckman JF. A family study of Gilles de la Tourette syndrome. Am J Hum Genet 1991; 48(1):154–163.
28. Pauls DL, Towbin KE, Leckman JF, Zahner GE, Cohen DJ. Gilles de la Tourette's syndrome and obsessive-compulsive disorder. Evidence supporting a genetic relationship. Arch Gen Psychiatry 1986; 43(12):1180–1182.
29. Walkup JT, Leckman JF, Price RA, Hardin M, Ort SI, Cohen DJ. The relationship between obsessive-compulsive disorder and Tourette's syndrome: a twin study. Psychopharmacol Bull 1988; 24(3):375–379.
30. Pauls DL, Cohen DJ, Kidd KK, Leckman JF. Tourette syndrome and neuropsychiatric disorders: Is there a genetic relationship? Am J Hum Genet 1988; 43(2):206–217.
31. Knell ER, Comings DE. Tourette's syndrome and attention-deficit hyperactivity disorder: evidence for a genetic relationship. J Clin Psychiatry 1993; 54(9):331–337.
32. Pauls DL, Leckman JF, Cohen DJ. Familial relationship between Gilles de la Tourette's syndrome, attention deficit disorder, learning disabilities, speech disorders, and stuttering. J Am Acad Child Adolesc Psych 1993; 32(5):1044–1050.
33. Egeland JA, Gerhard DS, Pauls DL, Sussex JN, Kidd KK, Allen CR, Hostetter AM, Housman DE. Bipolar affective disorders linked to DNA markers on chromosome 11. Nature 1987; 325(6107):783–787.
34. Kelsoe JR, Ginns EI, Egeland JA, Gerhard DS, Goldstein AM, Bale SJ, Pauls DL, Long RT, Kidd KK, Conte G, Housman DE, Paul SM. Re-evaluation of the linkage relationship between chromosome 11p loci and the gene for bipolar affective disorder in the Old Order Amish. Nature 1989; 342(6247):238–243.

35. Zhang H, Leckman JF, Pauls DL, Tsai CP, Kidd KK, Campos MR. Genome-wide scan of hoarding in sib pairs in which both sibs have Gilles de la Tourette syndrome. Am J Hum Genet 2002; 70(4):896–904.
36. van de Wetering BJ, Heutink P. The genetics of the Gilles de la Tourette syndrome: a review. J Lab Clin Med 1993; 121(5):638–645.
37. Boghosian-Sell L, Comings DE, Overhauser J. Tourette syndrome in a pedigree with a 7;18 translocation: identification of a YAC spanning the translocation breakpoint at 18q22.3. Am J Hum Genet 1996; 59(5):999–1005.
38. Kroisel PM, Petek E, Emberger W, Windpassinger C, Wladika W, Wagner K. Candidate region for Gilles de la Tourette syndrome at 7q31. Am J Med Genet 2001; 101(3):259–261.
39. Comings DE, Comings BG, Dietz G, Muhleman D, Okada TA, Sarinana F, Simmer R, Sparkes R, Crist M, Stock D. Linkage studies in Tourette syndrome. Am J Hum Genet 1986; 39:A151.
40. Donnai D. Gene location in Tourette syndrome. Lancet 1987; 1(8533):627.
41. Heutink P, van de Wetering BJ, Breedveld GJ, Weber J, Sandkuyl LA, Devor EJ, Heiberg A, Niermeijer MF, Oostra BA. No evidence for genetic linkage of Gilles de la Tourette syndrome on chromosomes 7 and 18. J Med Genet 1990; 27(7):433–436.
42. Petek E, Windpassinger C, Vincent JB, Cheung J, Boright AP, Scherer SW, Kroisel PM, Wagner K. Disruption of a novel gene (IMMP2L) by a breakpoint in 7q31 associated with Tourette syndrome. Am J Hum Genet 2001; 68(4):848–858.
43. Devor EJ, Magee HJ. Multiple childhood behavioral disorders (Tourette syndrome, multiple tics, ADD and OCD) presenting in a family with a balanced chromosome translocation (t1;8)(q21.1;q22.1). Psychiatr Genet 1999; 9(3):149–151.
44. Matsumoto N, David DE, Johnson EW, Konecki D, Burmester JK, Ledbetter DH, Weber JL. Breakpoint sequences of an 1;8 translocation in a family with Gilles de la Tourette syndrome. Eur J Hum Genet 2000; 8(11):875–883.
45. Taylor LD, Krizman DB, Jankovic J, Hayani A, Steuber PC, Greenberg F, Fenwick RG, Caskey CT. 9p monosomy in a patient with Gilles de la Tourette's syndrome. Neurology 1991; 41(9):1513–1515.
46. Singh DN, Howe GL, Jordan HW, Hara S. Tourette's syndrome in a black woman with associated triple X and 9p mosaicism. J Natl Med Assoc 1982; 74(7):675–682.
47. Veenstra-Vander Weele J, Kim SJ, Gonen D, Hanna GL, Leventhal BL, Cook EH Jr, Genomic organization of the SLC1A1/EAAC1 gene and mutation screening in early-onset obsessive-compulsive disorder. Mol Psychiatry 2001; 6(2):160–167.
48. Brett PM, Curtis D, Robertson MM, Dahlitz M, Gurling HM. Linkage analysis and exclusion of regions of chromosomes 3 and 8 in Gilles de la Tourette syndrome following the identification of a balanced reciprocal translocation 46 XY, t(3:8)(p21.3 q24.1) in a case of Tourette syndrome. Psychiatr Genet 1996; 6(3):99–105.

49. Brett P, Curtis D, Gourdie A, Schnieden V, Jackson G, Holmes D, Robertson M, Gurling H. Possible linkage of Tourette syndrome to markers on short arm of chromosome 3 (C3p21-14) [letter] [see comments]. Lancet 1990; 336(8722): 1076.
50. Heutink P, Sandkuyl LA, van de Wetering BJ, Oostra BA, Weber J, Wilkie P, Devor EJ, Pakstis AJ, Pauls D, Kidd KK. Linkage and Tourette syndrome [letter; comment]. Lancet 1991; 337(8733):122–123.
51. Sverd J. Tourette syndrome and autistic disorder: A significant relationship. Am J Med Genet 1991; 39(2):173–179.
52. Marriage K, Miles T, Stokes D, Davey M. Clinical and research implications of the co-occurrence of Asperger's and Tourette syndromes. Aust N Z J Psychiatry 1993; 27(4):666–672.
53. Baron-Cohen S, Scahill VL, Izaguirre J, Hornsey H, Robertson MM. The prevalence of Gilles de la Tourette syndrome in children and adolescents with autism: a large scale study. Psychol Med 1999; 29(5):1151–1159.
54. Comings DE, Comings BG. Clinical and genetic relationships between autism-pervasive developmental disorder and Tourette syndrome: a study of 19 cases. Am J Med Genet 1991; 39(2):180–191.
55. Ringman JM, Jankovic J. Occurrence of tics in Asperger's syndrome and autistic disorder. J Child Neurol 2000; 15(6):394–400.
56. Burd L, Fisher WW, Kerbeshian J, Arnold ME. Is development of Tourette disorder a marker for improvement in patients with autism and other pervasive developmental disorders? J Am Acad Child Adolesc Psych 1987; 26(2):162–165.
57. Hebebrand J, Martin M, Korner J, Roitzheim B, de Braganca K, Werner W, Remschmidt H. Partial trisomy 16p in an adolescent with autistic disorder and Tourette's syndrome [see comments]. Am J Med Genet 1994; 54(3):268–270.
58. Liu J, Nyholt DR, Magnussen P, Parano E, Pavone P, Geschwind D, Lord C, Iversen P, Hoh J, Ott J, Gilliam TC. A genomewide screen for autism susceptibility loci. Am J Hum Genet 2001; 69(2):327–340.
59. Philippe A, Martinez M, Guilloud-Bataille M, Gillberg C, Rastam M, Sponheim E, Coleman M, Zappella M, Aschauer H, Van Maldergem L, Penet C, Feingold J, Brice A, Leboyer M, van Malldergerme L. Genome-wide scan for autism susceptibility genes. Paris Autism Research International Sibpair Study. Hum Mol Genet 1999; 8(5):805–812.
60. Smalley SL, Kustanovich V, Minassian SL, Stone JL, Ogdie MN, McGough JJ, McCracken JT, MacPhie IL, Francks C, Fisher SE, Cantor RM, Monaco AP, Nelson SF. Genetic linkage of attention-deficit/hyperactivity disorder on chromosome 16p13, in a region implicated in autism. Am J Hum Genet 2002; 71(4):959–963.
61. Fisher SE, Francks C, McCracken JT, McGough JJ, Marlow AJ, MacPhie IL, Newbury DF, Crawford LR, Palmer CG, Woodward JA, Del'Homme M, Cantwell DP, Nelson SF, Monaco AP, Smalley SL. A genomewide scan for loci involved in attention-deficit/hyperactivity disorder. Am J Hum Genet 2002; 70(5):1183–1196.

62. Mundo E, Richter MA, Sam F, Macciardi F, Kennedy JL. Is the 5-HT(1Dbeta) receptor gene implicated in the pathogenesis of obsessive-compulsive disorder? Am J Psychiatry 2000; 157(7):1160–1161.
63. Mundo E, Richter MA, Zai G, Sam F, McBride J, Macciardi F, Kennedy JL. 5HT1Dbeta receptor gene implicated in the pathogenesis of obsessive-compulsive disorder: Further evidence from a family-based association study. Mol Psychiatry 2002; 7(7):805–809.
64. Quist JF, Barr CL, Schachar R, Roberts W, Malone M, Tannock R, Basile VS, Beitchman J, Kennedy JL. The serotonin 5-HT1B receptor gene and attention deficit hyperactivity disorder (ADHD). Mol Psychiatry, 2003; 8(1):98–102.
65. Swedo SE, Leonard HL, Kiessling LS. Speculations on antineuronal antibody-mediated neuropsychiatric disorders of childhood. Pediatrics 1994; 93(2):323–326.
66. Swedo SE, Leonard HL, Garvey M, Mittleman B, Allen AJ, Perlmutter S, Lougee L, Dow S, Zamkoff J, Dubbert BK. Pediatric autoimmune neuropsychiatric disorders associated with streptococcal infections: Clinical description of the first 50 cases. Am J Psychiatry 1998; 155(2):264–271.
67. Kiessling LS. Tic disorders associated with evidence of invasive group A β-hemolytic streptococcal disease. Dev Med Child Neurol 1989; 31(5 suppl 59):4848.
68. Morshed SA, Parveen S, Leckman JF, Mercadante MT, Bittencourt Kiss MH, Miguel EC, Arman A, Yazgan Y, Fujii T, Paul S, Peterson BS, Zhang H, King RA, Scahill L, Lombroso PJ. Antibodies against neural, nuclear, cytoskeletal, and streptococcal epitopes in children and adults with Tourette's syndrome, Sydenham's chorea, and autoimmune disorders. Biol Psychiatry 2001; 50(8): 566–577.
69. Singer HS, Giuliano JD, Hansen BH, Hallett JJ, Laurino JP, Benson M, Kiessling LS. Antibodies against human putamen in children with Tourette syndrome. Neurology 1998; 50(6):1618–1624.
70. Kiessling LS, Marcotte AC, Culpepper L. Antineuronal antibodies in movement disorders. Pediatrics 1993; 92(1):39–43.
71. Comings DE, Gursey BT, Hecht T, Blume K. HLA typing in Tourette syndrome. In: Friedhoff AJ, Chase TN, eds. Gilles de la Tourette Syndrome. New York: Raven Press, 1982:251–253.
72. Caine ED, Weitkamp LR, Chiverton P, Guttormsen S, Yagnow R, Hempfling S, Kennelly D. Tourette syndrome and HLA. J Neurol Sci 1985; 69(3):201–206.
73. Nishino S, Ripley B, Overeem S, Lammers GJ, Mignot E. Hypocretin (orexin) deficiency in human narcolepsy. Lancet 2000; 355(9197):39–40.
74. Barr CL, Shapiro CM. Current status of the genetics of narcolepsy. In: Wahlstrom J ed. Genetics and Psychiatric Disorders. Oxford: Elsevier Science Ltd., 1998:205–215.
75. Zai C, Wigg KG, Barr CL. Genetics and sleep disorders. Semin Clin Neuropsychiatry 2000; 5(1):33–43.
76. Lin L, Hungs M, Mignot E. Narcolepsy and the HLA region. J Neuroimmunol 2001; 117(1–2):9–20.
77. Lin L, Faraco J, Li R, Kadotani H, Rogers W, Lin X, Qiu X, de Jong PJ,

Nishino S, Mignot E. The sleep disorder canine narcolepsy is caused by a mutation in the hypocretin (orexin) receptor 2 gene. Cell 1999; 98(3):365–376.

78. Ripley B, Overeem S, Fujiki N, Nevsimalova S, Uchino M, Yesavage J, Di Monte D, Dohi K, Melberg A, Lammers GJ, Nishida Y, Roelandse FW, Hungs M, Mignot E, Nishino S. CSF hypocretin/orexin levels in narcolepsy and other neurological conditions. Neurology 2001; 57(12):2253–2258.
79. Peyron C, Faraco J, Rogers W, Ripley B, Overeem S, Charnay Y, Nevsimalova S, Aldrich M, Reynolds D, Albin R, Li R, Hungs M, Pedrazzoli M, Padigaru M, Kucherlapati M, Fan J, Maki R, Lammers GJ, Bouras C, Kucherlapati R, Nishino S, Mignot E. A mutation in a case of early onset narcolepsy and a generalized absence of hypocretin peptides in human narcoleptic brains. Nat Med 2000; 6(9):991–997.
80. Hungs M, Lin L, Okun M, Mignot E. Polymorphisms in the vicinity of the hypocretin/orexin are not associated with human narcolepsy. Neurology 2001; 57(10):1893–1895.
81. Hungs M, Mignot E. Hypocretin/orexin, sleep and narcolepsy. BioEssays 2001; 23(5):397–408.
82. Greer JM, Capecchi MR. Hoxb8 is required for normal grooming behavior in mice. Neuron 2002; 33(1):23–34.
83. Hess EJ, Jinnah HA, Kozak CA, Wilson MC. Spontaneous locomotor hyperactivity in a mouse mutant with a deletion including the Snap gene on chromosome 2. J Neurosci 1992; 12(7):2865–2874.
84. Hess EJ, Collins KA, Wilson MC. Mouse model of hyperkinesis implicates SNAP-25 in behavioral regulation. J Neurosci 1996; 16(9):3104–3111.
85. Heyser CJ, Wilson MC, Gold LH. Coloboma hyperactive mutant exhibits delayed neurobehavioral developmental milestones. Brain Res Dev Brain Res 1995; 89(2):264–269.
86. Washbourne P, Thompson PM, Carta M, Costa ET, Mathews JR, Lopez-Bendito G, Molnar Z, Becher MW, Valenzuela CF, Partridge LD, Wilson MC. Genetic ablation of the t-SNARE SNAP-25 distinguishes mechanisms of neuroexocytosis. Nat Neurosci 2002; 5(1):19–26.
87. Barr CL, Feng Y, Wigg K, Bloom S, Roberts W, Malone M, Schachar R, Tannock R, Kennedy JL. Identification of DNA variants in the SNAP-25 gene and linkage study of these polymorphisms and attention-deficit hyperactivity disorder. Mol Psychiatry 2000; 5(4):405–409.
88. Kustanovich V, Merriman B, Crawford L, Smalley S, Nelson S. An association study of SNAP-25 alleles shows evidence for biased paternal inheritance in attention deficit hyperactivity disorder. Am J Hum Genet 2001; 69(4):582.
89. Mill J, Curran S, Kent L, Gould A, Huckett L, Richards S, Taylor E, Asherson P. Association study of a SNAP-25 microsatellite and attention deficit hyperactivity disorder. Am J Med Genet 2002; 114(3):269–271.
90. Brophy K, Hawi Z, Kirley A, Fitzgerald M, Gill M. Synaptosomal-associated protein 25 (SNAP-25) and attention deficit hyperactivity disorder (ADHD): evidence of linkage and association in the Irish population. Mol Psychiatry 2002; 7(8):913–917.

91. Giros B, Jaber M, Jones SR, Wightman RM, Caron MG. Hyperlocomotion and indifference to cocaine and amphetamine in mice lacking the dopamine transporter. Nature 1996; 379(6566):606–612.
92. Cook EH Jr, Stein MA, Krasowski MD, Cox NJ, Olkon DM, Kieffer JE, Leventhal BL. Association of attention-deficit disorder and the dopamine transporter gene. Am J Hum Genet 1995; 56(4):993–998.
93. Waldman ID, Rowe DC, Abramowitz A, Kozel ST, Mohr JH, Sherman SL, Cleveland HH, Sanders ML, Gard JM, Stever C. Association and linkage of the dopamine transporter gene and attention-deficit hyperactivity disorder in children: Heterogeneity owing to diagnostic subtype and severity. Am J Hum Genet 1998; 63(6):1767–1776.
94. Gill M, Daly G, Heron S, Hawi Z, Fitzgerald M. Confirmation of association between attention deficit hyperactivity disorder and a dopamine transporter polymorphism. Mol Psychiatry 1997; 2(4):311–313.
95. Daly G, Hawi Z, Fitzgerald M, Gill M. Mapping susceptibility loci in attention deficit hyperactivity disorder: Preferential transmission of parental alleles at DAT1, DBH and DRD5 to affected children. Mol Psychiatry 1999; 4(2):192–196.
96. Campbell KM, de Lecea L, Severynse DM, Caron MG, McGrath MJ, Sparber SB, Sun LY, Burton FH. OCD-Like behaviors caused by a neuropotentiating transgene targeted to cortical and limbic D1+ neurons. J Neurosci 1999; 19(12): 5044–5053.
97. McGrath MJ, Campbell KM, Parks CR, Burton FH. Glutamatergic drugs exacerbate symptomatic behavior in a transgenic model of comorbid Tourette's syndrome and obsessive-compulsive disorder. Brain Res 2000; 877(1):23–30.
98. Hallett JJ, Harling-Berg CJ, Knopf PM, Stopa EG, Kiessling LS. Anti-striatal antibodies in Tourette syndrome cause neuronal dysfunction. J Neuroimmunol 2000; 111(1–2):195–202.
99. Taylor JR, Morshed SA, Parveen S, Mercadante MT, Scahill L, Peterson BS, King RA, Leckman JF, Lombroso PJ. An animal model of Tourette's syndrome. Am J Psychiatry 2002; 159(4):657–660.

19

Epidemiology of Tourette's Syndrome

Caroline M. Tanner
Parkinson's Institute
Sunnyvale, California, U.S.A.

INTRODUCTION AND GENERAL CONSIDERATIONS

Epidemiologists investigate the effects of a disorder within groups of people rather than in individuals. Through the application of epidemiological principles, we can learn about the magnitude and distribution of a disorder, evaluate the social and economic consequences of being affected, and develop and test theories about the cause of the disease. This chapter briefly introduces some epidemiological terms and provides a short review of epidemiological studies of tic disorders, particularly Gilles de la Tourette's syndrome (TS). Topics such as the genetic epidemiology of TS that might normally be considered in a chapter on epidemiology are covered in other chapters in this volume.

SOME EPIDEMIOLOGICAL CONCEPTS

Definitions

Incidence refers to the number of new cases of a disorder developing within a given time period in a specific community. For TS, incidence cannot be accurately determined from hospital or clinic records because not all persons with a disorder may seek medical attention. Rather, a survey of an entire population must be performed. Incidence is most commonly reported as the number of cases per unit population per year. Prevalence refers to the total number of cases in a specific community at a specified time (1). Like incidence, accurate determination of TS prevalence would require survey of an entire community. Prevalence is typically reported as the number of cases per unit population on a specific date.

Problems Specific to the Epidemiological Study of Tic Disorders

A major difficulty in the epidemiological study of tic disorders is the inability to definitely diagnose a true case. At present, there is no diagnostic test for TS, so diagnosis is dependent on clinical examination and history. The identification of a TS gene or genes using molecular genetic techniques may allow accurate diagnosis in the future, but until then, diagnostic errors may lead to erroneous conclusions about such important observations as the frequency, natural history, and clinical syndrome. Diagnosis is further confounded by the clinical characteristics of TS. First, tics typically occur less frequently in social situations, including those in which epidemiological investigations might occur. Thus tics may be missed if direct evaluation is in a setting likely to induce tic suppression. In addition, because of the characteristic waxing and waning of symptoms, if only a single examination is performed, some persons with TS may be misdiagnosed. The age of the subject may be a further critical modifier. Because tics are often most obvious in childhood, population studies may underestimate tics especially in those evaluated only as adults, when tic severity is typically less.

In studies in which examinations are not performed and cases are identified by history only, many cases may be missed because affected persons or their relatives may be unaware of the tics. For example, in a kindred of 159 members, 30% of 54 subjects with tics identified by examiners were not aware of tics (1). Only 18.5% of those affected had sought medical care for tics. Because diagnosis of TS requires multifocal tics, cross-sectional investigations may miss those with single tics at the time of the survey. On the other hand, when cases are identified only by interview, many cases may be missed because affected persons or their relatives may be unaware of the tics. Differences in interviewing techniques could also produce different estimates of disease.

Either overestimation or underestimation of disease may result from some methodological differences. For example, behavioral disorders such as attention-deficit disorder (ADD) and obsessive-compulsive disorder (OCD) appear to be associated with motor and vocal tics, but the relationship is not understood (2,3). As a result, when determining TS frequency, some investigators might include individuals with ADD, OCD, or simple tics, while others might include only those with motor or vocal tics. A second source of error arises if frequency of TS is determined only by interview, without a confirmatory examination. Differences in interviewing technique could produce inflated or deflated estimates of disease. In addition, tic severity typically varies with age, so an individual correctly classified as having TS in a survey during childhood might not be thus identified as an adult, when tic severity is typically less. Finally, tics are most common in male children (see below). Populations with many boys would be expected to have a greater frequency of tics than those with only a few. If population frequencies are used to calculate an estimated rate, without correction for age or sex, the rates may overestimate or underestimate disease frequency, depending on the demographic characteristics of the study population.

MAGNITUDE AND DISTRIBUTION

Incidence

Only one population-based study of TS incidence has been published. Annual incidence of the disorder was estimated for Rochester, Minnesota, as 4.6 per 1 million persons (4). Since this estimate was based on only three cases (all male) diagnosed during the 12-year period from 1968 to 1979, 95% confidence intervals are rather wide, ranging from 0.9 to 11.9/100,000. Extending this estimate to the entire U.S. population, the authors estimated an annual incidence rate of 1000 new cases of TS. In this study, cases were identified only if an individual was diagnosed as the result of seeking health care, and it is likely that only the most severely affected cases were identified in this way. Consequently, the actual incidence rate is likely greater. The fact that incidence rates were estimated using cases diagnosed during the time period 1968–1979, when physician awareness of TS was lower than at present (5), further suggests that this rate is an underestimation.

Prevalence

Several studies (6–19) have assessed the prevalence of tics in groups of young children in defined communities (Table 1). Ascertainment methods differed for each study, and diagnostic criteria were also often different. In the earliest studies, TS was not differentiated from simple tic (6,7), while later studies attempted to distinguish TS as a separate entity. Prevalence estimates for TS differ by a factor of 10, with the highest estimates found in special populations, such as children referred to psychiatrists or in special education classrooms, or when intensive ascertainment methods are used, including direct observation of children by a trained observer. Ascertainment using self-identification or physician identification results in much lower prevalence

Table 1 Some Studies Estimating Prevalence of Tics and TS in Children and Adolescen

Author, year	Base population size, age	Prevalence[a] per 10,000 TS	All tics
Boncour, 1910 (6)	1759 schoolchildren; ages 2–13	—	1940
Pringle et al., 1967 (7)	11,000 singletons; age 7	—	520 (by histor 400 (by exam)
Lapouse and Monk, 1964 (8)	482 schoolchildren; ages 6–12	—	12,000
Debray-Ritzen and Dubois, 1980 (9)	Parisian school children referred to psychiatrists	23	87
Burd et al., 1986 (10)	North Dakota children with TS found via patient registry or physician mail screen	5.2	—
Caine et al., 1988 (11)	Monroe County, New York, children aged 2–16 recruited by advertisement	2.9	—
Comings et al., 1990 (12)	Los Angeles school children referred to school psychologist	49.5	—
Apter et al., 1992 (13)	Israeli 16–17 year olds; national health exam	4.3	—
Landgren et al., 1996 (14)	Children aged 6–7 Identified by screening birth records in one hospital	34	
Costello et al., 1996 (15)	Community sample aged 9, 11, and 13 North Carolina	10	420
Verhulst et al., 1997 (16)	Community sample aged 13–18 Netherlands	10	400
Kurlan et al., 2001 (17)	School children aged 8.5–17.5 Rochester NY	150 80	2340 special ed. 1850 regular
Hornse et al., 2001 (19)	One English school children aged 13–14	185	
Khalifa et al., 2003 (18)	Children aged 7–15	60	660

[a] Because the underlying populations differ, direct comparison of these prevalence estimates is n appropriate.

estimates. For example, prevalence was estimated at 5.2/10,000 in North Dakota school-aged children (10) and 2.9/10,000 in children in Monroe County, New York (11).

Others estimated the incidence of TS in adolescent or adult populations. Burd et al. (20) surveyed North Dakota physicians and mental-health institutions and identified adult members of the statewide TS support group.

They estimated a total prevalence of 0.5/10,000 adults. Apter et al. (13) determined the prevalence of TS in Israeli adolescents undergoing a routine, nationwide health examination. All children were administered five screening questions about the presence or absence of any TS-like symptoms. Those answering positively were referred for a semistructured interview by a child psychiatrist and a final, structured diagnostic interview. A total of 9 boys and 3 girls with TS were identified from a total population of 18,364 males and 9673 females aged 16–17. Prevalence was estimated at 4.9/10,000 boys, 3.1/10,000 girls, and 4.3/10,000 total population aged 16–17. The resultant male/female ratio was 1.6:1. Rather than a low prevalence of TS, these results probably reflect, in part, the well-recognized decrease in severity of TS symptoms during adulthood (20–24). This age-associated decrease in symptoms is often accompanied by a decreased awareness of tics.

More intensive ascertainment methods have resulted in higher estimates of tic and TS prevalence. Costello et al. (15) used a two-stage design to ascertain cases of tic disorders and TS. First, the parents of a random sample of 4000 children aged 9, 11, and 13 years completed questionnaires about the child's behavior. The investigators next used direct interviews of children and parents in nearly 800 with behavioral problems and 260 with no behavioral problems, as identified by the parent questionnaire. They estimated prevalence of any tic disorder as 420 per 10,000 and TS as 10 per 10,000. Because children without disruptive behavior problems were not interviewed, tics in these children would have been missed. Using a similar study design, Verhulst et al. (16) had nearly identical results, estimating prevalence of all tic disorders at 400/10,000 and 10 cases per 10,000 for TS.

Direct screening of children in classroom settings using research technicians trained to identify tics along with interviews of parents and teachers has yielded even higher estimates of TS prevalence. Kurlan et al. (17) studied a random sample of children from special education classrooms and a comparison sample of children from regular education classrooms (frequency matched by age and gender). Research technicians trained to identify tics performed the standardized evaluations of each child. Teachers and parents were interviewed. For any tic disorder, weighted prevalence was 23.4% in special education and 18.5% in regular classrooms. Using DSM-IV diagnostic criteria, which require that tics cause significant impairment, TS frequency was 1.5% in special education and 0.8% for regular education classrooms. Excluding the impairment requirement, weighted prevalence was 7.8% for special education classrooms and 3.1% for regular education classrooms. In a systematic observation of 13- and 14-year-olds in ninth-grade classrooms followed by interviews and expert examination, TS prevalence was estimated at 1.85 % (18). A three-stage screen of Swedish school children (19) aged 7–15 using the more restrictive DMS-IV diagnostic criteria found TS in 0.6%, chronic motor tics in 0.8%, and chronic vocal tics in 0.5%. Transient tics were found in 4.8%.

Ascertainment through medical care systems rather than through community surveys may be particularly critical in determining the number of cases identified. More studies using direct observation to ascertain tics will be important to determine whether TS is a rare disorder, as has been believed, or a common disorder that only comes to medical attention when symptoms are severe.

This 100-fold difference in published estimates of TS prevalence highlights the challenge posed in the epidemiological investigation of tic disorders. The wide variation in these estimates of TS prevalence most likely represents differences in diagnostic criteria and in the methods used to identify affected persons. Studies determining the numbers of cases in a population by self-identified volunteers or by individuals seeking medical treatment for tics most likely underestimate prevalence, particularly for mild or infrequent tics. For example, a study of TS in a large kindred found that 30% were unaware of tics and only 18.5% had sought medical care (1). Characteristics such as age and possibly sex might influence severity of tics and thus the number of affected persons identified within a population surveyed. Other factors, such as socioeconomic and educational level, might affect awareness of tics and result in differences in reporting of symptoms. Studies using trained observers are most likely to identify mild and previously undiagnosed tics, but follow-up interviews and, ideally, multiple observation times for each subject are essential to avoid overestimation of rates.

The preceding considerations make it difficult to determine whether actual differences in TS frequency occur in the populations studied. In the absence of a diagnostic test for tics or TS, validation of any diagnostic approach is not possible. Until such a "gold standard" is available, the most intensive ascertainment methods, such as direct observation coupled with multiple interviews, combined with longitudinal follow-up will provide the most reliable and accurate estimates of the burden of disease.

Geographical Distribution

Tourette's syndrome appears to be worldwide in distribution. Clinical series and case reports have been published from numerous countries, including the United States (5), Europe (25,26), Japan (27), China (28), Hong Kong (29), the Middle East (13,30), and Brazil (31). Differences in disease frequency across populations are likely if TS is determined primarily by genetic factors, but the methodological difficulties discussed above and small numbers of population-based studies performed to date do not permit conclusions.

RISK FACTORS

Since few population-based studies of TS have been performed, risk factors for disease have been identified primarily from reviews of clinic-based surveys. The principal risk factors identified in this manner are male sex and heredity. In addition, severity of tics is typically greater during childhood and adolescence; as a result, those with TS might be most readily identified during childhood. Other risk factors may affect tic severity but are unlikely to be primary determinants of TS. Secondary tic disorders (34), such as those due to exposures to drugs, will not be considered here.

Gender

Tourette's syndrome is more common in males than in females in both clinical and community-based series (Table 2) (10–13,17,19,20,31). However, the frequent observation of obsessive-compulsive disorder in the female relatives of males with TS has prompted the suggestion that obsessive-compulsive disorder (OCD) may be a female-gender-determined expression of a common pathogenetic factor (32). Marcus and Kurlan (32) have suggested that rates in males and females may be similar if OCD were considered an alternate phenotype to TS. Younger age appears to be a risk factor for TS. While rare in the very young, school-aged children are more likely to be identified as having the symptoms of TS. However, few studies have assessed tics in adults. Follow-up studies of adults diagnosed as having TS in childhood generally find tics to be less severe in adults, particularly in women (22–25).

Table 2 Sex Distribution of Tourette Syndrome in Selected Studies[a]

Author, year	Location	Male/female
Burd et al., 1986 (10)	North Dakota	9.3:1 (Children), 3.4:1 (Adults)
Caine et al., 1988 (11)	Monroe County, New York	9.3:1 (Children)
Comings et al., 1990 (12)	Los Angeles, California	14:1 (Children)
Apter et al., 1992 (13)	Israel	1.6:1 (Adolescents)
Cardoso et al., 1996 (31)	Brazil	3:1
Kurlan et al., 2001 (17)	Rochester, New York	2:1 (Children)
Khalifa and von Knorring, 2003 (18)	Sweden	1.8:1 (Children)

[a] Crude ratios not adjusted for underlying population.

Ethnicity

Ashkenazi Jewish ancestry was once suggested to be a risk factor for TS (34), but subsequent studies (35) suggested that this represented characteristics of the populations attending specific clinics, rather than a true risk factor. As noted above, TS appears to occur worldwide, but differences in frequency cannot be determined due to the methodological variability of studies performed to date.

Heredity

Numerous studies suggest that the risk is higher in family members (2,11,21,32–35). Also supporting a genetic cause is the high concordance in monozygotic twins—100% if both tics and TS are considered (36). Yet despite the strong clinical evidence of a genetic cause of TS, a specific genetic determinant has yet to be identified. The genetics of TS are covered in detail in other chapters.

Group A Beta Hemolytic Streptococcal Infection

Swedo et al. (37) suggested that antecedent Group A beta hemolytic streptococcal (GABHS) infection is associated with a particularly malignant form of TS or OCD, with severe exacerbations poorly responsive to treatment. This has been termed "pediatric autoimmune neuropsychiatric disorders associated with streptococcal infection" or "PANDAS." GABHS infection is also believed to provoke the autoimmune reaction causing rheumatic fever, one feature of which may be a movement disorder (Sydenham's chorea) (38). Elevated expression of a B-lymphocyte surface marker has been associated with TS and OCD by some (39), and others have identified antineuronal antibodies in children fitting the clinical picture of PANDAS (40,41). While these observations provide indirect support for the proposed association of GABHS infection and TS or OCD, to date, a cause-and-effect relationship remains to be proven. Studies assessing this proposed association are in progress, promising improved understanding in the future (Kurlan, personal communication). PANDAS is covered in more detail in other chapters.

Perinatal and Growth Factors

Perinatal factors such as low birth weight, forceps delivery, and maternal stress have been proposed to increase severity of TS (42). Children with TS were more likely to have shorter stature in one clinical comparison (43). Because large, systematic, prospective population-based studies have not been conducted, however, it is possible that these associations are the result of methodological features such as recall or selection bias.

Stimulants

Centrally acting stimulants have been proposed to worsen existing TS. Because attention-deficit/hyperactivity disorder (ADHD) is comorbid with TS in a subgroup of persons, this possibility has caused concern. Recent studies do not support this association, suggesting that stimulants may be used in children with coexisting TS and ADHD without risk of worsening the tic disorder (44).

FUTURE DIRECTIONS

Much remains uncertain regarding the epidemiology of TS and tic disorders. Some progress has been made in determining the distribution of disease in populations. This recent work highlights the importance of population-based methods with intensive ascertainment to identify the broad range of tic disorders in a community. Use of a uniform diagnostic method and similar methods of ascertainment in populations worldwide will be essential to allow comparisons of disease frequency internationally. Population-based studies of the incidence of disease are nearly nonexistent. Incidence studies are critical for investigating the determinants of TS and tics, as well as risk factors influencing severity or persistence of tics. Importantly, longitudinal population-based studies (in contrast to studies of clinic-based populations) will be important to determine the significance of tics identified in childhood. Better description of the frequency and distribution of tics and related comorbid disorders such as OCD and ADHD will be essential in answering questions regarding the role of proposed risk or modifying factors. These answers, in turn, will lead to a better understanding of tic disorders and more effective approaches to treatment or even prevention.

REFERENCES

1. Kurlan R, Behr J, Medved L, Shoulson I, Pauls D, Kidd KK. Severity of Tourette's syndrome in one large kindred. Implication for determination of disease prevalence rate. Arch Neurol 1987; 44:268–269.
2. Pauls DL, Leckman JF. The inheritance of Gilles de la Tourette's syndrome and associated behaviors. N Engl J Med 1986; 315:993–997.
3. Comings DE, Comings BG. A controlled family history study of Tourette's syndrome, I: Attention-deficit hyperactivity disorder and learning disorders. J Clin Psychiatry 1990; 51:275–280.
4. Lucas AR, Beard CM, Rajput AH, Kurland LT. Tourette syndrome in Rochester, Minnesota, 1968–1979. Adv Neurol 1982; 35:267–269.
5. Shapiro AK, Shapiro ES, Bruun RD, Sweet RD. Gilles de la Tourette Syndrome. New York: Raven Press, 1978.

6. Boncour GP. Les tics chez l'6colier et leur interpretation. Prog Med 1910; 26:495–496.
7. Pringle, ML, Butler, NR, Davie, R. 11,000 Seven Year Olds. London, National Bureau for Cooperation in Childcare, 1967. Cited in Shapiro AK, Shapiro ES, Bruun RD, Sweet RD. Gilles de la Tourette Syndrome. New York: Raven Press, 1978:74, 422.
8. Lapouse R, Monk M. Behavior deviations in a representative sample of children: Variation by sex, age, race, social class and family size. Am J Orthopsychiatr 1964; 34:436–446.
9. Debray-Ritzen P, Dubois H. Maladies des tics de l'enfant. Rev Neurol 1980; 136:15–18.
10. Burd L, Kerbeshian J, Wikenheiser M, Fisher W. A prevalence survey of Gilles de la Tourette syndrome in North Dakota school-age children. J Am Acad Child Psych 1986; 25:552–553.
11. Caine ED, McBride MC, Chiverton P, Bamford KA, Rediess S, Shiao J. Tourette's syndrome in Monroe County school children. Neurology 1988; 38:472–475.
12. Comings DE, Himes JA, Comings BG. An epidemiologic study of Tourette's syndrome in a single school district. J Clin Psychiatry 1990; 51:463–469.
13. Apter A, Pauls D, Bleich A, Zohar AH, Kron S, Ratzoni G, Dycian A, Kotler M, Weizman A, Gadot N. A population-based epidemiologic study of Gilles de la Tourette syndrome in Israel. Arch Gen Psychiatry 1993; 50:734–738.
14. Landgren M, Petterson R, Kjellman B, Gillberg C. ADHD, DAMP, and other neurodevelopmental/psychiatric disorders in 6-year-old children epidemiology and co-morbidity. Dev Med Child Neurol 1996; 38:891–906.
15. Costello EJ, Angold A, Burns BJ, Stangl DK, Tweed DL, Erkanli A, Worthman CM. The Great Smoky Mountains study of youth: goals, design, methods, and the prevalence of DSM-III-R disorders. Arch Gen Psychiatry 1996; 53:1129–1136.
16. Verhulst FC, Van der Ende J, Ferdinand RF, Kasius M. The prevalence of DSM-III-R diagnoses in a national sample of Dutch adolescents. Arch Gen Psychiatry 1997; 54:329–336.
17. Kurlan R, McDermott MP, Deeley C, Como PG, Brower C, Eapen S, Andresen EM, Miller B. Prevalence of tics in schoolchildren and association with placement in special education. Neurology 2001; 57(8):1383–1388.
18. Khalifa N, von Knorring AL. Prevalence of tic disorders and Tourette syndrome in a Swedish school population. Dev Med Child Neurol 2003; 45:315–319.
19. Hornse H, Banerjee S, Zeitlin H, Robertson M. The prevalence of Tourette syndrome in 13–14-year-olds in mainstream schools. J Psychiatry Neurosci 2001; 26:417–420.
20. Burd L, Kerbeshian J, Wikenheiser M, Fisher W. Prevalence of Gilles de la Tourette's syndrome in North Dakota adults. Am J Psychiatry 1986; 143:787–788.
21. Zausmer DM. Treatment of tics in childhood. Arch Dis Child 1954; 29:537–542.

22. Goetz CG, Tanner CM, Stebbins GT, Leipzig G, Car W. Adult tics in Gilles de la Tourette syndrome: description and risk factors. Neurology 1992; 42:784–788.
23. de Groot CM, Bornstein RA, Spetie L, Burriss B. The course of tics in Tourette syndrome: a five year follow-up study. Ann Clin Psychiatry 1994; 64:227–233.
24. Burd L, Kkerbeshian PJ, Barth A, Klug MG, Avery PK, Benz B. Long-term follow-up of an epidemiologically defined cohort of patients with Tourette syndrome. J Child Neurol 2001; 16:431–437.
25. Lees AJ, Robertson M, Trimble MR, Murray NMF. A clinical study of Gilles de la Tourette syndrome in the United Kingdom. J Neurol Neurosurg Psychiatry 1984; 47:1–8.
26. Abuzzahab FS, Anderson FO. Gilles de la Tourette Syndrome: International Registry. St. Paul, MN: Mason Publishing, 1976.
27. Nomura Y, Segawa M. Tourette syndrome in oriental children: Clinical and pathophysiological considerations. In: Friedhoff AJ, Chase TN, eds. Gilles de la Tourette Syndrome. New York: Raven Press, 1982:277–280.
28. Bai CH, Han-Quin LF. Tourette syndrome: report of 19 cases. Chin Meal J 1983; 96:45–48.
29. Lieh F, Mak SY, Chung P, Lee S. Tourette syndrome in the Chinese: A follow-up of 15 cases. In: Friedhoff JA, Chase TN, eds. Gilles de la Tourette Syndrome. New York: Raven Press, 1982:281–284.
30. Robertson MM, Trimble MR. Gilles de la Tourette syndrome in the Middle East. Br J Psychiatry 1991; 158:416–419.
31. Cardoso F, Veado CC, deOliveira JT. A Brazilian cohort of patients with Tourette's syndrome. J Neurol Neurosurg Psychiatry 1996; 60:209–212.
32. Marcus D, Kurlan R. Tics and its disorders. Neurol Clinics 2001; 19:735–758.
33. Kurlan R, Behr J, Medved L, Shoulson I, Pauls D, Kidd JR, Kidd KK. Familial Tourette's syndrome: report of a large pedigree and potential for linkage analysis. Neurology 1986; 36:772–776.
34. Eldridge R, Sweet R, Lake CR, Ziegler M, Shapiro AK. Gilles de la Tourette syndrome: Clinical, genetic, psychologic and biochemical aspects in 21 selected families. Neurology 1977; 27:115–124.
35. Golden GS. Tourette syndrome in children: ethnic and genetic factors and response to stimulant drugs. Adv Neurol 1982; 35:287–289.
36. Walkup JT, Leckman JF, Price RA, Hardin M, Ort SI, Cohen DJ. The relationship between obsessive-compulsive disorder and Tourette's syndrome: a twin study. Psychopharmacol Bull 1988; 24:375–379.
37. Swedo SE, Leonard H, Garvey M, Mittleman B, Allen AJ, Perlmutter S, Lougee L, Dow S, Zamkoff J, Dubbert BK. Pediatric autoimmune neuropsychiatric disorders associated with streptococcal infections: clinical description of the first 50 cases. Am J Psychiatry 1998; 155:264–271.
38. Stollerman GH. Rheumatogenic streptococci and autoimmunity. Clin Immunol Immunopathol 1991; 61:131–142.
39. Swedo SE, Leonard HL, Mittleman BB, Allen AJ, Rapoport JL, Dow SP, Kanter ME, Chapman F, Zabriskie J. Identification of children with pediatric

autoimmune neuropsychiatric disorders associated with streptococcal infections by a marker associated with rheumatic fever. Am J Psychiatry 1997; 154:110–112.
40. Kiessling LS, Marcotte AC, Culpepper L. Antineuronal antibodies in movement disorders. Pediatrics 1993; 92:39–43.
41. Morshed SA, Parveen S, Leckman JF, Mercadante MT, Kiss MHB, Miguel EC, Arman A, Yazgan Y, Fujii T, Paul S, Peterson BS, Zhang H, King RA, Scahill L, Lombroso PJ. Antibodies against neural, nuclear, cytoskeletal and streptococcal epitopes in children and adults with Tourette syndrome. Sydenham's chorea and autoimmune disorders. Biol Psychiatry 2001; 50:566–577.
42. Leckman JF, Dolnansky ES, Hardin MT, Clubb M, Walkup JT, Stevenson J, Pauls DL. Perinatal factors in the expression of Tourette syndrome; an exploratory study. J Am Acad Child Adolesc Psychiatry 1990; 29:220–226.
43. Zelnik N, Newfield RS, Silman-Stolar Z, Goikhman I. Height distribution in children with Tourette syndrome. J Child Neurol 2002; 17:200–204.
44. Gadow KD, Sverd J, Sprafkin J, Nolan EE, Grossman S. Long-term methylphenidate therapy in children with comorbid attention-deficit hyperactivity disorder and chronic multiple tic disorder. Arch Gen Psychiatry 1999; 56:330–336.

20

The Treatment of Tics

Christopher G. Goetz and Stacy Horn
Rush University
Chicago, Illinois, U.S.A.

INTRODUCTION

The multidimensional elements of tic disorders and the frequent coexistence of other medical conditions make the management of Gilles de la Tourette's syndrome (TS) complex. As previous chapters have emphasized, accurate diagnosis and the definition of what behaviors represent tics and what behaviors are part of an adjustment reaction, attention-deficit/hyperactivity disorder (ADHD), obsessive-compulsive disorder (OCD) or other comorbidities are paramount to an appropriate treatment plan. With an accurate list of diagnoses, the clinician and patient can rank relative impairment from each and decide on the order of treatment priorities. This chapter deals with the treatment of tics themselves, and later chapters discuss the primary treatment of other comorbid conditions. Because the treatment of tics can affect these other conditions, however, mention of secondary influences of tic therapy on ADHD and OCD is addressed in this chapter.

Many tics do not need treatment. Because of the potency and the available medications, the risk of side effects, the fluctuating nature of the disease, and the overall good prognosis for tic disorders, before prescribing a treatment intervention, the clinician needs to distinguish between the presence of tics and the impairment that they cause. In the authors' view, impairment is best assessed by a review of four questions:

Do tics impact on the patient's achievement in school or work?
Do tics affect social interaction and integration in the classroom or workplace?
Do tics negatively affect home life?
Do tics cause any secondary neurological or medical problems?

Because the environment and adjustment capacities of each patient will be different, the frequency and intensity of tics are not of primary importance in treatment decisions. Rather, a treatment must be guided by the impairment caused by tics. For example, a child with eye blinks, neck-thrusting movements, and coughing tics, even if frequent, does not require treatment if tics do not cause disruption of his classroom, family structure, or friendships and do not cause a sore throat or tingling sensation as part of a compressive neuropathy in his neck. On the other hand, another child with the same symptoms, even if the tics are less frequent or intense, may require intervention if he has trouble focusing his eyes on reading materials, is teased by classmates, causes stress at home, or develops radicular symptoms from his neck tics. Using these four questions as the core of a treatment decision plan will allow the clinician to advise patients and families on treatments and avoid interventions and the risk of medication side effects in unnecessary situations.

The mainstays of treatment include education, behavioral therapies, medications, and, in rare instances, surgery. Combinations of therapy are often necessary for patients to maximize academic and social success and to transition into their roles as productive adults. The scientific data on these four modalities are unequally developed with very little controlled or randomized clinical trial information on education, behavioral therapies, or surgery. Available information is summarized in each category with additional suggestions for future research.

EDUCATION

The effectiveness of education in TS has not been extensively studied, but a review of psychological and educational resources has been published by Packer (1). A clear understanding of the disorder and the dispelling of incorrect assumptions are considered therapeutic pillars in clinical context. Effective education extends to family, teachers, and classmates or coworkers whose understanding of the involuntary nature and noncommunicability of the disorder may help to decrease the patient's ridicule, fear, punishment, and social isolation. It is especially important for patients and the community to understand that the exaggerated examples of TS shown on television or in movies are atypical and that most TS subjects have mild motor and vocal tics. Physicians can help with advocacy in the classroom by acknowledging that patients may need additional time to complete assignments due to their tics. An individual educational plan (IEP) can help to resolve some problems without lowering the academic or work standards. In addition, children with tics may find it helpful to sit near the door of the classroom and be allowed to reasonably leave the classroom to discharge tics and thus help to decrease classroom disruption (2). The Tourette Syndrome Association (TSA) can be a helpful educational resource that has both national and local chapters. The TSA can be contacted by writing to Tourette Syndrome Association, Inc., 42-40 Bell Boulevard, Bayside, New York 11361, 2861. Many local chapters offer support groups and other patient resources including teacher in-services, seminars, and educational advocacy services (1). Support groups can offer shared experiences and diminish social isolation by allowing patients to develop relationships. Lastly, celebrities have more recently begun to bring this illness to the limelight and serve as role models. The professional baseball player, Jim Eisenreich, has helped the public to understand that individuals afflicted with this illness can be successful, productive members of society.

BEHAVIORAL AND PSYCHOLOGICAL THERAPIES

Psychological or behavioral therapy is advocated to help control tics and diminish related impairments. These therapies have been advocated based on observations that stress and anxiety can exacerbate tics. Multiple case and open-label studies report on the impact of various forms of psychological or behavioral therapy on tics. A study by Peterson and Azrin (3) in 1992 compared three reportedly effective therapies: self-monitoring, relaxation training, and habit reversal. This study contained six subjects with TS and involved four phases given in randomized order, no intervention, self-monitoring, relaxation training, and habit reversal. Subjects were instructed in each therapeutic modality and then instructed to practice this method for 30 min following the initial instruction. Two trials of each method were completed. Patients were evaluated and videotaped before and after each treatment phase. During a 2.5-min rating period, subjects had a 44% reduction in tic frequency with self-monitoring, 32% reduction in tic frequency with relaxation training, and a 55% reduction in tic frequency with habit reversal over baseline. Each of these reductions was statistically significant in comparison with baseline status (3). There was a trend toward greater improvement in the second trial for habit reversal. This study also found a negative correlation between the no-intervention tic frequency scores and reduction of tics during all treatment phases (3). The small number of subjects involved in this study limits the interpretation of the results, but the findings suggest that behavioral therapy may be a useful therapeutic intervention with only modest instructions and training. A second study conducted by Bergin et al. (4) evaluated the effects of behavioral relaxation therapy on tic frequency and severity. This study included 23 subjects randomized to either control or treatment groups and stratified based on tic severity. Subjects were evaluated by blinded raters using videotapes and multiple rating scales including the Hopkins Motor and Vocal Tic Scale, Yale Global Tic Severity Scale, Tourette Syndrome Severity Scale, and the Goetz Videotape Scale. Subjects in each group were given 1-hr training sessions over 6 weeks with a psychologist with the treatment group being taught relaxation therapy modalities and the control group getting minimal therapy including listening to audiocassettes of music or environmental sounds. Subjects were rated at baseline, 6 weeks, and 3 months. Sixteen patients were able to complete this protocol. Subjects in the treatment group improved 71–100% at 6 weeks from baseline depending upon the evaluating rating scale as compared to the control group that improved 44–77% from baseline. The comparison between groups was not statistically significant. At 3 months, the treatment group had 57–71% improvement, while the control group had 44–55% improvement. Again, these results were not statistically significant. This study suggests that relaxation therapy has only limited utility in the treatment of tics. It emphasizes the importance of control group study design because of the implications of temporal fluctuations in tics. In spite of these findings, other authors advocate these modalities as adjunctive therapy for control of tics in select patients (5). Increased research efforts into the usefulness of behavioral therapies in tic control are needed. An important unanswered question is whether tic patients can be taught to enhance the volitional suppression of tics. Investigations need to address a larger body of patients with blinded evaluations to hopefully answer the usefulness of these treatment strategies in the future.

PHARMACOTHERAPY

Pharmacological agents should be considered when tics cause significant academic, social, or functional disability. The aim of medical intervention is a decrease in the number or intensity of tics and an improvement in the documented impairment that led to the medication intervention. As a rule, pharmacological agents should be used at the lowest dosages possible with tic reduction, not elimination, as the treatment goal. Based on the unified hypothesis that tics are related primarily to heightened activity of dopaminergic systems, most treatments focus on down-regulating dopaminergic function. The noradrenergic, glutaminergic, and nicotinic systems may also play ancillary roles in the pathophysiology of tic disorders. The final common pathway of the motor system involves the neuromuscular junction under cholinergic control. Pharmacological agents that have been used in the treatment of tics include α-adrenergic agonists, antipsychotic medications, benzodiazepines, tetrabenazine, dopamine agonists, botulinum toxin, and gamma-aminobutyric acid (GABA) agonists. Each agent is discussed in detail, and Table 1 lists the commonly used medications with typical starting dosages.

α-Adrenergic Agonists

α-Adrenergic agonists, clonidine and guanfacine, have been used for the treatment of tics in TS. As autoagonists that work primarily on presynaptic noradrenergic receptors at low doses, these drugs are thought to decrease release of norepinephrine centrally. These medications may be especially helpful in patients with ADHD and behavioral problems (6). Cohen et al. (7) reported a 70% global improvement in patients with TS in an open-label trial with clonidine. Cohen et al. suggested that this improvement was primarily the result of behavioral symptoms and not due to tic control. Clonidine was then evaluated in an open-label study of 20 patients with TS in 1982 by Bruun (8). Subjects that previously obtained no benefit from haloperidol were subsequently tried on clonidine. Subjects were started on 0.05 mg twice a day and optimized as tolerated to a maximum dosage of 0.4 mg a day. Six patients did not finish the study due to side effects or lack of benefit. Subjects were evaluated by subjective report and objective rating by the parents and physician. Ten of the 14 patients remaining in the study reported improvement in their symptoms, although with the dropout rate of 6 patients, this number represented only 50% of the enrolling population (8). Another open-label treatment study of clonidine was conducted in 1982 by Shapiro and Shapiro (9).

Table 1 Medications Frequently Used in the Treatment of TS

Medication	Typical starting dosage (mg/day)
Pimozide	1
Haloperidol	0.25
Risperidone	0.5
Clonidine	0.05
Guanfacine	0.5
Clonazepam	0.5
Tetrabenazine	25
Pergolide	0.05
Baclofen	5

This study evaluated clonidine in 36 patients, 28 patients on polytherapy with haloperidol and 8 patients on monotherapy. Patients were treated with an average of 0.3 mg a day over 3 months. The authors found 11% of subjects with at least a 70% improvement in tics, 14% of subjects with a 50–69% improvement in tics, 67% of subjects with no improvement or worsening, and 8% with an equivocal response (9). Singer et al. (10) published a retrospective study of haloperidol, fluphenazine, and clonidine in 1986. In this report of the 30 patients who received clonidine for the treatment of tics, 5 experienced good control, 9 experienced fair control, and 16 experienced poor control of tics with an overall improvement rate of 47% (10). Goetz et al. (11) published a double-blind crossover trial of clonidine in 1986. Thirty patients participated in this study over a 6-month period. Subjects were treated for 12 weeks with either clonidine or placebo and evaluated every 3 weeks with videotaping. The videotapes were blindly rated at the end of the study period. Patients were optimized to either 0.0075 or 0.015 mg/kg/day and maintained for 6 weeks. The authors did not find any statistically significant objective improvement in tic distribution, frequency, or severity. However, 13 patients reported subjective improvement in their tics and elected to stay on the medication after study completion (11). Leckman et al. (12) completed a 12-week randomized double-blind placebo-controlled trial of clonidine in 40 subjects with TS. Subjects were treated with placebo or up to 0.25 mg per day of clonidine. Subject's tics were evaluated at baseline, 6 weeks, and 12 weeks using the Tourette Syndrome Global Scale, the Shapiro Tourette Syndrome Severity Scale, and the Clinical Global Impression Scale for Tourette syndrome. Subjects taking clonidine were statistically improved over the placebo group. Total motor tic score showed the greatest effect with 35% improvement in the clonidine group compared with 8% improvement in the placebo group (12). A recent multicenter placebo-controlled double-blind clinical trial conducted by the Tourette's Syndrome Study Group involving 136 subjects confirmed that clonidine is effective in lessening tics, as measured by the Yale Global Tic Severity Scale and the Tic Symptom Self-Report Scale (13). The major side effects of clonidine include sedation, hypotension, and depression. Since the drug is typically well tolerated and does not aggravate ADHD or OCD, it is often used in practice as a first attempt to treat tic impairment.

Guanfacine, another α-adrenergic agonist, has been used in TS because of its longer duration of action and improved side-effect profile including less sedation and hypotension than clonidine. An open-label study was completed to evaluate the effectiveness of guanfacine in patient with tics and ADHD by Chappell et al. (14). Ten patients were studied for 4–20 weeks with patients taking an average of 1.5 mg a day. Tic ratings were assessed using the Yale Global Tic Severity Scale, the Tic Symptom Self-Report Scale, and the Conners Parent Rating Scale. This study found a significant decrease in the severity of motor and phonic tics (14). A double-blind placebo-controlled study of guanfacine for tics and ADHD was performed by Scahill et al. (15) in 2001. Thirty-four patients participated in this 8-week protocol and were randomly assigned to either treatment or placebo groups. Subjects were evaluated every 2 weeks. The authors found a statistically significant improvement in the guanfacine group with a 31% decrease in tic severity as compared to no improvement in the placebo group (15). This study suggests that guanfacine may be an effective treatment in some patients with TS, but larger double-blind studies are needed to confirm these results.

Antipsychotic Medications

The second class of drugs used for the treatment of tics in TS is the group of antipsychotic medications. The underlying mechanism of antipsychotic-induced tic improvement in TS is believed to be through dopaminergic receptor blockade. These medications include the typical neuroleptic antipsychotic medications, pimozide, haloperidol, fluphenazine, and trifluoperazine, as well as the atypical antipsychotic medications zisprasidone, quetiepine, olanzepine, risperidone, and clozapine.

The antipsychotic medications most frequently studied are haloperidol and pimozide. These medications have become standards of care mainly due to data derived from case reports and retrospective analysis. Multiple case studies reporting the effectiveness of haloperidol in the treatment of tics started to appear in 1961 (16–18). Haloperidol has been reported to be an effective agent in the treatment of disabling tics with an effectiveness reaching 80% (19). The drug is started at low dosages, usually 0.25 a day, and increased slowly. Side effects of haloperidol therapy include sedation, acute dystonic reactions, parkinsonism, akathisia, tardive dyskinesia, depression, and weight gain. Pimozide has also been used for the treatment of disabling tics and is the only FDA-approved antipsychotic for the treatment of tics. Pimozide appears to be equal to haloperidol in its effectiveness (19,20). A three-arm double-blind randomized crossover placebo-controlled study was conducted by Ross and Moldofsky (19) in 1978 to compare the effectiveness of placebo, haloperidol, and pimozide for the treatment of tics in nine subjects. Subjects were treated sequentially with either pimozide or haloperidol in random order for 12 days with a 6-day placebo period. Subjects were started on 2 mg a day of medication and escalated every second day by 2 mg until control of symptoms, side effects, or 12 mg a day. Subjects were evaluated at baseline and daily on days 5–33. The authors found significant improvement in tics among both groups with no significant difference between pharmacological agents (19). Pimozide was retrospectively studied in 31 patients over an average period of 9 months at doses ranging from 2 to 48 mg a day (20).

Twenty-eight patients (90.3%) reported subjective global improvement (20). A larger and longer retrospective study was published on 65 patients receiving pimozide for tic control (21). Subjects were followed in the outpatient clinic for 6–84 months on an average dosage of 0.5–9 mg daily. Forty-three patients (73%) experienced a favorable clinical response to pimozide with minimal side effects (21). Using a prospective and blinded study design, the Tourette Syndrome Study Group found pimozide to be effective in both short-term tic control and for the long-term prevention of tic exacerbations (22). The advantage of pimozide over haloperidol may be a lower propensity for adverse effects, especially sedation (20,23). Pimozide is typically started at 1 mg a day and slowly optimized to tic control. Potential side effects of pimozide include sedation, parkinsonism, akathisia, prolongation of the Q–T interval, tardive dyskinesia, depression, and weight gain. An electrocardiogram prior to the decision to institute pimozide therapy can determine if the Q–T interval is normal. Other typical neuroleptic medications have been used for the control of tics. These medications appear to have a relatively equal side effect profile and efficacy as compared to haloperidol (24). For patients who are unable or bothered by taking daily medication, fluphenazine decanoate can be given as an intramuscular injection once every 3 months.

Several atypical antipsychotic medications have been used for the control of tics because of their low side-effect profile in other patient groups and sometimes because of their reported benefit for treating conduct disorders that can be associated with tics. Risperidone has theoretical benefit for the treatment of OCD due to its high affinity for 5-HT receptors (25). An open-label 11-week trial evaluated the safety and efficacy of risperidone in seven tic patients (25). Using the Yale Global Tic Severity Scale, authors compared baseline and two follow-up visits. Subjects were started on risperidone 0.5 mg a day and increased to a maximum dosage of 2.5 mg a day. This study reported statistically significant amelioration of tics in the risperidone group with individual patients improving 18–66% compared to baseline. A second open-label study consisted of 38 patients with TS, rated at baseline and after 1 month of therapy using the Yale Global Tic Severity Scale (26). Subjects were started on 0.5 mg a day and increased by 0.5–1.0 mg a day until good control of symptoms or significant side effects. Eight patients withdrew from the trial due to intolerable side effects including lightheadedness, sedation, akathisia, and acute dystonic reactions. Twenty-two of the original 38 patients (58%) experienced improvement in their clinical symptoms (26). The results of these studies are encouraging for the use of risperidone for TS, but a large randomized double-blind placebo-controlled trial needs to be completed to confirm these results and define the extent and severity of adverse effects. The major side effects of risperidone include sedation, lightheadedness, akathisia, dystonia, depression, and weight gain. The use of quetiapine for tic control has been reportedly beneficial in case studies including small numbers of patients (27). Ziprasidone has been tested in a randomized double-blind placebo-controlled trial completed in 28 subjects over a 56-day period (28). Subjects in the treatment group were started on 5 mg a day of ziprasidone and titrated up to a maximum of 40 mg a day. Ziprasidone was found to significantly reduce tic frequency and count over placebo (28). The mean daily dosage of ziprasidone was 28 mg a day. Sleepiness was the most common side effect, but this medication was generally well tolerated.

Benzodiazepines

Benzodiazepines have been used in the treatment of TS, and the most frequently used chemical in the class is clonazepam (29). An open-label study was completed in 28 patients with a marked improvement in 9 patients (32%), a moderate improvement in 6 patients (21%), and therapeutic failure in the remaining 13 patients (46%) (29). Patients that responded to clonazepam were treated for a mean duration of 142.6 weeks with an average dosage of 4.8 mg a day. Open-label studies suggest that clonazepam may be beneficial in some patients who do not respond to other traditional medications or as adjunct therapy to other medications, but a double-blind placebo-controlled trial needs to be completed to define the effectiveness of this medication in TS. Clonazepam is typically started at 0.25–1 mg a day and increased up to 5 mg a day. The major side effect is sedation. Clonazepam should never be abruptly withdrawn in chronic therapy due to the possibility of withdrawal seizures.

Dopamine-Depleting Agents

Tetrabenazine has been used in the control of tics because it is a presynaptic depletor of monoamines that reduces dopamine levels and has dopaminergic receptor blocking properties. Tetrabenazine is not available for use in the United States but can be obtained from Canada and Europe for patient care. Sweet et al. (30) studied the effects of tetrabenazine in five patients in open-label fashion in 1974. Tetrabenazine was given in dosages up to 300 mg a day. Two patients had improvement in their clinical picture at dosages of 175–300 mg a day. The remaining patients did not have any significant clinical improvement, but did experience side effects. Jankovic and Beach (31) reported a 57.4% improvement in 47 patients with tics in an open-label study. Tetrabenazine can be used when other pharmacological agents fail. The major side effects of tetrabenazine include parkinsonism, sedation, akathisia, and depression.

Dopamine Agonists

On the premise that dopamine agonists in very low dosages preferentially act on the presynaptic receptors and thereby decrease dopamine release, pergolide has been studied for its effects on tics. In an open-label study of 32 patients, Lipinski et al. (32) found a 50% reduction in tics in 24 patients. Gilbert et al. (33) completed a randomized double-blind placebo-controlled crossover study using pergolide in 24 subjects with TS. Nineteen subjects completed the protocol and were given up to 0.3 mg per day of pergolide or placebo for 6 weeks with a 2-week washout and then crossed over to the other treatment group. The primary outcome measure was tic severity as measured by the Yale Global Tic Severity Scale. Subjects in the pergolide group had statistically significant reductions in their scale scores with few side effects. This study supports the possible effectiveness of pergolide in the treatment of TS and opens the field to larger clinical studies to test its efficacy as well as that of other dopamine agonists.

Talipexole, a dopamine autoagonist with preferential activity on the presynaptic dopamine receptors, was studied by Goetz et al. (34) in a double-blind placebo-controlled crossover study in 13 subjects with TS. Subjects were given two 12-week treatment regimens with a 2-week washout period. Subjects were given a maximum dosage of talipexole 2.4 mg per day. Eight subjects completed the study protocol. Of the 5 subjects that dropped out, 4 subjects experienced intolerable side effects, namely, sedation and dizziness. Blinded evaluation of videotapes failed to show any statistically significant improvement in tic frequency or severity. This medication is not recommended for standard treatment of TS due to its lack of efficacy and high propensity for side effects.

Botulinum Toxin

Botulinum toxin works at the neuromuscular junction to inhibit acetylcholine release. It is injected into selected muscles to produce mild weakness. This agent has been used to control phonic and motor tics that are restricted to isolated muscle groups. Case reports first began to appear in 1996 for the use of botulinum toxin to control vocal tics (35,36). Reports of improvement of phonic tics with laryngeal injections were favorable and led to larger studies. Jankovic (37) studied 10 patients in open-label fashion and found clinical improvement. Awaad (38) then studied 186 patients with botulinum toxin injections of the neck, face, vocal cords, and extremities. On average, patients were injected every 6–9 months, although the specifics of the injections including dosage were not detailed. Thirty-five patients experienced complete control of their motor tics, but less improvement of their vocal tics (38). In 2000, Kwak et al. (39) published an open-label study of 35 patients. Subjects were injected in their most affected sites and rated on a scale of 0–4 (0 = no improvement and 4 = marked improvement). Twenty-nine patients experienced improvement with botulinum toxin injections with 23 patients reporting a score of 3 or better. It is interesting to note that 25 patients had premonitory symptoms, and 84% of these patients reported improvement in their premonition with botulinum toxin injection. A randomized double-blind trial of the use of botulinum toxin in the treatment of simple motor tics was published in 2001 by Marras et al. (40). This study included 23 patients over a 3-year period with 18 patients completing the study protocol. This study found an overall reduced tic frequency and urge associated with the treated tic, but did not find an overall benefit in patient well being (40). The major side effects of botulinum toxin injection include weakness, soreness, and bruising. The treatment requires specialized training in injection techniques, available through training sessions sponsored by the American Academy of Neurology.

Gamma-Aminobutyric Acid Agonists and Analogs

Awaad (38) studied the effects of baclofen in 264 patients with tic disorders. Baclofen was given in dosages of 10–80 mg a day as open-label treatment, and improvement was reported in 250 patients. Patients were evaluated using the Yale Global Tic Severity Scale within 1–2 weeks of treatment. Patients experienced a statistically significant decrease in both motor and vocal tics (38). A double-blind randomized placebo-controlled crossover trial of baclofen at 60 mg a day was conducted by Singer et al. (41) in 2001 using 4-week treatment cycles with a 2-week washout period. Nine subjects completed the study and outcome measures were the Clinical Global Impression Scale and the Yale Global Tic Severity Scale completed at baseline, 28, 42, and 70 days. Baclofen treatment resulted in statistically significant reduction in total Yale Global Impression Scale scores. This improvement was not a reflection of tic reduction, but related to a reduction in the patients' impairment scores (41). The major side effects of baclofen include sedation and muscle weakness. Further trials with baclofen could focus on this discrepancy and define if the positive effects experienced with baclofen are due to features of tic disability other than actual tic frequency or severity. Because baclofen is a widely accepted treatment for dystonia, a clear definition of the medication's impact upon clonic vs. dystonic tics would be an important clinical study to perform.

SURGICAL THERAPY

When all other therapeutic modalities fail and tic impairment is severe, surgical therapy may be considered (see separate chapter on surgical approaches). Multiple case reports exist in the literature for the positive response of TS patients to surgical intervention, although these are all open-label reports (42–45). These surgical interventions have included multiple locations: the frontal lobes, limbic system, multiple sites, thalamus, and the cerebellum. Because no randomization, blinded rater evaluation, or large series has been reported in the surgical literature, no single procedure can be favored at the present time. Based on the success of surgical intervention in other movement disorders such as idiopathic Parkinson's disease, deep brain stimulation may be a promising area of surgical research in the future.

PRACTICAL ISSUES REVISITED

The treatment of motor and vocal tics in TS is necessary when disability develops. Educational efforts and the increased presence of the Tourette Syndrome Association may allow patients and families to have an image of TS that is more scientifically sound and devoid of mythological fears of a progressive and exotic bizarre disorder. Treatment options vary and should be directed to the control of target symptoms. Counseling and psychotherapy should not be viewed as a primary treatment of the neurochemical disorder, but may help some individual deal with issues of school, family, job, or social integration. If medications are needed, a careful analysis of the primary target symptoms to be abated will help select an appropriate pharmacological agent. It may be necessary to try more than one medication before control is achieved. It is also important to remember the variable nature of this disease and possibility of spontaneous improvement, so that trials of slow drug withdrawal should always be considered especially during times of a more relaxed schedule such as summer vacation. When treatment is necessary, therapies should be used to diminish symptoms, but not eliminate them completely. Medical therapies should be started at low dosages and optimized slowly to help prevent side effects. As further research helps to elucidate the underlying pathophysiology of this disorder, new medications can be developed and tested in double-blind randomized trials to target and treat TS.

REFERENCES

1. Packer LE. Social and educational resources for patients with Tourette syndrome. Neurol Clin 1997; 2:457–473.
2. Burd L, Kerbeshian J. Educational management of children with Tourette syndrome. In: Chase TN, Friedhoff AJ, Cohen DJ, eds. Advances in Neurology. New York: Raven Press, 1992:311–317.
3. Peterson AL, Azrin NH. An evaluation of behavioral treatments for Tourette syndrome. Behav Res Ther 1992; 30(2):167–174.
4. Bergin A, Waranch R, Brown J, Carson K, Singer HS. Relaxation therapy in Tourette syndrome: a pilot study. Pediatr Neurol 1998; 18(2):136–142.
5. Piacentini J, Chang S. Behavioral treatments for Tourette syndrome and tic

disorders: State of the art. In: Cohen DJ, Goetz CG, Jankovic J, eds. Tourette Syndrome. Philadelphia: Lippincott Williams and Wilkins, 2001:319–331.
6. Newcorn JH, Schulz K, Harrison M, DeBellis MD, Udarbe JK, Halperin JM. Alpha$_2$ adrenergic agonists: neurochemistry, efficacy, and clinical guidelines for use in children. Pediatr Clin North Am 1998; 45(5):1099–1122.
7. Cohen DJ, Detlor J, Young JG, Shaywitz BA. Clonidine ameliorates Gilles de la Tourette syndrome. Arch Gen Psychiatry 1980; 37:1350–1357.
8. Bruun RD. Clonidine treatment of Tourette syndrome. In: Friedhoff AJ, Chase TN, eds. Gilles de la Tourette Syndrome. New York: Raven Press, 1982:403–405.
9. Shapiro AK, Shapiro E. Clinical efficacy of haloperidol, pimozide, penfluridol, and clonidine in the treatment of Tourette syndrome. In: Friedhoff AJ, Chase TN, eds. Gilles de la Tourette Syndrome. New York: Raven, 1982:383–386.
10. Singer HS, Gammon K, Quaskey S. Haloperidol, fluphenazine and clonidine in Tourette syndrome: controversies in treatment. Pediatr Neurosci 1986; 12:71–74.
11. Goetz CG, Tanner CM, Wilson RS, Carroll MS, Como PG, Shannon KM. Clonidine and Gilles de la Tourette syndrome: double-blind study using objective rating methods. Ann Neurol 1987; 21(3):307–310.
12. Leckman JF, Hardin MT, Riddle MA, Stevenson J, Ort SI, Cohen DJ. Clonidine treatment of Gilles de la Tourette syndrome. Arch Gen Psychiatry 1991; 48:324–328.
13. The Tourette's Syndrome Study Group. Treatment of ADHD in children with tics. Neurology 2002; 58:527–536.
14. Chappell PB, Riddle MA, Scahill L, Lynch KA, Schultz R, Arnsten A, Leckman JF, Cohen DJ. Guanfacine treatment of comorbid attention-deficit hyperactivity disorder and Tourette syndrome: preliminary clinical experience. J Am Acad Child Adolesc Psych 1995; 34(9):1140–1146.
15. Scahill L, Chappell PB, Kim YS, Schultz RT, Katsovich L, Shepherd E, Arnsten AFT, Cohen DJ, Leckman JF. A placebo-controlled study of guanfacine in the treatment of children with tic disorders and attention deficit hyperactivity disorder. Am J Psychiatry 2001; 158(7):1067–1074.
16. Chapel JL, Brown N, Jankins RL. Tourette's disease: symptomatic relief with haloperidol. Am J Psychiatry 1964; 121:608–610.
17. Lucas AR. Gilles de la Tourette's disease in children: treatment with haloperidol. Am J Psychiatry 1967; 124(2):243–245.
18. Shapiro AK, Shapiro E. Treatment of Gilles de la Tourette's syndrome with haloperidol. Br J Psychiatry 1968; 114:345–350.
19. Ross MS, Moldofsky H. A comparison of pimozide and haloperidol in the treatment of Gilles de la Tourette's syndrome. Am J Psychiatry 1978; 135(5):585–587.
20. Shapiro AK, Shapiro E, Eisenkraft GJ. Treatment of Gilles de la Tourette syndrome with pimozide. Am J Psychiatry 1983; 140(9):1183–1186.
21. Regeur L, Pakkenberg B, Fog R, Pakkenberg H. Clinical features and long-term treatment with pimozide in 65 patients with Gilles de la Tourette's syndrome. J Neurol Neurosurg Psychiatry 1986; 49:791–795.
22. Tourette Syndrome Study Group. Short-term versus longer term pimozide therapy in Tourette's syndrome: a preliminary study. Neurology 1999; 52:874–877.

23. Shapiro E, Shapiro AK, Fulop G, Hubbard M, Mandeli J, Nordlie J, Phillips RA. Controlled study of haloperidol, pimozide, and placebo for the treatment of Gilles de la Tourette's syndrome. Arch Gen Psychiatry 1989; 46:722–730.
24. Goetz CG, Tanner CM, Klawans HL. Fluphenazine and multifocal tic disorders. Arch Neurol 1984; 41(3):271–272.
25. Lombroso PJ, Scahill L, King RA, Lynch KA, Chappell PB, Peterson BS, McDougle CJ, Leckman JF. Risperidone treatment of children and adolescents with chronic tic disorders: a preliminary report. J Am Acad Child Adolesc Psych 1995; 34(9):1147–1152.
26. Bruun RD, Budman CL. Risperidone as a treatment for Tourette's syndrome. J Clin Psychiatry 1996; 57(1):29–31.
27. Párraga HC, Párraga MI. Quetiapine treatment in patients with Tourette syndrome. Can J Psychiatry 2001; 46(2):184–185.
28. Sallee FR, Kurlan R, Goetz CG, Singer H, Scahill L, Law G, Dittman VM, Chappell PB. Ziprasidone treatment of children and adolescents with Tourette's syndrome: a pilot study. J Am Acad Child Adolesc Psych 2000; 39(3):292–299.
29. Truong DD, Bressman S, Shale H, Fahn S. Clonazepam, haloperidol, and clonidine in tic disorders. South Med J 1988; 81(9):1103–1105.
30. Sweet RD, Bruun R, Shapiro E, Shapiro AK. Presynaptic catecholamine antagonists as treatment for Tourette syndrome: effects of alpha-methyl-para-tyrosine and tetrabenazine. Arch Gen Psychiatry 1974; 31:857–861.
31. Jankovic J, Beach J. Long-term effects of tetrabenazine in hyperkinetic movement disorders. Neurology 1997; 48(2):358–362.
32. Lipinski JF, Sallee FR, Jackson C, Sethuraman G. Dopamine agonist treatment of Tourette disorder in children: results of an open-label trial of pergolide. Mov Disord 1997; 12(3):402–407.
33. Gilbert DL, Sethuraman G, Sine L, Peters S, Sallee FR. Tourette's syndrome improvement with pergolide in a randomized, double-blind, crossover trial. Neurology 2000; 54(6):1310–1315.
34. Goetz CG, Stebbins GT, Thelen JA. Talipexole and adult Gilles de la Tourette's syndrome: double-blind, placebo-controlled clinical trial. Mov Disord 1994; 9(3):315–317.
35. Scott BL, Jankovic J, Donovan DT. Botulinum toxin injection into vocal cord in the treatment of malignant coprolalia associated with Tourette's syndrome. Mov Disord 1996; 11:431–433.
36. Trimble MR, Whurr R, Brookes G, Robertson MM. Vocal tics in Gilles de la Tourette syndrome treated with botulinum toxin injections. Mov Disord 1998; 13(3):617–619.
37. Jankovic J. Botulinum toxin in the treatment of dystonic tics. Mov Disord 1994; 9:347–349.
38. Awaad Y. Tics in Tourette syndrome: new treatment options. J Child Neurol 1999; 14(5):316–319.
39. Kwak CH, Hanna PA, Jankovic J. Botulinum toxin in the treatment of tics. Arch Neurol 2000; 57:1190–1193.
40. Marras C, Andrews D, Sime E, Lang AE. Botulinum toxin for simple motor tics:

a randomized, double-blind, controlled clinical trial. Neurology 2001; 56:605–610.
41. Singer HS, Wendlandt J, Krieger M, Giuliano J. Baclofen treatment in Tourette syndrome: a double-blind, placebo-controlled, crossover trial. Neurology 2001; 56(5):599–604.
42. Mitchell-Heggs N, Kelly D, Richardson A. Stereotactic limbic leucotomy—A follow-up at 16 months. Br J Psychiatry 1976; 128:226–240.
43. Rauch SL, Baer L, Cosgrove GR, Jenike MA. Neurosurgical treatment of Tourette's syndrome: a critical review. Compr Psychiatry 1995; 36(2):141–156.
44. Kulisevsky J, Berthier ML, Avila A. Longitudinal evolution of prefrontal leucotomy in Tourette's syndrome. Mov Disord 1995; 10(3):345–348.
45. Robertson M, Doran M, Trimble M, Lees AJ. The treatment of Gilles de la Tourette syndrome by limbic leucotomy. J Neurol Neurosurg Psychiatry 1990; 53(8):691–694.

21

Obsessive-Compulsive Disorder in Tourette's Syndrome

Treatment and Other Considerations

Robert A. King, Diane Findley, Lawrence Scahill, Lawrence A. Vitulano, and James F. Leckman

Yale University School of Medicine
New Haven, Connecticut, U.S.A.

INTRODUCTION

Beginning with Gilles de la Tourette's (1) original description of the syndrome that bears his name, obsessive–compulsive symptoms (OCS) have been noted to be frequent concomitants of Tourette's syndrome (TS) and a common source of distress and/or impairment in individuals with TS.

The frequent co-occurrence of OC and tic symptoms appears to represent, in part, phenomenological overlap (such as that between "complex tics" or "simple compulsions"), as well as probable shared genetic and neurophysiological mechanisms. Although a wide range of obsessions and compulsions are found in individuals with TS, there appear to be distinctive features to the OC phenomena found in many individuals with TS. Consequently, a growing body of research has examined the hypothesis that, relative to non-tic-related OCD, tic-related OCD may constitute a distinctive "endophenotype" of OCD, characterized by earlier onset, greater male preponderance, denser family history of chronic tics, and poorer therapeutic response to monotherapy with serotonin-uptake inhibitors, as well as apparently distinctive patterns of symptom type, neurobiological features, and familial transmission. If distinctive features of tic-related OCD truly exist, better understanding this subtype of OCD will not only help to clarify the pathogenesis of TS and OCD, but also facilitate more effective treatments targeting tic-related obsession and compulsions.

This chapter reviews the clinical and descriptive aspects of tic-related OCD with attention to its potentially distinctive features and the implications of these findings for genetic studies and provides an overview of cognitive behavioral interventions suitable for addressing the range of obsessions and compulsions seen in tic disorders, as well as the psychopharmacology of this subtype of OCD.

PREVALENCE OF OBSESSIONS AND COMPULSIONS IN TS

Estimates of the prevalence of OCS in individuals with TS range from 11% to 80% in clinical and community samples, with prevalence rates varying with sample composition, means of assessment, and criteria used (2).

A representative picture of the frequency, type, and severity of obsessions and compulsions seen in TS is given by Robertson et al. (3), who assessed 57 young people with TS, age 4–15 years (mean 11.3 ± 2.4). One-quarter of the subjects had obsessional thoughts, including 12 of the sample whose obsessions involved intrusive violent scenes. Forty-one percent had compulsive rituals, 19% were excessively tidy, 30% had "evening-up" behaviors, and 60% had forced touching of objects, including, in a third of those cases, touching of dangerously hot objects. Twenty-three percent had obsessions or compulsions involving counting. However, only 9% of the subjects felt these symptoms were socially impairing.

NATURAL HISTORY

The natural history of obsessions and compulsions in individuals with TS is not well studied. Some early studies (4) concluded that OC symptoms in individuals with TS usually had their onset after the onset of tics or increased with duration of tics. However, more systematic prospective studies suggest that the appearance of OC symptoms often predate the onset of tics in children at risk for TS and in many cases may be the earliest harbinger of a tic disorder. For example, McMahon et al. (5) prospectively followed for up to 5 years 34 children of parents with TS, all from a single large pedigree. Although at entry at age 3–6 years, the children were free of tics or OC symptoms, during the follow-up period, 29.4% of the children had the onset of tics, 17.6% of the children developed OC symptoms that met full DSM-IV-TR criteria for OCD and an additional 14.7% developed subclinical OCD.

The mean age of onset for tics was 4.6 ± 2.1 and 3.8 ± 1.6 years for OCD or subclinical OCD. In contrast to a previous study (6), the age at onset of tics or OCD did not differ between children who had only one affected parent or those who had two.

Although tic severity and tic-related impairment often decrease substantially by late adolescence (7,8), the course of OC symptoms in TS is unclear. Bloch et al. (9) followed up 46 youngsters originally evaluated for TS at age 11.42 ± 1.59, and reinterviewed them an average of 7.6 years later, when they were all over 16 years of age. Only 35% of patients reported never having experienced OC symptoms. At follow-up, OC symptoms were reported as absent by 24 (52%) subjects, while mild symptoms (CY-BOCS < 10) were reported by 10 (22%) subjects, significant symptoms (CY-BOCS ≥ 10) by 9 (20%) subjects, and moderate symptoms (CY-BOCS ≥ 20) by 2 (4.3%) subjects (Children's Yale-Brown Obsessive Compulsive Scale; see Ref. 84). Worst-ever OC symptoms occurred on average at age 12.5 years, about 2 years later than worst-ever tic symptoms. IQ was significantly predictive of OCD severity at follow-up. Linear regression analysis was used to analyze association between brain volumes on MRI prior to age 14 and follow-up tic and OCD severity in late adolescence. Reduced caudate nucleus volumes were significantly associated with increased tic and OCD symptom severity at follow-up (10).

A prospective, longitudinal study of a large, community sample of children provides a picture of the relationship of tics, OC symptoms, and attention deficit hyperactivity disorder (ADHD) undistorted by the selection biases found in clinical samples (11). The presence of tics in childhood and early adolescence predicted the onset of OCS in late adolescence and adulthood. Childhood tics and separation anxiety in early adolescent predicted OCD symptoms in late adolescence. Tics and ADHD in late adolescence predicted greater OCD symptoms in adulthood. Older adolescents with OCD and tics were likely to have persistent tics in early adulthood. Higher IQ was associated with an increase in OCD symptoms from late adolescence to adulthood, a finding similar to that of Bloch et al. (9), who found IQ predicting the severity of OCD at follow-up in youngsters with TS.

CORRELATES OF OCD COMORBIDITY IN INDIVIDUALS WITH TIC DISORDER

How do those individuals with TS who develop OC symptoms differ from those who do not?

Santangelo et al. (12) found that perinatal complications appeared to be important predictors of comorbid OCD in individuals with TS. Probands with comorbid OCD were 8 times more likely to have a history of forceps delivery than were those without OCD. Fetal exposure to coffee, cigarettes, or alcohol was also a significant predictor of comorbid OCD.

Coffey et al. (13) compared adults with TS only, OCD only, and TS plus OCD. The TS plus OCD group differed from the TS-only and OCD-only groups in having significantly elevated rates of bipolar disorder, social phobia, body dysmorphic disorder, ADHD, and substance use disorders.

Children who have OCS in addition to TS are often more functionally impaired. Furthermore, comorbid OCS plus tics are often accompanied by other comorbid disorders, such as ADHD or anxiety disorders. Children with TS plus OCD may also manifest what Garland and Weiss (14) term "obsessive difficult temperament" with perseverativeness, inflexibility, intolerance of frustration, and difficulty shifting activities or tolerating changes in schedule (2). Sukhodolsky et al. (15) used hierarchical regression analysis to examine the predictors of social, adaptive, and emotional functioning in a group of 99 children (43 of whom also had ADHD and 48 of whom also had TS), 95 children with ADHD only, and 93 unaffected control children. After first entering the variables of TS, gender and age, the presence of OCD contributed significantly to poorer scores on the Vineland Adaptive Behavior Scales, the Child Behavior Check List (CBCL) Competency, Internalizing, and Externalizing Problem scales, the Children's Depression Inventory (CDI) scale, and the Children's Manifest Anxiety Scale-Revised. Added as a final variable, the presence of ADHD added still further to the poor scores on the Vineland Socialization Scale, the CBCL Social and School Competency scales, and the CDI.

In addition, compared to children with OCD but no ADHD, children with OCD plus ADHD had significantly higher rates of oppositional defiant disorder. This parallels the findings of Geller et al. (16,17) that, compared with children with OCD but no ADHD, comorbid ADHD plus OCD is associated with higher rates of impaired global functioning and educational problems.

Swerdlow et al. (18) found that compared with adult patients who had TS but no OCD, subjects with TS and even relatively mild OCD were more functionally impaired, with 2.5 times higher unemployment rates. The OCD symptoms of these subjects appear to have been even more disabling than their tics. Yale Global Tic Severity Scale (YGTSS) impairment scores for the OCD plus TS subjects were higher than those of subjects with TS alone and correlated significantly with scores on the Yale-Brown Obsessive Compulsive Scale (Y-BOCS).

The findings of Coffey et al. (13), Swerdlow et al. (18), and others raise the question of how to understand those cases where OCD and TS appear to overlap. Is the presence of OCD plus TS a marker for greater overall severity of illness, a "double hit" of vulnerability factors (whether genetic or environmental), or a condition different from either TS alone or OCD alone? Despite many ingenious studies, more work is needed to clarify whether it is more useful to think of a TS–OCD spectrum, with TS plus comorbid OCD representing an intermediate condition, or a series of discrete disorders or phenotypes.

DISTINGUISHING BETWEEN TICS AND COMPULSIONS

Many individuals with TS report obsessions or compulsions similar to those of individuals with OCD but no tics, such as contamination worries, compulsive cleaning, or repetitive checking. Along with the simple motor and vocal tics of TS, however, many patients with TS also report a spectrum of difficult-to-classify repetitive behaviors that defy easy dichotomization as either tics or compulsions. For example, patients with TS may not be able to give a motive for their repetitive touching or tapping or symmetrical arranging other than the urge to do it or to correct something not looking or feeling "just right." Unlike the anxiety-driven or harm-averting washing, checking, or avoidance of individuals with pure OCD, the repetitive actions of individuals with TS are most often not performed to avoid some feared consequence; rather, attempts to suppress the behavior produce a mounting sense of frustration or tension similar to that which accompanies the suppression of simple tics, while performance of the behavior produces an evanescent feeling of relief or completion.

Many tics are preceded by a premonitory urge or need to gain an elusive sense of completion by achieving some sort of tactile, somatosensory, or visual symmetry or order. Examples include having to "balance" touching or tapping by the right hand with a similar action with the left hand ("evening up"); needing to repeat an action an even or odd number of times; having to close a door repeatedly until it makes the right "clunk" with a corresponding "just right" sensation in the arm; or having to have parents answer repeated queries in just the right way. Not surprisingly, it is often impossible to determine whether a given repetitive behavior, taken in isolation, is best considered a complex tic or a simple compulsion.

Some patients with TS distinguish between tics and compulsions, regarding the former as prompted by or accompanied by a physical sensation, while the latter are prompted by some mental phenomenon (19). For example, one young adolescent with TS and OCS explained, "The tic is more of an itch, and a compulsion is a want. A tic is physical and the compulsion is a mental feeling." Similarly, an adult male noted, "The urge to tic is a release of a buildup of physical energy; the compulsive urge is a buildup of emotional energy" (20, p. 678). Many patients with TS, however, describe their premonitory urges as straddling the physical and mental (21).

Tic-Related OCD as a Distinct Endophenotype

A growing body of studies has examined the question of whether there are systematic phenomenological differences between the OCS of individuals with and without a personal or family history of TS (Table 1) (see Ref. 2 for older studies). Taken together, these studies suggest that compulsions to tap, touch, or rub are characteristic of tic-related OCD (and are found in 70–80% of patients with tics plus OCD, but only 5–25% of individuals with OCD but no tics). Similarly, violent or aggressive thoughts and images, religious and sexual preoccupations, and concerns about symmetry and exactness are found significantly more often in patients with tic-related OCD than in those with OCD but no tics. In contrast, contamination worries and cleaning compulsions are more frequently found in patients with non-tic-related OCD.

Factor-analytical studies have confirmed these general findings and also provide a robust quantitative method for studying the dimensional aspects of OC symptoms in various subject groups (for review, see Refs. 22,23). Following the seminal study of Baer (24), Leckman et al. (25,26) used 13 a priori categories to group the obsessions and compulsions as elicited with the Yale-Brown Obsessive Compulsive symptom checklist (Y-BOC-SC) in a sample of over 300 patients with OCD. Using the reported lifetime presence or absence of each group of obsessions or compulsions, principal components factor analysis yielded four factors accounting for over 60% of the variance in each of two separate samples (Fig. 1). Factor One included obsessions about aggression to self or others, sexual obsessions, moral or religious scrupulosity, and checking compulsions. Factor Two included obsessions concerning symmetry or exactness, repetitive rituals, counting compulsions, and ordering and arranging compulsions. Factor Three consisted of contamination obsessions and cleaning and washing compulsions. Factor Four included hoarding and collecting compulsions.

In all, close to a dozen studies have examined the factor structure of obsessions and compulsions in various samples of individuals with OCD (25,27–35) and found that 3–5 factors accounted for 48–81% of variance in the samples. In general, these studies have consistently replicated the dimensions of checking/washing, symmetry/ordering, and hoarding, but leave open whether the aggressive/checking and sexual/religious dimensions form a single unique factor or two separate dimensions (22).

The use of individuals' factor scores on these various OCD dimensions provides a useful quantitative trait method for genetic studies, an approach that may permit the teasing out of quantitative phenotypes or heritable components in complex heterogeneous disorders such as TS or OCD (22,36,37). This approach promises to be facilitated by the development of a dimensional version of the Yale-Brown Obsessive–Compulsive Scale (DYBOCS), which is now under way (22).

Table 1 Recent Studies of Tic-Related vs. Non-Tic-Related Obsessive–Compulsive Disorder (OCD)

	N	Sex (% female)	Onset	Distinctive symptoms
Petter et al. (1998) (117)				
OCD with tics	13			More intrusive nonviolent images; excessive concern for appearance; need for symmetry; touching and counting compulsions
OCD without tics	13			
Swerdlow et al. (1999) (18)				
OCD plus tics	18	28	9.39	More sexual obsessions; touching compulsions aggressive obsessions; intrusive violent images
OCD alone	46	50	13.02	
Mataix-Cols et al. (1999) (30)				
Tic-related OCD	46	35	12.5	More symmetry/ordering (difference accounted for by male subjects)
Non-tic-related OCD	127	53	16.9	
Cath et al. (2001) (42)				
OCD plus tics	10	50		More echophenomena
OCD, no tics	21	57		More counting
Grados et al. (2001) (115)				
Tic-related OCD probands	5	60	11.6	No difference between groups with respect to proportion of relatives with tics (inadequate power)
Non-tic-related OCD probands	72	51	11.5	
First-degree relatives with OCD + tics	8	NA		Earlier onset of OCD
First-degree relatives with OCD, no tics	42	NA		Later onset of OCD

Table 1 Continued

	N	Sex (% female)	Onset	Distinctive symptoms
Scahill et al. (2003) (116)				
Pediatric OCD plus tics	32	31	11.4	Repetition of routine behaviors, ordering and arranging compulsions; trend to more fear of acting on unwanted impulses or fear of harm to self/others, trend to more externalizing and attention problems
Pediatric OCD without tics	48	42	10.8	More contamination obsessions, washing, cleaning; compulsive requests for reassurance
Himle et al. (2003) (105)				
Tic-related childhood OCD	8	25	NA	Harm to others, repeating or checking
Non-tic-related childhood OCD	11	55	NA	Contamination/washing

Alsobrook et al. (38) used this approach to examine the scores of OCD probands and their relatives on Factor One (aggressive, sexual, religious obsessions/checking compulsions) and Factor Two (symmetry and ordering obsessions/compulsions). Probands with high scores on these factors were more likely to have relatives with OCD than did probands with low scores on these factors.

Using this approach with data from the Tourette Syndrome Association International Consortium for Genetics' Affected Sibling Pair Study, Leckman and colleagues (28) examined the quantitative OC symptom dimensions scores for 128 siblings with TS and their parents. Over half of the siblings had comorbid OCD, and there was a high correlation between siblings' scores for both Factor One (aggressive, sexual, religious obsessions/checking compulsions) and Factor Two (symmetry and ordering obsessions/compulsions). There was also a high correlation between the siblings' scores on these factors and those of their mothers, but not their fathers.

Rauch et al. (39) have utilized OCD dimensional factor scores to test a modular model of OCD, in which "dysfunction within separate (neurobio-

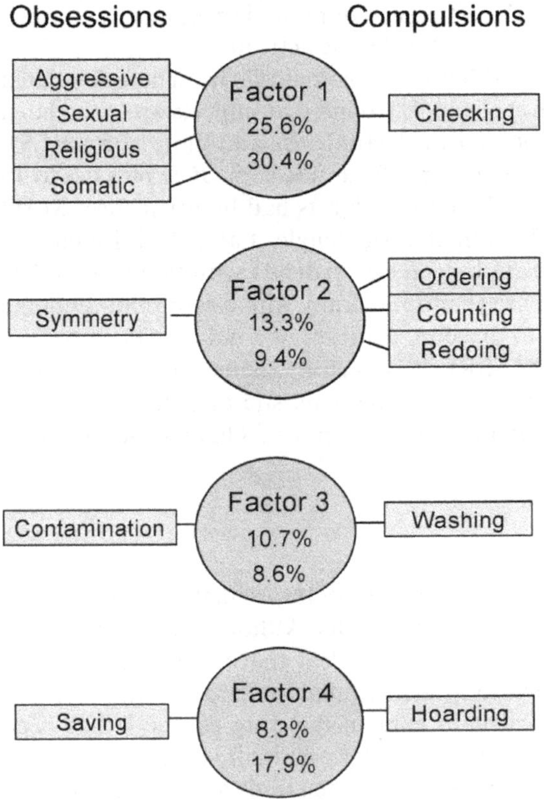

Figure 1 The four factors that accounted for over 60% of the variance in each of two separate samples.

logical) component systems may principally mediate independent symptom factors." In support of this notion, they examined the relative regional cerebral blood flow in 14 subjects with OCD using positron emission tomography (PET) during a continuous performance task. Factor One scores (religious/aggressive/sexual obsessions and checking) correlated with rCBF in the striatum bilaterally, with trends linking Factors Two and Three with other regions. Mataix-Cols et al. (31) used functional magnetic resonance imaging (fMRI) to examine the neural correlates of anxiety invoked in normal volunteers by means of viewing alternating blocks of pictures corresponding to neutral and normally aversive washing-relevant, checking-relevant, or hoarding-relevant images and imagining scenarios related to each picture type. Anxiety associated with the different symptom dimensions was associated with different patterns of cortical or limbic activation.

Tic-related OCD may also differ neurobiologically from non-tic-related OCD in other ways. Leckman et al. (40,41) found that subjects with tic-related OCD had higher afternoon plasma prolactin levels and more normal CSF oxytocin levels. Cath et al. (42) compared 21 adults with OCD plus tics to 15 subjects with OCD but no tics; the latter subjects had higher platelet MAO activity and whole-blood 5-HT. Finally, McDougle et al. (43,44) found that compared to patients with OCD but no tics, patients with tic-related OCD showed less therapeutic response to monotherapy with a serotonin-reuptake inhibitor (SSRI). Compared to placebo, addition of a neuroleptic improved the therapeutic response to the SSRI. It is unclear whether this less satisfactory response to SSRI monotherapy is characteristic of patients with tic-related OCD or a function of the specific types of OCD symptoms that characterized such patients.

PHARMACOTHERAPY

The selective serotonin-reuptake inhibitors (SSRIs) are first-line medications for the treatment of OCD in children and adults. Although their mechanism of action is not completely understood, it is clear that the SSRIs block the return of serotonin into the presynaptic neuron at the serotonin transporter. This action alone is not sufficient to explain the drug effects. It has been proposed that the blockade of the transporter eventually leads to a desensitization of the serotonin autoreceptors, which then leads to sustained increase in available serotonin (45).

A detailed meta-analysis of controlled studies in adults suggests a similar magnitude across the SSRIs including fluoxetine, fluvoxamine, sertraline, with a slightly larger effect size for clomipramine (46). Since the publication of this detailed meta-analysis, three other SSRIs—paroxetine, citalopram, and escitalopram—have been introduced into the U.S. marketplace. To date, paroxetine and citalopram have been studied and now are approved for the treatment of OCD in adults. Escitalopram, which is the single isomer presumed to be responsible for the citalopram's SSRI action, has been examined in depression, but not OCD (47).

A recent meta-analysis (118) of pharmacotherapy trials in pediatric OCD examined extant studies of paroxetine, fluoxetine, fluvoxamine, setraline, and clomipramine. Drug was significantly more effective than placebo, but the pooled standardized mean difference across all 12 studies was only 0.46, representing only a modest effect size. Clomipramine appeared significantly superior to each of the SSRIs, but the various SSRIs appeared comparably effective to one another.

Following the early clinical trials with clomipramine and fluoxetine in children and adolescents (48–50), three large placebo-controlled clinical trials in pediatric populations have been published (see Table 2; 51–53). SSRIs can be administered once a day, and, unlike clomipramine, they do not require blood level monitoring or ECGs. As shown in Table 2, the magnitude of effect is moderate [approximately a 3-point difference on the Children's Yale-Brown Obsessive–Compulsive Scales (CYBOCS) between active and placebo], with no appreciable differences between compounds.

A large-scale, open-label study with paroxetine involving 335 children and adolescents showed a response rate of 71% after 16 weeks of treatment (54). Positive response was defined as 25% reduction in the CYBOCS Total score and a score of "Much Improved" or "Very Much Improved" on the Improvement item of the Clinical Global Impression scale. The overall reduction was approximately 13 points on the CYBOCS. Clearly, this is a much higher change score than any of the placebo-controlled studies cited above. Given the open-label design, however, it is difficult to compare these results with those of double-blind studies. In a series of secondary analyses, the investigators showed that comorbidity attenuated the rate of positive response. The only exceptions to this general rule were separation anxiety and generalized anxiety, both of which showed a slightly higher positive response rate than patients with OCD alone.

Citalopram has been shown to effective for the treatment of OCD in adults (55). In that study, doses of 20, 40, or 60 mg/day were all superior to placebo. There was evidence of a dose response both with respect to benefit and adverse effects. To date, there are only two open-label studies with citalopram (56,57). Taken together, these two studies evaluated 38 subjects at doses ranging from 10 to 40 mg/day. The response rate was similar to the large

Table 2 Large-Scale Placebo-Controlled Studies in Childhood OCD

		CYBOCS change score		Rate of positive response (%)	
Drug [author/year]	*N*	Active	Placebo	Active	Placebo
Sertraline [March et al., 1998 (52)]	187	6.8	3.4	53	37[a]
Fluvoxamine [Riddle et al., 2001 (53)]	120	6.0	3.0	42	26[a]
Fluoxetine [Geller et al., 2001 (51)]	103	9.5	7.4	49	25[b]

[a] Defined as ≥25% decrease on CY-BOCS total score.
[b] Defined as ≥40% decrease on CY-BOCS total score.

open-label paroxetine study and the drug was well tolerated. Given the open-label design, however, the higher response rate in these open-label trials than the rate observed in the placebo-controlled studies should be interpreted with caution.

Some (43,44,58), but not all (e.g., Ref. 59) studies in adults have found that adult patients with a personal or family history of tics respond less well to monotherapy with an SSRI than do patients with non-tic-related OCD. If tic-related OCD is truly less responsive to SSRI monotherapy, it is not clear whether this is an intrinsic aspect of the TS diathesis, or whether it might be attributable to a greater proportion of SSRI-resistant subtypes of obsessions or compulsions (such as hoarding or somatic obsessions) in TS patients. Few data are available as to whether children with tic-related OCD are less responsive to SSRIs. An open trial of paroxetine in childhood OCD with response rates that were generally anomalously high found that children with comorbid tic disorders showed a 50% rate of positive response (which was significantly lower than that of children without tic disorder). This rate is virtually identical to that observed by Scahill et al. (60) in a smaller, placebo-controlled study of fluoxetine in children and adults with OCD and a chronic tic disorder. Other studies have observed no effect of fluoxetine on OC symptoms in children with a tic disorder (61,62).

Taken together, these data suggest that the SSRIs are generally well tolerated and modestly effective for the treatment of OCD in children, adolescents, and adults. However, the magnitude of response may not be as large in children as that observed in adults, with children with comorbid tic disorders being at apparently even higher risk for partial or nonresponse to an SSRI. For example, approximately 40% of the subjects in the multisite sertraline study showed less than a 25% improvement in obsessive–compulsive symptoms (52). Thus, clinicians and parents should be mindful that, by itself, SSRI treatment is unlikely to take away all OCD symptoms in children.

To manage partial response, the clinician and family often encounter the dilemma of whether to switch to another SSRI, try clomipramine or add an adjunctive medication. Although not well studied in children, a series of studies by McDougle et al. (44,58) have shown that the addition of low-dose antipsychotic medication (pimozide, haloperidol, or risperidone) can be effective in adults with refractory OCD. A few open trials of combination treatment adding another atypical, such as quetiapine (63) or olanzapine (64), to an SSRI have been reported, but there are no controlled studies. Although case reports suggest that the addition of clonazepam (65) or clomipramine (66) may be effective when combined with an SSRI, no other pharmacological augmentation strategies for refractory OCD have been shown to be effective in a controlled trial. Another strategy for refractory OCD is intravenous clomipramine or citalopram. To date, these approaches have been studied in only small number of patients (67–69).

In view of the inadequate support for combined pharmacotherapy and the potentially modest effects of SSRI monotherapy in children with OCD, cognitive–behavioral therapy (CBT) should be considered (70,71). Indeed, a recent multisite study in children and adolescents has shown that the combination of CBT, based on exposure and response prevention, and medication was more effective than either treatment alone (72). Further study of combined medication approaches with and without CBT for the treatment of children and adolescents with OCD are needed.

Clinical Management

The currently available SSRIs have relatively long half-lives, permitting single daily dosing in most instances. However, fluvoxamine, which has the shortest half-life of the currently available SSRIs, was given on a twice-daily schedule in the pediatric controlled studies (53,73). Citalopram and fluoxetine have the longest half-lives of currently available SSRIs, with estimates of 33 and 48–72 hr, respectively. In addition, fluoxetine has an active metabolite (norfluoxetine) with an elimination half-life of 7–14 days. To varying degrees, the SSRIs inhibit the activity of one or more hepatic enzymes responsible for metabolizing medications (74). Thus, attention to the possibility of drug interaction is warranted. For example, fluoxetine and paroxetine are potent inhibitors of CYP2D6. Thus, the level of any drug that relies on CYP2D6 (such as risperidone or fluphenazine) will rise when combined with fluoxetine or paroxetine. Citalopram also inhibits 2D6, but to a lesser extent. Fluvoxamine inhibits several CYP isoenzymes. By contrast, sertraline appears to exert little or no inhibition of CYP2D6 and only modest inhibition of CYP3A4. Inhibition of CYP3A4 is of particular concern for patients treated with drugs such as pimozide because pimozide relies on this pathway and can cause serious, even fatal, cardiac arrhythmias. Sudden death with the combination of pimozide and potent 3A4 inhibitors such as clarithromycin has been reported (75).

Given that in vitro studies suggest the possibility of interactions between pimozide and various SSRIs (76), great caution is indicated in their use in patients on pimozide. See Table 3.

Long-Term Treatment

One of the clinical dilemmas facing clinicians, families, and pediatric patients with OCD is how long to maintain the medication in the child who achieves clear benefit from an SSRI. That childhood-onset OCD can be a chronic condition is demonstrated by the follow-up study of 54 children and adolescents with OCD 2–7 years after participation in a medication trial (65). These investigators found that 70% (39/54) remained on medication for more than 2 years and only about 6% were remitted. Given the potential for chronicity in

Table 3 Dosing Guide for Antiobsessional Drugs Studied in Children and Adolescents

Drug	Typical starting daily dose (mg)	Typical maintenance daily dose (mg)
Clomipramine	25	75–150
Fluoxetine	5–10	10–40
Sertraline	12.5–25	75–200
Fluvoxamine	12.5–25	75–200
Paroxetine	5–10	10–40
Citalopram	5–10	10–40

childhood onset OCD, the question about duration of treatment warrants careful consideration. Two recent long-term studies suggest that drug treatment will result in gradual but continued improvement over 1-year follow-up in approximately 50% of cases (56,77). The relatively high rates of relapse of OCD symptoms seen following discontinuation of SSRI mediation provide another strong rationale for combined medication–CBT treatment.

Adverse Effects of the SSRIs

As a group, the SSRIs are generally well tolerated. Potentially serious side effects such as alterations in cardiac conduction times or seizures in the usual dose range have not been reported. The most common side effect of the SSRIs in children and adolescents appears to be behavioral activation—marked by insomnia, motor restlessness, and impulsive and disinhibited behavior. Activation most often occurs early in treatment or with dose increases (78). This observation underscores the importance of starting with low doses of SSRIs and increasing the dose slowly. Hypomania and mania have also been reported. For example, in a series of 33 children and adolescents being treated for depression, Tierney et al. (79) reported two cases of sertraline-induced mania. Other side effects include diarrhea, nausea, heartburn, decreased appetite, and fatigue. Sexual side effects, which are relatively common in adults, should also be considered in sexually active adolescents.

There have also been reports of suicidal ideation and self-injurious behavior with fluoxetine (80) and paroxetine (Food and Drug Administration website, 2003). Whether these reports are attributable to SSRIs, these specific SSRIs, or to all SSRIs is not clear. Thus, children and adolescents treated with an SSRI should be monitored for suicidal thought and self-injurious behavior.

A withdrawal syndrome characterized by dizziness, nausea, vomiting, myalgia, and fatigue has been reported with the shorter-acting SSRIs such as paroxetine, fluvoxamine, and sertraline (81,82). These reports have been confirmed by a controlled discontinuation study in 220 adults. In that study, Rosenbaum et al. (83) compared the effects of abrupt withdrawal of fluoxetine, paroxetine, and sertraline. Abrupt withdrawal of paroxetine and sertraline was associated with irritability, agitation, fatigue, insomnia, confusion, dizziness, and nervousness, but fluoxetine was not. The long half-life of fluoxetine and norfluoxetine presumably results in a gradual taper even when the oral dose is stopped abruptly. Based on these results, a slow withdrawal of the shorter acting SSRIs such as paroxetine, sertraline, and fluvoxamine is warranted. Citalopram has a half-life of 33 hr. In the absence of data on adverse effects of abrupt withdrawal, sudden discontinuation of citalopram should also be avoided.

Some controlled studies (60) have found no deleterious effect of SSRIs on tic severity in individuals with tic disorder. To the extent that SSRI treatment can reduce anxiety, depression, and obsessive–compulsive symptoms, it might be expected to have a beneficial effect on tic severity. Clinical experience, as well as some anecdotal case studies, however, suggests that in a few cases, SSRI administration can produce an increase in tics (or even de novo tics in previously unaffected individuals) (85,86).

COGNITIVE BEHAVIORAL TREATMENT FOR OCD

Cognitive behavioral treatment for obsessive–compulsive disorder has emerged as the most effective nonpharmacological treatment for adults as well as children and adolescents (87–89). This approach will be described, followed by the special considerations involved when treating individuals with comorbid tic disorders, especially children and adolescents.

Treatment generally begins with one or two sessions devoted to psychoeducation of the patient (and parents, in the case of children) about the nature of OCD. These sessions are intended to answer questions and clarify any misconceptions that may be held (90–92). For example, some patients may feel that they are "going crazy" because they are very aware of how unusual or bizarre some of their thoughts and feelings are. To some extent, normalization of intrusive thoughts and superstitious habits can be helpful. It should also be made clear that OCD is a biologically based disorder that, in a seeming paradox, can be positively impacted by purely cognitive–behavioral means (93). Also included in the psychoeducation phase is the rationale for treatment, which seems to be a critical component, as the patient will be asked to participate in the very activities he or she finds most distressing.

To begin, a hierarchy of the patients' symptoms is constructed by asking them to list their symptoms and rank them in order from least distressing to most distressing. In the following phase of treatment, exposure sessions are conducted generally beginning with a mildly to moderately distressing symptom and proceeding through the list, as tolerated, to the most distressing (92).

The behavioral component of the treatment package involves exposure and response (or ritual) prevention (ERP) (92,94). Exposure refers to arranging for the patients to confront situations which evoke their fear without being permitted to engage in the ritual that usually reduces the anxiety. Conceptually, a person has an intrusive thought (obsession) that is distressing and which the subject has great difficulty ignoring, creating high levels of anxiety. For example, a very common obsession is the excessive concern that one's hands are dirty and might lead to contracting an illness. The person then engages in some behavior (compulsion) that temporarily reduces the anxiety until the subject is once again confronted with the thought and the process continues. So, in our example, the person concerned about germs might engage in excessive hand washing. It also should be noted that the compulsive behavior might be the avoidance of the feared stimulus; e.g., the person might avoid touching doorknobs or other objects that could have germs.

In ERP, the person is exposed to the obsession then, by mutual consent, is not allowed to engage in the ritual (the response prevention component). A characteristic exposure/response prevention sequence, for example, might consist of rubbing the hands on the floor and then refraining from washing them for an agreed-upon period of time. During the therapy session, the patient is encouraged to observe and periodically rate the course of his or her anxiety while refraining from performing his or her usual ritual. Over the course of the session, the patient will experience a gradual decrease in anxiety as if he or she had engaged in the ritual, although the time required for the anxiety to decrease is likely to take much longer than if the person simply performed the ritual. Although not completely understood, this phenomenon is thought to be attributable to habituation of the anxiety (95,96); that is, one's level of arousal does not remain at that high level but will return to a homeostatic baseline.

Although ERP is generally considered a behavioral treatment, cognitive processing is also likely to be occurring such that new experiences are being encoded and stored and can be retrieved; learning is taking place. The individual is learning through his or her direct experience that the dreaded outcome does not occur when the ritual is not performed or the feared situation is not avoided. This is not to say that the individual will no longer have the obsessions, but rather that when they do occur, the anxiety will be much briefer, more tolerable, and quite possibly of less intensity. This gives the repeated opportunity for faulty appraisals to be disconfirmed (97).

To help augment compliance and tolerate the anxiety entailed, a whole tool-kit of adjunctive techniques have been developed to maximize the patient's involvement in exposure/response prevention work (91).

In some cases, specific cognitive strategies may be necessary to augment ERP (94). The importance one places on one's thoughts has been identified as a significant component of OCD and one that can interfere with treatment (98). Two common manifestations of this in OCD are thought suppression and thought–action fusion. Thought suppression refers to the phenomenon that the more one tries to suppress a thought (as someone with obsessions might attempt to do), the more it is likely that the subject will continue to have that thought (99,100). Thought–action fusion refers to the belief that thoughts have causal power (e.g., having the thought that a loved one will have an accident will cause it to actually happen) and that thinking about doing something is essentially the same as actually doing it (e.g., having a thought of stabbing a loved one is as terrible as actually doing it) (101,102).

Thus far, the discussion has focused on OCD in general, without any special consideration of subtypes. However, recent research strongly suggests that OCD is a heterogeneous disorder, with the corollary that a single psychosocial treatment approach may not be sufficient to produce meaningful symptom reduction in all cases of OCD (23,103). Although the approaches described here have been shown to be effective, in most reported studies treatment of cleaning compulsions have been overrepresented (104); as a result, there is relatively less information about the effectiveness of these procedures for counting, repeating, symmetry, and hoarding compulsions. This lack is of particular relevance to tic-related OCD, which, as discussed earlier, is characterized by higher rates of checking, counting, ordering, touching, and hoarding compulsions, as well as lower rates of cleaning compulsions than non-tic-related OCD (20,26). It would seem then that tic-related OCD would present special considerations when applying cognitive–behavioral treatments, although a recent uncontrolled trial comparing response to CBT in a small sample of children with tic-related and non-tic-related OCD showed no differences between the groups, with significant improvements reported for all subjects (105). On the other hand, in a study of predictors of response to CBT, Mataix-Cols et al. (103) found that, after controlling for symptom severity, higher scores on the sexual/religious obsessions factor predicted poorer outcome to CBT. In addition, high scorers on the "hoarding" dimension were relatively more likely to drop out of cognitive–behavioral treatment prematurely and benefit less.

It is often the case in tic-related OCD that compulsive behaviors do not occur in response to an anxiety producing obsession, but rather are performed in response to a perception of something not looking, feeling, or sounding "just right," or to an inexplicable urge to engage in the behavior (106). As discussed above, there is often no anxiety per se preceding such compulsions, but rather a feeling of inner tension (much like that which precedes a tic) (107). For example, an individual may feel the need to touch the wall in a particular way or to arrange items in a certain order, not to avoid some catastrophe but rather to relieve the tension from the urge to do so.

For these non-anxiety-driven symptoms, a behavioral treatment technique similar to ERP known as habit reversal training (HRT) (108) may be helpful. Habit reversal training has been used to treat tics, trichotillomania, and other habit disorders such as skin picking (109–111). The major components of HRT are self-awareness training, competing response training, and social support (112,113). In treating the compulsions of tic-related OCD, competing response training appears to be the most relevant component and is quite similar to ERP. A competing response is a behavior that the person performs rather than engaging in the usual behavior. For example, patients who experience strong urges to touch walls might be taught to clasp their hands together or put their hands in their pockets for a period of time when they experience the urge, instead of touching the wall. As in ERP, when the ritual is not performed, the patient is able to learn experientially in the therapy session that the urge decreases anyway, and with repeated practice, the urge to engage in the compulsive behavior decreases through habituation.

In implementing these above procedures with a child or adolescent, including a parent component is often necessary to ensure effectiveness. Along with the youngster receiving treatment, the parent should be provided with the basic facts about OCD and guidance in how to serve as natural resources during their child's recovery. Too often parents are worried that their child is "crazy" or that they have somehow caused the OCD. Collateral parent treatment sessions can help parents learn that OCD is a legitimate illness, that early diagnosis and treatment can save their child from progressive anguish and impairment, and most importantly that they are not alone. Because most ERP and habit reversal protocols involve homework assignments to practice the techniques learned in each session at home, parents also serve as an important resource in encouraging and monitoring the child's practicing these techniques. With the transition to adolescence, clinical judgment and frank discussion with both the youngster and parents are needed to determine what degree of parental involvement is optimal.

In their attempts to alleviate their child's distress, well-meaning parents can inadvertently reinforce OC ritual and avoidance symptoms, thereby making things worse. On the other hand, an abrupt unilateral withdrawal by a parent from involvement in a child's compulsive routines is usually not possible (or even productive) until the child (and the parent) feel that the child has available, through the therapy, alternative means of coping with his or her anxiety. A more complete understanding of behavioral treatment strategies will often allow parents to become active partners in the treatment of their children and to help their children to fend off compulsive urges at the very beginning of uncontrollable worrying and senseless ritualizing (114).

REFERENCES

1. Gilles de la Tourette G. Etude sur une affection nerveuse caracterisée par de l'incoordination motrice accompagnée d'echolalie et de copralalie. Arch Neurol (Paris) 1885; 9:19–42, 158–200.
2. King RA, Leckman J, Scahill L. Associated forms of psychopathology: obsessive–compulsive disorder, anxiety, and depression. In: Leckman JF, Cohen DJ, eds. Tourette's Syndrome—Tics, Obsessions, Compulsions: Developmental Psychopathology and Clinical Care. New York: John Wiley and Sons, 1999:43–62.
3. Robertson MM, Banerjee S, Eapen V, Fox-Hiley P. Obsessive compulsive behaviour and depressive symptoms in young people with Tourette syndrome. A controlled study. Eur Child Adolesc Psychiatry 2002; 11(6):261–265.
4. Jagger J, Prusoff B, Cohen DJ, Kidd KK, Carbonari CM, John K. The epidemiology of Tourette's syndrome: a pilot study. Schizophr Bull 1982; 8:267–277.
5. McMahon WM, Carter AS, Fredine N, Pauls DL. Children at familial risk for Tourette's disorder: child and parent diagnoses. Am J Med Genet 2003; 121B(1): 105–111.
6. McMahon WM, van de Wetering BJ, Filloux F, Betit K, Coon H, Leppert M. Bilineal transmission and phenotypic variation of Tourette's disorder in a large pedigree. J Am Acad Child Adolesc Psychiatry 1996; 35(5):672–680.
7. Leckman JF, Zhang H, Vitale A, Lahnin F, Lynch K, Bondi C, Kim Y-S, Peterson BS. Course of tic severity in Tourette's syndrome: the first two decades. Pediatrics 1998; 102:14–19.
8. Pappert EJ, Goetz CG, Louis ED, Blasucci L, Leurgans S. Objective assessments of longitudinal outcome in Gilles de la Tourette's syndrome. Neurology 2003; 61(7):936–940.
9. Bloch MH, Peterson BS, Otka J, Leckman JF. Clinical predictors of future tic and OCD severity in children with Tourette syndrome. Submitted.
10. Leckman J, Bloch MH, Peterson BS. Predictors on MRI of future tic severity in children with Tourette Syndrome. Abstract for ACNP meeting, Puerto Rico, December 2003.
11. Peterson BS, Pine DS, Cohen P, Brook JS. Prospective, longitudinal study of tic, obsessive–compulsive, and attention-deficit/hyperactivity disorder in an epidemiological sample. J Am Acad Child Adolesc Psychiatry 2001; 40:685–695.
12. Santangelo SL, Pauls DL, Goldstein J, Faraone SV, Tsuang MT, Leckman JF. Tourette's syndrome: What are the influences of gender and comorbid obsessive–compulsive disorder? J Am Acad Child Adolesc Psychiatry 1994; 33:795–804.

13. Coffey BJ, Miguel EC, Biederman J, Baer L, Rauch SL, O'Sullivan RL, Savage CR, Phillips K, Borgman A, Green-Leibovitz MI, Moore E, Park KS, Jenike MA. Tourette's disorder with and without obsessive–compulsive disorder in adults: are they different? J Nerv Ment Dis 1998; 186(4):201–206.
14. Garland EJ, Weiss M. Case study: obsessive difficult temperament and its response to serotonergic medication. J Am Acad Child Adolesc Psychiatry 1996; 35(7):916–920.
15. Sukhodolsky DG, Rosario-Campos MC, Scahill L, Katsovich L, Pauls DL, Peterson BS, King RA, Lombroso PJ, Findley D, Leckman JF. Adaptive and family functioning in children with obsessive–compulsive disorder with and without attention-deficit/hyperactivity disorder. Submitted.
16. Geller DA, Biederman J, Faraone SV, Cradock K, Hagermoser L, Zaman N, Frazier JA, Coffey BJ, Spencer TJ. Attention-deficit/hyperactivity disorder in children and adolescents with obsessive–compulsive disorder: fact or artifact? J Am Acad Child Adolesc Psychiatry 2002; 41(1):52–58.
17. Geller DA, Coffey B, Faraone S, Hagermoser L, Zaman NK, Farrell CL, Mullin B, Biederman J. Does comorbid attention-deficit/hyperactivity disorder impact the clinical expression of pediatric obsessive–compulsive disorder? CNS Spectrums 2003; 8(4):259–264.
18. Swerdlow NR, Zinner S, Farber RH, Seacrist C, Hartston H. Symptoms of obsessive–compulsive disorder and Tourette syndrome: a spectrum. CNS Spectrums 1999; 4:21–33.
19. Miguel EC, Coffey BJ, Baer L, Savage CR, Rauch SL, Jenike MA. Phenomenology of intentional repetitive behaviors in obsessive–compulsive disorder and Tourette's disorder. J Clin Psychiatry 1995; 56:246–255.
20. Leckman JF, Walker WK, Goodman WK, Pauls DL, Cohen DJ. "Just right" perceptions associated with compulsive behaviors in Tourette's syndrome. Am J Psychiatry 1994; 151:675–680.
21. Scahill L, Leckman JF, Marek KL. Sensory phenomena in Tourette's syndrome. In: Weiner WJ, Lang AE, eds. Advances in Neurology: Behavioral Neurology of Movement Disorders. New York: Raven Press, 1995:273–280.
22. Leckman JF, Mataix-Cols D, Rosario-Campos MC. Symptom dimensions in obsessive–compulsive disorder: developmental and evolutionary perspectives. In: Abramowitz JS, ed. Handbook of Obsessive–Compulsive Spectrum Disorders. New York: Kluwer. In press.
23. Mataix-Cols D, Rosario-Campos MC, Leckman JF. A multidimensional model of obsessive–compulsive disorder. Submitted.
24. Baer L. Factor analysis of symptom subtypes of obsessive–compulsive disorder and their relation to personality and tic disorders. J Clin Psychiatry 1994; 55:18–23.
25. Leckman JF, Grice DE, Boardman J, Zhang H, Vitale A, Bondi C, Alsobrook J, Peterson BS, Cohen DJ, Rasmussen SA, Goodman WK, McDougle CJ, Pauls DL. Symptoms of obsessive–compulsive disorder. Am J Psychiatry 1997; 154:911–917.

26. Leckman JF, Grice DE, Barr LC, deVries ALC, Martin C, Cohen DJ, Goodman WK, Rasmussen SA. Tic-related vs. non-tic related obsessive compulsive disorder. Anxiety 1995; 1:208–215.
27. Hantouche EG, Lancrenon S. Modern typology of symptoms and obsessive–compulsive syndromes: results of a large French study of 615 patients. Encephale 1996; 22:9–21.
28. Leckman JF, Pauls DL, Zhang H, Rosario-Campos MC, Katsovich L, Kidd KK, Pakstis AJ, Alsobrook JP, Robertson MM, Walkup JT, van de Wetering BJM, McMahon WM, King RA, Cohen DJ, and the Tourette Syndrome Association International Consortium for Genetics. Obsessive–compulsive symptom dimensions in affected sibling pairs diagnosed with Gilles de la Tourette syndrome. Am J Med Genet (Neuropsychiatric Genet) 2003; 116:60–68.
29. Summerfeldt LJ, Richter MA, Antony MM, Swinson RP. Symptom structure in obsessive-compulsive disorder: a confirmatory factor-analytic study. Behav Res Ther 1999; 37:297–311.
30. Mataix-Cols D, Rauch SL, Manzo PA, Jenike MA, Baer L. Use of factor-analyzed symptom dimensions to predict outcome with serotonin reuptake inhibitors and placebo in the treatment of obsessive–compulsive disorder. Am J Psychiatry 1999; 156(9):1409–1416.
31. Mataix-Cols D, Cullen S, Lange K, Zelaya F, Andrew C, Amaro E, Brammer MJ, Williams SC, Speckens A, Phillips ML. Neural correlates of anxiety associated with obsessive–compulsive symptom dimensions in normal volunteers. Biol Psychiatry 2003; 53(6):482–493.
32. Tek C, Ulug B. Religiosity and religious obsessions in obsessive–compulsive disorder. Psychiatry Res 2001; 104:99–108.
33. Cavallini MC, Di Bella D, Siliprandi F, Malchiodi F, Bellodi L. Exploratory factor analysis of obsessive–compulsive patients and association with 5-HTTLPR polymorphism. Am J Med Genet Neuropsychiatr Genet 2002; 114(3):347–353.
34. Foa EB, Huppert JD, Leiberg S, Langner R, Kichic R, Hajcak G, Salkovskis PM. The Obsessive–Compulsive Inventory: development and validation of a short version. Psychol Assess 2002; 14(4):485–496.
35. Feinstein SB, Fallon BA, Petkova E, Liebowitz MR. Item-by-item factor analysis of the Yale-Brown Obsessive Compulsive Scale Symptom Checklist. J Neuropsychiatry Clin Neurosci 2003; 15(2):187–193.
36. Leckman JF, Zhang H, Alsobrook JP, Pauls DL. Symptom dimensions in obsessive–compulsive disorder: toward quantitative phenotypes. Am J Med Genet (Neuropsychiatr Genet) 2001; 105:28–30.
37. Zhang H, Leckman JF, Tsai C-P, Kidd KK, Rosario-Campos MC. The Tourette Syndrome Association International Consortium for Genetics. Genome wide scan of hoarding in sibling pairs both diagnosed with Gilles de la Tourette syndrome. Am J Hum Genet 2002; 70:896–904.
38. Alsobrook JP II, Leckman JF, Goodman WK, Rasmussen SA, Pauls DL. Segregation analysis of obsessive–compulsive disorder using symptom-based factor scores. Am J Med Genet, Neuropsychiatr Genet 1999; 88:669–675.

39. Rauch SL, Dougherty DD, Shin LM, Baer L, Breiter HCR, Savage CR, Jenike MA. Neural correlates of factor-analyzed OCD symptom dimension: a PET study. CNS Spectrums 1998; 3:37–43.
40. Leckman JF, Goodman WK, North WG, Chappell PB, Price LH, Pauls DL, Anderson GM, Riddle MA, McSwiggan-Hardin MT, McDougle CJ, Barr LC, Cohen DJ. Elevated levels of CSF oxytocin in obsessive compulsive disorder: comparison with Tourette's syndrome and healthy controls. Arch Gen Psychiatry 1994; 51:782–792.
41. Leckman JF, Goodman WK, North WG, Chappell PB, Price LH, Pauls DL, Anderson GM, Riddle MA, McDougle CJ, Barr LC, Cohen DJ. The role of oxytocin in obsessive compulsive disorder and related normal behavior. Psychoneuroendocrinology 1994; 19:723–749.
42. Cath DC, Spinhoven P, Landman AD, van Kempen GM. Psychopathology and personality characteristics in relation to blood serotonin in Tourette's syndrome and obsessive–compulsive disorder. J Psychopharmacol 2001; 15(2):111–119.
43. McDougle CJ, Goodman WK, Leckman JF, Barr LC, Heninger GR, Price LH. The efficacy of fluvoxamine in obsessive compulsive disorder: effects of comorbid chronic tic disorder. J Clin Psychopharmacol 1993; 13:354–358.
44. McDougle CJ, Goodman WK, Leckman JF, Lee NC, Heninger GR, Price LH. Haloperidol addition in fluvoxamine-refractory obsessive–compulsive disorder: a double-blind, placebo-controlled study in patients with and without tics. Arch Gen Psychiatry 1994; 51:302–308.
45. Blier P, de Montigny C. Serotonin and drug-induced therapeutic responses in major depression, obsessive–compulsive and panic disorders. Neuropsychopharmacology 1999; 21(2 suppl):91S–98S.
46. Greist JH, Jefferson JW, Kobak KA, Katzelnick DJ, Serlin RC. Efficacy and tolerability of serotonin transport inhibitors in obsessive–compulsive disorder: a meta-analysis. Arch Gen Psychiatry 1995; 52(1):53–60.
47. Burke WJ, Gergel I, Bose A. Fixed-dose trial of the single isomer SSRI escitalopram in depressed outpatients. J Clin Psychiatry 2002; 63(4):331–336.
48. Leonard HL, Swedo SE, Rapoport JL, Koby EV, Lenane MC, Cheslow DL, Hamburger SD. Treatment of obsessive–compulsive disorder with clomipramine and desipramine in children and adolescents. A double-blind crossover comparison. Arch Gen Psychiatry 1989; 46(12):1088–1092.
49. DeVeaugh-Geiss J, Moroz G, Biederman J, Cantwell D, Fontaine R, Greist JH, Reichler R, Katz R, Landau P. Clomipramine hydrochloride in childhood and adolescent obsessive–compulsive disorder: a multicenter trial. J Am Acad Child Adolesc Psychiatry 1992; 31(1):45–49.
50. Riddle MA, Scahill L, King RA, Hardin MT, Anderson GM, Ort SI, Smith JC, Leckman JF, Cohen DJ. Double-blind, crossover trial of fluoxetine and placebo in children and adolescents with obsessive–compulsive disorder. J Am Acad Child Adolesc Psychiatry 1992; 31(6):1062–1069.
51. Geller DA, Hoog SL, Heiligenstein JH, Ricardi RK, Tamura R, Kluszynski S, Jacobson JG. Fluoxetine Pediatric OCD Study Team. Fluoxetine treatment for obsessive–compulsive disorder in children and adolescents: a placebo-controlled clinical trial. J Am Acad Child Adolesc Psychiatry 2001; 40(7):773–779.

52. March JS, Biederman J, Wolkow R, Safferman A, Mardekian J, Cook E, et al. Sertraline in children and adolescents with obsessive–compulsive disorder: a multicenter randomized controlled trial. J Am Med Assoc 1998; 280:1752–1756.
53. Riddle MA, Reeve EA, Yaryura-Tobias JA, Yang HM, Claghorn JL, Gaffney G, Greist JH, Holland D, McConville BJ, Pigott T, Walkup JT. Fluvoxamine for children and adolescents with obsessive–compulsive disorder: a randomized, controlled, multicenter trial. J Am Acad Child Adolesc Psychiatry 2001; 49:222–229.
54. Geller DA, Biederman J, Stewart SE, Mullin B, Farrell C, Wagner KD, Emslie G, Carpenter D. Impact of comorbidity on treatment response to paroxetine in pediatric obsessive–compulsive disorder: is the use of exclusion criteria empirically supported in randomized clinical trials? J Child Adolesc Psychopharmacol 2003; 13(1):S19–S29.
55. Montgomery SA, Kasper S, Stein DJ, Hedegaard KB, Lemming OM. Citalopram 20 mg, 40 mg and 60 mg are all effective and well tolerated compared with placebo in obsessive–compulsive disorder. Int Clin Psychopharmacol 2001; 16(2):75–86.
56. Thomsen PH, Ebbesen C, Persson C. Long-term experience with citalopram in the treatment of adolescent OCD. J Am Acad Child Adolesc Psychiatry 2001; 40(8):895–902.
57. Mukaddes NM, Abali O, Kaynak N. Citalopram treatment of children and adolescents with obsessive–compulsive disorder: a preliminary report. Psychiatry Clin Neurosci 2003; 57(4):405–408.
58. McDougle CJ, Epperson CN, Pelton GH, Wasylink S, Price LH. A double-blind, placebo-controlled study of risperidone addition in serotonin reuptake inhibitor-refractory obsessive–compulsive disorder. Arch Gen Psychiatry 2000; 57:794–801.
59. Erzegovesi S, Cavallini MC, Cavedini P, Diaferia G, Locatelli M, Bellodi L. Clinical predictors of drug response in obsessive–compulsive disorder. J Clin Psychopharmacol 2001; 21(5):488–492.
60. Scahill L, Riddle MA, King RA, Hardin MT, Rasmusson A, Makuch RW, Leckman JF. Fluoxetine has no marked effect on tic symptoms in patients with Tourette syndrome: a double-blind, placebo controlled study. J Child Adolesc Psychopharmacol 1997; 7:75–85.
61. Kurlan R, Como PG, Deeley C, McDermott M, McDermott MP. A pilot controlled study of fluoxetine for obsessive–compulsive symptoms in children with Tourette's syndrome. Clin Neuropharmacol 1993; 16:167–172.
62. Rosenberg DR, Stewart CM, Fitzgerald KD, Tawile V, Carroll E. Paroxetine open-label treatment of pediatric outpatients with obsessive–compulsive disorder. J Am Acad Child Adolesc Psychiatry 1999; 38(9):1180–1185.
63. Denys D, van Megen H, Westenberg H. Quetiapine addition to serotonin reuptake inhibitor treatment in patients with treatment-refractory obsessive–compulsive disorder: an open-label study. J Clin Psychiatry 2002; 63(8):700–703.
64. Bogetto F, Bellino S, Vaschetto P, Ziero S. Olanzapine augmentation of

fluvoxamine-refractory obsessive–compulsive disorder (OCD): a 12-week open trial. Psychiatr Res 2002; 96:91–98.
65. Leonard HL, Topol D, Bukstein O, Hindmarsh D, Allen AJ, Swedo SE. Clonazepam as an augmenting agent in the treatment of childhood-onset obsessive–compulsive disorder. J Am Acad Child Adolesc Psychiatry 1994; 33:792–794.
66. Figueroa Y, Rosenberg DR, Birmaher B, Keshavan MS. Combination treatment with clomipramine and selective serotonin reuptake inhibitors for obsessive–compulsive disorder in children and adolescents. J Child Adolesc Psychopharmacol 1998; 8(1):61–67.
67. Koran LM, Pallanti S, Paiva RS, Quercioli L. Pulse loading versus gradual dosing of intravenous clomipramine in obsessive–compulsive disorder. Eur Neuropsychopharmacol 1998; 8:121–126.
68. Pallanti S, Quercioli L, Koran LM. Citalopram intravenous infusion in resistant obsessive–compulsive disorder: an open trial. J Clin Psychiatry 2002; 63(9):796–801.
69. Sallee FR, Koran LM, Pallanti S, Carson SW, Sethuraman G. Intravenous clomipramine challenge in obsessive–compulsive disorder: predicting response to oral therapy at eight weeks. Biol Psychiatry 1998; 44:220–227.
70. Piacentini J. Cognitive behavioral therapy of childhood OCD. Child Adolesc Psychiatr Clin N Am 1999; 8(3):599–616.
71. King RA, Leonard H, March J. Practice parameters on the assessment and treatment of children with obsessive compulsive disorder. J Am Acad Child Adolesc Psychiatry 1998; 37(suppl):27S–45S.
72. March JS, Foa E, Franklin M, Leonard H. The Pediatric OCD Treatment Study (POTS): design and stage I outcomes. Annual Meeting of American Academy of Child and Adolescent Psychiatry, Miami, October 2003.
73. RUPP Anxiety Group. Fluvoxamine for the treatment of anxiety disorders in children and adolescents. The Research Unit on Pediatric Psychopharmacology Anxiety Study Group. N Engl J Med 2001; 344:1279–1285.
74. Osterheld JR, Flockhart DA. Pharmacokinetics II: cytochrome P450-mediated drug interactions. In: Martin A, Scahill L, Charney DS, Leckman JF, eds. Pediatric Psychopharmacology: Principles and Practice. New York: Oxford University Press, 2003:54–66.
75. Desta Z, Kerbusch T, Flockhart DA. Effect of clarithromycin on the pharmacokinetics and pharmacodynamics of pimozide in healthy poor and extensive metabolizers of cytochrome P450 2D6 (CYP2D6). Clin Pharmacol Ther 1999; 65:10–20.
76. Desta Z, Soukhova N, Flockhart D. In vitro inhibition of pimozide *N*-dealkylation by selective serotonin reuptake inhibitors and azithromycin. J Clin Psychopharmacol 2002; 22(2):162–168.
77. Wagner KD, Cook EH, Chung H, Messig M. Remission status after long-term sertraline treatment of pediatric obsessive–compulsive disorder. J Child Adolesc Psychopharmacol 2003; 13:53–60.
78. Riddle MA, King RA, Hardin MT, Scahill L, Ort SI, Leckman JF. Behavioral

side effects of fluoxetine in children and adolescents. J Child Adolesc Psychopharmacol 1991; 1:193–198.
79. Tierney E, Joshi PT, Linas JF, Rosenberg LA, Riddle MA. Sertraline for major depression in children and adolescents: preliminary clinical experience. J Child Adolesc Psychopharmacol 1995; 5:13–27.
80. King RA, Riddle MA, Chappell PB, Hardin MT, Anderson GM, Lombroso P, Scahill L. Emergence of self-destructive phenomena in children and adolescents during fluoxetine treatment. J Am Acad Child Adolesc Psychiatry 1991; 30:179–186.
81. Barr LC, Goodman WK, Price LH. Physical symptoms associated with paroxetine discontinuation. Am J Psychiatry 1994; 151:289289.
82. Louie AK, Lannon RA, Ajari LJ. Withdrawal reaction after sertraline discontinuation. Am J Psychiatry 1994; 151:450–451.
83. Rosenbaum JF, Fava M, Hoog SL, Ascroft RC, Krebs WB. Selective serotonin reuptake inhibitor discontinuation syndrome: a randomized clinical trial. Biol Psychiatry 1998; 44:77–87.
84. Scahill L, Riddle MA, McSwiggin-Hardin M, Ort SI, King RA, Goodman WK, Cicchetti D, Leckman JF. Children's Yale-Brown Obsessive Compulsive Scale: reliability and validity. J Am Acad Child Adolesc Psychiatry 1997; 36(6):844–852.
85. Delgado PL, Goodman WK, Price LH, Heninger GR, Charney DS. Fluvoxamine/pimozide treatment of concurrent Tourette's and obsessive compulsive disorder. Br J Psychiatry 1990; 157:762–765.
86. Fennig S, Naisberg S, Fennig M, Pato A. Emergence of symptoms of Tourette's syndrome during fluvoxamine treatment of obsessive–compulsive disorder. Br. J Psychiatry 1994; 164:839–841.
87. March JS, Franklin M, Nelson A, Foa E. Cognitive–behavioral psychotherapy for pediatric obsessive–compulsive disorder. J Clin Child Psychol 2001; 30: 8–18.
88. March JS, Leonard HL. Obsessive–compulsive disorder in children and adolescents: a review of the past 10 years. J Am Acad Child Adolesc Psychiatry 1996; 35:1265–1273.
89. Chambless DL, Ollendick TH. Empirically supported psychological interventions: controversies and evidence. Annu Rev Psychol 2001; 52:685–716.
90. Franklin ME, Tolin DF, March JS, Foa EB. Treatment of pediatric obsessive–compulsive disorder: a case example of intensive cognitive–behavioral therapy involving exposure and ritual prevention. Cogn Behav Pract 2001; 8:297–304.
91. March JS, Mulle K. OCD in Children and Adolescents: A Cognitive–Behavioral Treatment Manual. New York: Guilford, 1998.
92. Riggs DS, Foa EB. Obsessive compulsive disorder. In: Barlow DH, ed. Clinical Handbook of Psychological Disorders. New York: Guilford, 1993.
93. Schwartz JM. Neuroanatomical aspects of cognitive–behavioral therapy response in obsessive–compulsive disorder: an evolving perspective on brain behavior. Br J Psychiatry 1998; 173(suppl 355):38–44.
94. Sochting I, March JS. Cognitive aspects of obsessive compulsive disorder in

children. In: Frost RO, Skeketee G, eds. Cognitive Approaches to Obsessive and Compulsions: Theory, Assessment and Treatment. New York: Pergamon, 2002.
95. Mark IM. Fears, Phobias, and Rituals. New York: Oxford University Press, 1987.
96. Watson JP, Gaind R, Marks IM. Physiological habituation to continuous phobic stimulation. Behav Res Ther 1972; 10:269–278.
97. Salkovskis PM. Understanding and treating obsessive–compulsive disorder. Behav Res Ther 1999; 37(suppl 1):529–552.
98. Frost RO, Steketee G, eds. Cognitive Approaches to Obsessions and Compulsions: Theory, Assessment and Treatment. New York: Pergamon, 2002.
99. Tolin DF, Abramowitz JS, Przeworski A, Foa EB. Thought suppression in obsessive–compulsive disorder. Behav Res Ther 2002; 40:1255–1274.
100. Wenzlaff RM, Wegner DM. Thought suppression. Annu Rev Psychol 2000; 51:59–91.
101. Amir N, Freshman M, Ransey B, Neary E, Brigidi B. Thought–action fusion in individuals with OCD symptoms. Behav Res Ther 2001; 39:765–776.
102. Shafran R, Thordarson DS, Rachman S. Thought–action fusion in obsessive compulsive disorder. J Anxiety Disord 1996; 10:379–391.
103. Mataix-Cols D, Marks IM, Greist JH, Kobak KA, Baer L. Obsessive–compulsive symptom dimensions as predictors of compliance with and response to behaviour therapy: results from a controlled trial. Psychother Psychosom 2002; 71(5):255–262.
104. Ball SG, Baer L, Otto MW. Symptom subtypes of obsessive–compulsive disorder in behavioral treatment studies: a quantitative review. Behav Res Ther 1996; 34:47–51.
105. Himle JA, Fischer MSW, Van Etten ML, Janeck AS, Hanna GL. Group behavioral therapy for adolescents with tic-related and non-tic-related obsessive–compulsive disorder. Depress Anxiety 2003; 17:73–77.
106. Miguel EC, Baer L, Coffey BJ, Rauch SL, Savage CR, O'Sullivan RL, Phillips K, Moretti C, Leckman JF, Jenke MA. Phenomenological differences appearing with repetitive behaviors in obsessive–compulsive disorder and Gilles de la Tourette's syndrome. Br J Psychiatry 1997; 171:140–145.
107. Bullen JG, Hemsley DR. Sensory experience as a trigger in Gilles de la Tourette's syndrome. J Behav Ther Exp Psychiatry 1983; 14:197–201.
108. Azrin NH, Nunn RG. Habit-reversal: a method of eliminating nervous habits and tics. Behav Res Ther 1973; 11:619–628.
109. Wilhelm S, Deckersbach T, Coffey BJ, Bohne A, Peterson AL, Baer L. Habit reversal versus supportive psychotherapy for Tourette's disorder: a randomized controlled trial. Am J Psychiatry 2003; 160(6):1175–1177.
110. Woods DW, Miltenberger RG, eds. Tic Disorders, Trichotillomania, and Other Repetitive Behavior Disorders: Behavioral Approaches to Analysis and Treatment. Norwell, MA: Kluwer Academic Publishers, 2001.
111. Piacentini J, Chang S, Pearlman S, McCracken J. Behavioral treatment of childhood tic disorders. Presentation at Annual Meeting of American Academy of Child and Adolescent Psychiatry, Miami, October 2003.

112. Miltenberger RG, Fuqua RW, McKinley T. Habit reversal with muscle tics: replication and component analysis. Behavior Ther 1985; 16:39–50.
113. Woods DW, Miltenberger RG, Lumley VA. Sequential application of major habit-reversal components to treat motor tics in children. J Appl Behav Anal 1996; 29:483–493.
114. Wagner AP. What to Do When Your child Has Obsessive–Compulsive Disorder: Strategies and Solutions. Rochester, NY: Lighthouse Press, 2002.
115. Grados MA, Riddle MA, Samuels JF, Liang KY, Hoehn-Saric R, Bienvenu OJ, Walkup JT, Song D, Nestadt G. The familial phenotype of obsessive–compulsive disorder in relation to tic disorders: the Hopkins OCD family study. Biol Psychiatry 2001; 50(8):559–565.
116. Scahill L, Kano Y, King RA, Carlson A, Peller A, LeBrun U, Rosario-Campos MC, Leckman JF. Influence of age and tic disorders on obsessive–compulsive disorder in a pediatric sample. J Child Adolesc Psychopharmacol 2003; 13(S1): 7–18.
117. Petter T, Richter MA, Sandor P. Clinical features distinguishing patients with Tourette's obsessive-compulsive disorder without tics. J Clin Psychiatry 1998; 59(9):456–459.
118. Geller DA, Biederman J, Stewart SE, Mullen B, Martin A, Spencer T, Faraone SV. Which SSRI? A meta-analysis of pharmacotherapy trials in pediatric obsessive-compulsive disorder. Am J Psychiatry 2003; 160:1919–1928.

22

The Treatment of Comorbid Attention-Deficit Disorder and Tourette's Syndrome

Laurie Brown and Leon S. Dure
The University of Alabama at Birmingham
Birmingham, Alabama, U.S.A.

INTRODUCTION

One of the most difficult treatment scenarios for a clinician dealing with Tourette's syndrome (TS) is the patient with concomitant neuropsychiatric pathology requiring intervention. Behavioral comorbidities are common in TS, with attention-deficit disorder (with or without hyperactivity, henceforth referred to as ADHD) having the highest prevalence rates, estimated in the range of 35–70% (1). Recent epidemiological studies also indicate that TS is as common at 3% of school-age children, with an even higher percentage receiving special education services (2,3). Therefore, for the clinician caring for children with TS, it is likely that the combination of these two disorders will be encountered. The spectrum of TS symptoms poses different sets of problems to individuals and their families. Symptoms of ADHD may predate the onset of tics by an average of 2.5 years, and this may explain the often-reported association between therapy for ADHD and the appearance of tics. When considering the impact of various manifestations of TS and comorbid conditions, behavioral disorders may interfere more with daily living than motor or vocal tics. Inattention and distractibility often impair academic performance, and impulsivity can disrupt relationship with family and friends

(4). ADHD beginning early in childhood and continuing into adulthood can lead to the development of conduct disorder, substance abuse, anxiety, and affective disorder. Finally, there may be a mutually deleterious relationship with tic behaviors, as the mental effort required to suppress tics and premonitory urges may accentuate inattention.

TREATMENT ISSUES

The usual reason that patients with TS are brought to the attention of a neurological specialist is the presence of motor or vocal tics, and the initial focus is placed on the medical treatment of the tics. However, the spectrum of behavior problems that may be encountered can have more impact on family function, self-esteem, and potential for success in life. In terms of the relative impact of these conditions, a survey of families of 66 children with TS (5) showed that families considered ADHD and learning disabilities to be most significant, whereas motor and vocal tics were least important. In another study directly evaluating 128 child and adolescent ADHD patients over a 4-year period, it was determined in those with tics that there was no relationship between the courses of the two conditions (6). Similar findings have been reported in adults (7). Of 564 patients and controls, 36 of 312 adults with ADHD and 9 of 252 adults without ADHD had a tic disorder (12% vs. 4%). Of those combined 45 subjects with tic disorders, seven met diagnostic criteria for TS. The independent contribution of a tic disorder to a range of outcomes was assessed, demonstrating that comorbid tic disorders have a limited impact on the morbidity or dysfunction of ADHD in adults.

Treatment of ADHD itself can take the form of either pharmacological intervention and/or cognitive–behavioral approaches. Analysis of published studies is strongly indicative of the efficacy of psychostimulant medications, of which there are a variety of agents with differing pharmacokinetic profiles (Table 1) (8). Despite the evidence that ADHD may be associated with greater disability and impairment, practitioners have been hesitant to use stimulants in the setting of TS or other tic disorders after reports that tics worsened on stimulant therapy (9–13). In fact, the Physicians' Desk Reference as well as the package inserts for various stimulants list current or past history of tics, or even a family history of tics, as a contraindication for administration. Subsequent analyses, however, would suggest that such caution is in need of a reexamination.

A number of studies have addressed the effect of stimulant treatment for ADHD in the presence of tics, but not necessarily TS. In a study of 91 stimulant-naïve children with ADHD who were treated with methylphenidate (MPH) or placebo for 1 year (14), 27 subjects were noted to have comorbid

Table 1 Stimulants

Brand name	Generic name	How supplied	Daily dose (mg)	Doses per day
Ritalin	Methylphenidate	Tablets: 5, 10, and 20 mg	2.5–60	2–4
Focalin	D-methylphenidate	Tablets: 2.5, 5, and 10 mg	2.5–20	2
Concerta	OROS methylphenidate	Tablets: 18, 27, 36, and 54 mg	18–54	1
Metadate CD	Methylphenidate, extended release	Capsules: 20 mg	20–60	1
Ritalin LA	Methylphenidate, extended release	Capsules: 20, 30, and 40 mg	20–60	1
Adderall	D,L-amphetamine	Tablets: 5, 10, 20, and 30 mg	2.5–60	1–2
Adderal XR	D,L-amphetamine, extended release	Capsules: 5, 10, 15, 20, 25, and 30 mg	5–30	1
Dexedrine	Dextroamphetamine	Tablets: 5 mg	2.5–40	2–4
Dexedrine spansule	Dextroamphetamine, sustained release	Capsules: 5, 10, and 15 mg; tablets: 18.75, 37.5, and 75 mg	5–40	1
Cylert	Pemoline	Chewable tablets: 37.5 mg	18.75–112.5	1

tics, but did not satisfy criteria sufficient for a diagnosis of TS. In the treatment groups, 11 children with tics were included in the MPH group and 16 in the placebo group. Upon randomization, the dose of MPH/placebo was titrated to the same dose (0.5 mg/kg/day) in all patients, and parental and teacher tic ratings were made at baseline, after titration, and at 4, 8, and 12 months. A high attrition rate from the placebo group (27 of 45) was noted due to a lack of behavioral improvement, but not because of tics. These patients treated with placebo then were added to the MPH group. Interestingly, in this study, there were no differences between placebo and treatment groups with respect to appearance or exacerbation of tics. Nolan et al. (15) evaluated 19 patients with ADHD and chronic multiple tic disorder who had been treated with either MPH or dexedrine (DEX) for a minimum of 1 year. Patients were switched to placebo and assessed with direct observation and rating scales in double-blinded conditions. There was no evidence of tic exacerbation in a

2-week period of withdrawal from stimulants, nor upon return to maintenance treatment. Similarly, 34 patients with ADHD and chronic multiple tic disorder treated over 8 weeks in a double-blind, placebo-controlled trial with MPH were followed at 6-month intervals for 2 years as a prospective, nonblinded follow-up (16). Tics did not change in frequency or severity during treatment compared to initial evaluation or placebo evaluation.

In a study specifically addressing ADHD and TS, Castellanos et al. (17) studied the effects of stimulants (MPH and DEX) on tic severity in boys with ADHD and comorbid TS over 9 weeks in a placebo-controlled, double-blind crossover study. Twenty patients were studied for 3 weeks each on MPH, DEX, and placebo with escalating doses of each stimulant. At low or medium doses across all 20 patients, no change was observed in tic severity, but 14 of 20 at high dose showed worsening tics on DEX and MPH, with attenuation of the tics over time on MPH but not DEX. Finally, in the multicenter double-blind, placebo-controlled TACT (Treatment of ADHD in Tourette Syndrome) trial comparing MPH to the α_2-adrenergic agonist clonidine both alone and in combination, there was no significant difference between either drug alone or in combination compared to placebo with respect to worsening of tics (18). This study is one of the largest performed to date in children with TS, and the 4-month duration of the study would seem to further support the safety of stimulants in TS with comorbid ADHD.

SPECIFIC TREATMENT APPROACHES

Given a prevalence of ADHD in the general population ranging from 8% to 10% of school-age children, a recent practice guideline was issued by the American Academy of Pediatrics (19), and the overall paradigm for evaluation and management is of some use to the practitioner addressing TS with comorbid ADHD. The guideline enumerates the need for information regarding the child's behavior in multiple settings in order to make a diagnosis and to assess interventions. Moreover, this information should be derived from multiple observers, including parents, teachers, and other caregivers, to document the fulfillment of established criteria. The practitioner should be aware not only of the disorders commonly associated with ADHD, such as oppositional defiant disorder, conduct disorder, anxiety disorders, and depression, but also the other known comorbidities of TS, as all of these can complicate treatment decisions. Specifically relating to TS, it is especially important to rule out ruminative thoughts or obsessions and preoccupation with tic suppression, both of which may lead to inattention. Although the academy guideline does not endorse specific investigations, in the context of TS and depending on the experience of the practitioner, strong consideration should be given to a formal psychological evaluation in order to completely assess the emotional and behavioral makeup of the patient.

Pharmacological Management

Treatment of ADHD in the context of TS should be governed primarily by the degree of impairment. It is extremely important from the outset to distinguish the target symptoms and behaviors that need to be addressed, as well as to identify outcome goals. As mentioned above, it is imperative to distinguish true ADHD from other disorders that may render a child inattentive. If a therapeutic intervention is necessary, the practitioner should initially consider environmental and behavioral strategies that would be of benefit. A number of excellent resources are available from Children and Adults with Attention-Deficit Disorder (CHADD) and the Tourette Syndrome Association (TSA), and the reader is directed to these organizations for further information.

When the situation is one that demands a pharmacological intervention, it is difficult to ignore the demonstrated efficacy of stimulant medications for ADHD. An extensive literature review of controlled studies examining the response to stimulants revealed an overall beneficial response in 70% of patients (8). It is hoped that the preceding discussion of studies addressing tics and stimulant medications has made it clear that an empiric trial of such agents in TS with ADHD is warranted. This is not to say that there are no children whose tics worsen with stimulants, but that the response rate is such that stimulants should not be categorically avoided.

Since the first observations of stimulant responsiveness in ADHD to benzedrine (20), there have arisen a wide variety of agents approved for use. The most commonly prescribed compounds include methylphenidate (including a purified D-methylphenidate), dexedrine, and amphetamine salts (Table 1). Current studies indicate that of the different psychostimulant compounds, methylphenidate is the least likely to worsen tics. The psychostimulants effect an increase in dopamine and norepinephrine at neuronal synapses. Despite a lack of clear understanding of the mechanism of action in ADHD, a great deal of study has gone into the pharmacokinetics of the stimulants, and long-acting preparations of each type are available. The standard maxim when treating TS is to "start low, go slow," and this is decidedly true in the context of treating ADHD. It is usually recommended that a short-acting stimulant be used first, with a gradual increase in the dose, treating for effect. Subsequently, switching to a longer-acting preparation may be attempted after a good response is observed.

Adverse effects to stimulants include insomnia, irritability, headache, and weight loss, among others. In addition to these, the possibility of worsening of tics should be discussed with TS patients and their families, although there are some evidence that low doses of MPH can actually decrease some tic behaviors (21), and transient increases in tics have been observed that were not considered significant (17). In the case of persistent tics exacerbated by stimulants, it is very important to know if there has been any improvement in ADHD symptoms in guiding further therapy. Although no comparison studies have been performed in this population, it is the authors' experience that tic exacerbations do not occur with all stimulants, and switching to another agent or formulation should be attempted. Finally, a patient who has experienced an exacerbation related to stimulants may undergo reintroduction of the same stimulant without difficulties.

An alternative to the psychostimulants in TS and ADHD is the use of α_2-adrenergic agonists, namely clonidine and guanfacine. Although neither drug has Food and Drug Administration (FDA) approval for such a use, each has undergone study in controlled clinical trials that indicate some efficacy. Agonist activity at α_2 receptors inhibits the release of norepinephrine and dopamine. Given the role of the locus ceruleus in orienting behavior, there are some physiological bases for an effect on attention (22). A meta-analysis of published studies up to 1999 indicated that clonidine is a useful drug for the treatment of ADHD (23). However, the treatment effect is less than that of stimulants, and the side-effect profile is such that clonidine is considered a second-tier agent. In the context of TS, though, clonidine has been shown to have modest effects in reducing tics (24,25), so it has been considered an attractive alternative for TS with ADHD. Indeed, the TACT study demonstrated that clonidine was more effective than placebo with influences on ADHD equivalent to MPH. The study also found that the combination of MPH and clonidine was more effective than either MPH or clonidine alone for the treatment of ADHD and TS (18). One concern with this study, however, was the high rate of side effects in the clonidine-treated individuals, again underscoring the drawbacks of this agent.

Guanfacine is another α_2 agonist, but with reportedly less sedative effects than clonidine (22). In a placebo-controlled trial using guanfacine to treat ADHD in children with tic disorders, there was an improvement in ADHD over an 8-week period in treated children compared to controls (26). Interestingly, there was also an improvement in tic symptoms with guanfacine. Finally, examination of tolerability and effects on blood pressure demonstrated guanfacine to be an excellent alternative to psychostimulants or clonidine.

Similar to the caveats concerning stimulants, dosages of either clonidine or guanfacine should be low to begin with, and gradually increased for effect. Although each drug is classified as an antihypertensive, changes in blood pressure are modest in normotensive children at the usual doses (0.05–0.3 mg/

day for clonidine and 1–4 mg/day for guanfacine). Typical side effects include lethargy, somnolence, dry mouth, and irritability.

A number of other agents for the treatment of ADHD have been studied, including tricyclic antidepressants (8,27,28) and bupropion (29). Only two of these studies, both using desipramine, have addressed the problem of ADHD with comorbid TS (27,28), both indicating that desipramine may also be a safe and effective alternative to either stimulants or α_2 agonists. Despite the generally low incidence of side effects with desipramine, the risk of cardiotoxicity has limited its widespread use.

Behavioral Management

In 1999, the first results of the Multimodal Treatment Study of Children with ADHD (MTA Study) were published (30). In this multicenter trial, children with ADHD were randomized to receive medical management (using primarily psychostimulants), behavioral therapy, or a combination of the two, or they were referred back into the community for care. A total of 579 children were followed for 14 months, and evaluations were performed during and at the end of the study, which were comprehensive in scope and detail. Although only the first reports of the data have been published, the initial findings purported to show that medical management was superior to both community therapy and behavioral therapy. The combined therapy was only slightly superior to medical management alone. Interestingly, there have been alternative interpretations of the data from participating investigators (31), suggesting that behavioral approaches were not necessarily inferior to medical management, and perhaps even as effective.

Given this controversy and keeping in mind the risks of pharmacological intervention in the case of TS with comorbid ADHD, it is not unreasonable for the practitioner to be familiar with and consider behavioral approaches for these children. Potential behavioral interventions can be summarized as representing one or a combination of three approaches (32). One method, cognitive–behavioral therapy, involves the development of self-regulating strategies to overcome habits or behaviors that interfere with goal accomplishment. However, this method has not been shown to be particularly beneficial, perhaps because of the prerequisite necessity for attention and self-cognizance of behavior. A more promising technique has been clinical behavior therapy, which requires training of teachers and/or parents. In this type of program, contingency management strategies are implemented at home and at school, and there is coordination between parents and teachers to effect more desirable behaviors. This strategy was implemented as the behavior therapy arm of the MTA study and can be adapted for most school situations. Finally, the third method is contingency management, an approach that is more intensive and usually guided in the classroom by a trained individual. This would be considered the most intensive type of therapy, and requires significant expertise and cooperation. For an excellent review of the subject, the reader is directed to the review by Pelham and Gnagy (32).

The previous discussion has related primarily to ADHD alone, and there is a dearth of supporting evidence for behavioral management in TS plus ADHD. However, in approaching this problem, many of these strategies should be applicable to the TS population, and there is no known contraindication to their implementation (4). The thorough education of parents and families about the natural history of TS and associated comorbidities may be the first step in managing symptoms through behavior therapy. Families must be informed that tic severity may impact other dimensions of behavior, and that waxing and waning of tics are the natural course of the disorder, irrespective of therapy. Knowledge of the unpredictable course of TS may help to avoid calls for rapid medication changes or premature institution of a pharmacological intervention.

Education should not stop with the patient and family, as the focus of a child's problems tends to be in the school setting. The clinician should endeavor to provide instructional materials to school personnel, and a number of educator-specific materials are available from the TSA and other resources (33). Finally, given the type of expertise that may be required to institute a behavioral program in school or the home setting, it may be appropriate to refer the family to an experienced psychologist for management.

SUMMARY

In conclusion, treatment of comorbid ADHD in the child with TS can be complex, but there is good evidence of effective and safe therapy with conventional pharmacological agents. Although not definitively beneficial, behavioral strategies may have a role in the management of these children. It cannot be overemphasized that families, in concert with the treating physician and/or psychologist, need to identify appropriate treatment targets. In addition, there must be a well-defined and objective goal to assess treatment efficacy. With appropriate information regarding potential problems, irrespective of the treatment offered, children with TS and ADHD in combination can be expected to function appropriately and even exceptionally in the classroom and home setting.

For further information:

CHADD, 8181 Professional Place, Suite 201, Landover, MD 20785, USA. Tel.: (301) 306-7070; fax: (301) 306-7090

CHADD National Call Center. Tel.: (800) 233-4050
Tourette Syndrome Association, Inc., 42-40 Bell Boulevard, Bayside NY 11361, USA. Tel.: (718) 224-2999.

REFERENCES

1. Gadow KD, Sverd J. Stimulants for ADHD in child patients with Tourette's syndrome: the issue of relative risk. J Dev Behav Pediatr 1990; 11:269–271.
2. Mason A, Banerjee S, Eapen V, Zeitlin H, Robertson MM. The prevalence of Tourette syndrome in a mainstream school population. Dev Med Child Neurol 1998; 40:292–296.
3. Kurlan R, McDermott MP, Deeley C, et al. Prevalence of tics in schoolchildren and association with placement in special education. Neurology 2001; 57:1383–1388.
4. Peterson BS, Cohen DJ. The treatment of Tourette's syndrome: multimodal, developmental intervention. J Clin Psychiatry 1998; 59(suppl 1):62–72.
5. Dooley JM, Brna PM, Gordon KE. Parent perceptions of symptom severity in Tourette's syndrome. Arch Dis Child 1999; 81:440–441.
6. Spencer T, Biederman J, Coffey B, Geller D, Wilens T, Faraone S. The 4-year course of tic disorders in boys with attention-deficit/hyperactivity disorder. Arch Gen Psychiatry 1999; 56:842–847.
7. Spencer TJ, Biederman J, Faraone S, et al. Impact of tic disorders on ADHD outcome across the life cycle: findings from a large group of adults with and without ADHD. Am J Psychiatry 2001; 158:611–617.
8. Spencer T, Biederman J, Wilens T, Harding M, O'Donnell D, Griffin S. Pharmacotherapy of attention-deficit hyperactivity disorder across the life cycle. J Am Acad Child Adolesc Psychiatry 1996; 35:409–432.
9. Denckla MB, Bemporad JR, MacKay MC. Tics following methylphenidate administration. A report of 20 cases. JAMA 1976; 235:1349–1351.
10. Fras I, Karlavage J. The use of methylphenidate and imipramine in Gilles de la Tourette's disease in children. Am J Psychiatry 1977; 134:195–197.
11. Pollack MA, Cohen NL, Friedhoff AJ. Gilles de la Tourette's syndrome. Familial occurrence and precipitation by methylphenidate therapy. Arch Neurol 1977; 34:630–632.
12. Sleator EK. Deleterious effects of drugs used for hyperactivity on patients with Gilles de la Tourette syndrome. Clin Pediatr (Phila) 1980; 19:453–454.
13. Lowe TL, Cohen DJ, Detlor J, Kremenitzer MW, Shaywitz BA. Stimulant medications precipitate Tourette's syndrome. JAMA 1982; 247:1729–1731.
14. Law SF, Schachar RJ. Do typical clinical doses of methylphenidate cause tics in children treated for attention-deficit hyperactivity disorder? J Am Acad Child Adolesc Psychiatry 1999; 38:944–951.
15. Nolan EE, Gadow KD, Sprafkin J. Stimulant medication withdrawal during long-term therapy in children with comorbid attention-deficit hyperactivity disorder and chronic multiple tic disorder. Pediatrics 1999; 103:730–737.

16. Gadow KD, Sverd J, Sprafkin J, Nolan EE, Grossman S. Long-term methylphenidate therapy in children with comorbid attention-deficit hyperactivity disorder and chronic multiple tic disorder. Arch Gen Psychiatry 1999; 56:330–336.
17. Castellanos FX, Giedd JN, Elia J, et al. Controlled stimulant treatment of ADHD and comorbid Tourette's syndrome: effects of stimulant and dose. J Am Acad Child Adolesc Psychiatry 1997; 36:589–596.
18. Group TTsSS Treatment of ADHD in children with tics: a randomized controlled trial. Neurology 2002; 58:527–536.
19. Committee on Quality Improvement SoA-DHD Clinical practice guideline: diagnosis and evaluation of the child with Attention-Deficit/Hyperactivity Disorder. Pediatrics 2001; 105:1158–1170.
20. Spencer TJ. Attention-deficit/hyperactivity disorder. Arch Neurol 2002; 59:314–316.
21. Gadow KD, Nolan EE, Sverd J. Methylphenidate in hyperactive boys with comorbid tic disorder: II. Short-term behavioral effects in school settings. J Am Acad Child Adolesc Psychiatry 1992; 31:462–471.
22. Newcorn JH, Schulz K, Harrison M, DeBellis MD, Udarbe JK, Halperin JM. Alpha 2 adrenergic agonists. Neurochemistry, efficacy, and clinical guidelines for use in children. Pediatr Clin North Am 1998; 45(viii):1022–1099.
23. Connor DF, Fletcher KE, Swanson JM. A meta-analysis of clonidine for symptoms of attention-deficit hyperactivity disorder. J Am Acad Child Adolesc Psychiatry 1999; 38:1551–1559.
24. Leckman JF, Hardin MT, Riddle MA, Stevenson J, Ort SI, Cohen DJ. Clonidine treatment of Gilles de la Tourette's syndrome. Arch Gen Psychiatry 1991; 48:324–328.
25. Jimenez-Jimenez FJ, Garcia-Ruiz PJ. Pharmacological options for the treatment of Tourette's disorder. Drugs 2001; 61:2207–2220.
26. Scahill L, Chappell PB, Kim YS, et al. A placebo-controlled study of guanfacine in the treatment of children with tic disorders and attention deficit hyperactivity disorder. Am J Psychiatry 2001; 158:1067–1074.
27. Singer HS, Brown J, Quaskey S, Rosenberg LA, Mellits ED, Denckla MB. The treatment of attention-deficit hyperactivity disorder in Tourette's syndrome: a double-blind placebo-controlled study with clonidine and desipramine. Pediatrics 1995; 95:74–81.
28. Spencer T, Biederman J, Coffey B, et al. A double-blind comparison of desipramine and placebo in children and adolescents with chronic tic disorder and comorbid attention-deficit/hyperactivity disorder. Arch Gen Psychiatry 2002; 59:649–656.
29. Wilens TE, Spencer TJ, Biederman J, et al. A controlled clinical trial of bupropion for attention deficit hyperactivity disorder in adults. Am J Psychiatry 2001; 158:282–288.
30. Group TMC. A 14-month randomized clinical trial of treatment strategies for attention-deficit/hyperactivity disorder. Arch Gen Psychiatry 1999; 56:1073–1086.

31. Pelham W. The NIMH Multimodal Treatment Study for Attention-Deficit Hyperactivity Disorder: just say yes to drugs alone. Can J Psychiatry 1999; 44:981–990.
32. Pelham WJ, Gnagy E. Psychosocial and combined treatments for ADHD. Ment Retard Dev Disabil Res Rev 1999; 5:225–236.
33. Dornbush MP, Pruitt SK. Teaching the Tiger: A Handbook for Individuals Involved in the Education of Students with Attention Deficit Disorders, Tourette Syndrome or Obsessive–Compulsive Disorder. Duarte, CA: Hope Press, 1995.

23

The Neurosurgical Treatment of Tourette's Syndrome

Chris van der Linden and Henry Colle
St. Lucas Hospital Ghent
Ghent, Belgium

Elisabeth M. J. Foncke
Amsterdam Medical Center
Amsterdam, The Netherlands

Richard Bruggeman
University Hospital Groningen
Groningen, The Netherlands

INTRODUCTION

The treatment of Gilles de la Tourette's syndrome (TS) needs different approaches. In the first place, it is important to give detailed information to the patient, parents, school, or workplace. Generally, this information is sufficient for TS patients to cope with motor and vocal tics. Second, if tics interfere with social, school, and professional activities, pharmacological treatment may be necessary. Several classes of anti-tic medication are available, in particular the alpha-adrenergic drugs clonidine and guanfacine, neuroleptics such as haloperidol and pimozide, and more recently atypical antipsychotics such as risperidone (1). Third, recent studies have shown that behavioral therapy may, at least in part, control tics (2). Most patients with TS will have a significant reduction of tics by the time they reach adulthood (3). However, a small portion of TS patients continues to have bothersome tics with interfer-

Table 1 Brain Targets that Have Been Used for Lesioning for the Treatment of Tics in TS

Target	Ref.
Frontal cortex	5
Gyrus cinguli anterior	6
Limbic area	7,8
Thalamus	9,10
Infrathalamic area	11,12
Zona incerta	12
Nucleus dentatus	13

ence of both social and professional life despite adequate pharmacological treatment. In those patients, brain surgery has been employed since the early 1960s. Detailed data on the short- and long-term results are lacking and serious side effects have limited their general use. In fact, in the first edition of this Handbook, surgical treatment for tics is not mentioned, demonstrating the critical view of this form of treatment by TS specialists. Initially, neurosurgical procedures consisted of the destruction of various parts of the brain on the basis of empirical data. Most of the reported patients were operated on because of associated psychiatric disturbances, in particular obsessive–compulsive disorder (OCD) (4). Frequently, the tics were not responsive to the surgical procedure. If tics were reduced by the surgery, it was unclear which target was responsible for the reduction of tics because of the lack of selective lesions (4). In addition, the lesions were very large. Regions in the vicinity of the presumed target could have contributed to the reduction of tics. Table 1 shows an overview of the various presumed targets in recent publications. All authors report serious adverse events in several of the operated patients (5–13). Because of the serious morbidity, neurosurgery as a treatment option in TS was generally abandoned by most specialized TS centers. However, due to the refinement of the stereotactic technique and the safe procedure of deep brain stimulation (DBS) in other movement disorders, such as Parkinson's disease (PD), tremors and dystonia (14–16), neurosurgical treatment has received renewed attention.

PATHOPHYSIOLOGY

The growing knowledge of the pathophysiology of tics in TS has given us a better view of how to select a target for the stereotactic treatment of tics. To understand why a specific target for destruction or chronic stimulation could be used for tic control, a short simplified summary on the pathophysiology of tics in TS is given. For a more detailed description see Chapter 14.

The basal ganglia are probably the key structures in the pathophysiology of tics in TS (Fig. 1). Various circuits have been described in which activity originating from the frontal cortex leads back to the frontal cortex via the basal ganglia and thalamus, the so-called cortico–striato–thalamocortical loops (17,18). The various loops run parallel to each other and each have their own function, varying from a sensorimotor integration to a more complicated cognitive and behavioral function. These cognitive and behavioral loops probably play an important role in the pathogenesis of tics. All these circuits run through the internal pallidum (GPi), which serves as the major output structure of the basal ganglia. Via various thalamic nuclei, including the ventrolateral nucleus and the more median located nuclei such as the centromedian and parafascicular nuclei, the loops project back to the frontal cortex. Within the basal ganglia, two major pathways have been identified, the direct and the indirect, which connect the input and output of the basal ganglia. Using this simplified basal ganglia model one can hypothesize the pathogenesis of the various hypokinetic and hyperkinetic movement disorders. In TS, a typical hyperkinetic disorder, an altered modulation of the striatum, giving

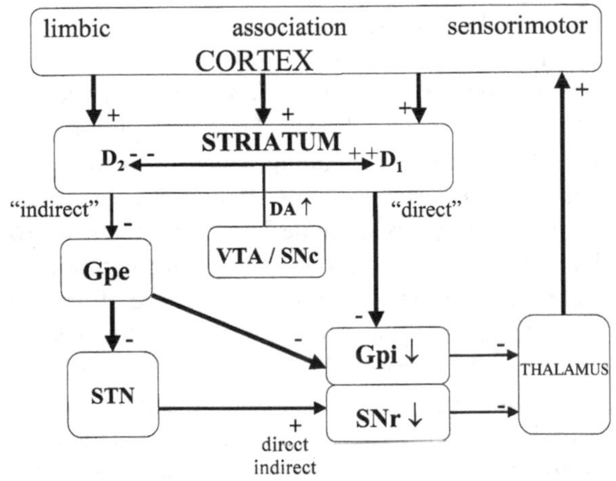

Figure 1 Schematic representation of the direct and indirect pathways. In Tourette's syndrome, a hyperdopaminergic state leads to inhibition of the indirect pathway and stimulation of the direct pathway, resulting in inhibition of the SNr and GPi. Inhibition of the SNr/GPi complex facilitates the thalamocortical projections. (From Ref. 1.)

rise to an increased inhibition of the GPi and disinhibition of the thalamocortical projection, may be involved in the pathogenesis. This altered inhibition of the GPi may be induced by abnormal activity originating from the prefrontal cortex (19). Moreover, animal experiments show that stereotypic behavior can be induced by abnormal activity of the striatum (20,21). Using PET and SPECT technology, in vivo studies reveal a disturbance of both the presynaptic and postsynaptic striatal dopamine receptors in patients with TS (22,23). Taking all those observations into account, altered modulation of the dopamine input seems important in the genesis of tics. This process had been hypothesized for decades by the notion that dopamine antagonists have a favorable effect in controlling tics (24). In addition, lesions in the mesencephalon, in which there is a large concentration of dopamine-containing neurons, have been described to cause tics (25).

NEUROSURGERY

Before the description of the cortico–striato–thalomocortical loops, neurosurgical procedures including thalamic lesioning and leucotomies were performed on an empirical basis. It was not until Hassler and Dieckman described their surgical cases of TS patients with intractable tics that specific regions of the brain were targeted for lesioning (10). They chose the medial thalamus as the main target, whereas Babel et al. (12) added the infrathalamic region on the basis of neurophysiological studies in TS. Side effects have limited this procedure. In a recent study, DBS was shown to be safer than lesioning in patients treated for tremor (15). Therefore, DBS was assumed the neurosurgical treatment of choice for intractable tics. The principle of electrical stimulation is believed to be similar to lesioning, since both methods inhibit the activity of the target. Vandewalle et al. reported on chronic bilateral medial thalamic stimulation in a 37-year-old male TS patient resistant to conventional therapy (26). The target was chosen on the basis of the reported lesioning by Hassler and Dieckman (10). Because of the multitude of lesions in Hassler and Dieckman's cases, the quadripolar electrode was placed in such a direction that many of their reported lesions could theoretically be involved in the stimulated area. The aforementioned cortico–striato–thalamocortical loops, including the medial thalamus with the centromedian nucleus as a possible source for the generation of tics, were taken into account. The safety of this procedure and the relief of the tics were demonstrated.

Similar procedures were carried out in two other adult male patients (ages 28 and 42) with medically intractable tics. The electrodes were placed bilaterally in the medial part of the thalamus, using the stereotactic approach. Van der Linden et al. (27) reported on the effects at long term in three patients with TS who underwent a bilateral thalamic stimulation. Tics were scored blindly using a 20-min videorecording with chronic stimulation and 12 hr after cessation of the stimulation. After a follow-up period of 5 years in patient 1, 1 year in patient 2, and 8 months in patient 3, there was a reduction of tics of 90.1%, 72.2%, and 82.6%, respectively. In the three patients, all major motor and vocal tics had disappeared. Moreover, there was a clear effect on associated behavioral disorders, consisting of compulsions in all three patients and automutilation in patient 2. No serious complications had occurred. When stimulation was applied at the voltage necessary to achieve an optimal result on the tics, a slight sedative effect was noted in all three patients. In patients 1 and 3 there were stimulation-induced changes in sexual behavior (28).

In a 27-year-old male TS patient, medial thalamic stimulation was compared to bilateral internal pallidal stimulation by placing one quadripolar electrode in each target bilaterally, thereby implanting a total of four intracerebral electrodes (29). Stimulation of the internal pallidum appeared to be more effective in reducing the tics than stimulation of the medial thalamus. Also in this patient there was a clear effect of the stimulation on associated compulsions. The ventrolateral part of the internal pallidum, the target used for the treatment of dystonia and for some patients with Parkinson's disease, was selected. Based on these results, the target to be used for chronic stimulation in the control of intractable tics remains to be determined.

METHODOLOGY OF DBS

DBS needs a multidisciplinary approach: a neurosurgeon specialized in the stereotactic technique, a neurologist specialized in movement disorders, a psychiatrist with interest in behavioral psychiatry, a neuroradiologist, a psychologist, and a specialized nursing staff. The neurologist is important for making a proper diagnosis and establishing a correct indication for surgery. The patient should be carefully evaluated by a psychiatrist to rule out any serious psychiatric comorbidity. The steps of the stereotactic procedure involve calculating the target with reference to a coordinate system using imaging techniques (MRI and CT-scan fusion), and determining the target point and the optimal trajectory using multiplanar (X-, Y-, and Z-axis system) brain images of the patient. With this method, the electrode can be placed according to the calculated trajectory and depth within 1 mm of the desired target). The methodology of DBS varies among centers, but all use the stereotactic approach for the introduction of the electrode to the desired target. The methodology used for the neurosurgical treatment of tics is similar for PD and other movement disorders, except that the desired target(s) may vary. One method consists of a combination of stereotaxy and neuronavigation: fiducials are placed at various strategic points on the skull for proper MRI/CT scan fusion; 1.5-mm T1-weighted MRI images with gadolinium are then taken. These images are fused using the fixed fiducials with the images of the CT scan taken on the day of the surgery with a stereotactic frame securely attached to the skull. MRI gives better resolution and quality of the brain structures, whereas CT scan has the advantage of a more precise geometric image with no distortion. The medial part of the thalamus was chosen by selecting the centromedian nucleus as the main target using the Schaltenbrand atlas and referring the target to the *X*-*Y*-*Z*-axis system. The target is calculated on a tridimensional reconstruction of the images with 0.1-mm precision in relation to the *X*, *Y*, and *Z* axes. Finally, an ideal trajectory is selected, thereby avoiding delicate brain structures such as blood vessels and ventricles. Because it is of utmost importance that the patient is fully immobile, the headframe is fixed to the operation table. The electrode is fixed to the frame and can only change its position according to a polar two-arc system. After making a burr hole, a test electrode is introduced, after which the patient is awakened. Perioperatively, propofol-tuned anaesthesia is used to perform a macroelectrode test stimulation in an awakened patient. During electrical test stimulation, a clinical response using low current is assessed and undesirable side effects are evaluated using higher currents. If no undesirable side effects are obtained with low current and a good clinical response is obtained, the test electrode is replaced by a flexible four-contact (quadripolar) electrode.

CONCLUSIONS

Review of the literature on the neurosurgical treatment of medication-resistant tics indicates that this treatment may result in relief. The lesioning technique is obsolete due to serious adverse events reported in most of the cases. The deep brain stimulation technique appears promising due to preliminary evidence of efficacy and safety in the four reported cases.

It remains to be determined which is the preferred target for optimal tic control. Based on the current understanding of the pathophysiology of TS, two targets (medial part of the thalamus and GPi) can be considered. Prospective studies are under way to evaluate the effect of stimulating these targets on tics and further evaluate the efficacy and safety of DBS for this condition.

ACKNOWLEDGMENTS

We thank Drs. Y. Temel and V. Visser-Vandewalle for their useful comments.

REFERENCES

1. Bruggeman R, Van der Linden C, Op den Velde W, et al. A comparative double-blind parallel group study of risperidone versus pimozide in Gilles de la Tourette's syndrome. J Clin Psychiatry 2001; 50–56.
2. Hoogduin CAL, de Haan E, Cath DC, van de Wetering BJM. Gedragstherapie. In: Buitelaar JK, van de Wetering BJM, eds. Syndroom van Gilles de la Tourette: een leidraad voor diagnostiek en behandeling. Assen: Van Gorkum, 1994: 61–67.
3. Leckman JF, Zhang H, Vitale A, et al. Course of tic severity in Tourette's syndrome: the first two decades. Pediatrics 1998; 102:14–19.
4. Rauch SL, Bear L, Cosgrove, Jenike M. Neurosurgical treatment of Tourette's syndrome: a critical review. Comp Psychiatry 1995; 36:141–156.
5. Baker EFW. Gilles de la Tourette syndrome treated by medial frontal leucotomy. Can Med Assoc J 1962; 86:746–747.
6. Kurlan R, Kersun J, Ballantine T, Caine ED. Neurosurgical treatment of severe obsessive–compulsive disorder associated with Tourette's syndrome. Mov Disord 1990; 5:152–155.
7. Sawle GV, Lees AJ, Hymas NF, Brooks DJ, Frackowiak RSJ. The metabolic effects of limbic leucotomy in Gilles de la Tourette syndrome. J Neurol Neurosurg Psychiatry 1993; 56:1016–1019.
8. Robertson M, Doran M, Trimble M, Lees AJ. The treatment of Gilles de la Tourette syndrome by limbic leucotomy. J Neurol Neurosurg Psychiatry 1990; 53:691–694.
9. Diviitis E, D'Errico, Cerillo A. Stereotactic surgery in Gilles de la Tourette syndrome. Acta Neurochir 1977; 24(suppl):7373.
10. Hassler R, Dieckmann G. Traitement stéréotaxique des tics et cris inarticulés ou coprolalique considérés comme phènoméne d'obsession motrice au cour de la maladies de Gilles de la Tourette. Rev Neurol (Paris) 1970; 123:89–100.
11. Leckman JF, de Lotbinière AJ, Marek K, et al. Severe disturbances in speech, swallowing, and gait following stereotactic infrathalamic lesions in Gilles de la Tourette's syndrome. Neurology 1993; 43:890–894.
12. Babel TB, Warnke PC, Ostertag CB. Immediate and long term outcome after infrathalamic and thalamic lesioning for intractable Tourette's syndrome. J Neurol Neurosurg Psychiatry 2001; 70:666–671.
13. Nadvornik P, Sramka M, Lisy L, Svicka J. Experiences with dentatomy. Confin Neurol 1972; 34:320–324.
14. Limousin P, Krack P, Pollack P, et al. Electrical stimulation of the subthalamic nucleus in advanced Parkinson's disease. N Engl J Med 1998; 330:1105–1111.
15. Schuurman PR, Bosch BA, Bossuyt PMN, et al. A comparison of continuous thalamic stimulation and thalamotomy for suppression of severe tremor. N Engl J Med 2000; 342:461–468.
16. Coubes P, Roubertie A, Vayssiere N, Hemm S, Echenne B. Treatment of DYT-1 generalized dystonia by stimulation of the internal globus pallidus. Lancet 2000; 355:2220–2221.
17. Alexander GE, Crutcher MD. Functional architecture of basal ganglia circuits: neural substrates of parallel processing. Trends Neurosci 1990; 13:266–271.

18. Groenewegen HJ. Bewegen: de rol van de basale ganglia. In: Wolters EC, van Laar T, eds. Bewegingsstoornissen. Amsterdam: VU Uitgeverij, 2002:3–34.
19. Leckman JF. Tourette's syndrome. Lancet 2002; 360:1577–1586.
20. Canales JJ, Graybriel AM. A measure of striatal functions predicts motor stereotypy. Nat Neurosci 2000; 3:377–383.
21. Graybiel AM, Canalis JJ. The neurobiology of repetitive behaviors: clues to the neurobiology of Tourette syndrome. Adv Neurol 2001; 85:123–131.
22. Ernst M, Zametkin AJ, Jons PH, et al. High presynaptic dopaminergic activity in children with Tourette's disorder. J Am Acad Child Adolesc Psychiatry 1999; 38:86–94.
23. Wolf SS, Jones DW, Knable MB, et al. Tourette syndrome: prediction of phenotypic variation in monozygotic twin by caudate nucleus D2 receptor binding. Science 1996; 273:1225–1227.
24. Challas G, Brauer W. Tourette's disease: relief of symptoms with R 1625. Am J Psychiatry 1963; 120:283–284.
25. Van der Linden C, Bruggeman R, Pengel J. Gilles de la Tourette syndrome in a patient with a mesencephalic lesion. Mov Disord 1994; 9:252.
26. Vandewalle V, van der Linden C, Caemaert J, Groenewegen HJ. Stereotactic treatment of Gilles de la Tourette syndrome by high frequency stimulation of thalamus. Lancet 1999; 353:724.
27. van der Linden C, Colle H, Vandewalle V, Alessi G, Rijckaert D, De Waele L. Chronic bilateral medial thalamic (MT) stimulation for the treatment of tics in 3 adult patients with Gilles de la Tourette syndrome. Mov Disord 2002;188(suppl).
28. Temel Y, van Lankveld JJDM, Boon P, Spincemaille GH, van der Linden C, Visser-Vandewalle V. Deep brain stimulation of the thalamus can influence penile erection. Int J Imp Res 2004; 16:91–94.
29. van der Linden C, Colle H, Vandewalle V, Alessi G, Rijckaert D, De Waele L. Successful treatment of tics with chronic bilateral internal pallidum (GPi) stimulation in a 27 year old male patient with Gilles de la Tourette's syndrome. Mov Disord 2002; 341(suppl).

24

Genetic Counseling

P. Michael Conneally
Indiana University School of Medicine
Indianapolis, Indiana, U.S.A.

INTRODUCTION

The term *genetic counseling*, coined by Reed (1) in 1955, does not have a precise definition. In broadest terms, it includes at least four activities: (1) establishment of a precise diagnosis, (2) estimation of recurrence risks, (3) determination of prognosis and burden on the family, and (4) proper communication of the above information to the patient and family members. In many instances, these goals are not attained. This is especially true of the last aspect—communication to individuals in terms that they understand and retain over a long period of time.

Genetic counseling is performed by many different kinds of health professionals, including geneticists, physicians in various disciplines, trained genetic counselors, nurses, and, in some cases, family members or friends. Over the last four decades, training centers for genetic counselors have been established across the United States. Students are given broad training in various aspects of genetic counseling, receive a master's degree, and usually are board-certified by the American Board of Medical Genetics. They normally work under the direction of a clinical geneticist.

MODELS OF GENETIC COUNSELING

Walker (2) suggests four models of genetic counseling. The eugenic model is based on the ideas of the eugenics movement beginning in the late 18th century and culminating with the Holocaust. The main reason for these movements was to "improve the human race" either by counseling families with a history of defective offspring not to reproduce, or to promulgate laws on sterilization, or, in the extreme, euthanasia. This has led to the "nondirective" approach to genetic counseling that prevails today. The second model is defined by Walker as the medical/preventive model. This was simply to attempt to offer families information based on empirical observations and offer the option to avoid childbearing. Fortunately, like the previous model, this one no longer prevails.

The decision-making model is due to the major advances in the field of genetics in the last 40 years. This allowed a more interactive type of counseling so that individuals were not only educated about their risks but also helped with the complex task of exploring issues about the disorder and aided in decisions on further testing and reproductive concerns. The final model proposed by Walker is the psychotherapeutic model. In this scenario, the counselor explores the counselee's emotional responses, goals, and cultural and religious beliefs, as well as other dynamics of the family. It is in this general area where the skills of an experienced genetic counselor come into play and is the optimum approach in helping families cope with a major crisis, including informing the individual with the necessary information as well as guiding the said individual through alternative decisions (3).

PREREQUISITES FOR GENETIC COUNSELING

The two most important prerequisites of counseling are a precise, confirmed diagnosis and an accurate pedigree (family history). In many situations, diagnosis is relatively straightforward. This is true when the basic defect is known and can be measured. However, in many disorders, there is genetic heterogeneity. There are two types of genetic heterogeneity. In the first, allelic heterogeneity, different mutations at the same locus can cause a disease (e.g., cystic fibrosis). Normally, this does not cause problems in counseling, but it can lead to difficulty in carrier detection and prenatal diagnosis if all mutations are not readily detectable.

The other type of genetic heterogeneity is locus heterogeneity, in which mutations at more than one locus can cause the disorder. An example is retinitis pigmentosa (RP), for which there are at least 12 autosomal dominant loci, 5 autosomal recessive loci, and at least 3 X-linked loci (4). Locus heterogeneity can be a major problem in genetic counseling. It is clear that if one is to properly counsel the parents of a child with RP, the mode of inheritance must be known because, for example, the risk to their grandchildren is very different if the disease is X-linked rather than autosomal recessive.

Sporadic cases can also be difficult to analyze. They may be due to new mutations or nonpaternity, or they may be phenocopies (i.e., caused by nongenetic factors). Thus, it is important to try to determine the origin of phenocopies; otherwise, the advice given may be totally misleading.

The second important aspect of counseling is the pedigree, or family history. Recording a precise family history can be time-consuming, but it is very important. Because many individuals are not familiar with the vital statistics or health status of members of their extended family, they need to be advised before the interview to seek this information from other relatives. A better method is the use of a family history questionnaire (5). This can be mailed to the individual at some point (usually a month) before the interview, allowing time for the said individual to obtain the necessary information from other family members. The questionnaire should be returned prior to the interview and a pedigree should be constructed. This has the advantage of providing more information beforehand, shortening the interview time and allowing for more specific questions to be asked during the interview. In interviewing an individual about the health status of relatives, it is important not to ask global questions such as "Do any of your brothers or sisters have health problems?" One needs to elicit specific information for each member (e.g., "Tell me about your brother John; does he have any health problems?"). Computerization of the pedigree allows for name searches to determine if any branch of the family is already in the database (6). This is especially useful for disorders that are rare or for which there is locus heterogeneity. In general, the larger is the pedigree, the more precise will be the diagnosis and mode of inheritance.

MOLECULAR GENETIC APPROACHES TO COUNSELING

The advent of recombinant DNA technology has revolutionized the field of medical genetics. The majority of major genetic disorders have been assigned a chromosomal location (mapped) and, in a large percentage of cases, the mutant gene has been cloned. These achievements have vastly broadened the scope of carrier detection and prenatal and presymptomatic diagnosis. Widespread carrier screening, especially for major genetic disease, is about to begin but the efficacy of such screening is being widely debated. It is clear, however, that in the near future, the majority of Mendelian disorders, especially those that are relatively common, will be amenable to prenatal or presymptomatic diagnosis for those who wish to know. Nonetheless, even in these situations, an accurate diagnosis and family history are essential.

COUNSELING IN TOURETTE'S SYNDROME (TS)

The previous discussion centered on inherited disorders with a simple Mendelian mode of inheritance. However, TS does not fit into this category.

Counseling in TS poses two major difficulties. The first is the definition of phenotype. The symptoms of TS are variable, encompassing a wide spectrum of motor and behavioral disturbances (7). The disorder is over three times as prevalent in males as in females. On the other hand, the frequency of obsessive–compulsive disorder (OCD) is significantly increased in families with TS and is more common in female members. Segregation analyses strongly suggest that OCD in families with TS is another manifestation of the same gene. This suggests that the risk to offspring of individuals with OCD is similar to the risk to their relatives with TS. Vertical transmission in families suggests that the disorder is due to an autosomal dominant gene. Segregation analysis strongly suggests the above mode of inheritance and is widely (8), although not universally, accepted (9).

Pauls (10), in a recent update on the genetics of TS, noted that there has been significant progress in understanding its genetic etiology. It would now appear from segregation analysis reported by Hasstedt et al. (11) and Pauls et al. (12) that the most parsimonious solution was an "intermediate" mode of inheritance. A major gene is undoubtedly involved, but other minor genetic contributions are also contributing to the phenotype. Concerted efforts to locate genes using linkage studies are underway, but results so far are not significant enough to warrant their usefulness in genetic counseling.

Probably the simplest approach is to assume a major dominant gene with decreased penetrance. Pauls and Leckman (13) estimated a penetrance of the TS gene in males to be approximately 100% and in females to be 70% when both TS and OCD are combined. In a later study, Price et al. (14) found penetrances of 80% in males and 70% in females. Therefore, an asymptomatic female (and possibly a male sib) of an affected individual from a family with TS may carry the gene for TS, and thus their child is at risk. This must be taken into account in counseling such individuals. The fact that penetrance is less than 100% will also decrease the risk to an offspring of an affected individual, but the difference from 50% is probably not significant, other than the fact that the phenotype can vary from mild OCD to severe TS.

As an example, we take the case of a female with OCD from a family with TS. Because we assume that OD is a manifestation of the TS gene (in families with TS) and that the disorders are inherited in an autosomal dominant fashion, the risk that her offspring will inherit the gene is 50%. Thus, if a child who inherits the gene is male, the likelihood of his having either TS (most likely) or OCD is approximately 100%. If the offspring receiving the mutant gene is female, the risk is approximately 70%, with OCD being much more likely than TS.

On the other hand, if we are counseling the above woman's sister who is asymptomatic, we must take into account the probability that she carries the TS gene. Because penetrance in females is approximately 70%, this probability is 30 × 50% (probability of inheriting the TS gene from her carrier parent), or 15%. If she carries the mutant gene, her risks are the same as those of her symptomatic sister.

Many of the difficulties in genetic counseling in TS will be overcome once the gene is mapped. For example, the mode of inheritance can then be precisely determined and nonpenetrant individuals will be more easily identified. Prenatal diagnosis will then be feasible although the demand may not be great. Locus heterogeneity can also be investigated. The above are, of course, interim benefits. The ultimate aim of molecular studies is the determination of the basic defect, with the most important goal of finding a definitive treatment for the disorder.

REFERENCES

1. Reed SC. Counseling in Medical Genetics. Philadelphia: WB Saunders, 1955.
2. Walker AP. The practice of genetic counseling. In: Baker DL, Schuette JL, Uhlmann WR, eds. A Guide to Genetic Counseling. New York: Wiley-Liss, 1998:1–20.
3. Begleiter ML. Science and society: training for genetic counsellors. Nat Rev Genet 2002; 3(7):557–561.
4. Nussbaum RL, McInnes RR, Willard HF. Genetics in Medicine. 6th ed. Philadelphia: WB Saunders, 2001:55.
5. Cole J, Conneally PM, Hodes ME, Merritt AD. Genetic family history questionnaire. J Med Genet 1978; 15(1):10–18.
6. Conneally PM. MEGADATS-3M in a medical genetics environment. Proc Eighteenth Int Conf Sys Sci 1985; III:2–8.
7. Kurlan R. The spectrum of Tourette's syndrome. Curr Opin Neurol Neurosurg 1988; 1:294–298.
8. Pauls DL, Towbin KE, Leckman JF, Zahner GEF, Cohen DJ. Tourette's syndrome and obsessive–compulsive disorder: evidence supporting a genetic relationship. Arch Gen Psychiatry 1986; 43:1180–1182.
9. Comings DE. Presidential address: the genetics of human behavior—lessons for two societies. Am J Hum Genet 1989; 44(4):452–460.
10. Pauls DL. Update on the genetics of Tourette Syndrome. In: Cohen DL, Goetz CG, Jankovic J, eds. Tourette Syndrome. Philadelphia: Lippincott, Williams and Wilkins, 2001:281–293.
11. Hasstedt SJ, Leppert M, Filloux F, van de Wetering BJM, McMahon WM. Intermediate inheritance of Tourette syndrome, assuming assortative mating. Am J Hum Genet 1995; 57(3):682–689.
12. Pauls DL, Raymond CL, Stevenson JM, Leckman JF. A family study of Gilles de la Tourette syndrome. Am J Hum Genet 1991; 48(1):154–163.
13. Pauls DL, Leckman JF. The inheritance of Gilles de la Tourette's syndrome and associated behaviors. Evidence for autosomal dominant transmission. N Engl J Med 1986; 315(16):993–997.
14. Price RA, Pauls DL, Kreyer SD, Caine ED. Family data support a dominant major gene for Tourette syndrome. Psychiatry Res 1988; 24:251–261.

[illegible]

25

The Child and Adolescent with Tourette's Syndrome

Clinical Perspectives on Phenomenology and Treatment

James F. Leckman and Donald J. Cohen †
Yale University School of Medicine
New Haven, Connecticut, U.S.A.

INTRODUCTION

In the simplest clinical situations, there is no distinction between the treatment of a discrete disorder and the care of a whole child. We skillfully suture a laceration, treat a sore throat, and send the child and family on their way. In clinical work with individuals with tic syndromes, however, these two clinical activities may become broadly divergent. Even when tics are the "chief complaint," the times when the clinician in a specialty practice of neurology or child psychiatry need attend only to the child's tics are rather few and far between. Indeed, the role of tics in the story of the child's life may be overshadowed by a decade or two of derailment in emotional, educational, and social development; by a saga of treatments tried and failed; by the emotional scarring of disappointments, alienation, and medical side effects; and by profound disruptions in family life and family economics. From these

†Deceased.

case histories, we can reconstruct the trajectory of a child's development from first tics to overwhelming obsessions and compulsions, from a childhood full of promise to chronic patienthood. The goal of clinical care of children with Tourette's syndrome (TS) today is not to eliminate tics but to help assure that development will move ahead as well as possible and to attempt to minimize the likelihood of the most adverse consequences of a chronic childhood illness.

The increasing recognition of multiple tic syndromes during the past decade has challenged clinicians with the task of defining the broad clinical spectrum of these disorders and the appropriate timing and use of varied modalities of intervention, including medication (1,2). For many children, the diagnosis of a tic syndrome or TS will require little more than reassurance, guidance, and availability over time. For others, the entire range of child psychiatric and neurological interventions are called upon—including psychological, familial, educational, and pharmacological approaches. The prevailing diagnostic criteria for TS have stood the test of time and research, but they do not convey the whole clinical story, including (1) the tremendous range of severity and impairment (from inconsequential to debilitating) and (2) the burden of other psychiatric difficulties related to the underlying diathesis or in response to the tic syndrome.

The decisions about whether to confer or defer a diagnosis of a tic disorder for a patient, which problems are most in need of clinical intervention, and the choice and staging of intervention require an understanding of the child's development as a full person and the complexities of natural history and associated features. Specifically, the decision to use medication for a child or adolescent with TS should be based on an assessment of subject's overall development—the child's emotional and social life and sense of self, as well as experiences at home, school, and in the community—and not just on the severity of the individual's tics, per se.

NATURAL HISTORY

Tics may not be the child's first difficulties, and his premorbid functioning may carry important prognostic significance. For many children who come to clinical care, behavioral difficulties, such as irritability, frustration intolerance, overactivity, or attentional problems, may have been apparent by nursery school, years before the appearance of tics. These problems may be prodromal of tics and reflect an early manifestation of the underlying diathesis in systems that subserve behavioral regulation (such as inhibition and sensory processing). Early behavioral symptoms may also be accompanied by a few tics that were overlooked until the emergence of the full-blown disorder. For children with severe troubles with attention-deficit hyperactivity disorder (ADHD), oppositional disorder, or aggression in the preschool years, the family milieu may already be tense and marked by ambivalent parental overconcern and anger before the onset of tics. These tensions set the stage for an escalation of familial anxiety, discord, and expressed negative emotion. That is, the tics may be seen by the family and child's teachers, and experienced by the child, within the framework of already problematic self-control and consequently be interpreted as willful acts of rude behavior.

For children with no previous difficulties, the first few episodes of transient tics may be accepted as merely childhood habits. They may elicit passing concern, or none at all. As the young child is less likely to be aware of his tics, their ultimate outcome may be appreciated only much later, when more persistent motor and vocal tics emerge. Some children are also aware of oddities in their sensory processing. They may be unusually sensitive to touch, to the feel of clothes, or to particular sensory experiences in their body or outside (e.g., they may feel that lights are too bright, sounds too loud).

When tics come in relentless cascades and take increasingly odd forms (jumping, twirling, throwing up arms, pulling weird faces, sticking out the tongue, chirping like a bird, howling) the child may feel that his mind has been invaded by demons he cannot defeat. These experiences are the fantasies of which nightmares are constructed. No matter how much his parents explain, plead, or punish, he knows that he cannot control the tics for long, if at all. Yet he knows, in a deep and often guilty fashion, that the urges and actions are his, that they do come from within himself, and that there are moments when he can suppress them. There is no denying, as much as he would like to do so, that he is the author of the alien and odd impulses he expresses and that make him stand out in a crowd, subject to disapproving glances. He may feel the need to defend himself from ridicule, including self-ridicule; he may sense he is both the perpetrator and the victim of his own inner workings. As his parents also do not understand what the child is experiencing, they may scold and cajole; they may punish or deprive the child of treats; they may try to ignore the tics or the child himself; and they may banish the child from their sight. Even if they do understand, they may not be able to disguise fully their grief and upset. Yet these varied forms of behavioral modification are generally unsuccessful. The major result of this negative, intrusive interaction between parents and child may be to make both the child and the parents feel ashamed and estranged (3). Although there are many parallels, we can imagine how different it is for the child who develops diabetes, arthritis, or another serious medical disorder. In such cases, parents may blame themselves; they may suffer neurotic guilt and depression; but they do not plead with the child to heal himself.

Over the course of a few years, the child may focus increasing time and energy on his bodily urges, the tics that pop out of him or the acts and sounds that, in a fashion, are his actions. His internal direction of attention will increase with the progressive awareness experienced by most patients of bodily sensations that precede the tic actions. These "premonitory urges" are unpleasant sensory experiences located in particular bodily sites (particular muscle groups, in the throat, on the surface of the skin); these feelings tend to start as mild tensions and build up to a crescendo of tension, which is reduced only when the patient performs a particular tic (4–6). Patients thus are not caught unawares and are not merely passive in relation to their tics: an uncomfortable feeling state (a tension or anxiety) is ameliorated by an unacceptable but gratifying action (tic, complex movement, dystonic posture, loud noise, etc.). Patients describe the sensory experience by analogy to a sneeze that starts at the periphery of consciousness as a tingle in the nasal passageways and mounts to a demand for explosive discharge. Through self-observation, reflections in the responses of others, and phenomena such as premonitory urges, a child will become more aware of the tics he has at any time, how "bad" his tics are at that period, and which tics are most embarrassing. As he matures, the child will work, to a greater or lesser degree, on holding back or camouflaging tics. He will become an expert on recognizing the impact of symptoms on others and he will find safe places where he can "let go."

To a far greater extent than normal, the child with TS will monitor his bodily states of tension and the self-generated gratification when tics are executed "just right" (7). He will also be sensitive to the nuances of how others react to him. Through the reactions of others and his own self-criticism, he may start to feel that he is conspiring with the compelling urges to tic, surrendering to their demands rather than bravely resisting, and satisfying himself rather than choosing the moral high road of abstinence. A child may begin to feel not only burdened but guilty, as he recapitulates, many times a day, the cycle of impulse, tic, or other action that reduces the tension, remorse, and return of the internal tension. Thus, the child may feel disloyal to his family, which he can see is distressed by his symptoms, and to himself, for giving in to the pressures rather than conquering them. The child may feel angry at his body for what it has done to him; at the same time, he may feel angry at his parents whom he may feel have not been able to help rid him of his troubles. Through all these processes, the child's self-image becomes blemished by what he suffers in the privacy of his mind and in the overtly public displays of his body.

Motor and phonic tics occur in bouts over the course of a day, and wax and wane in severity over the course of weeks to months (8). The bouts are characterized by brief periods of stable intra tic intervals (i.e., time between successive tics) of short duration, typically 0.5–1.0 sec. Less well known is the "self-similarity" of these temporal patterns across different time scales (9). Over the course of minutes to hours, this means that the bouts of tics themselves occur in bouts. Over the course of days and weeks, these bouts-of-bouts of tics also occur in bouts, as do the bouts-of-bouts-of-bouts. Knowledge of the temporal patterning of tics is fundamental for the practitioner as it informs decisions about when to initiate anti-tic medications, when to change medications, and when to be patient and simply provide close monitoring and support to the family. A deeper understanding of the multiplicative processes that govern these timing patterns may clarify both microscopic neural events occurring in millisecond time scales as well as macroscopic features of the natural history of tic disorders that occur over decades.

Along with other children who have chronic illnesses, the child with TS irrationally may feel guilty for having the disorder, as if he brought it on himself by something he thought or did, and for the troubles it brings his family, but, in contrast with children with most other conditions, the child with tics may feel the additional guilt that accompanies the sense that he has a hand, however weak, in its expression.

The child's sensory experiences and tuning in on the functioning of his body, and his attempts to understand and control his symptoms, may make him more introspective in general than other children his age. While healthy children take their bodies for granted, and are called upon to describe their inner states only in relation to the ordinary events of daily life ("Are you hungry?" "Tired?") or when occasionally ill ("Where does it hurt? Is it a sharp or throbbing pain?"), children with TS are constantly assaying their thoughts, feelings, and acts, trying to discern small differences and convey them to their parents and physicians. They develop tropes for describing different types of tics, odd thoughts, and compulsive actions, and try to use descriptive words to convey what it feels like to have a tension or discomfort take a bodily part as a hostage and demand, without compromise, a grotesque action as a ransom for freedom, however brief.

Thus, recurrent, multiple tics may become a distorting influence on a child's sense of his body as a source of pleasure and his mind as the agent for shaping and controlling instinctual urges. Some children identify with the impulsivity and the rudeness. In varied and individualized ways, tics become enmeshed in his relations with family and peers, in the inner world of fantasy, and in the child's sense of himself as an autonomous individual whose desires are balanced by values and controls (10,11). This formulation is consistent with empirical research that their peers see children with TS as withdrawn and less popular than others (12), and as socially immature by their parents (13,14).

No domain of symptoms reveals the internal split within the child's self between agent and object more graphically than self-injurious behavior. Fortunately, less than 5% of patients seen in specialty clinics have some degree of self-inflicted injury. But they are among the most distressing patients for clinicians and families; they arouse both pity and anger; they evoke our wish to be physicianly healers and frustrate our narcissism when we fail. There are multiple forms of self-injurious symptoms: skin-picking, eye gouging, head banging, face slapping, poking at the skin with objects, scratching, etc. The symptoms may ostracize a person with TS, increase his self-loathing, and lead to serious medical problems, including blindness or fractures. Here the border with other "compulsive" actions, such as hair-pulling (trichotillomania), nail-biting, stereotypic self-injury of patients with pervasive developmental disorder, and wrist slashing of borderline patients, may be hard to define and the concept of "tic" seems stretched to its limit.

Tics involving self-injury raise very interesting questions about the nature of sensory gating and the experience of pain in various psychiatric disorders, including TS (15). What might be the motivation, psychological or physiological, that drives a patient to overcome the natural instinct for self-preservation that may lead him to mercilessly beat himself into a bloody mess? For some patients, the pain during self-injury seems muted, or at least less intense than one might anticipate; for others, the pain seems tolerated as the price for the relief; for others, the experience during the "act" that causes the tic is not of pain, but pain follows the physical insult; still, for others, there seems to even be a desire for the pain, an attachment to it, and a requirement for pain as a condition for satisfaction of the internal demand. The torture inflicted by the patient on his body is thus experienced as horrible and yet gratifying, masochistic, just deserts for secret pleasures. There are patients who experience these episodes in quasi-dissociated states, as if they were standing outside their bodies and sadistically attacking the flesh of the other. Families and physicians may be more overwhelmed than the patient.

Thus, the natural history and clinical manifestations of TS are far richer and variegated than may be conveyed by diagnostic criteria. While the paradigmatic case is easily described (recurrent motor and vocal tics, starting at age 5–7) (16), the range of severity of tic symptoms among patients with TS is enormously broad. Most children with TS have generally mild tic symptoms; they never come for clinical diagnosis and generally do not require therapeutic intervention. For those who are diagnosed, the severity of the motor and vocal tic typically peaks early in the second decade with many patients showing a marked reduction in tic severity by the age of 19 or 20 (17). However, ultimate social adaptation may be a function more of behavioral and attentional difficulties than of tic-symptom severity. Many patients with severe tics achieve adequate social adjustment in adult life, although usually with considerable emotional pain. The factors that appear to be of importance with regard to social adaptation include the patient's level of self-confidence, the seriousness of attentional problems, school achievement, intelligence, degree of family support, and severity of complex motor and phonic symptoms. While the majority of TS patients have no or little impairment from their self-limited symptoms, for other patients the disorder takes over their entire lives and they become, in the fullest sense, "victims of TS" (10).

ASSOCIATED CONDITIONS—COMORBIDITY

There are many pathways of connection between tic disorders and other psychiatric, behavioral, and developmental disorders. Experienced clinicians, along with parents and teachers, have often described children with tics as being more sensitive, high-strung, and emotional. Along with others, we have seen studious, high-achieving boys and girls (both in the clinic and in daily life) who would support such a stereotype. Since the very first descriptions of TS more than a century ago, patients have been described with varied and severe psychiatric disturbances. Until the last few decades, when TS has become more broadly recognized by clinicians, patients with TS were often diagnosed as psychotic, schizophrenic, and, of course, obsessive–compulsive. The identification of a genetic basis for TS has added new interest to trying to understand the relations among tic disorders and other psychiatric and behavioral disorders (18,19).

In clinic populations, including our own, up to half of the patients with TS have behavioral difficulties that would earn another psychiatric diagnosis in addition to a tic syndrome (20,21). These other diagnoses include attentional disorders (ADHD) and learning difficulties, obsessive–compulsive symptoms (OCS) and disorder (OCD), anxiety disorders, personality disorders, and affective illnesses (14,22). When an individual has more than one condition, the term comorbidity is often used descriptively. However, there are different ways in which a tic disorder may be related to other problems and disorders; also, there are complex factors that may lead to an overrepresentation of the most difficult cases in specialty clinics. We will note three broad types of associations that can lead to the clinical appearance of comorbidity: (1) associations that reflect the result of having a chronic disorder, (2) associations that reflect the pathways into treatment, and (3) associations that reflect the varied manifestations of an underlying cause.

Developmental and Reactive Associations

There are multiple stresses related to a chronic medical condition (such as diabetes or TS) and its treatment. These stresses include social stigma, restrictions on autonomy, the intrusion of the illness or treatments on normal functioning, limitation of opportunities for being with others or going places, medications involved in treatment, and the like. Thus, patients with TS, just like those with other chronic medical illness, may develop or be more vulnerable to other problems (such as depression) because of multiple acute stresses and persistent, chronic trauma. For decades, clinicians have known that children with diabetes are likely to have difficulties during the course of development (e.g., with achieving adolescent autonomy) and that children with severe asthma may be prone to anxiety or personality difficulties. Being sick, especially when young, may affect many spheres of personal development. Serious tic disorders are like other diseases in this sense: they are burdens on children and families and are thus risk factors for other types of emotional, developmental, and behavioral disorders.

The presence of a severe tic disorder in a child may be a risk factor for emotional difficulties in a parent or sibling. Just as the birth of a defective child may lead to parental discord and depression, the onset of TS and the years of severe symptoms may be a risk factor for parental depression, escape into alcohol, or other forms of psychopathology. Thus, when we find parents who are unhappy, distracted, or avoidant of their child, it is important to recognize that this may be a reaction to the child's difficulties and years of coping with the stress of a chronic disorder.

Ascertainment and Triage

Tic disorders may seem to be particularly related to other mental or behavioral difficulties because of the ways in which patients are referred or decide to come for treatment. Here, comorbidity may be a reflection of the ways in which individuals with problems become defined clinical cases.

Severity and Life-Adjustment Difficulties

Individuals with the worst overall problems—the patient whose brittle diabetes leads to coma, the asthmatic who goes into status—are more likely to come to medical attention than those with milder problems. The patient whose TS is more severe is most likely to have other life problems; these life-adjustment difficulties and severe TS symptoms increase the probability of clinical recognition and going for treatment. In our family studies and in formal epidemiological research, it appears that only a small minority of TS patients (perhaps 10–20%) is diagnosed as such. Undiagnosed patients tend to be those with milder tic syndromes and with less likelihood of having any additional psychiatric problems (23).

Multiplicity of Difficulties, Particularly Those That Disturb Others

When a child has two or more medical problems, he is more likely to be referred for medical attention (e.g., the learning-disabled boy who is also very active is probably more likely to be diagnosed than the quiet, polite fourth-grade girl who seems like such a sweet youngster). Thus, the TS patient with impulsive and rude behavior is more likely to come for care than one with fewer difficulties.

Amplification of the Primary Disorder by the Presence of a Second

Having a second problem may make the first condition more severe and/or more difficult to manage: obesity complicates hypertension; the tensions surrounding severe school problems and failure may exacerbate tics. The compounding of a child's difficulties may reduce resilience and decrease the availability of compensatory processes; these vulnerabilities may lead to increased severity of tics. Just as with Job, when a child has more than one difficulty, he is likely to have three or four: grief begets grief, problems build upon problems, and as the child is worn down, everything becomes worse for him and his family.

Vulnerability and Phenocopies

Tic symptoms are common in patients with other neurological and developmental disorders, such as children with mental retardation, pervasive developmental disorders, and other forms of trauma to the central nervous system (CNS). Such cases of "comorbidity" are increasingly being recognized. A neurological insult may "unmask" a latent vulnerability or may lead to tics in children who have no family history of tics and who might not have developed them. The presence of neurological difficulty also may convert the tendency to have a mild tic disorder (such as recurrent transient tics) into a full-blown case of TS. These tic disorders may be understood as "phenocopies" of TS, or they may actually express the same underlying genetic diathesis.

Variant and Associated Manifestations

Theoretically, the most interesting types of comorbidity are those in which two apparently distinct disorders are intrinsically related to a shared, underlying etiology. An individual patient may have one or both disorders; also, the two disorders may be found in different individuals as "alternative" manifestations of the etiology. In general medicine, comorbidity of this type is common. The associations reflect the expression of the underlying pathogenic mechanism in different tissues [e.g., the expression of autoimmune phenomena in joints, liver, and kidney (as in lupus); the expression of a genetic lesion in muscle and brain (as in muscular dystrophy)]. For tic syndromes, we should thus not be surprised if the underlying genetic and neurobiological vulnerability is expressed in varying motor, vocal, and behavioral manifestations.

Genetic evidence suggests that, at the least, obsessions and compulsions, including OCD, are an alternative manifestation of some of the putative TS vulnerability "genes" (18).

Perhaps 40% of TS patients suffer from obsessions and compulsions, and may be diagnosed as having OCD (24). Family members also have a marked increase in the frequency of OCD, both with and without concomitant tics. Thus, TS and OCD may be comorbid (in the same individual) and may be expressed as variant manifestations of the diathesis in different patients. The genetic association between TS and OCD represents, we believe, one of the most interesting findings of the genetics of psychiatric disorders: the association between the hyperexcitable phenomena of tic disorders and the overly reflective, inhibitory phenomena of OCD. Nowhere in psychiatry are we given a more dramatic example of the psychoanalytical propositions that relate opposite phenomena to a disturbance in an underlying regulatory process, such as the modulation of impulses.

Half of the children with TS seen by us and other clinicians have ADHD (20,21). These common behavioral disturbances relate to the regulation of attention and activity. The symptoms of distractibility, impulsivity, and hyperactivity may originate early in the preschool years and precede the onset of tics. We have felt that the difficulties with inattention appear to reflect the underlying psychobiological dysfunctions involving inhibition in TS and may be exacerbated by the strain in attending to the outer world while working hard to remain quiet and still. We are not sure, however, precisely how the tic disorders and attentional problems are related. There is some evidence that some type of ascertainment bias may be at work: children who have serious overactivity and tics are more likely to be referred for evaluation than children with tics alone. But this is not likely to be the whole story. As clinicians, we are tempted to think that there is some deeper commonality; working in the clinic consulting room and hearing the ways in which overactive children go on to develop tic disorders, we do not feel that ADHD is merely an accidental accompaniment of a tic disorder. The central role of broadly distributed cortical regions and their basal ganglia connections in both TS and ADHD may lead to multiple ways in which these conditions may be related at a neurobiological level (25–28).

As many as one-third of children receiving treatment for TS have serious handicaps in school performance that may justify special intervention. More recent studies from our group have also shown that TS patients with ADHD are far more likely to have serious social troubles. For example, we have found that children with TS and ADHD are, as a group, more than 2 standard deviations below the normal levels for socialization on the Vineland Adaptive Behavior Scales (14). This discrepancy may reflect aspects of their social isolation, adverse experiences, style of care giving they have received, or other manifestations of their underlying diathesis. As a group, children with TS are at risk for school and social troubles; yet many are successful, especially those without ADHD, learning disorders, or personality difficulties (21,22).

Thus, for many reasons, we are likely to see patients in specialty clinics who have serious problems and more than one problem: these children are both (1) more likely to be detected and then (2) more likely to be brought or to come for care. To address their most serious needs, the full range of the patient's difficulties must be assessed. Treatment must be aimed at the most impairing aspects of their problems, which may not be their tic disorder as such.

ASSESSMENT

Clinical evaluation of the child with tics should include an assessment of the child or adolescent as a whole person and not only as someone with tics. In the process of evaluation, the full range of difficulties and competencies can be charted. During the process of evaluation, the clinician, family, and child collaborate in the reconstruction of the child's history, tic symptomatology (onset, progression, waxing and waning, and factors that have worsened or ameliorated tic status), and current functioning. A critical question is the degree to which tics are interfering with the child's emotional, social, familial, and school experiences. To determine this, it is useful to monitor symptoms over a few months in order to assess their severity and fluctuation, impact on the family, and the child's and family's adaptation. This monitoring can be facilitated by the family's keeping records or using standard forms.

The deeply distressed family may emphasize the child's tics; the clinician must recontextualize these symptoms with respect to the child and his overall development (3). Before receiving a diagnosis, the child and family may think the child is "going crazy." By the time of evaluation, the child may be extremely upset by his experiences and by criticism from parents who have scolded, threatened, and perhaps beaten him to stop his strange behavior. A central task of evaluation is to explicate, clarify, and address family issues, including parental guilt. Diagnostic evaluation is closely connected with the first steps of treatment. During the process of clinical inquiry, the physician can approach sensitive issues through clarification, education, and an opening therapeutic discussion with the child and family.

As with other children with school-performance problems, the child with TS requires a careful assessment of cognitive functioning and school achievement. Children with TS tend to have difficulties in attentional deployment, perseverance, and ability to keep themselves and their work organized. Many have poor penmanship. Schoolwork may be impaired by compulsions, such as the need to scratch out words or return to the beginning of a sentence. Some school problems can be handled as academic or remedial issues (e.g., through the use of a typewriter, oral reports, untimed exams, or permission to leave the classroom when tics are severe).

The neurological examination of a child with TS does not often greatly contribute to diagnosis or treatment. Some severely affected patients have immaturities or atypicalities on the neuromaturational examination (so-called soft signs). These may suggest disturbances in the body schema and in the integration of motor control, but their relevance is not really clear. Electroencephalography and structural magnetic resonance imaging are generally normal and are not yet of proven clinical use (except where there are other neurological suspicions). Similarly, laboratory studies may establish a child's general health profile and assist in differential diagnosis of other movement disorders, but there are no laboratory tests for the positive diagnosis of TS or other tic disorders.

A careful assessment will allow the clinician to learn about the fluctuation of symptoms. As the child becomes more comfortable, he will show his symptoms with less suppression or inhibition. Only with trust in the doctor is a child or adult likely to acknowledge the most frightening, ego-dystonic symptoms (e.g., bathroom rituals or aggressive thoughts). Also, a patient or family members may recognize a symptom as a tic after they have been educated about possible symptoms.

The history of patients with long-standing TS is often confused by the use of medications. Often, medications have been stopped because they were thought to have been useless or to have caused side effects. The history of treatments and what they have meant to the child and family can be pieced together during the evaluation. Also, the clinician can learn why earlier therapeutic attempts were not useful. It is common for consulting clinicians to see children and families who have had bad luck with other physicians; these patients present themselves for a new consultation burdened by past failures and with ambivalent (sometimes idealizing but also skeptical) attitudes about what this current consultation will achieve. The consultant gains little from accepting the family's criticism of previous therapists at face value: he may very well join them in the patient's history at some time in the future. Nor should he dismiss previous problems either. Rather, the assessment provides an opportunity to reconstruct the child's past encounters with medical professionals, with the goal of achieving a shared sense of realistic expectations of the current one.

When the child or adolescent and his parents are given enough time, over the course of several sessions, to narrate their experiences, sadness, and disappointments, they may feel that their full story has finally been heard, perhaps for the first time after having seen many physicians. This process of rethinking the past and integrating disparate threads of experience can be therapeutically useful in its own right and may help ease the immediate crisis that led to the consultation. The experience of the therapeutic encounter, of being understood through the diagnostic process, is reassuring. Many patients and families often feel supported, understood, and reassured by hearing a more or less detailed account of our emerging understanding of the pathogenesis and natural history of TS. Knowing that their experience is similar to that of other families and that many of the most puzzling features of the disorder are typical (such as waxing and waning, symptom variation, suppressibility, and premonitory urges) can be enormously reassuring to families.

The current and past impact of medication especially complicates assessment. Today, many children are seen while on medication of various types. The clinician must decide whether more or less medication, or some other medication, is needed. In evaluating a patient who is having severe troubles while on a "lowish" level of a medication, it is difficult to decide whether to increase the dose or stop and observe. The problems are more difficult when the patient has benefited to some degree and is having moderately severe problems that are threatening his retention in school, for example.

Discontinuation of antipsychotics, typical or atypical, may lead to exacerbations or withdrawal-emergent worsening of symptoms for 1 or 2 months or longer. Thus, the child's "real" clinical status may not be visible for quite a while. Some children improve for a few weeks after an antipsychotic medication has been discontinued; they generally then have an exacerbation after another week or so. Side effects, such as cognitive blunting, dullness, amotivational states, fearfulness, social phobias, excessive appetite, and sedation, may lift rather quickly, over days to several weeks; this may happen while emergent tic symptoms remain or become worse.

"Cold-turkey" or rapid withdrawal from clonidine is contraindicated because there may be rebound in both blood pressure and behavioral activity (29). Gradual withdrawal from clonidine and guanfacine over the course of a few weeks is usually not associated with any rebound phenomena.

The decision to discontinue medication is often more difficult than the one to initiate it. Withdrawal must be planned so as to disrupt the child's life as little as possible. Often, families and children will have great difficulty in tolerating the discontinuation and will need the physician's emotional support. We frequently face this problem in adolescents who have been well controlled on medication for several years; they may be anxious about stopping the medication but also eager to see how they are and whether they need medication before going to college. Very often, discontinuation proceeds easily and the patient is gratified to discover that he no longer needs it.

When symptoms are poorly controlled at the time of evaluation, a clinician will have to decide whether to try to "clean out" a child by discontinuing all medications or to change dosages. The presence of serious side effects would probably lead us to attempt detoxification, but only careful assessment of the child's and family's coping and response to intervention can guide the clinician in proceeding down either path.

TREATMENT GUIDELINES AND OPTIONS

The decision about whether to treat will depend not only on the primary diagnosis but on the degree to which the varied tic symptoms interfere with the child's normal development (30). The primary emphasis should be to help the child navigate the normal tasks of development, or the school-aged child to feel competent in school, make friendships, feel trust in his parents, and enjoy life's adventures. Many children with multiple tics or TS do well in moving forward in their development. For them, treatment for tics is generally not indicated. Natural parental upset about the tics requires lengthy, calm discussion and education about available treatments. If treatment is decided upon by the child, family, and physician, developmental issues must constantly be reassessed. A child's tics may be stopped by medication; but, too often, so are his progress in school and achievements in sports. Nothing is gained when unhealthy development is the price for tic amelioration.

Local chapters of patient advocacy organizations such as the Tourette Syndrome Association can play an enormously supportive role by putting families of newly diagnosed children in contact with more experienced families. Parents should be encouraged to build on their child's strengths.

Monitoring

Unless there is an emergency, such as self-injurious behavior or suspension from school because of tics, the clinician can usually follow a patient for several months before a specific treatment plan is instituted. Several goals of this first stage of treatment are to: (1) establish a baseline of symptoms; (2) define associated difficulties in school, family, and peer relationships; (3) obtain medical and psychological tests; (4) monitor the range and fluctuations in symptoms and the contexts of greatest difficulty; (5) and establish a relationship.

Reassurance

It may become apparent that the child's tics are of minimal functional significance. Even if a child satisfies the criteria for TS, he may have good peer relationships, school achievement, and sense of himself, and no treatment may be needed. If parents have read about TS, they may be worried about the child's future. In general, by the time a child has had TS for 2–3 years, one can guess with some degree of accuracy how severe the disorder ultimately will be. Thus, for a 13-year-old boy with mild TS that first appeared at age 7, one can reassure the family that it probably will become no worse than what they have already seen. On such occasions, we tend to tell families that their child's TS is unlikely to be as severe or take the same form as TS cases they might have heard about. For transient single tics, such reassurance is fully appropriate. Because of the clear genetic factors involved in TS, families deserve to be advised of the emerging knowledge in this area even if they are reassured about the nature of their child's disorder.

Psychotherapy

Individual psychotherapy may be useful for children with TS, just as for children with other medical problems who have personality and adjustment difficulties, difficult peer relationships, depression, anxiety, etc. As a rule, tics are not responsive to psychotherapy and should not be the target of treatment. Parent support groups and family therapy may help families of children with TS. In addition, investigators have used a number of specific behavioral techniques (e.g., habit reversal, hypnotherapy, relaxation, and biofeedback techniques), and there is a growing utilization of alternative treatments (e.g., acupuncture and dietary supplements). These interventions may be useful for some individuals, but systematic clinical trials have not been undertaken. Specific cognitive behavioral techniques (e.g., exposure and response prevention training) have proven to be useful for selected patients with TS who present with OCD.

School Interventions

Children with attentional and learning problems require educational interventions similar to those used in the treatment of other forms of ADHD and learning disabilities. TS patients may benefit from tutoring, a learning laboratory, a self-contained classroom, or a special school, depending on the severity of academic and associated behavioral problems. Since TS is uncommon, school personnel need to be informed about the symptoms of TS, the child's inability to suppress symptoms, the ways in which he might deal with bouts of tics (e.g., by leaving the room), the use of prosthetic devices (such as a computer for poor handwriting), and the puzzling nature of OCD symptoms, which may block or interfere with a child's performance. Over the past several years, internet web sites have also appeared that contain valuable compilations of recommendations for parents and teachers including "Tourette Syndrome 'Plus'" developed by Leslie E. Packer, Ph.D., and located at:

<http://www.tourettesyndrome.net/> and "Tourette, Now What?" located at <http://tourettenowwhat.tripod.com/>. *Teaching the Tiger: A Handbook for Individuals Involved in the Education of Students with Attention Deficit Disorder, Tourette Syndrome or Obsessive Compulsive Disorder* (Hope Press, 1995) is an excellent resource for parents and educators.

Children with TS are sometimes forced to be homebound because their symptoms (e.g., coprolalia, explosive yelling, touching others) are too disruptive for the classroom. Phonic and behavioral symptoms are most difficult for schools. Being homebound is an emergency situation and demands medical and legal intervention. When a child is at home and deprived of school, his TS symptoms are likely to be further exacerbated; the child may exert less control over his symptoms, feel bored without outside diversion, and become locked in heatedly ambivalent interactions with parents. A chain reaction may be ignited: bad symptoms lead to worse symptoms and increasing isolation from normal forces of socialization. Even more than tics, school difficulties and appropriate school placement require prompt clinical intervention, sometimes including hospitalization.

Hospitalization

Short-term hospitalization may be useful during extreme crises. However, TS patients may be unwelcome on an inpatient neurology or psychiatry service because of their disruptive and bizarre behavior. The availability of an inpatient service willing to accept a TS patient in crisis can be reassuring for both the patient and the physician. It is nice to have such a unit in reserve when one is managing the reduction of medication or working with a particularly behaviorally disordered adolescent.

Pharmacotherapy

Many cases of uncomplicated TS can be successfully managed with just these interventions and do not require anti-tic medication. When patients present with coexisting ADHD, OCD and/or depression, it is often better to treat these "comorbid" conditions first, as successful treatment of these disorders will often diminish tic severity.

Ideal anti-tic treatments are not currently available. None of the agents or techniques can be effectively used just when tics are at their worst. Most of the available pharmacological agents require long-term treatment, and many have potentially serious side effects. Indeed, for some medications, it is much easier to commence their use than to stop them. The natural waxing and waning pattern of tics frequently confounds the results of medication trials. Even without intervention, periods of severe tics will be followed by a period of spontaneous waning. Because tic-suppressant medication often requires several weeks to have its full effect, it is often difficult to distinguish a therapeutic response to medication from a spontaneous waning of symptoms. As a result, it is usually best to avoid beginning or increasing medication as soon as an exacerbation begins. There are several partially effective pharmacological treatments for tic disorders and associated conditions. In deciding on the use of medication, the benefits for the child in relation to the reduction of tics must be weighed against short- and long-term problems, both biological and developmental, to which medication may expose him.

Nonetheless, the presence of severe tics may limit the child's social world, impair his sense of control over what is inside, and lead to painful social and emotional scarring. The use of medication may have considerable positive impact on the child's feelings of self-control, self-esteem, and social acceptance. Yet medication may also alter how a child's body feels to him and how he experiences the working of his mind, single out a child in school, alter his daily schedule, and focus parental and other adult concern on small changes in symptoms and side effects.

Two general classes of medication are most widely used to control tics associated with TS—α_2-adrenergic agonists and antipsychotics. Guanfacine and clonidine are two α_2-adrenergic agents originally developed as antihypertensive agents in adults. In low doses, clonidine reduces central noradrenergic activity by stimulating presynaptic α_2-adrenergic autoreceptors; guanfacine is believed to act more selectively on postsynaptic α_2-adrenergic receptors in the prefrontal cortex. First introduced in 1979 (31), the use of these agents is supported by randomized, placebo-controlled clinical trials (32–34). However, this support is not uniform (35,36). Although they are generally not as potent as the antipsychotics in suppressing tics, guanfacine and clonidine are more benign in terms of potential short- and long-term side effects and are often the first choice in previously untreated individuals, especially those with mild-to-moderate symptoms. Treatment with these agents is usually initiated at a low dose and gradually titrated upward. Beginning with a morning dose of 0.025 or 0.05 mg of clonidine, additional doses are added at 3- to 4-hr intervals. The size of each dose may be gradually titrated upward to a total dose of 0.2–0.3 mg daily. Although the effect of each individual dose of clonidine appears to wear off after about 3–5 hr, the full tic-suppressant effects of the regimen may require 10–12 weeks to be apparent. Guanfacine is longer acting than clonidine but is titrated in a similar fashion in a range of 0.25–1.0 mg two or three times a day. The principal side effect of clonidine and guanfacine in the recommended dose range is sedation, sometimes accompanied by irritability. This unwanted effect may require dose reduction or a change of medication. Reversible cardiac arrhythmias have been infrequently reported with clonidine; however, the need for electrocardiographic studies at baseline and once a stable dose level is reached remains controversial. Hypotension has not been a common problem in children taking these agents. If a decision is made to discontinue these medications, gradual tapering over a week or two is advisable to avoid tic flare-ups or rebound hypertension.

Several typical and atypical antipsychotics are commonly used for treating TS, especially those patients with more severe tics or those whose tic symptoms are unresponsive to an adequate trial with an α_2-adrenergic agonist. The efficacy of antipsychotic agents appears to be related to their potency in blocking postsynaptic dopamine-2 (D2) receptors. Pimozide, haloperidol, and tiapride are the most commonly used typical neuroleptic antipsychotics, while risperidone and ziprasidone are two atypical antipsychotics with demonstrated tic-suppressant efficacy (37–43). It is best to start out with a low daily dose and gradually titrate upward. The use of high doses of these agents rarely produces additional improvement in tics and very often produces bothersome side effects. Withdrawal from antipsychotics can produce tic exacerbations and dyskinesias that may be delayed in onset by several weeks. Although antipsychotics are widely prescribed for patients with TS, many patients are noncompliant. The most common, dose-related side effects are sedation or dysphoria. Weight gain is also a problem with most of these agents, especially risperidone. Some children taking antipsychotics develop de novo separation anxiety and school refusal. Although the atypical antipsychotics are believed to have a lower risk of tardive dyskinesia, acute extrapyramidal reactions (e.g., torticollis, oculogyric crisis, akathisia) may occur and may require anticholinergic medication. Because of potential QT changes, baseline and follow-up electrocardiography is recommended for risperidone, ziprasidone, and pimozide. It is also essential for the prescribing clinician to be familiar with potential cytochrome P-450-related drug interactions, because fatal interactions have occurred with pimozide- and erythromycin-related antibiotics.

Nicotinic agents, particularly in combination with antipsychotic medication, have shown some promise in clinical trials (44,45). Other agents with some promise include low doses of pergolide, a mixed D1–D2–D3 dopamine receptor agonist (46), as well as locally injected dilute botulinum toxin (47). Remarkably, some patients report a marked reduction in the premonitory sensory urges following local injections of botulinum toxin.

The treatment of ADHD in patients with a personal history of tics is common, complex, and controversial. In addition to classroom and behavioral interventions at home (e.g., parent management training and behavioral management is often very important especially when the child manifests disruptive behavioral problems), clinicians often find medications to be helpful in treating this condition. Psychostimulants, such as methylphenidate, dextroamphetamine, and related agents, are the most effective agents for uncomplicated ADHD. Although these drugs may be used with impunity in some individuals with tics, in a small percentage of cases, they can precipitate de novo tics or exacerbate pre-existing tics in some individuals with TS. Consequently many clinicians will begin with clonidine or guanfacine, which, although not as potent as the stimulants, appear less prone to exacerbating tics (32–34). One recent large-scale, double blind clinical trial found that the combination of clonidine and methylphenidate was most efficacious in treating ADHD (34). Of interest, this study reported that these two agents had differential effects—with clonidine being most helpful for impulsivity and hyperactivity, and methylphenidate being most helpful for symptoms of inattention.

Serotonin-reuptake inhibitors are often useful in treating the OCD symptoms found in TS, but may not produce as full a therapeutic response (48). Augmentation with a low dose of an antipsychotic may increase these agents' antiobsessional efficacy (49,50). At higher dose levels, the serotonin-reuptake inhibitors may occasionally precipitate or exacerbate tics.

Although it has been proposed that some cases of TS may be a sequela of group A beta-hemolytic streptococcus infections, this connection remains controversial and is likely to be a contributing mechanism in only a minority of TS cases (51). Antibiotic prophylaxis and arduous investigational interventions such as plasma exchange or intravenous immunoglobulins have been successfully used in a small number of cases with well-documented exacerbations following streptococcal infection (52,53). Such measures should be considered only with expert child psychiatric and pediatric consultation. At present, the principal mandate for the clinician is to be vigilant in assessing children with pharyngitis or those exposed to streptococcus and vigorously treating and following up those with positive throat culture results.

The decision to stop medication is as important and complex as the decision to start. Many factors need to be considered: the child's short- and long-term response, the side-effect profile, the severity of tics and associated symptoms, school performance, social relationships, the level of current chronic and acute stressors, and patient and parental attitudes about the medication. Generally, if a child has had an adequate response to a medication and side effects are minimal, we consider dosage reduction or discontinuation after a full year or 18 months on a medication. A shorter duration of treatment may not give the child time to make the social, academic, and emotional gains that may be possible following medication-induced reduction of symptoms.

CONCLUSIONS

From the clinical perspective, particularly the view from the child psychiatric specialty clinic, TS can be conceptualized as a persistent and often lifelong disorder that places a child at developmental risk for other emotional, behavioral, and developmental difficulties. Simple motor and phonic tics generally interfere less with development than complex tics and associated obsessive–compulsive, attentional, and behavioral problems. TS is a serious disorder and deserves the kind of meticulous, intensive evaluation that physicians offer to other children with very long-term disturbances. Clinical evaluation must include careful attention to the way the child is developing as a whole person at home, in school, and in his personal, emotional life. The process of evaluation is closely related to the design of a systematic intervention. The major goal of intervention is not solely to ameliorate tics, but to help the child and family maintain a positive outlook and sustain the child's normal developmental trajectory insofar as is possible. The whole range of child psychiatric modalities may be enlisted for children and their families: education, reassurance and support, guidance and advocacy in relation to appropriate school placement, psychotherapy, and medication if needed. In conducting an assessment and guiding a child's treatment, target symptoms should include not only motor and phonic symptoms but the child's and adolescent's full range of functioning and development. The major goal of treatment is to help the child succeed in moving along the various lines of development. The use of medication that interferes with these achievements runs the risk of creating patients who are socially more disadvantaged than had they been left untreated. Taking psychoactive medications for many years poses many medical and behavioral toxicological risks.

Family therapy, psychotherapy, and behavior modification approaches have limited value in regard to the motor and phonic tics. They may be invaluable in helping children deal with the behavioral and psychological problems that may compound TS, or be elicited in a family because of the stress of living with a beloved child who is suffering from a chronic neuropsychiatric disorder. As with any chronic disorder, periods of exacerbation are likely to lead to anxiety, stress, and lowered mood, which may further exacerbate the condition. The clinician's availability and a long-standing relationship are especially important at such times. One reassuring fact for families and patients with TS is that the disorder has become an area of active clinical research interest. The detection, cloning, and understanding of the gene(s) underlying TS will lead to profound increases in our knowledge of the pathogenesis and treatment of this complex developmental disorder. As our understanding increases, the clinician who works with individual families will continue to play important roles as educator, guide, and translator of research into clinical practice. The clinician will also help advance the field of knowledge by careful clinical description of natural history, asking questions of researchers, and testing out new hypotheses about the nature and treatment of TS in the actual experience of clinical work.

ACKNOWLEDGMENTS

This chapter is dedicated to the memory of Donald J. Cohen and his tireless efforts on behalf of children with Tourette's syndrome. Donald's voice and wisdom echo through the prose of this chapter. He was a passionate man who cared deeply about the need to see the child, despite the tics and other behavioral problems. We are most appreciative of our patients who have taught much of what we know of this condition, and our colleagues in the Child Study Center Tic Disorder Specialty Clinic, particularly the clinicians who provide continuity of care including Drs. Diane Findley, Larry Scahill, Robert King, Paul Lombroso, and Ms. Eileen Hanrahan. The research was supported by the National Institutes of Health (MH-49351, MH-30929, and RR-00125). We are particularly grateful for the support of the Gateposts Foundation and the Tourette Syndrome Association.

REFERENCES

1. Leckman JF, Cohen DJ. Tourette's Syndrome: Tics, Obsessions, Compulsions—Developmental Psychopathology and Clinical Care. New York: John Wiley and Sons, 1998.
2. Cohen DJ, Goetz C, Jankovic J, eds. Tourette Syndrome. New York: Lippincott, Williams & Wilkins, 2001.
3. Cohen DJ, Ort SI, Leckman JF, Riddle NM, Hardin MT. Family functioning in Tourette's syndrome. In: Cohen DJ, Bruun RD, Leckman JF, eds. Tourette's Syndrome and Tic Disorders: Clinical Understanding and Treatment. New York: Wiley, 1988:179–196.
4. Bliss J. Sensory experiences in Gilles de la Tourette's syndrome. Arch Gen Psychiatry 1980; 37:1343–1347.
5. Kurlan R, Lichter D, Hewitt D. Sensory tics in Tourette's syndrome. Neurology 1989; 39:731–734.
6. Leckman JF, Walker DE, Cohen DJ. Premonitory urges in Tourette's syndrome. Am J Psychiatry 1993; 150:98–102.
7. Leckman JF, Walker WK, Goodman WK, Pauls DL, Cohen DJ. "Just right" perceptions associated with compulsive behaviors in Tourette's syndrome. Am J Psychiatry 1994; 151:675–680.
8. Lin HQ, Yeh C-B, Peterson BS, Scahill L, Grantz H, Findley D, Katsovich L, Otka J, Lombroso PJ, King RA, Leckman, JF. Assessment of symptom exacerbations in a longitudinal study of children with Tourette syndrome or obsessive–compulsive disorder. J Am Acad Child Adolescent Psychiatry. In press.
9. Peterson BS, Leckman JF. Temporal characterization of tics in Gilles de la Tourette's syndrome. Biol Psychiatry 1998; 44:1337–1348.
10. Cohen DJ. Tourette's Syndrome: Developmental Psychopathology of a Model Neuropsychiatric Disorder of Childhood. 27th Annual Institute of Pennsylvania Hospital Award Lecture in Memory of A. Edward, Strecker, 1990.

11. Cohen DJ. Finding meaning in one's self and others: clinical studies of children with autism and Tourette's syndrome. In: Kessel F, Bornstein M, Sameroff A, eds. Contemporary Constructions of the Child: Essays in Honor of William Kessen. Hillsdale, NJ: Lawrence Eribaurn Associates, 1991:159–175.
12. Stokes A, Bawden HN, Carnfield PR, Backman JE, Dooley JM. Peer problems in Tourette's disorder. Pediatrics 1991; 87(6):936–942.
13. Bawden HN, Stokes A, Camfield CS, Camfield PR, Salisbury S. Peer relationship problems in children with Tourette's disorder or diabetes mellitus. J Child Psychol Psychiatry 1998; 39(5):663–668.
14. Carter AS, O'Donnell DA, Schultz RT, Scahill L, Leckman JF, Pauls DL. Social and emotional adjustment in children affected with Gilles de la Tourette's syndrome: associations with ADHD and family functioning. J Child Psychol Psychiatry 2000; 41:215–223.
15. Swerdlow NR, Karban B, Ploum Y, Sharp R, Geyer MA, Eastvold A. Tactile prepuff inhibition of startle in children with Tourette's syndrome: in search of an "fMRI-friendly" startle paradigm. Biol Psychiatry 2001; 50(8):578–585.
16. Leckman JF, King RA, Cohen DJ. Tics and tic disorders. In: Leckman JF, Cohen DJ, eds. Tourette's Syndrome Tics, Obsessions, Compulsions—Developmental Psychopathology and Clinical Care. New York: John Wiley and Sons, 1998:23–42.
17. Leckman JF, Zhang H, Vitale A, Lahnin F, Lynch K, Bondi C, Kim Y-S, Peterson BS. Course of tic severity in Tourette's syndrome: the first two decades. Pediatrics 1998; 102:14–19.
18. Pauls DL, Leckman JF. The inheritance of Gilles de la Tourette syndrome and associated behaviors: Evidence for autosomal dominant transmission. N Engl J Med 1986; 315:993–997.
19. Kurlan R, Behr J, Medved L, Shoulson I, Pauls D, Kidd KK. Severity of Tourette's syndrome in one large kindred. Implication for determination of disease prevalence rate. Arch Neurol 1987; 44(3):268–269.
20. Spencer T, Biederman J, Harding M, O'Donnell D, Wilens T, Faraone S, Coffey B, Geller D. Disentangling the overlap between Tourette's disorder and ADHD. J Child Psychol Psychiatry 1998; 39(7):1037–1044.
21. Sukhodolsky DG, Scahill L, Zhang H, Peterson BS, King RA, Lombroso PJ, Katsovich L, Findley D, Leckman JF. Disruptive behavior in children with Tourette's syndrome: association with ADHD comorbidity, tic severity and functional outcome. Submitted.
22. Peterson BS, Pine DS, Cohen P, Brook JS. Prospective, longitudinal study of tic, obsessive–compulsive, and attention-deficit/hyperactivity disorders in an epidemiological sample. J Am Acad Child Adolesc Psychiatry 2001; 40(6):685–695.
23. Hornse H, Banerjee S, Zeitlin H, Robertson M. The prevalence of Tourette syndrome in 13–14-year-olds in mainstream schools. J Child Psychol Psychiatry 2001; 42(8):1035–1039.
24. King RA, Leckman JF, Scahill LD, Cohen DJ. Obsessive–compulsive disorder, anxiety, and depression. In: Leckman JF, Cohen DJ, eds. Tourette's Syndrome

Tics, Obsessions, Compulsions—Developmental Psychopathology and Clinical Care. New York: John Wiley and Sons, 1998:43–62.

25. Leckman JF, Riddle MA. Tourette's syndrome: when habit forming units form habits of their own? Neuron 2000; 28(2):349–354.
26. Peterson BS, Skudlarski P, Anderson AW, Zhang H, Gatenby JC, Lacadie CM, Leckman JF, Gore JC. A functional magnetic resonance imaging study of tic suppression in Tourette syndrome. Arch Gen Psychiatry 1998; 55:326–333.
27. Peterson BS, Staib L, Scahill L, Zhang H, Anderson C, Leckman JF, Cohen DJ, Gore JC, Albert J, Webster R. Regional and ventricular volumes in Tourette syndrome. Arch Gen Psychiatry 2001; 58:427–442.
28. Peterson BS, Thomas P, Kane MJ, Scahill L, Zhang H, Bronen R, King RA, Leckman JF, Staib L. Basal ganglia volumes in Tourette syndrome. Arch Gen Psychiatry. In press.
29. Leckrnan JF, Ort SI, Cohen DJ, Caruso KA, Anderson GM, Riddle MA. Rebound phenomena in Tourette's syndrome after abrupt withdrawal with clonidine: Behavioral, cardiovascular and neurochemical effects. Arch Gen Psychiatry 1986; 43:1168–1176.
30. Cohen DJ, Leckman JF, Shaywitz BA. The Tourette syndrome and other tics. In: Shaffer D, Ehrhardt A, Greenhill L, eds. The Clinical Guide to Child Psychiatry. New York: The Free Press, 1985:3–28.
31. Cohen DJ, Young JG, Nathanson JA, Shaywitz BA. Clonidine in Tourette's syndrome. Lancet 1979; ii:551.
32. Leckman JF, Hardin MT, Riddle MA, Stevenson J, Ort SI, Cohen DJ. Clonidine treatment of Tourette's syndrome. Arch Gen Psychiatry 1991; 48, 324–328.
33. Scahill L, Chappell PB, Kim YS, Schultz RT, Katsovich L, Shepherd E, Ansten AF, Cohen DJ, Leckman JF. Guanfacine in the treatment of children with tic disorders and ADHD: a placebo-controlled study. Am J Psychiatry 2001; 158:1067–1074.
34. Tourette Syndrome Study GroupTreatment of ADHD in children with tics: a randomized controlled trial. Neurology 2002; 58:527–536.
35. Goetz CG, Tanner CM, Wilson RS, Carroll VS, Como PG, Shannon KM. Clonidine and Gilles de la Tourette's syndrome: double-blind study using objective rating methods. Ann Neurol 1987; 21:307–310.
36. Singer HS, Brown J, Quaskey S, Rosenberg LA, Mellits ED, Denckla MB. The treatment of attention-deficit hyperactivity disorder in Tourette's syndrome: a double-blind placebo-controlled study with clonidine and desipramine. Pediatrics 1995; 95:74–81.
37. Shapiro AK, Shapiro E. Controlled study of pimozide vs. placebo in Tourette's syndrome. J Am Acad Child Psychiatry 1984; 23:161–173.
38. Eggers C, Rothenberger A, Berghaus U. Clinical and neurobiological findings in children suffering from tic disease following treatment with tiapride. Eur Arch Psychiatry Neurol Sci 1988; 237:223–229.
39. Shapiro E, Shapiro AK, Fulop G, Hubbard M, Mandeli J, Nordlie J, Phillips RA. Controlled study of haloperidol, pimozide and placebo for the treatment of Gilles de la Tourette's syndrome. Arch Gen Psychiatry 1989; 46:722–730.

40. Sallee FR, Nesbitt L, Jackson C, Sine L, Sethuraman G. Relative efficacy of haloperidol and pimozide in children and adolescents with Tourette's disorder. Am J Psychiatry 1997; 154:1057–1062.
41. Sallee FR, Kurlan R, Goetz CG, Singer H, Scahill L, Law G, Dittman VM, Chappell PB. Ziprasidone treatment of children and adolescents with Tourette's syndrome: a pilot study. J Am Acad Child Adolesc Psychiatry 2000; 39:292–299.
42. Bruggeman R, van der Linden C, Buitelaar JK, Gericke GS, Hawkridge SM, Temlett JA. Risperidone versus pimozide in Tourette's disorder: a comparative double-blind parallel-group study. J Clin Psychiatry 2001; 62:50–56.
43. Scahill L, Leckman JF, Schultz RT, Katsovich L, Peterson BS. A placebo-controlled trial of risperidone in Tourette syndrome. J Am Acad Child Adolesc Psychiatry. In press.
44. Silver AA, Shytle RD, Philipp MK, Wilkinson BJ, McConville B, Sanberg PR. Transdermal nicotine and haloperidol in Tourette's disorder: a double-blind placebo-controlled study. J Clin Psychiatry 2001; 62:707–714.
45. Silver AA, Shytle RD, Sheehan KH, Sheehan DV, Ramos A, Sanberg PR. Multicenter, double-blind, placebo-controlled study of mecamylamine monotherapy for Tourette's disorder. J Am Acad Child Adolesc Psychiatry 2001; 40:1103–1110.
46. Gilbert DL, Sethuraman G, Sine L, Peters S, Sallee FR. Tourette's syndrome improvement with pergolide in a randomized, double-blind, crossover trial. Neurology 2000; 54:1310–1315.
47. Marras C, Andrews D, Sime E, Lang AE. Botulinum toxin for simple motor tics: a randomized, double-blind, controlled clinical trial. Neurology 2001; 56:605–610.
48. McDougle CJ, Goodman WK, Leckman JF, Barr LC, Heninger GR, Price LH. The efficacy of fluvoxamine in obsessive–compulsive disorder: effects of comorbid chronic tic disorder. J Clin Psychopharmacol 1993; 13:354–358.
49. McDougle CJ, Fleischmann RL, Epperson CN, Wasylink S, Leckman JF, Price LH. Haloperidol addition in fluvoxamine-refractory obsessive–compulsive disorder. A double-blind, placebo-controlled study in patients with and without tics. Arch Gen Psychiatry 1994; 51:302–308.
50. McDougle CJ, Epperson CN, Pelton GH, Wasylink S, Price LH. A double-blind, placebo-controlled study of risperidone addition in serotonin reuptake inhibitor-refractory obsessive–compulsive disorder. Arch Gen Psychiatry 2000; 57:794–801.
51. Singer HS, Giuliano JD, Zimmerman AM, Walkup JT. Infection: a stimulus for tic disorders. Pediatr Neurol 2000; 22:380–383.
52. Perlmutter SJ, Leitman SF, Garvey MA, Hamburger S, Feldman E, Leonard HL, Swedo SE. Therapeutic plasma exchange and intravenous immunoglobulin for obsessive–compulsive disorder and tic disorders in childhood. Lancet 1999; 354:1153–1158.
53. Garvey MA, Perlmutter SJ, Allen AJ, Hamburger S, Lougee L, Leonard HL, Witowski ME, Dubbert B, Swedo SE. A pilot study of penicillin prophylaxis for neuropsychiatric exacerbations triggered by streptococcal infections. Biol Psychiatry 1999; 45:1564–1571.

26

Tourette's Syndrome

A Human Condition

Oliver Sacks
Albert Einstein College of Medicine
Bronx, New York, U.S.A.

When I went to the First International Scientific Symposium on Tourette Syndrome in 1981, I went with a patient [whom I wrote about in "Witty Ticcy Ray" (1)]—a patient who over the years had become a friend. "That's terrific stuff they're presenting," he said to me at the end of the first day, "but it gives *no idea* of what Tourette's is actually like" (2).

I had (and expressed) somewhat similar thoughts myself, when I was invited to the Second International Scientific Symposium in Boston this year. There have been astounding advances in chemistry, pharmacology, neuroimaging, and genetics—and all of these were potently synthesized at the symposium. And yet, it seemed to me, there were other, no less essential, aspects of Tourette's syndrome that were completely ignored, and this became apparent whenever one encountered, among the throng of researchers on Tourette's, an occasional person who actually *had it*. I spent hours surreptitiously glancing at one such person—a colleague, as it turned out, a surgeon with Tourette's (but one who shows not a trace of it, has no impulse to it, when he is operating). I wished I knew more of him, because he himself showed me, showed us, by the sheer density of his presence, what Tourette's was actually like—and how thin and reductive our formulations were.

Gilles de la Tourette himself, and his teacher Charcot, a century ago, were intensely aware of the complexity of phenomenal reality—they did not limit their observations to the "pathognomonic" or the "diagnostic"; they were not constrained by DSM-III criteria—they tried to see everything, every phenomenon, that occurred in Tourette's syndrome; and they were prepared, in principle, to go outside the clinic, to see how life actually appeared to, and was lived by, a person with Tourette's. And they expressed their observations in beautiful, clear language—above all, in *narratives*, because one requires a narrative (as opposed to an itemization or checklist) to convey the full complexity and vicissitudes of a life.

These great lessons are all but forgotten today. The great neuropsychologist A. R. Luria, who was born at the turn of the century, born into a great clinical tradition, was extremely conscious of the change in medicine that had occurred in his lifetime, and spoke of it poignantly in the last year of his life (3):

> Since the beginning of this century there has been enormous technical progress, which has changed the very structure of the scientific enterprise.... Reductionism, the effort to reduce complex phenomena to their elementary particles, became the leading principle of scientific efforts. In psychology, it seemed that by reducing psychological events to elementary physiological ones, we could attain the ultimate explanation of human behavior.... In this atmosphere, the rich and complex picture of human behavior which had existed in the nineteenth century disappeared....The physicians of our time, having a battery of auxiliary aids and tests, frequently overlook clinical reality.... Physicians who are great observers and great thinkers have gradually disappeared.... In the previous century, when auxiliary laboratory methods were rare, the art of clinical observation and description reached its height. One is not able to read the clinical descriptions of the great physicians J. Lourdat, A. Trousseau, P. Marie, J. Charcot, Wernicke, Korsakoff, Head and A. Meyer, without seeing the beauty of the art of science. Now this art of observation and description is nearly lost.

All this seems to me very pertinent to what one could observe at the Second International Scientific Symposium, and what, by and large, has distinguished the current explosion in our knowledge and understanding of Tourette's. We have made enormous advances in the "hard science" of Tourette's, but we have almost lost sight of the overall picture—which Ben van de Wetering expresses so well when he calls Tourette's not just a disease, but "a whole mode of being" (personal communication).

If one is to really understand Tourette's (short of having it, like my surgeon colleague, when one *really* understands it), one must take off one's white coat, and go out of the clinic, and share some real life—as a participant-observer—with a Touretter.* Then, at once, one sees many other things, one appreciates that there is not only a neuroanatomy of Tourette's, but a neuroanthropology as well—and one that is no less important, no less scientific, than the neuroanatomy. If one spends time with Touretters, one may observe that they face special difficulties and challenges in boundary situations—entering or leaving houses, bathrooms, cars, etc. One cannot comprehend this without analyzing the nature of "inside" and "outside," of personal "place" and "boundary," and what these may mean for a human being. Thus, for example, if one dines with a Touretter, one may observe, perhaps, that he has to sit in a corner—and that if he does not, he is not merely uncomfortable, but may reach out violently, "ticcily," convulsively, to try to touch people sitting behind him, to bridge the space between him and them. One sees that situatedness in physical and social space has an enormous influence on Tourette's, that Tourette's is partly *about* just this, and one's reactions to the remoteness or proximity of other objects and (especially) people. Thus one is forced to give up the pathologizing notion that Tourette's is merely "tics," produced by short circuits or sparks in the brain, and to see it as a complex behavior—a behavior that may be of great ontogenetic and phylogenetic antiquity.

One may see, in relaxed social settings, innumerable forms of Tourettic humor, clowning, and play; a certain phantasmagoric license or playfulness is of the essence of Tourette's, and well described in autobiographical accounts such as "Les confidences d'un ticqueur" (5)—but it is not something that is likely to occur in the severe and test-oriented setting of a clinic. This play, which may reach surrealistic heights, while it has a perseverative quality reminiscent of *witzelsucht*, has a complex psychological structure akin to that of wit and dreams, and requires an analysis no less complex than they do.

Such an analysis cannot be merely psychodynamic or Freudian, for although the phenomena of Tourette's are sometimes Freudian, they are never merely so. The neurodynamics of Tourette's are no less important—and are characteristically (as Luria has remarked of such processes) accelerated, unselective, highly stimulus-bound, perceptually driven, and field-dependent. One has to observe every tic, every touch, every movement, every noise, every (enacted) perception and mental process, as a *reaction*, however accelerated and distorted, to some outer or inner stimulus impinging upon the sensorium or psyche of the Touretter. This may involve observing dozens of reactions at

*I did, subsequently, spend several days with my Tourettic colleague, and have written about him and his life at length (4).

once, proceeding in functional dissociation and simultaneously, and sometimes in a time frame to be measured in a few hundredths of a second. Such observation is obviously beyond the unaided perceptual and memory capacities of an observer—and it is necessary, therefore, to supplement these by high-speed videotaping or cinematography, and to examine the resultant record frame by frame, in order to miss nothing of the complexity involved. With this, one may achieve a microscopy of mind such as Freud and Luria dreamed of, but never achieved. Tourette's makes such a microscopy possible (see also Ref. 6).

What we may see, in the more extravagant sorts of Tourettic play, is something akin to a public dream—a continuous incorporation of sights, sounds, noises, and words from the outside, and their reciprocal projection, oneirically and Tourettishly transformed, *upon* the outside. One patient, a young woman in Holland, told me, "There is something primal, something Ur, in Tourette's—whatever I perceive or think or feel is instantly transformed into movements and sounds." She enjoyed this rushing stream; she felt it was "like life itself," but acknowledged that it could cause much trouble in social settings.

Indeed, Tourette's, in its effects, is never confined to the person, but spreads out and involves others, and their reactions; and they in turn exert pressure—often disapproving, sometimes violent—on those with Tourette's. Tourette's cannot be studied or understood in isolation, as a "syndrome" confined to the person of those affected; it invariably has social consequences, and comes to include and incorporate these, as part of itself. What one sees finally, therefore, is not just some sort of neurological emission (like chorea), but a complex negotiation between the affected individual and his world, a form of adaptation sometimes humorous and benign, at other times charged with conflict, pain, anxiety, and rage.

One could multiply such observations a thousandfold; the phenomenology of Tourette's is limitless. What is crucial, to my mind, is that the observer–thinker confront the *whole* picture, which is never just a mass of symptoms, dispositions, or behaviors, but an entire identity—an identity that may have been present since earliest life, that has wound itself around and interwoven itself in personal identity, to such an extent that it is no longer clear, sometimes, what is Tourette's, what is person; the Tourette's may be personalized, the person Tourettized. (This is so, to some extent, with all illness and dispositions.)

And these reactions and interactions, these identity formations, are not just intrapsychic—they affect the families, the friends, the communities of Touretters; thus the would-be neuroanthropologist of Tourette's must study not just an individual, but a whole society, the attitudes and reactions of which get internalized in each patient. When one young woman I know with

Tourette's finds herself under increasing social pressure, she yells, "Hurry up! Hurry up!," and even when the external pressure is over, she continues to yell this, Tourettishly—the hurry of the world now a part of her Tourette's. Thus, it is not sufficient to look just at "Tourette's syndrome," as a cluster of neurological or neuropsychiatric abnormalities; one has to examine the Tourettic *life*, the totality of all that it involves and produces and inflicts; one must see it not only in neurological, but in human and existential terms.

Luria liked to speak of "classical" vs. "romantic" science; classical scholars, he writes (3):

> look upon events in terms of their constituent parts. . .single out important units and elements until they can formulate abstract, general laws. . .. One outcome of this approach is the reduction of living reality with all its richness of detail to abstract schemas. The properties of the living whole are lost. . ..Romantic scholars' traits, attitudes and strategies are just the opposite. . .. [They] want neither to split living reality into its elementary components, nor to represent the wealth of life's concrete events in abstract models that lose the properties of the phenomena themselves. It is of the utmost importance to romantics to preserve the wealth of living reality, and they aspire to a science that retains this richness.

Luria wondered, throughout his life—he died in 1977—whether any conjunction could be made between the classical and the romantic approaches. Sadly, he did not live to see this occur. But in the last 15 years, at every level from cosmology to chaos theory to paleontology to Edelman's theory of neural Darwinism, there has been the emergence of a new sort of science, a global science, a science of complexity, which endeavors to avoid a bit-by-bit reductionism, and to see complex processes, and living processes, in their full interactive complexity, as a whole. This is the prospect, I think, that now faces all of us who are interested in Tourette's—we must continue a meticulous investigation of its chemical and physiological and genetic determinants, but see it also in its full complexity, as a mode of being, as a form of life, as a whole. We must see Tourette's as a window, not merely on the pathophysiology of the basal ganglia and diencephalon, but on what it means to be human, and to live in the world.

REFERENCES

1. Sacks O, Witty Ticcy Ray. The Man who Mistook his Wife for a Hat. New York: Summit Books, 1986.
2. Sacks OW. Acquired Tourettism in adult life, presented at First International

Scientific Symposium, New York, 1981. In: Friedhoff AJ, Chase TN, eds. Gilles de la Tourette Syndrome. New York: Raven Press, 1982.
3. Luria AR. In: Cole M, Cole S, eds. The Meaning of Mind. Cambridge: Harvard University Press, 1979.
4. Sacks O. A surgeon's life. The New Yorker. March 16, 1992; 85–94.
5. Meige H, Feindel E. Les Tics et leur Traitement. Paris: Masson, 1902.
6. Sacks O. Neuropsychiatry and Tourette's. In: Mueller J, ed. Neurology and Psychiatry: A Meeting of Minds. Basel: Karger, 1989.

27

The Tourette Syndrome Association, Inc.

Sue Levi-Pearl
Tourette Syndrome Association, Inc.
Bayside, New York, U.S.A.

INTRODUCTION

For over two decades, the Tourette Syndrome Association (TSA) has not only worked to improve the lives of people with Tourette's syndrome (TS), but has carefully nurtured a productive working partnership with both the physicians who treat people with TS and the scientists engaged in TS research. Close cooperation among professional health organizations established and directed by patient families not only can make a significant contribution to the well being of patients and their families, but at the same time provide valuable assistance to clinicians and researchers dedicated to helping those patients.

Uniquely American, there is a long tradition of voluntary health organizations founded and supported by patients and their families. All share a common objective, namely, to help people suffering from a variety of disorders and diseases. The evolution of the TSA is typical of those groups.

In 1972, the distraught father of a young boy who had received a diagnosis of TS wrote to the editor of a New York City newspaper calling for a response from anyone else who had ever received the diagnosis of this extremely rare movement disorder. At that time, it was generally believed that only 50 cases of this disorder had ever been reported in all of recorded medical history. A handful of families responded to the letter. They met, and, with a courageous spirit and deep commitment, set out to improve conditions for people everywhere who suffer from TS.

THE COMMITMENT

Because of the highly unusual and sometimes socially unacceptable range of TS symptoms, the founders were determined to send a clear message to the general public: no matter what the symptoms looked like, the root causes of the disorder were physical in nature and not psychologically caused. Simply put, the symptoms of TS are involuntary, not purposeful. Because their loved ones were suffering from painful social stigma in schools, on the job, and in public places, those TSA volunteers were determined to educate people everywhere about the disorder. By battling ignorance, they hoped to change the misconception that people with TS were mentally ill, or less capable and intelligent than the rest of society. The founders were convinced that, through their efforts, the lives of their children and their grandchildren would be made easier, more fulfilling, and worthwhile. Indeed, as TS symptoms have become better understood, children and adults with TS are being accepted more readily in our society. The vast majority of patients can and do lead normal productive lives.

THE PROCESS

Because so little was known about the ailment, the founding group had committed itself to a very long and complex process of medical and public education. First, the TSA needed to find the undiagnosed and misdiagnosed patients, and then refer them to a handful of physicians who, at that time, knew how to provide treatment. Today, 20 years later, diagnoses of TS are commonly made by neurologists, psychiatrists, pediatricians, and general practitioners. Often, referrals to doctors are made by educators, social workers, and psychologists. The ability of all these professionals from different fields to recognize the symptoms of TS is direct testimony to the effectiveness of the work of the association.

Back in the early 1970s, scientific investigations into the causes and treatment of the disorder were all but nonexistent. The TSA leadership quickly sought ways to capture the attention, interest, and talent of the broad scientific community. In 1984, to encourage research activity in fields relevant to TS, they generously contributed funds to establish a TSA Permanent Research Fund. For the past 8 years, this program has been providing seed money in support of scores of clinical and preclinical investigators interested in the disorder.

In the early years, all the activities of the TSA were carried out on a strictly volunteer basis, primarily out of the homes of its founding members. Those who remember this period fondly call it "the era of the kitchen table." Patients and their families diligently compiled mailing lists and developed, printed, and distributed the only informational materials about TS available anywhere in the world. They convinced expert psychiatrists, neurologists, researchers, and educators to volunteer their time and professional expertise by serving on two very important national committees: a Medical Committee, responsible for guiding and advising on matters of clinical care, and a Scientific Advisory Board, charged with reviewing research applications and recommending for funding only the best among them. To this day, those two professional advisory committees remain key elements in the association's successful efforts to help people with TS.

ACHIEVING OBJECTIVES

Publicity

One of the TSA's most successful efforts has been the accurate communication of its message through the media—television, radio, and print. At considerable expense, the organization has produced several 30-second public service announcements for TV and radio, featuring nationally known athletes with TS and personalities from the entertainment world who explain the involuntary nature of the symptoms and encourage greater tolerance for people who are different from the general public. Viewers are encouraged to contact the association. Moreover, people with TS, together with our medical advisors, have appeared on several widely viewed TV programs. Over the years, hundreds of articles and several dramatizations about the disorder have appeared on TV, in magazines, and in local newspapers. This wide media attention has brought about countless numbers of new diagnoses, helped the TSA increase its membership, and, above all, fostered greater tolerance, acceptance, and respect for all people with TS.

Legislation

By intelligently bringing the problems of patients to the attention of elected officials, the TSA has significantly increased support for broader patients' rights and increased government funding for scientists working in areas relevant to this disorder. TSA spearheaded and successfully brought about the passage of the Orphan Drug Act, which today permits the economical development and speedy Food and Drug Administration (FDA) approval of new medications for patients with rare diseases. The very first medication to receive approval under the Orphan Drug Act was pimozide, a medication now used by many TS patients. Our own modest grant awards (US$25,000 being the top level) have helped TS researchers with innovative ideas gather valuable pilot data. The organization is particularly gratified by the fact that subsequent to receiving grant awards from the association, several TSA-funded researchers have gone on to receive major National Institutes of Health (NIH) grants to continue their TS investigations.

Credibility

By cooperating closely and learning from our volunteer medical advisors, the TSA has earned a reputation among professionals as a patient group that always advocates for its members in a responsible manner. For example, all the association's medical and scientific literature is reviewed by our professional advisors prior to publication. Despite its modest size, the organization is well known and respected. This credibility makes it much easier to bring attention to patients' needs and, ultimately, to effect positive change.

By collaborating with larger and more powerful coalitions with similar concerns, problems, and interests, the TSA has strengthened its ability to help not only people with TS, but the professionals working in the field as well. The TSA is a member of the National Organization for Rare Diseases; several groups working to increase government funding for all biomedical research; an organization struggling to educate the public about the critical need for the continued humane use of animals in research; and another coalition working to improve the inadequate system of health insurance coverage in the United States.

Present Status

The TSA files contain countless letters of gratitude from individuals who discovered, to their astonishment, that their long-endured and often-ridiculed "bizarre habits" were actually caused by an imbalance in the chemistry of their brain environment that makes them less able than the rest of us to inhibit their body movements and behaviors.

Although the TSA leadership continues to remain in the hands of its active board of directors, all functioning on a "volunteer" basis, the association has grown considerably and now employs a paid staff of 16. A quarterly newsletter reaches a readership of 30,000, and there are 45 affiliated chapters nationwide. The TSA also cooperates closely with patients and doctors in 12 other countries. Each month, more than 1000 physicians, other professionals, and families contact the national offices. These inquiries come about either through media attention or from patients who have been referred by their physicians.

SERVING THE PROFESSIONAL AND THE PATIENT

By far, the vast majority of requests for help are related to either medical or school problems. Despite national legislation guaranteeing a free and appropriate education to all, it is still common to hear of TS children being expelled from classes or prohibited from riding schoolbuses because it is believed that they are "purposely" disturbing everyone with their symptoms. However, a variety of TSA literature and videofilms specifically written for educators have proven effective in helping to resolve such situations. Once educators become informed, there is usually a vast improvement in the general acceptance of the child by both teachers and peers. Generally, when caring physicians and mental health counselors are willing to take the time to directly intercede with the schools or employers on behalf of their patients, the situation improves.

Each year, the TSA budgets thousands of dollars to cover the expenses of providing informational exhibits at a variety of medical, scientific, and professional meetings. Local volunteers—both patients and their families—are always present to answer questions. Up-to-date information on TS treatment, management, and current research is provided. Invariably, participants are eager to receive those materials, which they find very useful in treating patients. Typically, the TSA underwrites exhibits at the annual meetings of adult and child psychiatrists, neurologists, neuroscientists, geneticists, school nurses, social workers, and special education teachers. This investment of resources has proven valuable as we see the continuing significant increase in the number of diagnoses and research investigations in the field.

THE TSA AND THE RESEARCH SCIENTIST

Molecular Genetics

One of the most promising areas of current research involves the discovery of specific gene defects that cause inherited disorders. To successfully carry out family linkage studies, there must be close and continuing cooperation among clinicians, basic scientists, and the participating patient families. Each party plays a crucial role because without cooperation, these studies cannot succeed.

When the association discovered that large families with multiple affected generations were needed for genetic research, it advertised in its newsletters and searched its database for appropriate families. The TSA interviewed dozens of potential participants, and eventually referred many of them to interested geneticists.

Voluntary health organizations are in a unique position to greatly facilitate progress in genetic research. Since 1985, the TSA has sponsored a highly effective, multinational collaborative effort among six laboratories, all seeking a marker for the TS gene. The TSA continues to provide genetic researchers with the single most important element necessary for advancing linkage studies—ongoing, personal communication among all the collaborators. The TSA not only contributes funding to the participating groups, but every 6–8 months sponsors a genetic workshop where attendees have an opportunity to come together with our scientific advisors and informally discuss their progress and plans for future research directions. The association then publishes an up-to-date progress report that is circulated among interested investigators.

When the TSA leadership learned that a serious risk to carrying out any linkage study is the imprecise definition of the phenotype, the TSA convened a consensus group of expert clinicians to develop a TS unified rating scale and diagnostic criteria. These research tools are now being validated and will be published and made available to clinical geneticists as well as all other interested researchers worldwide. The quality of all TS clinical studies will be greatly improved once these scales are universally employed.

OTHER CLINICAL AND PRECLINICAL AREAS OF STUDY

Recently, a researcher at the National Institute of Mental Health who was keenly interested in carrying out a very costly and comprehensive study of twins with TS contacted the association. Once again, the TSA advertised vigorously and 54 sets of TS twins have been referred and studied. Only with the help of a patient organization and its registry could those subjects have been located.

In 1986, the TSA's scientific advisors informed the organization that technological advances in neuropathology held great promise for improving the understanding of the basic etiology of the disorder. Unfortunately, there was not one TS brain specimen available for scientific study. The TSA launched a costly campaign among its members to educate them on the importance of this area of research, and encouraged members to register with the Brain Bank program. An educational videofilm on the subject was created, and the program is regularly promoted in newsletters. Currently, Brain Bank registrations have doubled. Efficient distribution of this rare and valuable material is being closely monitored by knowledgeable members of the TSA's Scientific Advisory Board.

SUMMARY

To best achieve its stated goals of public and professional education, patient advocacy, and research support, the watchwords of the TSA leadership have been responsibility and dedication—responsibility in the way its activities are conducted and dedication to all those who depend on the association's programs to help them cope with living with TS.

Members of the board of directors have often said that it is their fondest dream to find a cure and then be able to close the association's doors forever. Until that time, the TSA will continue to be at the service of the people who have this disorder as well as all those who endeavor to help them.

Editor's note: Interested readers can contact the Tourette Syndrome Association, Inc., at 42-40 Bell Boulevard, Bayside, New York 11361-2861, USA. Tel.: (718) 224-2999, (800) 237-0717; fax: (718) 279-9596.

Index

About the Editor

Roger Kurlan is Professor of Neurology, Chief of the Cognitive and Behavioral Neurology Unit, and Director of the Tourette's Syndrome Clinic at the University of Rochester Medical Center, Rochester, New York. He is the author or coauthor of numerous articles published in highly regarded journals of neurology and psychiatry. Actively researching Tourette's syndrome and Parkinson's disease, Dr. Kurlan is also a frequent presenter at national conferences on movement disorders and cognitive and behavioral disorders. He received the M.D. degree from Washington University School of Medicine, St. Louis, Missouri.

Milton Keynes UK
Ingram Content Group UK Ltd.
UKHW020006071024
449327UK00031B/2669